BIOLOGY OF THE SYNOVIAL JOINT

BIOLOGY OF THE SYNOVIAL JOINT

Edited by

Charles W. Archer, Bruce Caterson,
Michael Benjamin and James R. Ralphs

Cardiff School of Biosciences
University of Wales, Cardiff, UK

harwood academic publishers
Australia • Canada • China • France • Germany • India
Japan • Luxembourg • Malaysia • The Netherlands
Russia • Singapore • Switzerland

Amsteldijk 166
1st Floor
1079 LH Amsterdam
The Netherlands

British Library Cataloguing in Publication Data

A catalogue record for this book is available from the British Library.

ISBN 90-5702-327-X

Contents

Preface

This book is based around contributions to the symposium 'The Biology of the Synovial Joint' held at the University of Wales, Cardiff from 30 June–2nd July 1996. The idea for the symposium came from an earlier one-day meeting on synovial joints that we held at Cardiff under the auspices of the Anatomical Society of Great Britain and Ireland in 1993. Both meetings stemmed from our belief that joints need to be seen as whole organs – a number of very different tissues/structures act together to produce a functional unit. Thus, pathological change or injury to one part would be expected to affect the others. Because of the complexity of joints, most workers have concentrated on a single tissue – e.g. cartilage, bone, ligament or synovium. What we attempted to do in the symposium was to bring together specialists in all of the component tissues of joints to get a unique overview of our current state of knowledge. There are frequent international meetings on the individual components of joints e.g. articular cartilage or bone, but as far as we are aware this was the first large scale international meeting dedicated to the biology of the joint as a whole.

The contributors were chosen for their wide range of expertise, so that both the symposium and this book could reflect the range of research currently in progress on the synovial joint and its component tissues. Thus, contributions range from the molecular and biochemical, through development and cell biology, to histological, anatomical and clinical studies. All authors were given the remit of writing a review article on their subject area, illustrated where appropriate with their own work. We hope that this unique collection of review articles will serve as a useful source of reference for anyone interested in the biology of joints. Abstracts of the symposium presentations and associated posters have already been published in *Connective Tissue Research* **36**, 85–149 (1997).

The meeting was generously supported by The Arthritis and Rheumatism Council; Anachem Ltd; Beckman Instruments (UK) Ltd; Ciba-Geigy Corporation; Dupont Merck; Glaxo Wellcome Research and Development; Howmedica Inc.; Lab Impex; Life Sciences International (UK) Ltd; Osteonics; Oxford GlycoSystems; Roche Bioscience; Hoechst, Smith and Nephew; and The Wellcome Trust.

We would like to thank the School of Molecular and Medical Biosciences, University of Wales, Cardiff for allowing us to run the meeting in the School. We are especially grateful for the help of a number of individuals without whom the meeting could not have taken place. Thus, we thank Sue O'Brien, Glynis Hudson, and the postgraduate and postdoctoral researchers in the Connective Tissue Biology Laboratory. Thanks are also due to the staff at Harwood Academic Publishers for their support, encouragement and patience during the production of this book.

C.W. Archer, B. Caterson, M. Benjamin and J.R. Ralphs
Cardiff School of Biosciences
University of Wales, Cardiff, UK

Contributors

Archer, C.W.
Connective Tissue Biology Labs
Cardiff School of Biosciences
University of Wales Cardiff
Museum Avenue
Cardiff, CF1 3US
UK

Banes, A.J.
Department of Orthopaedics
School of Medicine
University of North Carolina
Chapel Hill, NC 27599–7055
USA

Benjamin, M.
Connective Tissue Biology Labs
Cardiff School of Biosciences
University of Wales Cardiff
Museum Avenue
Cardiff, CF1 3US
UK

Billingham, M.E.J.
Rheumatology Laboratories
OSCOR Facility
University Veterinary School
Southwell Street
Bristol, BS2 8EJ
UK

Boitano, S.
Cell Biology and Anatomy
School of Medicine
UCLA
Los Angeles, CA 90095–1361
USA

Brown, T.
Department of Orthopaedics
College of Medicine
University of Iowa
Iowa City, IA 52242
USA

Buckwalter, J.A.
Department of Orthopaedics
College of Medicine
University of Iowa
Iowa City, IA 52242
USA

Burt, J.
Physiology Department
College of Medicine
University of Arizona
Tuscon, AZ 85721
USA

Caterson, B.
Connective Tissue Biology Labs
Cardiff School of Biosciences
University of Wales Cardiff
Museum Avenue
Cardiff, CF1 3US
UK

Coleman, P.J.
Department of Physiology
St George's Hospital Medical School
Cranmer Terrace
London, SW17 0RE
UK

Cowell, S.
Strangeways Research Labs
Worts' Causeway
Cambridge, CB1 4RN
UK

Duance, V.C.
Connective Tissue Biology Labs
Cardiff School of Biosciences
University of Wales Cardiff
Museum Avenue
Cardiff, CF1 3US
UK

Edwards, J.C.W.
Rheumatology Unit
Arther Stanley House
Tottenham Street
London, W1P 9PG
UK

Evanko, S.P.
Department of Pathology
School of Medicine
University of Washington
Seattle, WA 98195
USA

Feikes, J.
Department of Engineering Science
University of Oxford
Parks Road
Oxford, OX1 3PJ
UK

Flannery, C.R.
Connective Tissue Biology Labs
Cardiff School of Biosciences
University of Wales Cardiff
Museum Avenue
Cardiff, CF1 3US
UK

Francis-West, P.
Department of Craniofacial Development
United Medical and Dental Schools
Floor 28, Guy's Tower
London Bridge
London, SE1 9RT
UK

Gill, H.S.
Department of Engineering Science
University of Oxford
Parks Road
Oxford, OX1 3PJ
UK

Golden, E.B.
Department of Anatomy and Histology
School of Dental Medicine
University of Pennsylvania
Philadelphia, PA 19104–6003
USA

Handley, C.J.
School of Human Biosciences
La Trobe University
Bundoora
Victoria 3083
Australia

Hascall, V.C.
Department of Biomedical
  Engineering, WB3
Cleveland Clinic Foundation
Cleveland, OH 44195
USA

Havelka, S.
Institute of Rheumatology
Na slupi 4
CZ-12850
Prague
Czech Republic

Hembry, R.M.
Strangeways Research Labs
Worts' Causeway
Cambridge, CB1 4RN
UK

Hiscock, D.R.R.
Connective Tissue Biology Labs
Cardiff School of Biosciences
University of Wales Cardiff
Museum Avenue
Cardiff, CF1 3US
UK

Horesovsky, G.
Molecular Pharmacology
Glaxo Wellcome
Research Triangle Park
NC 27709
USA

Horn, V.
Tissue Bank
University Hospital
Brno
Czech Republic

Hughes, C.E.
Connective Tissue Biology Labs
Cardiff School of Biosciences
University of Wales Cardiff
Museum Avenue
Cardiff, CF1 3US
UK

Hunziker, E.B.
Muller Institute
Bern
Switzerland

Kenamond, C.
Department of Orthopaedics
School of Medicine
University of North Carolina
Chapel Hill, NC 27599–7055
USA

Kirsch, T.
Department of Anatomy and Histology
School of Dental Medicine
University of Pennsylvania
Philadelphia, PA 19104–6003
USA

Knäuper, V.
Strangeways Research Labs
Worts' Causeway
Cambridge, CB1 4RN
UK

Koyama, E.
Department of Anatomy and Histology
School of Dental Medicine
University of Pennsylvania
Philadelphia, PA 19104–6003
USA

Kwan, A.P.L.
Connective Tissue Biology Labs
Cardiff School of Biosciences
University of Wales Cardiff
Museum Avenue
Cardiff, CF1 3US
UK

Lawrence, W.T.
Department of Surgery
School of Medicine
University of Massachusetts Medical Center
Worcester, MA 01655
USA

Leardini, A.
Department of Engineering Science
University of Oxford
Parks Road
Oxford, OX1 3PJ
UK

Leatherman, J.L.
Department of Anatomy and Histology
School of Dental Medicine
University of Pennsylvania
Philadelphia, PA 19104–6003
USA

Levick, J.R.
Department of Physiology
St George's Hospital Medical School
Cranmer Terrace
London, SW17 0RE
UK

Little, C.B.
Connective Tissue Biology Labs
Cardiff School of Biosciences
University of Wales Cardiff
Museum Avenue
Cardiff, CF1 3US
UK

Lu, T.-W.
Department of Engineering Science
University of Oxford
Parks Road
Oxford, OX1 3PJ
UK

Ligten, F.P.
Bone Research Branch
National Institute of Dental Research
National Institutes of Health
Bethesda, MD 20892–1188
USA

Mason, R.M.
Department of Biochemistry
Charing Cross and Westminster
 Medical School
Fulham Palace Road
London, W6 8RF
UK

McNeilly, C.
Connective Tissue Biology Labs
Cardiff School of Biosciences
University of Wales Cardiff
Museum Avenue
Cardiff, CF1 3US
UK

Messner, K.
Sports Medicine
Faculty of Health Sciences
University of Linköping
581 85 Linköping
Sweden

Miller, L.
Molecular Pharmacology
Glaxo Wellcome
Research Triangle Park
NC 27709
USA

Mulligan, P.J.
Research and Teaching Centre
Royal Orthopaedic Hospital
The Woodlands
Northfield
Birmingham, B31 2AP
UK

Murphy, G.
Strangeways Research Labs
Worts' Causeway
Cambridge, CB1 4RN
UK

Nalin, A.M.
Department of Orthopaedics
University of Washington
Seattle Veterans Affairs Medical Center
Seattle, WA 98108
USA

Newell, R.L.M.
Connective Tissue Biology Labs
Cardiff School of Biosciences
University of Wales Cardiff
Museum Avenue
Cardiff, CF1 3US
UK

O'Connor, J.J.
Oxford Orthopaedic Engineering Centre
Nuffield Orthopaedic Centre
Oxford, OX3 7LD
UK

Pacifici, M.
Department of Anatomy and Histology
School of Dental Medicine
University of Pennsylvania
Philadelphia, PA 19104–6003
USA

Pitsillides, A.A.
The Department of Veterinary
  Basic Sciences
The Royal Veterinary College
Royal College Street
London, NW1 0TU
UK

Ralphs, J.R.
Connective Tissue Biology Labs
Cardiff School of Biosciences
University of Wales Cardiff
Museum Avenue
Cardiff, CF1 3US
UK

Riley, G.
Rheumatology Research Unit
PO Box 194
Addenbrooke's Hospital
Cambridge, CB2 2QQ
UK

Robbins, J.R.
Arthritis Research
149 The Navy Yard
Massachusetts General Hospital East
Charlestown, MA 02129
USA

Sandell, L.J.
Department of Orthopaedics, ORT 112
University of Washington
VA Puget Sound Health Care Systems
1660 S. Columbian Way
Seattle, WA 98108
USA

Sandy, J.D.
Shriners Hospital for Crippled Children
Tampa Unit
12502 North Pine Drive
Tampa, FL 33612–9499
USA

Scott, D.
Department of Physiology
St George's Hospital Medical School
Cranmer Terrace
London, SW17 0RE
UK

Tsuzaki, M.
Department of Orthopaedics
School of Medicine
University of North Carolina
Chapel Hill, NC 27599–7055
USA

Vaughan-Thomas, A.
Connective Tissue Biology Labs
Cardiff School of Biosciences
University of Wales Cardiff
Museum Avenue
Cardiff, CF1 3US
UK

Vogel, K.G.
Department of Biology
University of New Mexico
Albuquerque, NM 87131
USA

Wardale, R.J.
Connective Tissue Biology Labs
Cardiff School of Biosciences
University of Wales Cardiff
Museum Avenue
Cardiff, CF1 3US
UK

Weinhold, P.
Department of Orthopaedics
School of Medicine
University of North Carolina
Chapel Hill, NC 27599–7055
USA

Wilson, D.R.
Department of Engineering Science
University of Oxford
Parks Road
Oxford, OX1 3PJ
UK

Wotton, S.F.
Connective Tissue Biology Labs
Cardiff School of Biosciences
University of Wales Cardiff
Museum Avenue
Cardiff, CF1 3US
UK

Zavatsky, A.B.
Department of Engineering Science
University of Oxford
Parks Road
Oxford, OX1 3PJ
UK

Zhu, Y.
Department of Orthopaedics
University of Washington
Seattle Veterans Affairs Medical Center
Seattle, WA 98108
USA

1 An Introduction to Synovial Joints

M. Benjamin

Connective Tissue Biology Labs, Cardiff School of Biosciences,
University of Wales Cardiff, PO Box 911,
Museum Avenue, Cardiff CF1 3US, UK

The purpose of this chapter is to give a brief overview of the basic structure and variety of synovial joints for orthopaedic researchers whose expertise is not centred around morphology. The account is not intended to cover new or original work.

WHAT IS A SYNOVIAL JOINT?

A *joint* (also known as an *arthrosis* – hence 'arthrology' the study of joints) is a union between two or more parts of the skeleton – typically bones, but also cartilages earlier in development. A *synovial* joint (also known as a *diarthrosis*) is one that has a joint cavity that is enclosed by a fibrous capsule linking the skeletal elements (Figure 1.1). The capsule is lined by a synovial membrane that secretes a lubricating and nutritive fluid. The opposing surfaces of the bones are covered with articular hyaline cartilage (usually) or fibrocartilage (occasionally).

It is important to realise that not all joints are synovial and that not all joints permit movement! Non-synovial joints are collectively called *synarthroses*. These include *fibrous joints* where the skeletal elements are directly linked by fibrous tissue (e.g. the sutures between the bones in the skull cap where no movement is allowed) and *cartilaginous joints* where two bones are linked by cartilage (e.g. the joints between the vertebral bodies where limited movement is permitted). Synovial joints are typical of the limbs and have evolved to promote movement. This is clearly facilitated by their joint cavity.

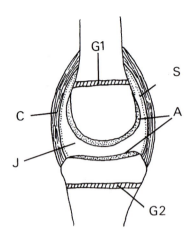

FIGURE 1.1   A generalised diagram of a synovial joint. The bones are covered with articular cartilage (A) and separated by a joint cavity (J). They are connected by a fibrous capsule (C), lined by a synovial membrane (S) that is responsible for secreting synovial fluid. Note that the synovial membrane does not cover the articular surfaces of the joint. The site of attachment of the capsule determines whether or not a growth plate lies inside (G1) or outside (G2) the joint.

GENERAL PRINCIPLES OF STRUCTURE

ARTICULAR CARTILAGE

Bones can be classified developmentally as cartilage bones or membrane bones – only the former are preceded by a hyaline cartilage model in the early foetus. All the limb bones are cartilage bones, but certain others (e.g. the clavicle) are membrane bones. Where synovial joints have developed between cartilage bones, the bones in the adult are covered with *hyaline* cartilage (e.g. the knee, hip and shoulder). This cartilage represents that which has 'escaped' endochondral ossification. Where the bones in a synovial joint are membrane bones, they are covered by *fibro*cartilage formed by the periosteum (e.g. the clavicle in sterno-clavicular joint). Articular cartilage is an avascular and aneural tissue that provides a wear-resistant surface with low frictional properties for the joint. It is well suited for withstanding compression and shear and may be up to 7 mm thick in larger joints. Variations in thickness across the joint can improve the congruity of the bones beyond that which might be anticipated from examining a dried skeleton. The deep part of the cartilage is calcified and has an irregular interface with the underlying bone that is important in holding the two tissues together. Articular cartilage does not show up on a radiograph and thus the joint space looks bigger than it really is.

CAPSULE AND LIGAMENTS

The capsule is a fibrous connective tissue that is attached to the skeletal elements of a joint beyond their articular surfaces. In the small bones of the hands and feet, it is often attached immediately beyond the articular cartilages, but in the long bones it may be fixed further away – presumably to promote a greater range of movement. Where the capsule links two long bones, its line of attachment relative to the position of the growth plate is important (Figure 1.1). Although the growth plate is a barrier to infection, if it lies within the joint, infections on the metaphyseal side of the long bone (the *metaphysis* is the flared region between the shaft or *diaphysis* and the expanded end or *epiphysis*) can spread into the joint, or fractures of the metaphysis can directly affect the joint itself.

Most capsules are strengthened by local thickenings called *ligaments* – though it does not follow that all ligaments associated with a joint are part of the joint capsule. Additional or *accessory ligaments* may be found inside (e.g. the cruciate ligaments of the knee joint) or outside (e.g. the lateral collateral ligament of the knee joint) the joint capsule (Figure 1.2). Ligaments permit free movements when they are lax, but can prohibit unwanted movements when tight – by virtue of their high tensile strength. Occasionally, capsules are strengthened by tendons, e.g. the extensor tendon in the finger joints.

The capsule and its associated ligaments serve to hold the bones together and to guide and limit joint movements. Because they are richly endowed with nerve fibres, their stretching can initiate active muscle contractions that prevent them from being over-stretched. Thus, the capsule and its ligaments play an active part in maintaining joint stability beyond their ability to resist stretch. They are also well endowed with pain fibres so that twisting/stretching of joint capsules or ligaments is very painful, and have autonomic nerve fibres that supply their blood vessels. As a general rule, the nerves supplying a joint also supply the muscles acting on the joint and the skin over it (this is known as Hilton's law).

ARTICULAR DISCS, MENISCI AND LABRA

In several important joints in the body, the joint cavity is partly or completely subdivided into two compartments by fibrous or fibrocartilaginous structures that are often attached to the capsule and are called articular discs (e.g. in the wrist and sternoclavicular joints) or menisci (e.g. in the knee joint; Figure 1.2). Their functions have long been debated and

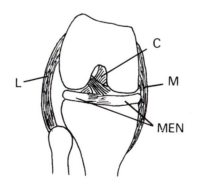

FIGURE 1.2   The knee joint provides a good example of different types of ligament. It has one that fuses with the capsule (the medial collateral ligament, M) and others that are completely independent of the capsule and lie either inside (cruciate ligaments, C) or outside (lateral collateral ligament, L) the joint. In addition, its joint cavity is partly subdivided by two menisci (MEN).

numerous suggestions include (a) improving the congruity of badly-fitting joints (although it seems unlikely that some joints are so 'badly designed' that they need additional spacers to make them work properly), (b) distributing weight over large articular surfaces, (c) acting as shock absorbers, (d) allowing rolling movements of a joint, (e) promoting separate movements in the two halves of the joint cavity that result from the presence of a disc, and (f) spreading synovial fluid and thus contributing to joint lubrication. Related in structure to articular discs and menisci, and also providing an additional articular surface are *labra*. These are fibrocartilaginous rims that extend the periphery of articular surfaces and are best documented in the shoulder and hip joints.

SYNOVIUM

The synovial membrane lines the non-articular surfaces of a joint (e.g. capsule, ligaments) but stops short of the articular surfaces themselves – including those provided by articular discs or menisci (Figure 1.1). It is responsible both for secreting and absorbing synovial fluid. This is a dialysate of blood plasma with added hyaluronan that contributes significantly to its viscoelastic and thixotropic characteristics. Synovial fluid lubricates the joint and provides at least partly for the nutrition of articular cartilage, discs and menisci. Typically, a synovial membrane consists of 1–3 layers of cells (synoviocytes), supported by a vascular connective tissue. It frequently extends into the joint cavity as small projections called villi or as larger and fatty folds. Fatty folds are called *articular fat pads* and are relatively common features of joints – they are well documented, for example, in the knee joint. Because fatty tissue is bulky and the lipid in the cells is fluid at body temperatures, it provides an extremely compliant and space-filling tissue surrounding articular surfaces that can readily accommodate to joint movements.

MOVEMENTS AT SYNOVIAL JOINTS

Essentially, all movements can be reduced to spinning, rocking or sliding movements or a combination of all three (Figure 1.3), but a wide variety of more specific terms are widely used in orthopaedics and the major ones are briefly explained below.

It is conventional to describe movements of the body as occurring around one or more of three planes or axes – horizontal (transverse), sagittal and coronal (frontal; Figure 1.4a,b). *Flexion* occurs in the sagittal plane, e.g. bending the forearm at the elbow joint (Figure 1.4c) or the leg at the knee joint. The opposite movement of straightening a bent limb is *extension* (Figure 1.4c). When you move an arm or leg away from the midline of the body, in the coronal plane, you are performing the movement of *abduction* (Figure 1.4d). *Adduction* is the converse (Figure 1.4d). *Circumduction* occurs when the movements of flexion, extension, abduction and adduction occur in sequence. If you are *rotating* a limb, you are turning it around its long axis. *Medial* or *internal rotation* is an inward turning movement, and *lateral* or *external rotation* an outward movement (Figure 1.4e). Certain additional terms are used to describe particular movements that are characteristic of certain joints only. There are many examples of

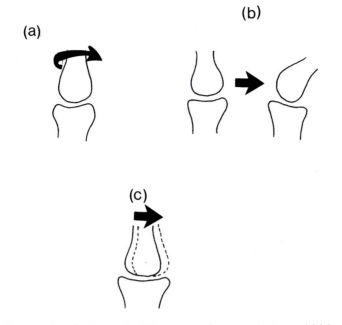

FIGURE 1.3 There are three fundamentally different types of movements at synovial joints, (a) spinning, (b) rocking, (c) sliding. Modified after Rogers A.W. (1992) *Textbook of Anatomy*, Churchill Livingstone, Edinburgh.

these that have to be learned as and when they arise, but among those that may be of special concern to those involved in orthopaedic research are *supination* and *pronation* – lateral and medial rotation respectively of the forearm (Figure 1.4f), whereby the palm of the hand is made to face forwards or backwards, *dorsiflexion* and *plantarflexion* (pointing the foot upwards or downwards; Figure 1.4g) and *inversion* and *eversion* – movements of the foot beyond the level of the ankle joint, where the sole of the foot is turned inwards or outwards respectively (Figure 1.4h).

The range of movement that a joint permits is limited by a variety of factors:

1. Muscles – the tightness of the hamstrings often limits flexion at the hip joint
2. Ligaments – the strong ligaments at the sides of the finger joints (collateral ligaments) that prevent abduction and adduction from occurring
3. Contact of opposing fleshy parts – flexion of the elbow joint is limited by contact between the muscles on the front of the forearm and arm.

A distinction can be made between *active movements* of a joint that result from muscle contraction and *passive movements* produced by gravity or by an examiner when the patient's muscles are relaxed. The range of passive movement is generally greater than the range of active movement and some passive movements cannot be performed actively, e.g. pulling joint surfaces slightly apart (*distraction*) or the passive rotation of a finger (interphalangeal) joint, when there are no muscles capable of producing such

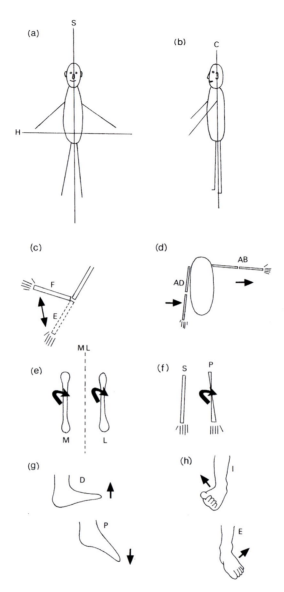

FIGURE 1.4 Movements at synovial joints – arrows indicate directions of movement. (a) The sagittal (S) and horizontal (H) planes of reference. (b) The coronal (C) or frontal plane of reference. (c) Flexion (F) and extension (E) as shown at the elbow joint. Flexion is bending the limb; extension is straightening it. (d) Abduction (AB) and adduction (AD) as shown at the shoulder joint. When the arm is abducted, it is moved away from the body and from the midline; when it is adducted, it is moved towards the midline. (e) Rotation of a long bone. In medial rotation (M), the bone (e.g. femur or humerus) rotates around its long axis towards the midline (ML). In lateral rotation (L), the bone rotates around its long axis away from the midline. (f) Supination (S) and pronation (P) of the right forearm. When the forearm is pronated, the radius and ulna twist around each other, turning the palm of the hand over so that it faces backwards. (g) Dorsiflexion (D) involves pointing the foot upwards and plantarflexion (P) involves pointing the foot downwards. (h) When the foot is inverted (I), the medial ('inner') side is turned upwards and when it is everted (E), the lateral border of the foot is turned upwards.

a movement. Because movements at a synovial joint may be so varied and extensive, the joints are often supplied by a complex anastomosing network of arteries. This ensures that one vessel or other is always open, no matter what the position of the joint.

Finally, it is important to appreciate that joints seldom move alone and most movements of the body involve more than one joint. Many joints, for example, work together in controlling body posture – so injury to one may produce a compensatory change in another. Certain pairs of joints are unavoidably linked. Thus, movement at the superior radioulnar joint in the forearm cannot occur independent of movement at the inferior radioulnar joint.

JOINT STABILITY

The stability of a joint is determined by the shape and arrangement of the articular surfaces and the ligaments and muscles associated with a joint. The ball and socket arrangement of the hip joint (see below) is a prime example of how the shape of the bones is important for joint stability. In marked contrast, the stability of the acromioclavicular joint (the small joint between the collar bone and the shoulder blade) largely depends on the strength and arrangement of its ligaments, and that of the shoulder joint rests heavily on its well-known rotator cuff muscles. Joints are usually most stable in what is called the *close-packed position* – where there is maximal contact area between the bones. Significantly, this is where the capsule and ligaments are usually most tense. The close-packed position lies at one extreme of the range of movement – e.g. the position of full extension of the knee joint. Joints are prone to dislocate when their protective mechanisms are caught off guard – e.g. when muscles are relaxed, or by leverage in the most vulnerable direction.

CLASSIFICATION OF SYNOVIAL JOINTS

Synovial joints can be classified according to whether they allow movement in one plane only (*uniaxial joints*), or in two (*biaxial joints*) or three (*multiaxial joints*) planes independently. What at first sight may look to be a simple movement occurring in a single plane is often more complex. For example, the hinge-like movement of the knee joint is actually accompanied by rotation of either the tibia or femur around its own longitudinal axis. Because this rotation does not occur independently, the knee joint is still regarded as uniaxial. Synovial joints have also been classified according to the shape of their articular surfaces and the types of movements they allow.

UNIAXIAL JOINTS

Plane joints (Figure 1.5a)

These are usually small and the articular surfaces flat and approximately equal in size. They permit gliding or slipping movements in any direction, or twisting of one bone on

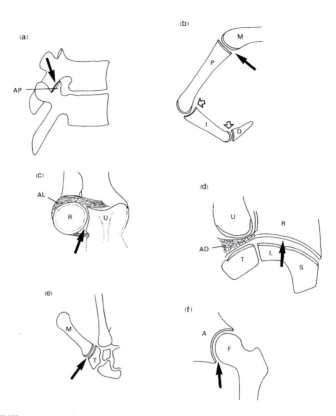

FIGURE 1.5 Different types of synovial joints. (a) *Plane* – e.g. the zygapophysial joints (arrow) between the articular processes (AP) of adjacent vertebrae. (b) *Hinge* – e.g. the interphalangeal joints of the fingers (open arrows) between the proximal (P), intermediate (I) and distal (D) phalanges, and *Condyloid* – e.g. the meta-carpophalangeal joint of the fingers (solid arrow) between the metacarpal bone (M) and proximal phalanx (P). (c) *Pivot* – e.g. the superior radioulnar joint (arrow) between the head of the radius (R) and the bony-ligamentous ring formed by the anular ligament (AL) and the ulna (U). (d) *Ellipsoid* – e.g. the wrist joint (arrow), where the radius (R) and articular disc (AD) overlying the head of the ulna (U) articulate with the proximal row of carpal bones (triquetral T, lunate L and scaphoid S). (e) *Saddle joint* – e.g. the metacarpophalangeal joint of the thumb (arrow) between the 1st metacarpal (M) and the triquetral (T). (f) *Ball and socket joint* – e.g. the hip joint (arrow) between the head of the femur (F) and the acetabulum (A). Figures b, c and d are redrawn after *Sobotta Atlas of Human Anatomy*, vol. 1, eds Putz R. and Pabst R., 12th edn, Urban & Schwarzenberg.

another. They include various small joints in the wrist (carpal joints) and the joints between the articular processes of adjacent vertebrae (zygapophysial joints).

Hinge joints (Figure 1.5b)

These permit hinge-like movements of flexion and extension only, and have strong liga-ments at the sides of the joint (i.e. collateral ligaments) that prevent other movements. The interphalangeal joints of the fingers are a good example.

Pivot joints (Figure 1.5c)

Here, a pivot formed by a bone is encircled by a ring formed by both a bone and a liga-ment. Either (1) the pivot rotates within the ring as in the forearm, where the radius rotates around the ulna within the confines of the anular ligament, or (2) the ring rotates around the bone, e.g. at the base of the skull, where the atlas and transverse ligaments rotate around the peg-like odontoid process of the axis, when you turn your head to one side.

BIAXIAL JOINTS

Condyloid joints (Figure 1.5b)

These allow independent movements in two axes at right angles to each other. The principal movements are flexion-extension and abduction-adduction. A pair of convex condyles (a 'condyle' is a general term for a rounded swelling on a bone) on one side of the joint fit into a complementary pair of concave surfaces on the other. The knuckle (metacarpophalangeal) joints are a good example.

Ellipsoid joints (Figure 1.5d)

An oval convex surface on one side of the joint fits into an elliptical concavity on the other – as in the wrist joint. These joints allow flexion-extension and abduction-adduction.

MULTIAXIAL JOINTS

Saddle joints (Figure 1.5e)

Here, the articular surfaces are reciprocally concavo-convex – like a horse's saddle. The best known example is the metacarpophalangeal joint at the base of the thumb. It allows flexion-extension, abduction-adduction and rotation.

Ball and socket joints (Figure 1.5f)

These are joints where a rounded ball or 'head' of a bone (e.g. on the femur) fits into a cup (e.g. acetabulum) on the other side of the joint. They are the most freely mobile of all synovial joints and allow flexion-extension, abduction-adduction and rotation.

Section 1
Development of Synovial Joints

2 The Development of Joints and Articular Cartilage

Charles W. Archer[1] and Philippa Francis-West[2]

[1]*Connective Tissue Biology Labs, Cardiff School of Biosciences,*
University of Wales, Cardiff, Museum Avenue,
Cardiff CF1 3US, UK;
[2]*Department of Craniofacial Development, United Medical and*
Dental Schools, Floor 28, Guy's Tower, London Bridge,
London SE1 9RT, UK

INTRODUCTION

Little is known of the mechanisms of joint formation including the development of articular cartilage. This paucity in knowledge is surprising considering the number of skeletal dysplasias which involve joints and because of the predisposition of articular cartilage to degenerative diseases the onset of which can be precocious in the event of dysplasia. The genetic basis of many skeletal malformations have now been identified (Vandenberg *et al.*, 1991; Kingsley *et al.*, 1994; Li *et al.*, 1995) yet the downstream molecular and cellular events surrounding or regulating a number of key processes remain to be elucidated. Some of these processes include the specification of the joint, mechanisms of joint cavitation (see Chapter 4 by Pitsillides), the specification and origin of articular cartilage and its mechanism of growth. Here, we will outline some of our studies addressing these problems.

We have utilized the embryonic chick as a model to study early events in joint formation. However, because of its fibrous articular surface (Craig *et al.*, 1987), the chick is an inappropriate model to study the development of hyaline articular cartilage present in most synovial joints of mammals. We have, therefore, chosen the marsupial *Monodelphis domestica* as a model to study articular cartilage development. This is because it combines the advantages of relatively easy colony establishment and maintenance together with a characteristic of marsupials in parturition at much earlier stages than eutherian mammals such as rats, mice or rabbits. For example, at birth, the hindlimbs are still limb buds at the early stages of chondrogenesis (equivalent to stage 25/26 of the chick; Hamburger and Hamilton, 1951) and are thus accessible to experimental investigations.

EARLY JOINT FORMATION

Histologically, the formation of joints in a number of species have been well documented in the earlier literature. Larger joints of the limb have been studied most extensively and appear to develop in a similar manner. These joints include the hip (Gardner and Gray, 1950; Andersen, 1962), knee (O'Rahilly, 1951; Andersen, 1961; Gardner and O'Rahilly, 1968), elbow and shoulder (Gray and Gardner, 1951; Gardner and Gray, 1953) in addition to the joints of the carpal and tarsal elements. In essence, at the histological level the joint is first discernible as a flattening of cells within the early cartilage anlagen. Subsequently, this region can be resolved into three layers; two 'chondrogenous' layers associated with the epiphyses comprising more rounded cells and a central layer of flattened cells of high cell density. Once resolved, this region becomes known as the joint interzone although its precise morphology varies with some joints showing just a single or double layer of flattened cells (see above refs. and Edwards *et al.*, 1994). Nevertheless, it is in this region that cavitation occurs which is covered in some detail by Pitsillides (Chapter 4). Concomitant with the formation of the interzone, we have previously shown that there is a transition in matrix synthesis from that of a chondrogenic nature to a non-chondrogenic type I collagen secreting interzone (Craig *et al.*, 1987). Thus, in essence, in the case of long bone elements at least, the skeleton develops as continuous (and in the case of elements such as the femur, tibia and fibula also branching) rods of cartilage which subsequently segment and cavitate into separate elements (Craig *et al.*, 1987).

In addition to its role in delineating the presumptive joint line and possible roles during cavitation, it is becoming evident from *in situ* hybridisation studies that the interzone may have many other roles. For example, Storm *et al.* (1994) have demonstrated that the TGFβ like factor GDF-5 (growth and differentiation factor) is differentially expressed within the interzone in a temporal manner. Furthermore, null mutations of this factor in mice produce the same phenotype as that of *brachypodia* mutation whereby the elements of the appendicular skeleton are shortened, especially more distal elements. Other factors which have been reported to be differentially expressed in the interzone include BMP4 (personal observation, P. F-W), BMP-2 (Macias *et al.*, 1997) and *ck-erg* (Ganan *et al.*, 1996).

Gain-of-function studies can complement loss-of-function experiments achieved through homologous recombination of stem cells. The chick embryo is a particularly useful model since it can be transfected with replication-competent retroviruses carrying the requisite gene at an early stage. Earlier studies by us showed that using the R-CAS retroviral system, transfected fibroblasts over-expressing both BMP-2 and BMP-4 and implanted into early forelimb buds resulted in massive chondrogenesis leading to highly dysplastic limbs which also lacked many joints (Duprez *et al.*, 1996). We have utilised a similar approach in relation to GDF5. Figure 2.1 shows the normal expression pattern of GDF-5 in the developing limb. The resulting changes due to overexpression again showed chondrogenic stimulation leading to a larger skeleton but was not as dysplastic as those observed for BMP-2 and -4 overexpression. Furthermore, joint definition was well developed with the occasional partial fusion (Figures 2.2 and 2.3). However, both the

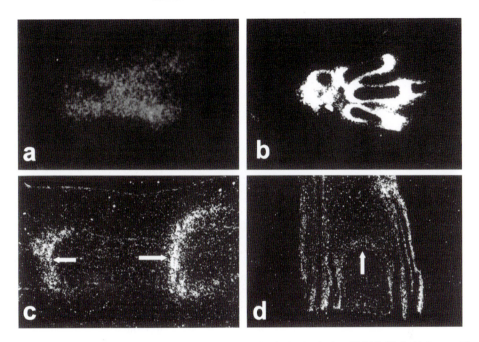

FIGURE 2.1 *In situ* hybridisation of GDF-5 mRNA expression in the developing chick hindlimb. (a) At stage 25, expression of GDF-5 can be detected throughout the prechondrogenic condensations of the tibia and fibula. (b) By stage 30, high levels of expression are restricted to the joint interzones involving long bone elements and the phalanges. (c) Stage 34 metatarsophalangeal joint showing restriction of GDF-5 expression to the joint interzone (arrows) and occasionally to the epiphyseal perichondrium (upper right of micrograph). (d) In the stage 36 metatarsophalangeal joint (just prior to the onset of cavitation), expression is reduced at the interzone (arrow).

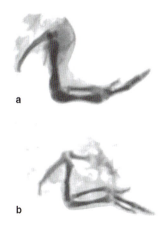

FIGURE 2.2 Overexpression of GDF-5 in chick wings. cDNA sequences encoding mouse GDF-5 were inserted into the replication-competent retrovirus RCASBP(A) in the sense orientation or as negative controls the antisense orientation. Chick fibroblasts were transfected with virus and implanted into the distal tip of stage 18–20 wing buds as previously described (Duprez *et al.*, 1996). (a) Whole-mount wing of chick subjected to GDF-5 over-expression. (b) Contralateral control. Note in (a) the larger skeleton with a 50% increase in length of distal elements in some specimens.

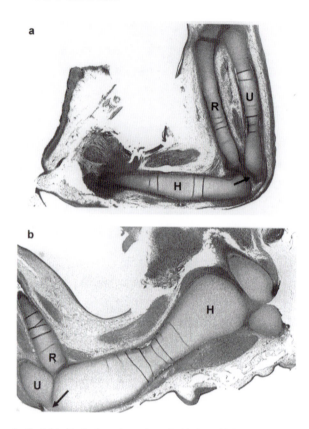

FIGURE 2.3 Longitudinal histological sections through 10-day chick wings in which GDF-5 has been over-expressed. (a) In the control wing the 'elbow' joint between the humerus (H), radius (R) and ulna (U), the interzone can be discerned as a three-layered structure comprising two chondrogenous layers and an inter-mediate fibrous layer (arrow). (b) In the over-expressed wing it can be seen that the humeral element is much larger than the control side. Note also the lack of a three-layered interzone in the 'elbow' joint. A chondrogenic bridge can be seen linking the ulna and humerus (arrow). Trichrome stain.

brachypodia mutation studies and the complementary studies on GDF-5 overexpression do indicate that the joint interzone may be an important signalling centre which can regu-late early chondrogenic growth prior to the establishment of an epiphyseal growth plate. Similar approaches on other differentially expressed factors within the joint interzone will further define the role of this important region in skeletogenesis.

ARTICULAR CARTILAGE DEVELOPMENT

The situation in relation to the development of articular cartilage is very similar to that pertaining to the joint as a whole; we know very little. Classic studies by Mankin (1962) concluded that articular cartilage grew by a combination of appositional and interstitial growth. Using tritiated thymidine incorporation as a marker for chondrocyte proliferation, he detected in the immature rabbit knee cartilage two bands of proliferative activity. The first lay just beneath the articular surface whilst the second was detected above the basal hypertrophying chondrocytes (Mankin, 1962). As indicated in the introduction, we are using the marsupial *Monodelphis domestica* to investigate further articular cartilage development. Again, there are a number of important questions which remain to be resolved. These include the precise mechanisms of growth and how the structure of cartilage is generated. For example, is the gross collagenous structure (Benninghoff's arcades; Benninghoff, 1925) specified mechanically or genetically or a combination of both? At a finer level, how is the structure of chondrons regulated? The answers to these questions are central if we are to accurately reproduce the structure of articular cartilage during repair.

GROWTH FACTOR EXPRESSION IN DEVELOPING ARTICULAR CARTILAGE

Using a panel of antibodies to insulin-like growth factors I and II (IGF I and II) and to three isoforms of transforming growth factor β (TGFβ 1, 2 and 3), we have mapped the spatio-temporal patterns of these factors in the knee of *Monodelphis* from parturition to the skeletally mature animal (8 months). We have correlated these data with that obtained using an antibody to proliferating cell nuclear antigen (PCNA) as a marker of proliferative chondrocytes.

   All of the factors studied showed similarities in the patterns of distribution throughout development. In the neonate, growth factor expression was extensive throughout the cartilage element with IGFs additionally labelling hypertrophic chondrocytes. With continued development, there is a gradual restriction of labelling to the cartilaginous epiphyses. At two months, the secondary centre of ossification begins to form and the epiphyseal cartilage can be delineated from the articular cartilage proper. At this stage, again, labelling for all the growth factors is extensive through the articular cartilage. However, further development sees a continued restriction of labelling pattern towards the articular surface. Consequently, by 4 months post-partum, labelling is restricted to the chondrocytes occupying the surface-most two or three cell layers of the cartilage. In general, after the formation of the secondary centre of ossification, the pattern of PCNA labelling is similar to that observed for both IGFs and TGFβs (Figure 2.4). This pattern of labelling remains essentially unchanged until adulthood at 8 months.

   The above data is consistent with the notion that once the secondary centre of ossification begins to develop, then growth (as assessed by growth factor and proliferative chondrocyte localisation) of the presumptive articular cartilage becomes increasingly appositional (Figure 2.5). From the latter figure, if one considers growth between 2 and 6 months, the articular cartilage will have replaced itself (with the exception of the articular surface). The tissue, therefore, grows in a manner which is similar to the epiphyseal growth plate; being renewed at or near the articular surface and being resorbed at the base through endochondral ossification during the establishment of the sub-chondral bone and, finally, sub-chondral plate. Further indirect evidence for such a mechanism comes from blocking chondrocyte proliferation with bromodeoxyuridine (BrDU). Knee joints of 3-month animals were given injections of BrDU (30 mg/ml, 20 µl per joint) at two-day intervals for 14 days and the effects monitored histologically after a further two months. In many

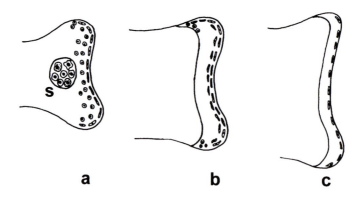

FIGURE 2.4   Diagrammatic representation of the expression of growth factors (IGFs and isoforms of TGFβ) together with proliferating chondrocytes in the developing articular cartilage of Monodelphis. (a) At two months positive chondrocytes can be detected throughout the epiphyses and in the case of IGFs hypertrophic chondrocytes in the secondary centre of ossification were also immunopositive. By 3 months (b) and at skeletal maturity (8 months; c) there is a gradual restriction to the surface-most chondrocytes of the tissue.

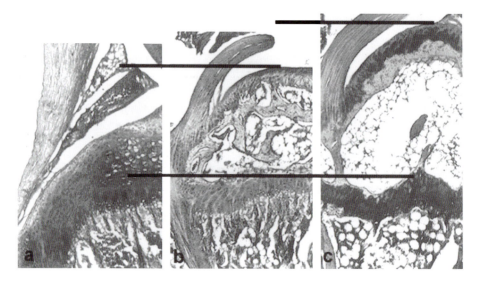

FIGURE 2.5   Micrograph showing longitudinal section through the posterior aspect of the tibial plateau in a 2-month (a), 4-month (b) and 6-month (c) Monodelphis knees. The insertion of the posterior cruciate ligament has been used as a topographical reference point. The top of the epiphyseal growth plate, which will not move in relative terms, has been aligned (basal line traversing the three micrographs). It can be seen that between 2 and 4 months and 4 and 6 months, the articular cartilage has been replaced during development (upper lines).

parts of the joint, the transitional layer had been abolished completely (not shown). Thus, the cartilage comprised a superficial layer and a basal hypertrophic layer.

Short-term studies on rabbit articular cartilage also support indirectly an appositonal growth mechanism. It has been reported that in the rabbit femoral trochlear, cell density and tissue thickness both declined between weeks 6 and 8, but the decline in cell density was most marked in the surface zone (Oreja *et al.*, 1995). Our own preliminary stereo-logical studies on *Monodelphis* articular cartilage also concur with the above data on rabbit cartilage.

One ramification of such a growth mechanism is that it would rely on an articular cartilage progenitor cell or 'stem' cell residing within the articular surface. Additionally, work from other groups has suggested that articular cartilage can be delineated from epiphyseal cartilage early in development even before cavitation of the joint. In this context, it is interesting that a number of ECM molecules are differentially expressed at the presumptive articular surface. In *Monodelphis*, these include fibromodulin and biglycan (Archer *et al.*, 1996) and in the rabbit, type V collagen (Bland and Ashhurst, 1996). It is possible, therefore, that articular cartilage has a lineage quite distinct from that of epiphyseal cartilage and we are conducting studies to investigate this possibility further.

CARTILAGE DEVELOPMENT, DISEASE AND REPAIR

It is well established that cartilage has a poor intrinsic reparative potential. However, during degenerative change or upon wounding, cartilage displays responses which may be interpreted as reparative. These include elevated matrix synthesis and renewed chondrocyte proliferation (see Archer, 1994 for review). It is evident that these responses are insufficient to heal even limited lesions particularly under functional loading. Consequently, a number of strategies have been devised in order to promote or augment cartilage repair. The most common strategy is the implantation of chondrocytes usually within a carrier vehicle (polymers or biopolymers) into an experimental defect within articular cartilage (see Chapter 13 by Buckwalter). Whilst this strategy is not new (stemming from early work by Bentley and colleagues; Bentley and Greer, 1971) it has become increasingly popular. Overall, however, longer-term results are ambiguous (Messner and Gilquist, 1996).

The above data and ideas have ramifications in relation to cartilage repair strategies. Since articular cartilage grows from the surface region, there is likely to be an 'articular cartilage progenitor' in that region, which is responsible for the generation of the tissue. Interestingly, during degenerative disease, chondrocytes at the articular surface either die or are sloughed off during fibrillation. It is possible, therefore, that the cells which may possess the developmental repertoire to regenerate articular cartilage rather than hyaline cartilage *per se,* are lost during the disease process. It is also possible that once articular cartilage matures, then the cells responsible for its growth lose the capacity for further tissue regeneration.

Another common approach to many articular cartilage repair strategies is the use of cartilage progenitor cells from a number of sources which include the marrow cavity (Shapiro *et al.*, 1993), perichondrium (Homminga *et al.*, 1990) and periosteum (Lorentzon *et al.*, 1996). In all these cases, progenitor cells have been used in attempts to augment repair in drill-hole defects within load bearing joints. Whilst copious amounts of hyaline cartilage is often produced within these defects, there is seldom evidence of the defined architecture characteristic of articular cartilage. We would argue that such cells do not have the developmental programme to regenerate articular cartilage.

SUMMARY

Little detail is known about the cell and molecular events which control the development of joints and articular cartilage. In early joint development, it is becoming apparent that the interzone is an important signalling region which may have its immediate effects on regulating the growth of the early cartilage elements. We are accumulating data on the growth mechanisms of articular cartilage. Indications are that articular cartilage, once formed, grows by apposition from the articular surface in a mechanism not dissimilar to the epiphyseal growth plate. Such a mechanism would require the existence of an articular cartilage progenitor or 'stem' cell to reside at the articular surface. We hypothesise that articular cartilage has a lineage quite distinct from embryonic epiphyseal cartilage. The above ideas have ramifications to our current thinking on strategies of articular cartilage repair.

ACKNOWLEDGEMENT

The authors gratefully acknowledge the Arthritis and Rheumatism Council for financial support.

REFERENCES

Andersen, H. (1962) Histochemical studies of the development of the human hip joint. *Acta Anat.*, **48**, 258–292.

Archer, C.W., Morrison, H. and Pitsillides, A. (1994) Cellular aspects of the development of diarthrodial joints and articular cartilage. *J. Anat.*, **184**, 447–456.

Archer, C.W. (1994) Skeletal development and osteoarthrtis. *Ann. Rheum. Dis.*, **53**, 624–630.

Benninghoff, A. (1925) Form und Bau der Gelenkknorpel in ihren Beziehungen zur Function Z. *Zellforsch mikrosk Anat.*, **2**, 783–862.

Bentley, G. and Greer, R. (1971) Homotransplantation of isolated epiphyseal and articular chondrocytes into the joint surfaces of rabbits. *Nature*, **230**, 385–388.

Bland, Y. and Ashhurst, D. (1996) Development and ageing of the articular cartilage of the rabbit knee joint: distribution of fibrillar collagens. *Anat. Embryol.*, **194**, 607–619.

Brittberg, M., Lindahl, A., Nilsson, A., Ohlsson, C., Isaksson, O. and Peterson, L. (1994) Treatment of deep cartilage defects in the knee with autologous chondrocyte transplantation. *N. Eng. J. Med.*, **331**, 889–895.

Buckwalter, J.A. (1992) In: Mechanical injuries of articular cartilage (ed. Finerman, G.). *Biology and Biomechanics of the Traumatized Synovial Joint*, pp. 83–96. Park Ridge IL: American Academy of Orthopaedic Surgeons.

Calandruccio, R.A. and Gilmer, W.S. (1962) Proliferation, regeneration and repair of articular cartilage of immature animals. *J. Bone Joint Surg.*, **44A**, 431–455.

Caplan, A., Goto, T., Wakitani, S., Pineda, S., Haynesworth, S. and Goldberg, V. (1992) In: Mechanical injuries of articular cartilage (ed. Finerman, G.). *Cell based technologies for cartilage repair*, pp. 111–122. Park Ridge IL: American Academy of Orthopaedic Surgeons.

Caterson, B., Mahmooodian, F., Sorrell, J., Hardingham, T., Bayliss, M. *et al.* (1991) Modulation of native chondroitin sulphate structuers in tissue development and disease. *J. Cell Sci.*, **97**, 411–417.

Craig, F., Bentley, G. and Archer, C.W. (1987) The temporospatial distributions of collagen types I and II and keratan sulphate in the developing metatarsophalangeal joint of the chick. *Development*, **99**, 383–391.

DePalma, A.F., McKeever, C. and Subin, D. (1966) Process of repair of articular cartilage demonstrated by histology and autoradiography with tritiated thymidine. *Clin. Orthop.*, **48**, 229–242.

Duprez, D., de Bell, E., Richardson, M., Archer, C.W., Wolpert, L., Brickell, P. and Francis-West, P. (1996) Overexpression of BMP-2 and BMP-4 alters the size and shape of developing skeletal elements in the chick limb. *Mechanisms of Development*, **57**, 145–157.

Edwards, J., Wilkinson, L., Jones, H., Soothill, P., Henderson, K., Worral, J. and Pitsillides, A. (1994) The formation of human joint cavities: a possible role for hyaluronan and CD44 in altered interzone cohesion. *J. Anat.*, **185**, 355–367.

Francis-West, P., Richardson, M., Bell, E., Chen, P., Luyten, F., Brickell, P., Wolpert, L. and Archer, C.W. (1996) The effect of over expression of BMP-4 and GDF-5 on the development of limb skeletal elements. *Trans. Orthop. Res. Soc.*, **21**, 62.

Ganan, Y., Macias, D., Duterque-Coquillaud, M., Ros, M. and Hurle, J. (1996) Role of TGFβs and BMPs as signals controlling the position of the digits and the areas of cell death in the developing chick limb autopod. *Development*, **122**, 2349–2357.

Gardner, E. and Gray, D.J. (1950) Prenatal development of the human hip joint. *Am. J. Anat.*, **87**, 163–212.

Gardner, E. and Gray, D.J. (1953) Prenatal development of the human shoulder and acromioclavicular joint. *Am. J. Anat.*, **92**, 219–276.

Gardner, E., O'Rahilly, R. (1968) The early development of the knee joint in staged human embryos. *J. Anat.*, **102**, 289–299.

Gray, D.J. and Gardner, E. (1951) Prenatal development of the human elebow joint. *Am. J. Anat.*, **88**, 429–469.

Harrington, E., Fanidi, A. and Evan, G. (1994) Oncogenes and cell death. *Current Opinion in Genetics and Development*, **4**, 120–129.

Homminga, G., Bulstra, S., Bouweester, P. and van der Linden, A. (1990) Perichondrial grafting for cartilage lesions of the knee. *J. Bone Joint Surg.* (Br), **72**, 1003–1007.

Ishizaki, Y., Burne, J. and Raff, M. (1994) Autocrine signals enable chondrocytes to survive in culture. *J. Cell Biol.*, **126**, 1069–1077.

Joseph, J., Thomas, G. and Tynan, J. (1961) The reaction of the ear cartilage of the rabbit and guinea-pig to trauma. *J. Anat.*, **95**, 564–568.

Kingsley, D., Bland, A., Grubber, J., Marker, P., Russell, L., Copeland, N. and Jenkins, N. (1992) The mouse *short ear* skeletal morphogenesis locus is associated with defects in a bone morphogenetic memeber of the TGFβ superfamily. *Cell*, **71**, 399–410.

Li, Y., Lacerda, D.A., Warman, M.L., Beier, D., Yoshioka, H., Ninomiya, Y., Oxford, J., Morris, N., Andrikopoulos, K., Ramirez, T., Wardell, B., Lifferth, G., Teuscher, C., Woodward, S., Taylor, B., Seegmiller, R. and Olsen, B. (1995) A fibrillar collagen gene Col IIaI is essential for skeletal morphogenesis. *Cell*, **80**, 423–430.

Lorentzon, R., Hildingsson, C. and Alfredson, H. (1996) Treatment of deep cartilage defects with periosteum transplantation. Swedish Orthop. Ass. Meeting, Karlstad, September 1996.

Macias, D., Ganan, Y., Sampath, T.K., Piedra, M., Ros, M. and Hurle, J.M. (1997) Role of BMP-2 and OP-1 (BMP-7) in programmed cell death and skeletogenesis during chick limb development. *Development*, **124**, 1109–1117.

Mankin, H.J. (1962) Localisation of tritiated thymidine in articular cartilage of rabbits. I Growth in immature cartilage. *J. Bone Joint Surg.*, **44A**, 682–688.

Messner, K. and Gillquist, J. (1996) Cartilage repair. A critical review. *Acta Orthop. Scand.*, **67**, 523–529.

O'Rahilly, R. (1951) The early prenatal development of the human knee joint. *J. Anat.*, **85**, 135–194.

Oreja, M., Rodriguez, M., Abelleira, A., Garcia, M., Garcia, M.A. and Barreiro, F. (1995) Variation in articular cartilage in rabbits between weeks six and eight. *Anat. Rec.*, **241**, 34–38.

Sailor, L., Hewick, R. and Morris, E. (1996) Recombinant human bone morphogenetic protein-2 maintains the articular chondrocyte phenotype in long-term culture. *J. Orthop. Res.*, **14**, 937–945.

Shapiro, F., Koide, S. and Glimcher, M. (1993) Cell origin and differentiation in the repair of full-thickness defects of articular cartilage. *J. Bone Joint Surg.*, **75A**, 532–553.

Silver, F. and Glasgold, A. (1995) Cartilage wound healing. *Otolaryngologic Clinics of North America*, **28**, 847–864.

Stockwell, R.A. (1979) *Biology of Cartilage Cells*. Cambridge University Press, Cambridge.

Storm, E. and Kingsley, D. (1997) Joint patterning defects caused by single and double mutations in members of the bone morphogenetic protein family. *Development*, **122**, 3969–3979.

Storm, E., Huyth, T., Copeland, N., Jenkins, N. and Kingsley, D. (1994) Limb alterations in brachypodism mice due to muations in a new memeber of the TGFβ superfamily. *Nature*, **368**, 639–643.

Vandenberg, P., Khillan, J., Prockop, D.J., Helminen, H., Kontusaari, S. and Alkokko, L. (1991) Expression of a partially-deleted gene of human type II procollagen (COL2A1) in transgenic mice produces a chondrodysplasia. *Proc. Nat. Acad. Sci. USA*, **88**, 7640–7644.

Wakitani, S., Kimura, T., Hirooka, A., Ochi, T., Yoneda, M., Yasui, N., Owaki, H. and Ono, K. (1989) Repair of rabbit articular surfaces with allograft chondrocytes embedded in collagen gel. *J. Bone Joint Surg.*, **71B**, 74–80.

Walmesley, R. and Bruce, J. (1938) The early stages of the replacement of the semi-lunar cartilages of the knee joint in rabbits after operative excision. *J. Anat.*, **72**, 260–263.

3 Involvement of Tenascin-C and Syndecan-3 in the Development of Chick Limb Diarthrodial Joints

Maurizio Pacifici*, Eiki Koyama, Thorsten Kirsch,
Judith L. Leatherman and Eleanor B. Golden

*Department of Anatomy and Histology, School of Dental Medicine,
University of Pennsylvania, Philadelphia, PA 19104-6003, USA*

INTRODUCTION

The limb continues to represent a favoured experimental system to study problems of skeletal patterning and morphogenesis and skeletal cell differentiation. Limb skeleto-genesis begins with the emergence of mesenchymal cell condensations in its core region and proceeds in a proximal-to-distal and posterior-to-anterior fashion (Hinchliffe and Johnson, 1980; Duboule, 1994). For example, in the chick embryo leg bud, the first condensation becomes recognizable around Day 3 of embryogenesis (approximately stage 22; Hamburger and Hamilton, 1951), and by stage 24 it displays its characteris-tic uninterrupted Y shape. The rod-like proximal part of the Y-shaped condensation represents the presumptive femur while the distal arms represent presumptive tibia and fibula, all fused together at the site of the future knee joint of which there is no obvious sign at this stage. By stage 26, additional condensations emerge beyond the forked distal end of the Y-shaped condensation and represent tarsal and digit elements (Thorogood and Hinchliffe, 1975). In similar proximal-to-distal and posterior-to-anterior fashions, the condensations undergo cytodifferentiation and give rise to chondrocytes; the first cartilage matrix producing cells become evident in the most proximal condensation around stage 24–25 (Oettinger *et al.*, 1985). The chondrocytes located in the future dia-physeal region of each skeletal element are then the first to undergo maturation and

* Corresponding author.

hypertrophy; the maturation process spreads toward the epiphyses with further development and culminates with erosion of the hypertrophic cartilage and deposition of subperiosteal bone.

The joints connecting the limb skeletal elements are diarthrodial synovial joints. These joints develop from the so-called interzone and include articular cartilage, synovial tissue, menisci, ligaments and a surrounding fibrous capsule (Holder, 1977; Mitrovic, 1977). The interzone is the mesenchymal tissue that comes to separate the early skeletal elements from each other. In some condensations such as the proximal Y-shaped and tarsophalangeal condensations, their uninterrupted nature initially gives rise to a continuous cartilaginous structure. Subsequent joint development involves a more complex process (Thorogood and Hinchliffe, 1975; Smith, 1978; Craig et al., 1987; Archer et al., 1994). The chondrocytes located in the presumptive joint area become flattened and lose their characteristic metachromatic matrix. Surrounding mesenchymal cells then migrate into the joint area and, possibly together with the flattened 'dedifferentiated' chondrocytes, give rise to the interzone. Once formed, the interzone is the source of precursor cells that give rise to the various joint structures. Joint development is brought to conclusion with the cavitation process which creates a fluid-filled movable synovial cavity (Persson, 1983; Craig et al., 1987).

While the above morphological aspects of limb skeletal development have been thoroughly studied and are well documented, the underlying mechanisms of regulation remain poorly understood. Thus, we know little about how the precartilaginous condensations form and differentiate into chondrocytes, how the uninterrupted cartilaginous anlagens become separated by the interzone at the sites of future joints, how the interzone itself forms and gives rise to the various joint structures, and how the most epiphyseal chondrocytes of each skeletal element acquire the capacity to become permanent articular chondrocytes while the remaining epiphyseal, metaphyseal and diaphyseal transient chondrocytes undergo maturation into hypertrophic chondrocytes and are eventually replaced by bone cells.

To address these and related important questions, we have carried out studies over the last few years on the possible roles of the extracellular matrix component tenascin-C and a cell surface receptor syndecan-3 in skeletal development and, in particular, joint development (Pacifici et al., 1993; Koyama et al., 1995, 1996; Pacifici, 1995; Shimazu et al., 1996). The possibility that these macromolecules may have roles in these processes was based on several previous findings and considerations, including the following. First, tenascin-C had been found to be particularly rich at boundaries between different adjacent tissues and structures in the embryo (Chiquet and Fambrough, 1984; Erickson and Bourdon, 1989). Joint development, particularly in the case of uninterrupted chondrocytic anlagens, does involve formation of a tissue 'barrier' (i.e. the interzone), resulting in the creation of two contiguous but distinct skeletal elements. Thus, we reasoned that tenascin-C may have a role in establishing such a 'barrier'. Second, tenascin-C had been found to act as an anti-adhesive agent and to maintain a variety of cultured cell types in a round configuration (Chiquet-Ehrismann et al., 1988). In early cartilaginous skeletal elements, the most epiphyseal chondrocytes, which will give rise to articular cartilage, do display a round configuration and are morphologically distinct from the underlying chondrocytes in the growth plate which are flat and irregularly shaped

(Lutfi, 1974; Howlett, 1979). Thus, we reasoned that tenascin-C may also have a role in maintaining developing articular chondrocytes in a round configuration and help them become distinguished from non-articular chondrocytes. Third, tenascin-C had been found to interact with a variety of receptors at the cell surface, including integrins and syndecans (Salmivirta *et al.*, 1991; Prieto *et al.*, 1993; Sriramarao *et al.*, 1993; Grumet *et al.*, 1994). Thus, if tenascin-C were indeed involved in joint development, cell surface receptors interacting with the protein may have to be involved as well. We focused on syndecan-3 because this cell surface component had already been shown to be expressed by limb prechondrogenic cell condensations and thus to be involved in skeletogenesis (Gould *et al.*, 1992).

TENASCIN-C

Tenascin-C belongs to a family of large extracellular matrix macromolecules including tenascin-X and tenascin-R (Bristow *et al.*, 1993) and consists of six identical subunits associated into a disulfide-bonded hexabrachion structure (Erickson and Iglesias, 1984). Each subunit of the hexabrachion displays a complex structure and contains structural domains homologous to those of other proteins including several epidermal growth factor-like domains comprising the N-terminal half of the protein, several fibronectin type III repeats comprising most of the C-terminal half, and a fibrinogen-like Ca^{2+}-binding domain at the C-terminal end. Tenascin-C variants differing in molecular size have been described in mammals and avians. They are the product of alternative splicing and differ in the number of fibronectin type III repeats (Jones *et al.*, 1989; Saga *et al.*, 1991). In the chick, the largest variant has subunits of 230 kDa, each containing 11 fibronectin type III repeats (TnC230); smaller variants containing 9 or 8 repeats display subunit sizes of 200 kDa (TnC200) and 190 kDa (TnC190), respectively.

In vivo studies have shown that tenascin-C is present in a highly restricted number of embryonic and adult tissues and is particularly prominent at tissue–tissue boundaries (Erickson and Bourdon, 1989). Studies with cultured cells have indicated that tenascin-C often acts as an anti-adhesive agent and interferes with attachment and spreading of many cell types (Chiquet-Ehrismann *et al.*, 1988), suggesting that tenascin may exert a 'barrier' function *in vivo* by limiting cell adhesion. This possibility would correlate with the finding that tenascin-C is transiently expressed by migrating, possibly loosely-attached cells during morphogenesis *in vivo* (Chuong *et al.*, 1987). On the other hand, tenascin-C has also been shown to exert pro-adhesion effects on certain cell types such as endothelial cells (Sriramarao *et al.*, 1993). As revealed by experiments with tenascin-C fragments, the anti-adhesion properties of the protein probably reside in the N-terminal half while the pro-adhesion activity is probably located in the C-terminal half (Spring *et al.*, 1989).

The diverse effects of tenascin-C on cell behavior are probably mediated by its interactions with different cell surface receptors and other extracellular components. The protein has in fact been found to interact with several integrins and cell surface-associated proteoglycans such as neurocan, phosphocan and syndecan-1 (Prieto *et al.*, 1993; Sriramarao *et al.*, 1993; Grumet *et al.*, 1994; Salmivirta *et al.*, 1991).

SYNDECAN-3

Syndecan-3 is a member of a family of proteoglycans intimately associated with the cell surface and all bearing heparan sulfate chains (Bernfield *et al.*, 1992; Gould *et al.*, 1992). The core proteins of these proteoglycans contain a hydrophobic region through which these macromolecules remain anchored to the cell surface as integral membrane components, and a cytoplasmic domain which may interact with cytoplasmic proteins including the cytoskeleton. Because of their location at the cell surface, heparan sulfate-rich proteoglycans were originally suggested to serve as structural and functional links between the cell surface and surrounding microenvironmental components (Pacifici and Molinaro, 1980; Moscatelli, 1987). Indeed, syndecans are now known to interact with several pericellular matrix macromolecules (Koda and Bernfield, 1984; Sun *et al.*, 1989; Salmivirta *et al.*, 1991). They also interact with powerful growth factors including fibroblast growth factors, vascular endothelial cell growth factor, and epidermal growth factor (Moscatelli, 1987; Ornitz and Leder, 1992; Gitay-Goren *et al.*, 1992, Higashiyama *et al.*, 1991; Chernousov and Carey, 1993). In fact, the interaction of growth factors such as fibroblast growth factor with syndecans is required for biological activity; that is, the factor must interact with the heparan sulfate chains of the syndecans before it can interact with its tyrosine kinase-containing receptor, which transduces the signal intracellularly.

Syndecan-3 is a typical member of the syndecan family. cDNA and protein analyses in the chick (Gould *et al.*, 1992, 1995) have shown that its core protein is 383 amino acids long and has a predicted molecular size of about 42 kDa. The extracellular domain is 325 amino acids long and contains a total of eight potential sites for attachment of glycosaminoglycan chains, and the cytoplasmic domain is 33 amino acids long and is potentially capable of interactions with the cytoskeleton. Electrophoretic analysis of purified syndecan-3 following treatment with heparinase or chondroitinase has shown that syndecan-3 contains heparan sulfate chains but not chondroitin sulfate chains. Comparison of these features and other core protein characteristics among known syndecan family members show that syndecan-3 is most closely related to syndecan-1 (Saunders *et al.*, 1989; Gould *et al.*, 1995).

TENASCIN-C, SYNDECAN-3 AND CHONDROGENIC CELL DIFFERENTIATION

Both tenascin-C and syndecan-3 have been found to be associated with chondrogenesis in the developing chick embryo (Mackie *et al.*, 1987; Gould *et al.*, 1992). Both macromolecules become particularly prominent in limb prechondrogenic mesencymal cell condensations *in vivo* but are barely visible in the surrounding mesenchyme. As the condensations differentiate into chondrocytes, expression of these macromolecules decreases markedly but remains significant in the perichondral mesenchymal cells immediately adjacent to the differentiated chondrocytes (Hoffmann *et al.*, 1988; Prieto *et al.*, 1990; Vakeva *et al.*, 1990; Tucker 1993). Studies with prechondrogenic mesenchymal cells in micromass culture have shown that exogenous tenascin-C stimulates chondrogenic cell differentiation in limb cell micromass cultures whereas treatment with anti-tenascin antibodies inhibits it (Mackie *et al.*, 1987; Chuong *et al.*, 1993). Similar experiments using antisera to syndecan-3 or exogenous syndecan-3 have not yet been reported. Taken together, the above data have led to the conclusion that tenascin-C and syndecan-3 participate in the cytodifferentiation of chondrocytes and most likely promote this process. The macro-molecules would have a similar positive role in chondrogenesis even when they relocalize to the perichondrium; in this location, they have been suggested to favor the differentia-tion of perichondral mesenchymal cells into chondrocytes, thus contributing to the initial appositional growth of the cartilaginous models.

EXPRESSION OF TENASCIN-C AND SYNDECAN-3 DURING JOINT DEVELOPMENT

The first clue that tenascin-C may also play roles in joint development is to be found in the seminal work of Chiquet and Fambrough (1984). These authors found that in early chick embryos tenascin-C was particularly obvious in the perichondrium along the incip-ient diaphysis of limb cartilaginous skeletal elements. With further development, the pro-tein appeared also at the epiphyses where it delineated in a striking and clear manner the contour of adjacent skeletal elements along their joint boundary. Based on this and other findings (see above), we carried out *in situ* hybridization and immunohistochemical stud-ies to determine more closely the gene expression of tenascin-C as well as syndecan-3 during limb skeletal development in chick embryos, aiming to uncover the possible involvement and roles of these macromolecules in joint development and function (Pacifici *et al.*, 1993; Koyama *et al.*, 1995, 1996; Pacifici, 1995). Some of our key find-ings are described below.

In stage 28–29 chick embryos (Day 6–6.5 of embryogenesis), the metacarpal and digit elements are still ill-defined morphologically but are already cartilaginous. *In situ* hybridization on tissue sections using a ^{35}S-labelled type II collagen riboprobe revealed the presence of abundant transcripts encoding this typical cartilage matrix macromolecule in these elements and depicted their morphology (Figure 3.1A). When we examined syndecan-3 gene expression in companion sections, we found that this macromolecule was strongly expressed by cells at the outer border of the elements, particularly by the perichondral cells forming a thick mesenchymal tissue around the incipient diaphysis (Figure 3.1B). A positive but fainter signal was also present in epiphyseal chondrocytes and surrounding adjacent mesenchymal cells but no signal was appreciable in diaphyseal chondrocytes (Figure 3.1B). In comparison, tenascin-C gene expression was in general weaker than that of syndecan-3 and was particularly evident only in the inner layer of diaphyseal perichondrium (Figure 3.1C, arrowhead); expression was also appreciable but diffuse at each epiphysis (Figure 3.1C). Immuno-histochemical analysis using monospecific or monoclonal antibodies to tenascin-C and syndecan-3 revealed that the distribution of the proteins was superimposable to that of their respective mRNAs (not shown). The level of immunolabelling observed was, however, not very strong, par-ticularly when compared with that obtained at later developmental stages (see below);

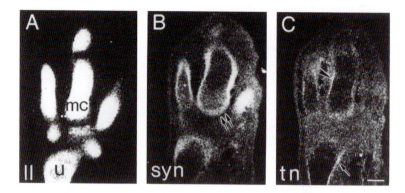

FIGURE 3.1   *In situ* hybridization analysis of the distribution of transcripts encoding type II collagen (A), syndecan-3 (B) and tenascin-C (C) in serial sections of stage 28 (Day 6) chick embryo metacarpal elements. In (B), double arrow points to the epiphysis of the metacarpal (mc) element rich in syndecan-3 transcripts. In (C) arrowhead points to the tenascin-C-rich inner layer of diaphyseal perichondrium of metacarpal element, and arrow points to tenascin-C-rich metaphyseal perichondrium of ulna (u). Bar, 175 μm.

this indicated that at these earlier stages the amounts of syndecan-3 and tenascin-C were relatively low.

With further development and elongation of the skeletal elements, we observed that the expression of syndecan-3 and tenascin-C decreased along the diaphysis while increasing at the epiphyses and the developing joints. *In situ* hybridization at the level of the joint between the proximal phalange (pp) and distal phalange (dp) in stage 36 chick embryos revealed that each epiphysis contained abundant levels of syndecan-3 mRNA, particularly in the cells at the very extremity of each element along the incipient articulating border (Figure 3.2A and 2C, double arrow). Conversely, tenascin-C mRNA was very prominent at the periphery of each epiphysis (Figure 3.2E, arrowhead) and was gradually reduced along the articulating line (Figure 3.2E).

Strikingly, when we examined the joint between the proximal phalange and the metacarpal element (which is developmentally older than the joint between proximal and distal phalanges) in the same stage 36 embryos, different expression patterns were observed (Figures 3.2B, 3.2D and 3.2F). Most notably, the overall syndecan-3 expression pattern, while largely unchanged topographically, appeared to have diminished quantitatively (Figure 3.2D), as compared to that in the younger joint (Figure 3.2C). In contrast, tenascin-C expression was extremely prominent and characterised all of the most epiphyseal chondrocytes and adjacent interzone cells along the articulating surface and epiphyseal contour (Figure 3.2F, double arrow). Also of interest is the fact that the interzone cells located in between the opposing elements appeared to express very low levels of both tenascin-C and syndecan-3 (Figures 3.2E–3.2F, double arrow), creating a multi-layered structure reminiscent of a typical three-layered interzone (Haines, 1947).

Together, the above results indicate that tenascin-C and syndecan-3 are first strongly but distinctly expressed along the diaphysis of long bone cartilaginous models. In this location, they are probably involved in the development and function of the diaphyseal

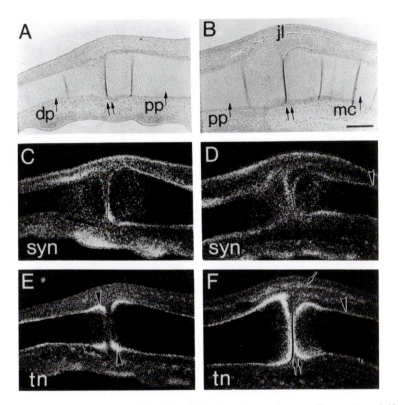

FIGURE 3.2   *In situ* hybridization analysis of the distribution of transcripts encoding syndecan-3 (C–D) and tenascin-C (E–F) in serial sections of joints between the metacarpal (mc) element and proximal phalange (pp), and between the proximal phalange and distal phalange (dp) in stage 36 (Day 10) chick embryo. (A) and (B) are corresponding phase micrographs. In (D) and (F), arrowheads point to metaphyseal perichondrium, single arrow points to joint ligament (jl), and double arrow points to most-epiphyseal chondrocytes and intervening joint interzone. In (E), arrowheads point to peripheral epiphyseal chondrocytes and adjacent cells rich in tenascin-C transcripts. Bar, 175 μm.

perichondral collar, long recognised to be instrumental in the morphological definition of the diaphysis (Fell, 1925). The subsequent increases in the expression of both molecules at the epiphyses are probably linked to the genesis of the interzone, the full separation of contiguous opposing elements, and the development of epiphyseal chondrocytes.

It should be noted that at the above stages, the syndecan-3- and tenascin-C-expressing epiphyseal chondrocytes have not yet been separated into a population of most-epiphyseal permanent articular chondrocytes and an underlying population of growth plate chondrocytes extending into the metaphysis. Indeed, we have found that the entire population of epiphyseal chondrocytes is actively proliferating (see Figure 3.5A). This confirms previous results obtained in mammalian embryos (Mankin, 1962; Archer *et al.*, 1994) and sustains the view that these proliferating chondrocytes are responsible for the initial lengthening of the cartilaginous models before this function is taken over by the growth plate at later stages.

DEVELOPMENT OF ARTICULAR CARTILAGE AND GROWTH PLATE

Given the above results and interpretations, it was of interest to assess the expression of syndecan-3 and tenascin-C at later stages when articular and growth plate chondrocytes emerge at the epiphyses (Pacifici, 1995). To this end, we carried out an immuno-histochemical analysis of the distribution of these macromolecules in stage 46 (approx. Day 18) chick embryo long bone models. Longitudinal sections of tibia stained with the M1 monoclonal antibody to tenascin-C (Chiquet and Fabrough, 1984) and polyclonal antibodies to syndecan-3 (Gould *et al.*, 1992) revealed that tenascin-C was now extremely abundant but confined to articular chondrocytes (Figures 3.3A and 3.3D) and associated structures, such as fibrocartilage and menisci (not shown).

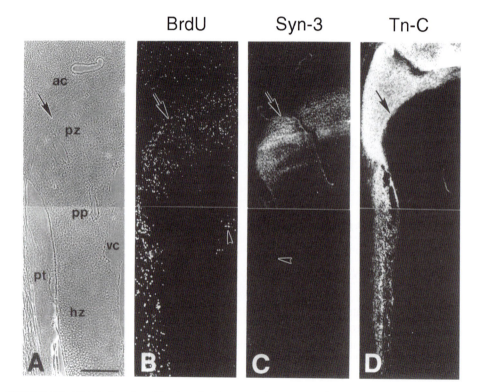

FIGURE 3.3   Distribution of proliferating chondrocytes (B), syndecan-3 (C) and tenascin-C (D) in Day 18 chick embryo tibia. Longitudinal sections of the proximal portion of tibia from bromodeoxyuridine (BrdU)-labeled embryos were processed for immunofluorescence using a monoclonal antibody to BrdU. Similar serial sections form unlabeled embryos were processed directly for immunohistochemistry. Note that the BrdU-rich chondrocytes in (B) correspond to those containing high levels of syndecan-3 in (C). Note also that the prolifer-ating syndecan-3-rich chondrocytes lie immediately below the tenascin-C-rich articular chondrocytes, thus cre-ating a striking boundary (arrow in A through D) between these two populations of cells. Arrowhead in (B) points to blood vessel-associated proliferating cells; arrowhead in (C) points to syndecan-3-containing peri-chondral tissue. ac, articular cartilage; pz, proliferative zone; pp, post-proliferative pre-hypertrophic zone; hz, hypertrophic zone; vc, vascular canal; and pt, perichondral tissue. Bar, 250 μm.

We and others have shown that tenascin-C remains an abundant component of adult articular cartilage (Pacifici *et al.*, 1993; Savarese *et al.*, 1996). In contrast, syndecan-3 was virtually undetectable in articular chondrocytes and was restricted to proliferating chondrocytes in the top zone of the growth plate lying immediately below the articular cartilage (Figures 3.3A and 3.3C). That the syndecan-3-rich chondrocytes represented proliferating chondrocytes was confirmed by pulse-labeling with 5-bromo-2'-deoxy-uridine (BrdU) *in vivo* (Wilson, 1992) followed by immunodetection of incorporated BrdU on tissue sections (Figure 3.3B). Neither syndecan-3 nor tenascin-C was detectable in the remainder of the growth plate chondrocytes, including hypertrophic chondrocytes.

Thus, a dramatic change in distribution and levels of tenascin-C and syndecan-3 accompanies the emergence of articular and growth plate chondrocytes in the epiphysis and metaphysis of long bone models.

TENASCIN VARIANTS

The three splice variants of chick tenascin-C, TnC230, TnC200 and TnC190, display tissue-specific distributions *in vivo* (Prieto *et al.*, 1990; Chiquet-Ehrismann *et al.*, 1991). Thus, we asked whether different tenascin-C variants are present in the different joint tissues. Longitudinal sections of Day 19 chick embryo knee were processed for immuno-histochemistry using the monoclonal antibodies anti-Tn26, anti-Tn32 and M1 (kindly provided by Dr. R. Chiquet-Ehrismann) which can distinguish among the three variants. We found that the most peripheral articular chondrocytes in the tibial plateau contained both TnC200 and TnC190 whereas the bulk of the articular tissue contained the smallest variant only, TnC190. In contrast, other joints tissues such as cruciate ligament and meniscus contained all three tenascin-C variants (Pacifici *et al.*, 1993). Thus, different tenascin-C variants are present in different joint tissues.

SYNDECAN-3 AND CHONDROCYTE PROLIFERATION

The above *in vivo* data demonstrate that there is a coincidence between syndecan-3 expression and chondrocyte proliferation. To obtain evidence for a causal relationship, we carried out experiments with chondrocytes isolated from the entire cartilaginous sternum of Day 13–14 chick embryos (Leboy *et al.*, 1989). As we showed previously, the sternum at this stage contains in large part resting and immature chondrocytes which, once reared in standard serum-containing culture conditions, will initiate a phase of rapid cell proliferation followed by maturation into hypertrophic chondrocytes. We asked whether the sternum-derived cells expressed syndecan-3 and whether interference with syndecan-3 structure and function by heparinase treatment would affect their proliferative behavior in response to treatment with fibroblast growth factor-2 (FGF-2). The premise of these experiments is the fact that, as discussed above, growth factors such as FGF-2 must interact with heparan sulfate chains on the cell surface before they can elicit a proliferative response in cells (Moscatelli, 1987; Ornitz and Leder, 1992).

Accordingly, the freshly-isolated sternal chondrocytes were first grown for about 1 week in monolayer in complete medium containing 10% fetal calf serum, which caused stimulation of proliferation. Northern and western blot analyses showed that the 1 week-old cultures expressed large amounts of syndecan-3 (Shimazu *et al.*, 1996). Cultures were then switched to a medium containing 0.3% serum for 1 day to induce mitotic quiscence. Over the following 24 h, cultures were treated with various amounts of FGF-2; during the last 2 h of incubation, they were pulse-labeled with ^{3}H-thymidine. Doses as little as 0.1 to 0.3 ng/ml FGF-2 induced a strong proliferative response in the chondrocyte cultures, with maximal effects observed at about 5 ng/ml (Figure 3.4A, open squares). However, when the cultures were co-treated with FGF-2 and 1 unit/ml of heparinase I or heparinase III, the proliferative response was essentially prevented, even at high FGF-2 doses (Figure 3.4A, open and closed circles). In complementary experiments, the cultures were treated with the same dose of FGF-2 (1 ng/ml) and increasing amounts of heparinases (Figure 3.4B). We observed a clear dose-dependent inhibition of triated thymidine incorporation, with appreciable inhibition starting at enzyme concentrations as little as 0.05 units/ml (Figure 3.4B).

Clearly, heparan sulfate-rich proteoglycans associated with the surface of chondrocytes mediate the proliferative response of the cells to growth factors, such as FGF-2.

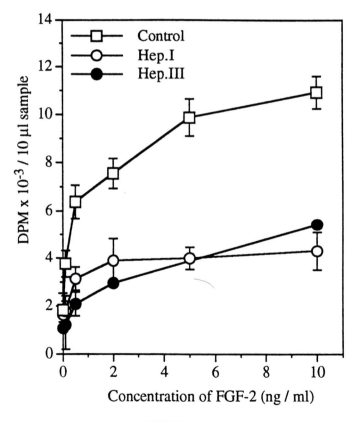

FIGURE 3.4A

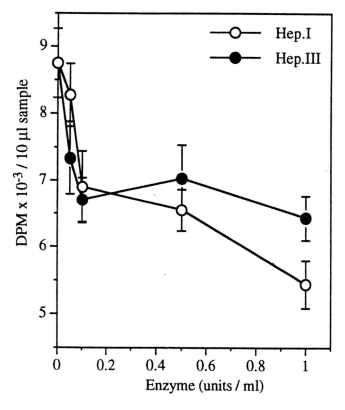

FIGURE 3.4B

FIGURE 3.4   Effects of FGF-2 and heparinase treatment on chondrocyte proliferation. (A) One week-old cultures of Day 13–14 chick embryo sternal chondrocytes were reared for 24 h in medium containing 0.3% serum to induce mitotic quiescence. During the following 24 h, the cultures were treated with increasing amounts of FGF-2 in the absence (control; open squares) or presence of heparinase I (open circles) or heparinase III (closed circles). During the last 2 h of incubation, cultures were pulse-labeled with triated thymidine and incorporated radioactivity was determined by scintillation counting. (B) Similar cultures were co-treated with 1 ng/ml FGF-2 and increasing amounts of heparinase I (open circles) or heparinase III (closed circles) for 24 h. During the last 2 h of incubation, the cultures wer pulse-labeled with tritiated thymidine and incorporated radioactivity determined as above.

CONCLUSIONS AND IMPLICATIONS

The results of our recent studies (Pacifici *et al.*, 1993; Koyama *et al.*, 1995, 1996; Pacifici, 1995; Shimazu *et al.*, 1996) summarized above and schematically represented in Figure 3.5 have provided clear evidence that tenascin-C and syndecan-3 participate in the development of diathrodial joints in the chick limb. The macromolecules appear to be closely associated with the initial process of definition of the outer contour of the cartilaginous elements and subsequently with the structural and functional definition of the epiphyseal ends.

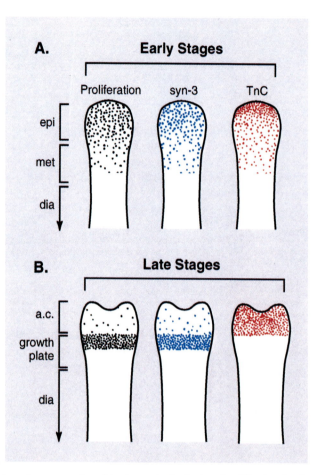

FIGURE 3.5   Schematic representation of the changes in distribution of proliferating chondrocytes (black), syndecan-3 (blue) and tenascin-C (red) in skeletal elements at early and late stages of embryogenesis. (A) At early stages (see Figures 3.1 and 3.2 above), there is a near coincidence between proliferating chondrocytes (which occupy the entire epiphysis and extend into the underlying metaphysis) and the gene expression patterns of syndecan-3 and tenascin-C. Note that at these stages tenascin-C gene expression is particularly strong at the most-epiphyseal border. (B) At late stages (see Figure 3.3 above), however, the proliferating chondrocytes form the top proliferating zone of growth plate, which extends from the metaphysis toward the diaphysis (dia); only syndecan-3 gene expression characterizes proliferating chondrocytes while tenascin-C gene expression is restricted to, and extremely abundant in, the entire population of epiphyseal articular chondrocytes.

What specific roles do these macromolecules play in such complex processes? Our current results allow us only to partially answer this question but suggest interesting possibilities. Syndecan-3 is a cell surface component which is likely able to interact with and react to a number of other macromolecules and growth factors (Bernfield *et al.*, 1992). Likewise, tenascin-C is a large multi-domain protein which can interact with a number of macromolecules and cell surface receptors, and exerts a number of effects on cell behaviour, including anti-adhesive effects (Spring *et al.*, 1989). Given their multiple potentials, syndecan-3 and tenascin-C could exert multiple effects during skeletogenesis.

For instance, our results have shown that syndecan-3 and to a lesser extent tenascin-C are expressed at the very onset of joint development when surrounding mesenchymal cells seem to be in the process of invading the future joint space (Koyama *et al.*, 1995). It is thus possible that the macromolecules could aid the migration of the mesenchymal cells. Syndecan-3 could mediate the interactions with or effects of factors, such as scatter factor (Takebayashi *et al.*, 1995), which are present at the sites of developing joints and may direct and stimulate cell migration. Tenascin-C could aid this process by virtue of its anti-adhesive properties; the protein has indeed been shown to be closely associated with migrating cells *in vivo* and *in vitro* (Chuong *et al.*, 1987; Chung *et al.*, 1996). The slow but steady increase of tenascin-C gene expression and levels along the epiphyseal contour (Chiquet and Fambrough 1984; Koyama *et al.*, 1995) with time would then lead to completion of interzone delineation and would fully separate the opposing elements with the establishment of a possibly non-adhesive 'barrier'.

Our data show that as interzone development is in progress, gene expression of tenascin-C and syndecan-3 becomes increasingly preponderant in the entire population of epiphyseal chondrocytes in each element and that this population is entirely mitotic (Figure 3.5A). With further development, however, expression of these macromolecules undergoes radical quantitative and qualitative changes; tenascin-C becomes restricted to and is extremely abundant in the most-epiphyseal articular chondrocytes, while syndecan-3 comes to characterize only the underlying growth plate proliferative chondrocytes (Figure 3.5B). We believe these changes in macromolecular distribution and levels are important and possibly instrumental for the structural and functional definition of epiphyseal and metaphyseal chondrocytes. Based on our evidence (Shimazu *et al.*, 1996) that syndecan-3 may regulate chondrocyte proliferation (Figure 3.4), we propose that syndecan-3 may contribute to the proliferative status of the entire epiphyseal chondrocyte population at the earlier stages (Figure 3.5A), when tenascin-C levels are still relatively low. As the amounts of tenascin-C increase markedly at the epiphyseal extremity, the local chondrocytes would substantially decrease their proliferative activity, decrease their expression of syndecan-3, and eventually become permanent postmitotic articular chondrocytes. Tenascin-C could exert these changes by virtue of its ability to bind to and possibly compete with cell surface receptors (including syndecans), to maintain cells in a phenotypically stable round configuration, and to influence cell behaviour and fate. The underlying tenascin-C-poor chondrocytes would then be able to remain in a proliferative state, maintain high levels of syndecan-3 expression, and become recognisable as the top proliferative zone of the growth plate. In support of these speculations, we should reiterate that the neoforming articular chondrocytes at the epiphyses of long bone models indeed display a round cell configuration while the underlying proliferative chondrocytes are irregularly shaped and flat to oval (Lutfi, 1974; Howlett, 1979). In addition, tenascin-C has been shown to maintain cells in a round cell configuration (Spring *et al.*, 1989).

In closing, we may ask how tenascin-C and syndecan-3 can exert different functions at different developmental stages and sites that we attribute to them above. We have proposed that these macromolecules may be able to exert multiple functions because of their complex multidomain structure. Another possible answer can be found in the fact that different tenascin-C variants with possibly different functions (Zisch *et al.*, 1992; Chung and Erickson, 1994) are expressed at different developmental stages and different sites during skeletogenesis. We have shown that in the knee joint of late chick embryos, the articular chondrocytes produce for the most part the smallest variant, TnC190, while the adjacent ligaments and menisci contain a mixture of all three variants (Pacifici *et al.*, 1993). With regard to syndecan-3, isoforms or variants of this macromolecule have not been described yet. Still, specificity of syndecan-3 action may derive from other means. First, syndecan-3 is expressed at different levels at different sites, and the resulting quantitative differences *per se* could contribute to specificity. Second, syndecan-3 may be able to mediate unique or characteristic processes depending on the nature of the cell's microenvironment, the composition of the cell surface, and the available specific signalling mechanisms. For example, we have shown that syndecan-3 is expressed in both the proliferative zone of growth plate and perichondrial tissue of the day 18 embryo tibia. *In situ* hybridization studies by others have shown that developing cartilage expresses fibroblast growth factor receptors 1 and 3 (FGF-R1 and FGF-R3) while perichondrial tissue expresses FGF-R2 and syndecan-2 (Peters *et al.*, 1993; David *et al.*, 1993). Thus, different complements of syndecans and FGF-Rs in different cells and tissues could mediate site- and time-specific effects. Lastly, the fine structure of the heparan sulfate chains has been shown to affect biological function (Sanderson *et al.*, 1994). Thus, the syndecan-3 molecules produced by different cells, including perichondrial cells and growth plate chondrocytes, may bear structurally different heparan sulfate chains with distinct biological properties.

ACKNOWLEDGEMENT

We thank Dr. Ruth Chiquet-Ehrismann for providing antibodies to chick tenascin-C isoforms and Dr. Robert Kosher for the antiserum to chick syndecan-3. The original work was supported by grants from the National Institutes of Health and the University of Pennsylvania Research Foundation.

REFERENCES

Archer, C.W., Morrison, H. and Pitsillides, A.A. (1994) Cellular aspects of the development of diarthrodial joints and articular cartilage. *J. Anat.*, **184**, 447–456.

Bernfield, M., Kokenyesi, R., Kato, M., Hinkes, M.T., Spring, J., Gallo, R.L. and Lose, E.J. (1992) Biology of the syndecans: a family of transmembrane heparan sulfate proteoglycans. *Annu. Rev. Cell Biol.*, **8**, 365–393.

Bristow, J., Tee, M.K., Gitleman, S.E., Melton, S.H. and Miller, W.L. (1993) Tenascin-X: a novel extracellular matrix protein encoded by human XB gene overlapping P450c21B. *J. Cell Biol.*, **122**, 265–278.

Chernousov, M.A. and Carey, D.J. (1993) N-syndecan (syndecan 3) from neonatal rat brain binds basic fibroblast growth factor. *J. Biol. Chem.*, **268**, 16810–16814.

Chiquet, M. and Fambrough, D.M. (1984) Chick myotendinous antigen. I. A monoclonal antibody as a marker for tendon and muscle morphogensis. *J. Cell Biol.*, **98**, 1926–1936.

Chiquet-Ehrismann, R., Kalla, P., Pearson, C.A., Beck, K. and Chiquet, M. (1988) Tenascin interferes with fibronection action. *Cell*, **53**, 383–390.

Chiquet-Ehrismann, R., Matsuoka, R., Hofer U., Spring, J., Bernasconi, C. and Chiquet, M. (1991) Tenascin variants: differential binding to fibronectin and distinct distribution in cell cultures and tissues. *Cell Reg.*, **2**, 927–938.

Chung, C.Y. and Erickson, H.P. (1994) Cell surface annexin II is a high affinity receptor for the alternatively spliced segment of tenascin-C. *J. Cell Biol.*, **126**, 539–548.

Chung, C.Y., Murphy-Ullrich, J.E. and Erickson, H.P. (1996) Mitogenesis, cell migration, and loss of focal adhesion induced by tenascin-C interacting with its cell surface receptor, annexin II. *Mol. Biol. Cell*, **7**, 883–892.

Chuong, C-M., Crossin, K.L. and Edelman, G.M. (1987) Sequential expression and differential functions of multiple adhesion molecules during the formation of cerebellar cortical layers. *J. Cell Biol.*, **104**, 331–342.

Chuong, C-M., Widelitz, R.B., Jiang, T.X., Abbott, U.K., Lee, Y.S. and Chen, H.M. (1993) Roles of adhesion molecules NCAM and tenascin-C in limb skeletogenesis: analysis with antibody perturbation, exoenous gene expression, Talpid[2] mutants and activin stimulation. In *Limb Development and Regeneration* (eds J.F. Fallon, P.F. Goetinck, R.O. Kelley and D.L. Stocum), pp. 465–474. Wiley-Liss, New York.

Craig, F.M., Bentley, G. and Archer, C.W. (1987) The spatial and temporal pattern of collagen I and II and keratan sulfate in the developing chick metatarso-phalangeal joint. *Development*, **99**, 383–391.

David, G., Bai, X.M., Van der Schueren, B., Marynen, P., Cassiman, J-J. and Van der Berghe, H. (1993) Spatial and temporal changes in the expression of fibroglycan (syndecan-2) during mouse embryonic development. *Development*, **119**, 841–854.

Duboule, D. (1994) How to make a limb? *Science*, **266**, 575–576.

Erickson, H.P. and Bourdon, M.A. (1989) Tenascin: an etracellular matrix protein prominent in specialized embryonic tissues and tumors. *Annu. Rev. Cell Biol.*, **5**, 71–92.

Erickson, H.P. and Iglesias, J.L. (1984) A six-armed oligomer isolated from cell surface fibronectin preparations. *Nature*, **311**, 267–268.

Fell, H.B. (1925) The histogenesis of cartilage and bone in the long bones of the embryonic fowl. *J. Morphol. Physiol.*, **40**, 417–459.

Gitay-Goren, H., Soker, S., Vlodavsky, I. and Neufeld, G. (1992) The binding of vascular endothelial growth factor to its receptor is dependent on cell surface-associated heparin-like molecules. *J. Biol. Chem.*, **267**, 6093–6098.

Gould, S.E., Upholt, W.B. and Kosher, R.A. (1992) Syndecan-3: a member of the syndecan family of membrane-intercalted proteoglycas that is expressed in high amounts at the onset of chicken limb cartilage differentiation. *Proc. Natl. Acad. Sci. USA*, **89**, 3271–3275.

Gould, S.E., Upholt, W.B. and Kosher, R.A. (1995) Characterization of chicken syndecan-3 as a heparan sulfate proteoglycan and its expression during embryogenesis. *Dev. Biol.*, **168**, 438–451.

Grumet, M., Milev, P., Sakurai, T., Karthikeyan, L., Bourdon, M., Margolis, R.K. and Margolis, R.U. (1994) Interactions with tenascin and differential effects on cell adhesion of neurocan and phosphocan, two major chondroitin sulfate proteoglycans of nervous tissue. *J. Biol. Chem.*, **269**, 12142–12146.

Haines, R.W. (1947) The development of the joints. *J. Anat.*, **81**, 33–55.

Hamburger, V. and Hamilton, H. (1951) A series of normal stages in the development of the chick embryo. *J. Morphol.*, **88**, 49–92.

Higashiyama, S., Abraham, J.A., Miller, J., Fiddes, J.C. and Klagsbrun, M. (1991) A heparin-binding growth factor secreted by macrophage-like cells that is related to EGF. *Science*, **251**, 936–939.

Hinchliffe, J.R. and Johnson, D.R. (1980) In *The Development of the Vertebrate Limb*, Oxford University Press, New York, pp. 76–83.

Hoffman, S., Crossin, K.L. and Eddelman, G.M. (1988) Molecular forms, binding functions, and developmental expression of cytotactin and cytotactin-binding proteoglycan, an interactive pair of extracellular matrix molecules. *J. Cell Biol.*, **106**, 519–532.

Holder, N. (1977) An experimental investigation into the early development of the chick elbow joint. *J. Embryol. Exp. Morphol.*, **39**, 115–127.

Howlett, C.R. (1979) The fine structure of the proximal growth plate in the avian tibia. *J. Anat.*, **128**, 377–399.

Jones, F.S., Hoffman, S., Cunningham, B.A. and Edelman, G.M. (1989) A detailed structural model of cytotactin: protein homologies, alternative splicing, and binding regions. *Proc. Natl. Acad. Sci. USA*, **86**, 1905–1909.

Koda, J.E. and Bernfield, M. (1984) Heparan sulfate proteoglycans from mouse mammary epithelial cells: basal extracellular proteoglycan binds specifically to native type I collagen fibrils. *J. Biol. Chem.*, **259**, 11763–11770.

Koyama, E., Leatherman, J.L., Shimazu, A., Nah, H-D. and Pacifici, M. (1995) Syndecan-3, tenascin-C, and the development of cartilaginous skeletal elements and joints in chick embryos. *Dev. Dynam.*, **203**, 152–162.

Koyama, E., Shimazu, A., Leatherman, J.L., Golden, E.B., Nah, H-D. and Pacifici, M. (1996) Expression of syndecan-3 and tenascin-C: possible involvement in periosteum development. *J. Orthop. Res.*, **14**, 403–412.

Leboy, P.S., Vaias, L., Uschmann, B., Golub, E., Adams, S.L. and Pacifici, M. (1989) Ascorbic acid induces alkaline phosphatase, type X collagen, and calcium deposition in cultured chick chondrocytes. *J. Biol. Chem.*, **264**, 17281–17286.

Lutfi, A.M. (1974) The ultrastructure of cartilage cells in the epiphyses of long bones in the domestic fowl. *Acta. Anat.*, **87**, 12–21.

Mackie, E.J., Thesleff, I. and Chiquet-Ehrismann, R. (1987) Tenascin is associated with chondrogenic and osteogenic differentiation *in vivo* and promotes chondrogenesis *in vitro*. *J. Cell Biol.*, **105**, 2569–2579.

Mankin, H.J. (1962) Localisation of tritiated thymidine in articular cartilage of rabbits. I. Growth of immature cartilage. *J. Bone. Joint Surg.*, **44A**, 682–688.

Mitrovic, D.R. (1977) Development of the metatarsalphalangeal joint in the chick embryo: morphological, ultrastructural and histochemical studies. *Am. J. Anat.*, **150**, 333–348.

Moscatelli, D. (1987) High and low affinity binding sites for basic fibroblast growth factor on cultured cells: absence of a rolefor low affinity binding in the stimulation of plasminogen activator production by bovine capillary endothelial cells. *J. Cell Physiol.*, **131**, 123–130.

Ornitz, D.M. and Leder, P. (1992) Ligand specificity and heparin dependence of fibroblast growth factor receptors 1 and 3. *J. Biol. Chem.*, **267**, 16305–16311.

Oettinger, H.F., Thal, G., Sasse, J., Holtzer, H. and Pacifici, M. (1985) Immunological analysis of chick notochord and cartilage matrix development with antisera to cartilage matrix macromolecules. *Dev. Biol.*, **109**, 63–71.

Pacifici, M. (1995) Tenascin-C and the development of articular cartilage. *Matrix Biol.*, **14**, 689–698.

Pacifici, M., Iwamoto, M., Golden, E.B., Leatherman, J.L., Lee, Y-S. and Chuong, C-M. (1993) Tenascin is associated with articular cartilage development. *Dev. Dynam.*, **198**, 123–134.

Pacifici, M. and Molinaro, M. (1980) Developmental changes in glycosaminoglycans during skeletal muscle cell differentiation in culture. *Exp. Cell Res.*, **126**, 143–152.

Persson, M. (1983) The role of movements in the development of sutural and diathrodial joints tested by long-term paralysis of chick embryo. *J. Anat.*, **137**, 591–599.

Peters, K.G., Ornitz, D., Werner, S. and Williams, L.T. (1993) Unique expression patterns of the FGF receptor 3 gene during mouse organogenesis. *Dev. Biol.*, **155**, 423–430.

Prieto, A.L., Edelman, G.M. and Crossin, K.L. (1993) Multiple integrins mediate cell attachment to cytotactin/tenascin. *Proc. Natl. Acad. Sci. USA*, **90**, 10154–10158.

Prieto, A.L., Jones, F.S., Cunningham, B.A., Crossin, K.L. and Edelman, G.M. (1990) Localization during development of alternatively spliced forms of cytotactin mRNA by *in situ* hybridizations. *J. Cell Biol.*, **111**, 685–689.

Saga, Y., Tsukamoto, T., Jing, N., Kusakabe, M. and Sakakura, T. (1991) Murine tenascin: cDNA cloning, structure and temporal expression of isoforms. *Gene*, **104**, 177–185.

Salmivirta, M., Elenius, K., Vainio, S., Hofer, U., Chiquet-Ehrismann, R., Thesleff, I. and Jalkanen, M. (1991) Syndecan from embryonic tooth mesenchyme binds tenascin. *J. Biol. Chem.*, **266**, 7733–7739.

Sanderson, R.D., Turnbull, J.E., Gallagher, J.T. and Lander, A.D. (1994) Fine structure of heparan sulfate regulates syndecan-1 function and cell behavior. *J. Biol. Chem.*, **269**, 13100–13106.

Saunders, S., Jalkanen, M., O'Farrell, S. and Bernfield, M. (1989) Molecular cloning of syndecan, an integral membrane proteoglycan. *J. Cell Biol.*, **108**, 1547–1556.

Savarese, J.J., Erickson, H. and Scully, S.P. (1996) Articular chondrocyte tenascin-C production and assembly into de novo extracellular matrix. *J. Orthop. Res.*, **14**, 273–281.

Shimazu, A., Nah, H-D., Kirsch, T., Koyama, E., Leatherman, J.L., Golden, E.B., Kosher, R.A. and Pacifici, M. (1996) Syndecan-3 and the control of chondrocyte proliferation during endochondral ossification. *Exp. Cell Res.*, **229**, 126–136.

Smith, A.R. (1978) Digit regeneration in the amphibian, *Triturus cristatus*. *J. Embryol. Exp. Morphol.*, **44**, 105–112.

Spring, J., Beck, K. and Chiquet-Ehrismann, R. (1989) Two contrary functions of tenascin: dissection of the active sites by recombinant tenascin fragments. *Cell*, **59**, 325–334.

Sriramarao, P., Mendler, M. and Bourdon, M.A. (1993) Endothelial cell attachment and spreading on human tenascin is mediated by a_2b_1 and a_vb_3 integrins. *J. Cell Sci.*, **105**, 1001–1012.

Sun, X., Mosher, D.F. and Rapraeger, A. (1989) Heparan sulfate-mediated binding of epithelial cells to thrombospondin. *J. Biol. Chem.*, **264**, 2885–2889.

Takebayashi, T., Iwamoto, M., Jikko, A., Matsumura, T., Enomoto-Iwamoto, M., Myoukai, F., Koyama, E., Yamaai, T., Matsumoto, K., Nakamura, T., Kurisu, K. and Noji, S. (1995) Hepatocyte growth factor/scatter factor modulates cell motility, proliferation, and proteoglycan synthesis of chondrocytes. *J. Cell Biol.*, **129**, 1411–1419.

Thorogood, P.V. and Hinchliffe, J.R. (1975) An analysis of the condensation process during chondrogenesis in the embryonic chick hind limb. *J. Embryol. Exp. Morphol.*, **33**, 581–606.

Tucker, R.P. (1993) The *in situ* localization of tenascin splice variants and thrombospondin 2 mRNA in the avian embryo. *Development*, **117**, 347–358.

Vakeva, L., Mackie, E., Kantomaa, T. and Thesleff, I. (1990) Comparison of the distribution patterns of tenascin and alkaline phosphatase in developing teeth, cartilage and bone of rats and mice. *Anat. Rec.*, **228**, 69–76.

Wilson, G.D. (1992) Cell kinetic studies using a monoclonal antibody to bromodeoxy-uridine. In *Methods in Molecular Biology*, *vol. 10*; *Immunochemical Protocols* (ed M. Manson), pp. 387–398. The Humana Press, Totowa, NJ.

Yokouchi, Y., Sasaki, H. and Kuroiwa, A. (1991) Homeobox gene expression correlated to the bifurcation process of limb cartilage development. *Nature*, **353**, 443–445.

Zisch, A.H., D'Alessandri, L., Ranscht, B., Falchetto, R., Winterhalter, K.H. and Vaughan, L. (1992) Neuronal cell adhesion molecule contactin/F11 binds to tenascin via its immunoglobulin-like domain. *J. Cell Biol.*, **119**, 203–213.

4 The Role of Hyaluronan in Joint Cavitation

Andrew A. Pitsillides

The Department of Veterinary Basic Sciences, The Royal Veterinary College, Royal College Street, London NW1 0TU, UK

INTRODUCTION

Many observations support the view that there is a dynamic relationship between the structural characteristics of connective tissues and their prevailing mechanical environment. Similarly, the morphology of different types of joint in the musculo-skeletal system is closely related to the degree of movement which they facilitate. Consequently, three fundamental types of articulation are observed: synarthroses and fibrous joints, which facilitate only a small degree of movement, and diarthrodial joints, which are distinguished on the basis that they provide an extensive range of friction-free movement and they contain cavities between the opposed articular cartilage elements which are lined by synovium (Nomina Anatomica, 1950).

Synovium's facilitation of efficient joint and tendon movement in adults has long been recognised, as have the many situations in which this is compromised. The failure to provide appropriate synovial function is evident in a range of clinical problems, including adhesive shoulder capsulitis, post-operative failures in mobilisation and around joint replacement prostheses. Paradoxically, there are also instances, such as loosening around prosthetic stems, where undesired 'synovial-like' separation is apparent. Synovial joints are also susceptible to a number of diseases, including rheumatoid arthritis (RA) and degenerative osteoarthritis which produce a loss of joint mobility associated with alterations in the synovium.

As emphasised by Fassbender (1982), the characteristic destruction of articular cartilage in RA occurs from the edges of the cartilage directly opposed to the synovial lining. Moreover, he found that cultured synovial lining cells isolated from patients with RA, but not those isolated from normal subjects, were capable of rapidly removing both the proteoglycans and collagen from cartilage matrix *in vitro*, whilst in contrast, blood monocytes removed only the proteoglycans very slowly. These observations led to the suggestion that such RA-associated cartilage destruction is mediated by a population of immature synovial lining cells and that synovium may be considered the primary target tissue in RA. This point has been emphasised by the studies of Chayen and co-workers, in which it has been shown that resident synovial lining cells show the earliest evidence of joint pathology (Chayen and Bitensky, 1982).

Despite the obvious functional importance of synovial lining cells in maintaining joint function, the biochemical characteristics which are responsible for promoting their normal role remain ill-defined. By establishing the mechanisms which regulate both formation and subsequent maintenance of the synovial joint cavity, our aims are: first to establish how synovial lining cells contribute to friction-free movement, and second to define how this fails in joints functionally compromised by disease, thus providing a cellular basis for the restoration of joint function where it would otherwise remain compromised.

MORPHOGENESIS OF SYNOVIAL JOINTS

Most studies in limb development have addressed the mechanisms controlling temporospatial patterning of skeletal elements within the conceptual framework of positional information (Wolpert, 1989), but have not addressed the morphogenetic events directly. It has been shown that these patterning processes involve dynamic reciprocal relationships between a thickened region of the embryonic ectoderm (apical ectodermal ridge; AER) and the most distal mesenchyme within the limb. Such interactions result in the maintenance of this mesenchyme in a proliferative, undifferentiated state (the progress zone) which is responsible for limb outgrowth (Summerbell, 1977).

As a consequence of continuing outgrowth, cells depart from the AER's influence, and as they do so, they appear to become committed to particular fates. This commitment seems to depend on the specific time and location at which cells leave the progress zone, and a series of elegant studies have identified several key regulatory genes which appear to control such skeletal patterning (Izpisua-Belmonte and Duboule, 1992; Storm et al., 1994; Tickle, 1995; Duprez et al., 1996). However, whilst these studies have provided some knowledge of the organisational mechanisms which may control the location of distinct structures, few have addressed the cellular basis by which the morphogenetic changes associated with joint cavity formation are controlled.

During development, synovial joint cavities form by a process involving the separation of predetermined opposed cartilaginous elements, producing non-adherent articular surfaces and associated synovial structures. A convenient model for considering this morphogenic process has involved its division into two continuous phases: the initial formation and configuration of cartilaginous anlagen, and the subsequent formation of a cavity within an apparently uninterrrupted extracellular matrix (Bernays, 1878; Andersen and BroRasmussen, 1961; O'Rahilly and Gardner, 1978).

Many histological studies have described the morphological changes occurring within developing synovial joints in several species, and these suggest that fundamentally similar processes are involved (Bernays, 1878; Gardner and Gray, 1950; Andersen, 1962; Mitrovic, 1977, 1978; O'Rahilly and Gardner, 1978). The one major anatomical difference between chicks and mammals, is that the developing articular surface in chicks is largely fibrocartilaginous, whereas in mammals this surface is cartilaginous. Nonetheless, in all species examined the elements are laid down and subsequently develop in a proximo-distal sequence (Saunders, 1948).

The origins of a synovial joint become defined within an area of early blastemal mesenchyme found between the developing cartilaginous skeletal condensations, which are initially avascular and enveloped by the perichondrium. Subsequently, these cartilaginous condensations in opposing anlagen expand rapidly by chondroblastic apposition from the perichondrial inner surface, and by both extracellular matrix (ECM) production and cell division. Concomitantly, the presumptive joint becomes increasingly more defined as a transverse region of persisting densely-packed flattened cells, representing the remains of the primitive blastema, forming the early interzone (Bernays, 1878). As development proceeds and the cartilaginous cores expand further, this interzonal area becomes increasingly attenuated and flattened. Later, the peripheral presumptive joint capsule/synovium, initially continuous with this interzone, becomes vascularised and subsequently tissue separation occurs within the avascular central region by an, as yet, undetermined mechanism. Therefore, with time and continued cartilaginous expansion, the ever-decreasing relative proportion of blastemally-associated mesenchymal cells within the limb will contribute directly to the initial tissue separation at the joint line, as well as the establishment of the synovial lining surface.

Consequently, the precise differentiation required for the acquisition of a cellular phenotype associated with 'synovialisation', or joint tissue separation, can be addressed readily. Further, interventional studies which have predominantly used embryonic chick limb development as the model system, enable the relationship between these phenotypic characteristics, as well as their potential contribution to joint formation, to be investigated. With specific reference to the possible role of hyaluronan (HA), this chapter focuses on local changes occurring at the site of this initial separation, as well as addressing the regulatory role of movement in maintaining a fluid-filled space between opposed diarthrodial joint articular elements.

CHEMICAL AND PHYSICAL PROPERTIES OF HYALURONAN

HA was first isolated from the vitreous body of the eye over 60 years ago (Meyer and Palmer, 1934). It is a ubiquitous component of the ECM, found at highest concentrations in Wharton's jelly of the umbilical cord, rooster comb, vitreous humour of the eye and in synovial joint fluid (Laurent and Fraser, 1992). All of these, as well as particular strains of streptococci (Kendall *et al.*, 1937), have been used for the isolation of HA (Meyer, 1947; Laurent and Fraser, 1986). Using enzymatic digestion followed by chemical analyses of isolated oligosaccharides, it has been shown that HA is composed of repeating disaccharide units of D-glucuronic acid linked to N-acetyl-D-glucosamine (Rapport *et al.*, 1951). These repeating units are usually linked to form a negatively charged, high Mr polysaccharide member of the hexosamine-containing glycosaminoglycan (GAG) family of molecules.

As alluded to above, the synovial fluid of normal diarthrodial joints contains particularly high concentrations of high molecular weight HA (Sundbland, 1953; Balazs *et al.*, 1967). However, the characteristics of HA which relate to its functional role in diarthrodial joints are not yet fully defined. HA differs from other GAGs in that it lacks covalently-linked polypeptide and is unsulphated, and it is well-established that tissues in which HA is present at high concentrations are all relatively soft. Further, in comparison to tissues with higher tensile strength which contain higher proportions of sulphated GAGs and quantitatively predominant collagen fibrils, these softer tissues also contain relatively little collagenous matrix (Laurent, 1989). Indeed, synovial fluid is completely liquefied and its functional properties are, for the most part, independent of collagen. Thus, the initial elaboration and subsequent conservation of a synovial 'fluid'-filled joint cavity appears to provide an ideal circumstance in which the functionally-appropriate features of HA structure and the mechanisms controlling its synthesis to be elucidated.

Extracted HA has a polydisperse molecular mass (usually several million kDa), and early rheological studies suggested that HA could form extensive branched complexes (Blumberg and Ogston, 1958; Preston *et al.*, 1965). Later, using electron microscopic (EM) studies dependent on the binding of basic cytochrome c molecules to negatively charged molecular constituents, it was shown that HA appeared as a linear polymer (Fessler and Fessler, 1966). However, as pointed out by Scott *et al.* (1991), the first metallic shadowing EM study of HA suggested that HA could exist in an 'anastomosing fibrous structure', and recent X-ray diffraction and spectroscopy studies appear to support this original notion (Heatley and Scott, 1988; Scott, 1989). Furthermore, there is now a molecular basis to underpin this view.

Individual HA molecules seem to be stabilised by hydrogen bonds parallel to the chain axis. Thus, HA in aqueous solution obtains a helical co-operative arrangement, in which water molecules produce a bridge between neighbouring sugar residues (Scott, 1989). This model of HA structure also proposes the formation of large hydrophobic clusters which, when repeated at regular intervals on alternate sides of large Mr HA 'tape-like' molecules, provide a basis for interchain association and offer persuasive evidence supporting HA self-aggregation (Preston *et al.*, 1965). Indeed, computer simulation showed that HA duplexes were energetically and sterically feasible, whilst rotary shadowing EM showed that pure HA in solution could certainly aggregate to form large irregularly branched meshworks (Scott *et al.*, 1991). Importantly, it was shown that networks formed at concentrations as low as 1 µg/ml, that they existed as 'sheets' at 1 mg/ml, and that their branching potential was also related to HA's molecular weight.

These properties of HA appear to provide it with several physical characteristics which may facilitate friction-free joint movement. For example, HA solutions are extremely viscous, and HA is responsible for the visco-elastic behaviour of synovial fluid. The viscosity of synovial fluid, or its shear resistance, decreases as shear rate increases, and is a function of both HA's concentration and Mr (Balazs, 1974). Thus, HA may function as a joint lubricant (Ogston and Stanier, 1953) and, therefore, HA at the developing joint line may facilitate efficient sliding between forming and newly-formed surfaces.

In addition, high concentrations of high Mr HA may not require other mechanically functional ECM components (e.g. fibrous collagen) to facilitate its proposed role as an elastic shape-forming gel. As such meshworks are dependent on the Mr of HA, modest

enzymatic HA cleavage in existing meshworks, or a reduction in the Mr of newly synthesised HA, may produce marked decreases in the functional competence of such
gel-like fluids. Further, HA's stiffened coil structure exhibits non-ideal osmotic behaviour
capable of producing large swelling potential (Oster *et al.*, 1985) and highly-hydrated
domains effectively 'shielding' water by virtue of its extensive negative-charge (Laurent,
1989). This results in HA's action as an osmotic buffer as well as the relatively slow diffusion from the site of its synthesis (Ogston and Stanier, 1953). Further, HA may act to
sterically exclude other macromolecules and limit their diffusion into the HA-rich synovial joint space (Ogston and Stanier, 1953), and its large osmotic swelling potential-
dependent, shape-forming gel-like properties may result in the separation between
neighbouring tensile components of the ECM, and also result in the formation of cell-free
spaces.

HYALURONAN SYNTHESIS

Hyaluronan biosynthesis appears to differ fundamentally from that of other GAGs, which
are synthesised in the Golgi complex. HA is synthesised at the plasma membrane, and is
apparently extruded directly into the ECM (Prehm, 1984). Despite much debate and some
discrepancy in a series of elegant studies (Prehm, 1989; Prehm and Mausolf, 1986; Mian,
1986), it is now accepted that the reducing end of nascent HA chains is elongated by
alternate addition of sugar residues derived from UDP-glucuronate and UDP-N-acetyl
glucosamine, by the enzyme HA-synthase (Prehm, 1983). The activity of HA-synthase is
associated with several processes, including: mitosis (Brecht *et al.*, 1986); cell growth
(Hronowski and Anastassiades, 1980); differentiation; and metastasis (Toole *et al.*,
1979). Further, a number of growth factors, such as TGFb, have been shown to stimulate
HA synthesis *in vitro* (Toole *et al.*, 1989). However, the mechanisms regulating HA
synthesis are obscure, and it remains possible that the supply of monosaccharides
constitutes a key point of regulation.

   All GAG monosaccharides are synthesised by enzymatic interconversion between
nucleotide sugars (Ginsburg, 1964; Phelps, 1973). Uridine diphospho (UDP)-glucose
dehydrogenase (UDPGD, EC. 1.1.1.22) is responsible for the conversion of UDP-glucose
to UDP-glucuronate, and it has been suggested that UDPGD activity is an irreversible,
rate-limiting step in UDP-glucuronate production (Molz and Danishefsky, 1971;
McGarry and Gahan, 1985). Using enzymes isolated from epiphyseal plate cartilage and
cornea, DeLuca *et al.* (1975, 1976) showed that UDPGD may have a pivotal role in
controlling the type of monosaccharides produced by UDP-glucose utilisation. They also
showed that increasing the ratio of NADH to NAD appeared to inhibit this UDPGD
activity, and that this redox-related inhibition was most marked at pH values near
neutrality (De Luca and Castellani, 1984). Handly and Phelps (1972) showed that the
availability of UDP-amino sugars (such as UDP-N-acetyl glucosamine of HA) does not
normally appear to limit the rate at which GAGs are synthesised. Consistent with these
observations we have shown that UDPGD activity may constitute a key regulatory branch
point in GAG synthesis (Hickery *et al.*, 1993; Pitsillides *et al.*, 1993b).

Assessment of the site and activity of a specific enzyme in individual cells within a heterogeneous tissue, such as the developing limb bud, is difficult to achieve using conventional biochemical techniques (Kulyk and Kosher, 1987). Quantitative cytochemistry, or *in situ* biochemistry, coupled with scanning and integrating microdensitometry has been developed as a quantitative procedure to achieve these aims (Chayen, 1984; Chayen and Bitensky, 1992). Fortunately, a quantitative assay for UDPGD activity was recently developed (Mehdizadeh *et al.*, 1991). Using this assay we showed that UDPGD activity in fibroblast-like intimal synoviocytes was six or more times higher than in the synovial subintimal fibroblasts (Pitsillides and Blake, 1992; Pitsillides *et al.*, 1993a), suggesting that measurement of UDPGD activity may reflect their ability to synthesise the high local concentrations of synovial fluid HA.

EXTRACELLULAR AND CELLULAR ASPECTS OF JOINT CAVITATION

Although many hypotheses, including necrotic cell death, vascular ingression, cellular migration, apoptosis, and increased breakdown of ECM components, have been implicated in the cavity formation process (Mitrovic, 1971, 1974, 1977; Milaire, 1947; Andersen, 1963; Nalin *et al.*, 1995), the mechanisms essential for the generation and subsequent maintenance of fully functional diarthrodial joint cavities remain enigmatic. It is evident that cavity formation must involve a local and precisely defined loss of tensile properties within the matrix. Thus, it is likely that this may be mediated by mechanically or enzymatically-related degradation of coherent matrix elements, by changes in local synthesis and secretion of non-coherent ECM components with low tensile strength, or by a combination of such factors.

EXTRACELLULAR MATRIX CHANGES AT THE SITE OF JOINT CAVITY FORMING

Consistent with the notion that joint cavitation involves local alterations in ECM components, several findings suggest a role for changes in GAG synthesis and secretion in this process. Andersen and BroRasmussen (1961) described the presence of a metachromatic substance in developing interdigital zone ECM. Initially, Munaron (1954) had suggested that such metachromasia, which was lost from sections pretreated with a hyaluronidase, may be due to HA. These conclusions were subsequently discounted by Andersen (1962), who showed that the particular hyaluronidase used was not specific for HA, suggesting that the amorphous ECM at the presumptive joint line was predominantly chondroitin 4-sulphate or chondroitin 6-sulphate.

However, studies using radiolabelled precursors (autoradiography and biochemical analysis of isolated macromolecules) have shown that HA constitutes a major component of material extracted from newly formed spaces at another embryonic site, into which neural crest cells migrate during craniofacial development (Pratt *et al.*, 1975). Additionally, HA is considered an essential component of cell-free, highly hydrated matrices responsible for facilitating cell invasion, as well as the separation of cellular or fibrous tissues (Toole, 1982; Fisher and Solursh, 1977).

Using immunolabelling for ECM components in sections of developing chick joints, Craig *et al.* (1987) also proposed that cavities may be produced as a result of differential matrix turnover. Their findings indicated a loss of type II collagen from the joint inter-zone, and its replacement by type I collagen, concomitant with cavitation. This conver-sion, however, seemed to relate more closely to formation of fibrocartilaginous articular surfaces, than to the line of initial joint separation itself (Craig *et al.*, 1987). Labelling for keratan sulphate (KS)-containing proteoglycans was found throughout the joint before cavitation, and similarly, as cavitation progressed this was lost from the interzone, but maintained (with type II collagen) in epiphyses (Archer *et al.*, 1994).

Recently, these findings were elegantly extended by Nalin *et al.* (1995). Using *in situ* hybridisation they showed that transient procollagen type IIA mRNA expression, as well as consistent expression of type I collagen mRNA, was present in interzonal cells prior to cavitation. At cavitation, chondrocytes express mRNA for type IIB procollagen; however, a second layer of fibroblastic chondroprogenitors nearer the joint continues to express type IIA mRNA, whilst type I collagen synthesis was observed only in the interzone domain (Nalin *et al.*, 1995). Such changes in collagen protein and mRNA expression may lead to the speculation that such fibrous collagenous components would have to be removed for cavitation to occur at the forming joint line.

However, evidence supporting the localised enzyme-mediated degradation of such ECM components at the forming joint line is limited. Increases in the activity of lysoso-mal acid phosphatase have previously been described within the developing interzone (Milaire, 1947); however, our own qualitative investigations in developing human joints suggest that such increases, if at all present, are only minor (Edwards *et al.*, 1994). Currently, collagen removal processes have focussed on the involvement of matrix metal-loproteinases (MMPs; Murphy and Reynolds, 1993). However, Edwards *et al.* (1996) failed to show immunocytochemical evidence for increased local levels of MMPs I, II, III or IX, or differential expression of the tissue inhibitor of MMPs (TIMP) at the developing joint line in embryonic human limbs. Nevertheless, observations regarding differential collagen expression and synthesis may provide useful insights into the changing struc-tural characteristics of the joint line ECM.

Using biotinylated HA-binding region link-protein complex, we and others have demonstrated the appearance of staining for free HA at the joint line, concomitant with the first signs of overt cavitation (Craig *et al.*, 1990; Pitsillides *et al.*, 1995). It was postu-lated by Craig *et al.* (1990) that HA may be produced locally and secreted into the presumptive joint space, and that unlike the HA and proteoglycans present in opposing epiphyseal cartilage, the absence of a collagen network in the presumptive cavity may allow this HA to achieve its natural swelling potential (Oster *et al.*, 1985; Laurent, 1989).

However, these observations have several limitations: firstly, HA staining using biotinylated HA-binding region (HABr) may not produce a meaningful measure of local HA concentration at particular sites; secondly, staining may be absent from areas in which the HA is saturated with proteoglycan monomer, or is otherwise occupied, resulting in a lack of available binding sites for HABr; and finally, the site and dynamics of HA synthesis remain purely speculative. Thus, the presence of staining for HA in embryonic spaces may indicate that local synthesis of HA is intimately involved in the genesis of the space, or alternatively, that HA diffuses into a space already formed by other mechanisms.

CHANGES IN HA SYNTHESIS AND CELLULAR BEHAVIOUR ASSOCIATED WITH JOINT FORMATION

Using the novel application of an *in situ* biochemical method for UDPGD activity to developing embryonic limbs; together with immunolabelling using a monoclonal antibody raised against streptococcal HA-synthase (see Klewes *et al.*, 1993) and autoradiography for radiolabelled sulphate incorporation, we evaluated the role of local cells in the synthesis of HA during joint cavitation. Our results indicated that prior to, and concomitant with the separation of cartilaginous elements, higher UDPGD activities/cell, and relatively rich HA-synthase immunolabelling, were both evident in cells within the interzone. In fully-cavitated joints, these phenotypic characteristics were maintained in all cells directly bordering the joint cavity. Interestingly, the peak in UDPGD activity/cell was apparent at the exact site and in synchrony with the first signs of overt cavity formation, and the level of HA synthase expression was increased at these same sites (Pitsillides *et al.*, 1995). Thus, it appears that the differentiation of cells bordering sites of active separation in developing joints may involve alterations associated specifically with differential synthesis of HA.

The immediate product of UDPGD activity, namely UDP-glucuronate, has three possible fates: (i) it may be decarboxylated to UDP-xylose (initiates sulphated GAG chain elongation); (ii) it may be used as a constituent monosaccharide of sulphated GAGs (Roden, 1980; Hascall *et al.*, 1991); or (iii) used in synthesis of HA (unsulphated). Thus, our conclusions are consistent with the observation that cells in presumptive interzones also incorporate markedly reduced levels of radiolabelled sulphate than their neighbouring epiphyseal chondrocytes (Hinchcliffe, 1977; Pitsillides *et al.*, 1995). This may indicate that cells at presumptive sites of tissue separation utilise UDP-glucuronate preferentially in the synthesis of HA, rather than sulphated GAGs. This conclusion is also in accord with our recent findings, using the 'critical electrolyte method' of Scott and Dorling (1965) to differentiate between alcian blue staining for various GAG species. These provide preliminary evidence that cells in chick knee joint interzones are associated with histochemical staining consistent with the predominance of HA at these sites (Ward and Pitsillides, 1998).

Interestingly, the UDPGD gene in group A streptococci appears to be mapped to a locus required for HA synthesis, and it is closely linked to a mutation which inactivates HA-synthase (Dougherty and van de Rijn, 1993). Although we cannot exclude the possibility that UDPGD activity in cells within the interzones may be controlled by post-translational modification, our studies suggest that coordinately-controlled transcription of UDPGD and HA-synthase may be involved in the regulation of HA synthesis at the presumptive space. However, whilst these findings suggest that HA present at these sites of separation may facilitate efficient sliding between newly-formed surfaces, and that cells directly bordering these sites may be responsible for this increased HA production, they do not necessarily establish that HA is responsible for joint 'space' generation.

It is possible that the joint 'space' is produced by some, as yet, unidentified mechanism, and that as a consequence HA is synthesised locally so as to effectively fill this newly formed cavity.

Indeed, HA has been implicated directly in the generation of similar fluid-filled spaces during embryonic development (see Toole, 1982). For example, it has been suggested that HA may be involved in the formation of a space between the external corneal epithelium and endothelium in the embryonic chick (Toole and Trelstad, 1971). Similarly, HA has been implicated in epithelial movement evident during the formation of semi-circular canals in the inner ear of Xenopus (Haddon and Lewis, 1991). Our studies suggest that during diarthrodial joint formation, local cells have a role in the synthesis of HA produced during the development of fluid-filled synovial joint cavities, and that after cavity formation, continued synthesis of HA is required for the joint's functional competence.

As in many connective tissues, the cells which populate synovium's characteristic non-adherent intimal surface have been considered, by many, to be of two distinct classes. Although, it has been suggested that these may be interchangeable, it is convenient to classify these as resident fibroblast-like synovial lining cells (synoviocytes) responsible for ECM (and HA) synthesis, and leucocyte-derived macrophages (Pitsillides and Blake, 1992; Wilkinson et al., 1992; Pitsillides et al., 1993a).

In this regard, in order to establish the type of cell involved in joint formation, our studies using embryonic human limbs have shown that cells of the macrophage lineage (CD68 positive) are present prior to overt cavitation, but only in vascularised peripheral regions (identified using Factor VIII-related antigen), and not in the avascular joint interzone. In contrast, using antibodies specific to CD44 (a cell surface-associated HA-binding protein; Aruffo et al., 1990), we found that CD44 was expressed by interzone cells which contain high UDPGD activity, at all stages of cavitation (Edwards et al., 1994). Therefore, it is apparent that macrophages have little, if any, role in the early stages of joint cavity formation, and that synoviocyte-like fibroblastic cells may be intimately involved in generating the initial joint line. This may depend upon their expression of an HA-binding protein and appears to involve their differential synthesis of increased levels of HA.

THE ROLE OF CELL-ASSOCIATED HA-BINDING PROTEINS AND THEIR CYTOSKELETAL LINKING ELEMENTS IN JOINT CAVITY FORMATION

Previous studies suggested that HA in conjunction with cell surface-associated HA-binding proteins (HABPs) was capable of facilitating cell separation in vitro (Toole, 1981). It was also suggested that variations in local HA concentration may modulate cell–cell interaction. Briefly, it was postulated that low concentrations of HA may promote aggregatory/cohesive interactions between adjacent HABP-expressing cells. Conversely, increased local HA concentrations may promote cell–cell separation, by a process involving saturation of their cell surface-associated HABPs (Toole, 1982). As discussed, our findings suggested that cells immediately bordering sites of joint tissue separation showed evidence for: (i) increased HA synthesis, (ii) an association with HA-rich ECM (Pitsillides et al., 1995), and (iii) at least in human joints, also expressed CD44

(Edwards *et al.*, 1994). Consequently, it was hypothesised that these characteristics are a primary influence in the creation of a joint cavity, and that thereafter, their continued interactive relationships are also required for the maintenance of functionally appropriate diarthrodial joint cavities.

HA is capable of binding to both matrix-associated and cell surface-associated HA-binding proteins, and their structure and role in many cellular processes has been elegantly reviewed by many authors (Toole, 1990; Underhill, 1992; Knudson and Knudson, 1993; Sherman *et al.*, 1994). It has been proposed that members of these two groups should be termed hyaladherins (Toole, 1990). Of the many matrix-associated hyaladherins described, the best-characterised are aggrecan and link protein of articular cartilage (Hardingham *et al.*, 1976). Their interaction with HA is mediated by a common protein domain (Link module; Perkins *et al.*, 1989; Neame and Barry, 1993), which appears in all matrix hyaladherins as well as in some cell-surface hyaladherins, including CD44 (see Toole, 1990; Hardingham and Fosang, 1992).

CD44 was originally described as a lymphocyte differentiation marker, and is now defined as a transmembrane hyaladherin and the principal cell-surface receptor for HA (Aruffo *et al.*, 1990; Lesley *et al.*, 1993). CD44 can bind to a region of HA containing only six sugar residues, but this interaction is weak when compared to its much greater affinity for larger HA molecules. It also binds, via its chondroitin sulphate side chains to other ligands, including collagen type I and VI (Wayner and Carter, 1987; Underhill, 1992). In addition, CD44 which is apparently quiescent with respect to HA-binding can achieve full HA-binding status following phorbol ester treatment (Liao *et al.*, 1993), suggesting that CD44's ability to bind HA can be modified. Although paradoxical evidence has been presented, CD44's HA-binding appears to be modulated by the interaction of its 70 amino acid cytoplasmic tail with the actin cytoskeleton (Lacy and Underhill, 1987; Isacke, 1994; Murakami *et al.*, 1994; Perschl *et al.*, 1995), as well as by its degree of clustering on the cell surface (Underhill, 1989). This, along with distinct post-translational glycosylation and alternative transcriptional splicing patterns, provides a system by which HA-binding can be regulated.

It has been proposed that the definition of a hyaladherin should be extended to include HABPs which are cell surface-expressed, but do not necessarily contain a 'link module' (Knudson and Knudson, 1993). Of these, the best-characterised was originally isolated by Turley and co-workers from migrating rabbit fibroblasts *in vitro*. This receptor for HA-mediated motility (RHAMM) is a 58-kDa HA-binding component of a receptor complex (containing four proteins), which can either bind HA at the cell surface, or is released as soluble proteins (Turley, 1989; Turley *et al.*, 1991; Hardwick *et al.*, 1992).

RHAMM does not contain a link module, but it and all other hyaladherins do appear to share a common HA-binding amino acid sequence. Importantly, binding to HA via such sequences differs fundamentally from that mediated by link modules on the basis that the latter are sensitive to reducing conditions (see Toole, 1990). However, like CD44, RHAMM has also been shown to co-localise with the ends of actin stress fibres during cell migration (see Sherman *et al.*, 1994). There are other members of this group which are recognised in chick tissues by the IVd4 antibody. This was raised against an epitope present in embryonic chick brain and was capable of blocking isolated brain extract cellular HA-binding capacity (Banerjee and Toole, 1991) which appears to be necessary for pericellular coat formation by chondrocytes, fibroblasts and endothelial cells *in vitro* (Banerjee and Toole, 1992; Yu *et al.*, 1992).

The relationship between various cell surface hyaladherins is not known; however, many examples are available where they are associated with localised HA degradation (Knudson and Toole, 1985). Nevertheless, observations indicating that high exogenous HA concentrations appear to decrease HA synthesis by chondrocytes *in vitro*, suggested that cell surface-associated hyaladherin occupancy, or more precisely saturation of these sites, may inhibit HA synthesis (Mason *et al.*, 1989). Moreover, it has been proposed that chain length-selective termination of nascent HA elongation may also regulate HA synthesis (Prehm, 1989). Thus, it is conceivable that these hyaladherins may indirectly control the concentration and molecular weight of HA in the ECM.

Our recent findings demonstrate that several cell surface-associated hyaladherins, namely CD44, RHAMM and epitopes recognised by IVd4, may all be present at sites of joint cavity formation in chick limbs. Of these, CD44 shows the most marked joint-line selective differential labelling at all stages of the cavitation process (Dowthwaite *et al.*, 1998). This CD44 labelling has a marked pericellular distribution and was most intense in cells at presumptive joint interzone, and later in cells in developing articular surfaces, whilst in comparison neighbouring epiphyseal chondrocytes labelled weakly for CD44. In contrast, cells at these developing surfaces which express RHAMM and the IVd4 receptor, do so with a marked intracellular localisation.

Whilst immunocytochemical studies may describe hyaladherin distribution, they provide little information on their functional HA-binding status. Using biotin-labelled HA we have shown that cells within developing joint interzones, but not those in fibrocartilaginous articular surfaces of fully cavitated joints, do indeed show evidence for HA-binding ability (Dowthwaite *et al.*, 1998). This agrees with our previous findings concerning the distribution of free HA. We showed that labelling of fibrocartilaginous articular surfaces was virtually nonexistent, whilst all other tissues lining developing joint cavities were intensely labelled (Pitsillides *et al.*, 1995).

Thus, cells associated with the loss of cohesion at the developing joint line show: abundant expression of hyaladherins (particularly CD44), possess functional HA-binding capacity and are also associated with an ECM containing an abundance of free-HA. In contrast, cells within the structurally coherent fibrocartilaginous articular surface of established joints appear to have some hyaladherin expression, without the functional capacity to actively bind HA, and are associated with an ECM possessing little free HA. This suggests that HA present within the fibrocartilage is insufficient to cause cell–cell separation, that HA synthesised in these sites may be actively excluded by some as yet unidentified mechanism, and that the separation evident at the joint line may be mediated by HA by some hyaladherin-dependent mechanism.

Many observations have demonstrated that interactions between actin cytoskeletal elements and cell-surface hyaladherins appears to be a prerequisite for effective ligand binding (Isacke, 1994). Further, this binding may also be regulated by a family of actin-capping CD44-linking proteins, namely ezrin, radixin and moesin, collectively known as the ERM proteins (Sato *et al.*, 1992; Tsukita *et al.*, 1994). Our immunolabelling studies show that interzone cells at the developing joint space label strongly with a pan-specific antibody to these actin-capping ERM proteins. Further, using specific monoclonal antibodies to individual ERM members, we have established that moesin appears to show the most marked differential expression at the presumptive and forming joint-line (Dowthwaite et al., 1997; 1998).

Our confocal microscopic studies using FITC conjugated phalloidin also revealed a specific alignment of polymerised filamentous actin parallel to developing joint surfaces. The intensity of staining and the degree of specific alignment was most obvious within cells directly bordering sites of recently formed cavities and at sites of presumptive cavitation. In contrast, neighbouring epiphyseal chondrocytes showed markedly reduced levels of actin staining which lacked this regular specific alignment. Previous studies have established that CD44 can exist in any one of three distinct HA-binding states, these are: inactive, activatable, and constitutively active (Perschl et al., 1995). Thus, the presence of polymerised actin and the concomitant co-distribution of ERM family members, particularly moesin, at sites of joint cavity formation in developing limbs, appears to suggest that any CD44 present at these sites is likely to be functionally engaged in binding to HA.

These results also imply that structurally predefined sites of potential separation may exist within the presumptive interzone prior to overt cavitation. These appear to be associated with the specific alignment of polymerised actin within cells at presumptive joint lines, which in conjunction with moesin and CD44 may facilitate cell adhesion in one plane, whilst allowing a loss of cohesion in the opposite plane. Further, it is possible that local changes in HA synthesis between these 'potential cleavage planes' may then promote the loss of cohesion required for cavitation to occur, without the necessity for any widespread interzone matrix degradation.

Nevertheless, it has been suggested that sites of potential cavitation are genetically determined, whilst the initial separation and subsequent maintenance of functionally competent joints is dependent on movement (Fell and Canti, 1934). Although we have described many cellular characteristics consistent with the hypothesis that HA has a central role in the cavitation process, it is apparent that we cannot exclude the possibility that these events are all dependent on mechanically-induced signals. Therefore, it remains possible that all these HA-related cellular characteristics associated with the initial loss of cohesion, may reflect a dynamic relationship between the structural characteristics of these tissues and the degree of movement which they facilitate, or what we may consider to be their prevailing mechanical environment.

THE ROLE OF MOVEMENT

Many studies have emphasised the essential role of movement in the processes contributing to both the formation of joint cavities and their subsequent maintenance (Fell and Canti, 1934; Hamburger and Waugh, 1940; Lelkes, 1958; Drachmann and Sokoloff, 1966; Murray and Drachmann, 1969; Mitrovic, 1971; Yasuda, 1973; Mitrovic, 1974; Ruano-Gil et al., 1980; Mitrovic, 1982). In essence, these studies have shown that the eradication of a movement-induced mechanical stimulus either by limb removal and maintenance in organ culture, or by in ovo immobilisation using botulinum toxin, decamethonium bromide (DMB), succinylcholine or neurectomy, results in the prevention of cavity formation in, as yet, un-cavitated joints, and the regression of previously cavitated joints.

However, whilst these elegant studies provided excellent analogous extensions to the original paradigm, concerning movement's role in joint cavitation, they do not necessarily provide an understanding of its mechanistic role in producing functionally appropriate synovial joint structure. Although our current findings appear to suggest that HA-related changes may be a component of the mechanism by which initial separation is controlled, there appear to be at least three possibilities by which movement might contribute to such cavitation events, by inducing: (i) disruption at the joint line, (ii) differential patterns of growth, or (iii) alterations in local ECM metabolism.

Firstly, it has been suggested that muscular contraction may produce mechanical forces at the joint line which directly disrupt cell–cell cohesion (Drachmann and Sokoloff, 1966; Murray and Drachmann, 1969; Mitrovic, 1982). However, the preceding morphogenetic events appear to indicate that cells at the presumptive joint are intrinsically predetermined, and it would appear developmentally superfluous to define specific populations at such sites, if they were not to contribute directly to the cavitation process. Further, the evident precision with which initial separation is coordinated, in diverse diarthrodial joint structures, may suggest that such seemingly imprecise disruptive forces alone will not accurately define the joint line.

Secondly, it is possible that joint line separation may be promoted by differential patterns of growth. Indeed, it was shown by Lewis (1977) that limbs removed from chicks exposed to tritiated thymidine (before cavitation) and subsequently grafted onto unlabelled (growing and developing) host chicks, failed to show evidence for growth in joint interzonal areas, whilst dilution of labelled cells in the cartilaginous anlagen indicated division and growth in these areas. Our own studies in human developing joints similarly show that interzone cells express only very low levels of labelling for the proliferation cell nuclear antigen, Ki67, when compared to neighbouring chondrogenic regions (Edwards et al., 1994).

However, Drachmann and Sokoloff (1966) showed that three-day paralysis prevented initial formation of cavities in developing chick joints, whilst morphogenesis in the joint region proceeded up to the point when cavitation should occur, and apart from shortening of the upper beak and inducing skeletal distortions, such DMB-induced paralysis had only a small effect on growth. In fact, only a slight delay in development was evident in long-term (days 7–19) botulinum toxin-induced immobilisation in chicks, in which almost all joints failed to form cavities (Murray and Drachmann, 1969). Therefore, although differential growth may be responsible, in part, for the cavitation process, it alone would appear insufficient to control joint cavity formation.

Finally, it is possible that movement-induced mechanical stimuli alter local ECM turnover, and that this leads to the observed halting of joint cavitation in immobilised limbs. Consistent with this hypothesis, the seminal studies of Fell and Canti (1934) described chondrification in joint tissues in cultured chick limbs. Later, many authors have observed that articular surfaces unite and can undergo fibrous, cartilaginous or bony 'fusion', indicating an immobilisation-induced alteration in ECM turnover.

This suggests that movement may indeed contribute to the altered ECM synthesis which normally accompanies tissue separation at these sites. Consequently, we examined the effects of immobilisation on HA synthesis at initial sites of joint tissue separation. We found that DMB-induced immobilisation resulted in a failure to form joint cavities, and involved merging of fibrocartilaginous articular surfaces and interzone layers to form a homogeneous rounded cell zone continuous with both opposed cartilages (Ward and Pitsillides, 1998; Ward *et al.*, in preparation). We also showed that this was associated with decreased UDPGD activity in cells in these joint tissues. Further, in such 'fused' DMB-treated joints, there was no discernible difference in the UDPGD activity in cells within this 'new' fusion tissue and those in the 'original' cartilage of the anlagen (Ward *et al.*, in preparation). It is, therefore, tempting to speculate that movement contributes to joint formation by stimulating differential HA synthesis in cells at the joint line, and that withdrawal of this mechanical stimulus results in the synthesis of ECM matrix inappropriate for friction-free movement at this site.

However, it is evident that these 'fusion' tissues in which HA synthesis appears to be decreased, all have relatively high tensile strength in comparison to the fluid-like matrix which normally fills this space in mobile limbs. This may suggest that these replacement 'fusion' tissues have adapted their structural characteristics to their novel, prevailingly immobile mechanical environment, in which friction-free movement is not required. Alternatively they may indicate that movement is essential for the differential HA-related ECM synthesis at the developing joint line, and is a pre-requisite for normal functionally-appropriate joint structure.

FUNCTION OF SYNOVIAL LINING CELLS IN NORMAL AND DISEASED JOINTS

Our embryological studies provide novel insights into how functional competence of joints is established and conserved in developing limbs. The rationale for these studies is that they will provide a cellular basis for the restoration of joint function where it is compromised by diseases such as RA. The maintenance of friction-free movement is at least to some extent dependent on the chemical and physical characteristics of HA of particularly high concentrations and high molecular weights (see above and also chapters by Levick and Mason herein). It is also well-established that both HA's concentration and Mr are decreased in the synovial fluid of functionally compromised RA joints (Sundbland, 1953; Balazs *et al.*, 1967). Additionally in RA joints treated with intra-articular corticosteroids, in which many of the properties associated with efficient joint functional integrity are transiently re-established, there is a restoration of synovial fluid (and serum) HA concentrations toward normal levels (Pitsillides *et al.*, 1994). Despite these facts, until recently it has been difficult to describe, in precise quantifiable terms, a relevant functional activity which indicates a role of synovial lining cells in the synthesis of these HA levels in their adjacent synovial fluid.

Using a quantitative cytochemical assay for UDPGD activity we have shown that in non-inflamed synovium, UDPGD activity in synovial lining cells (SLC) is six or more times higher than in other fibroblasts within the tissue (Pitsillides *et al.*, 1993a). Further, by applying such cytochemical techniques in combination with immunolabelling for 'markers' classically-associated with macrophage-like cells (non-specific esterase and CD68), we have shown that in non-inflamed, rheumatoid and also osteoarthritic synovia, cells with high UDPGD activity were predominantly fibroblast-like synovial intimal (type B) cells, and not (type A) macrophages (Wilkinson *et al.*, 1992; Pitsillides *et al.*, 1993a).

Similarly, it is apparent that changes associated with differential HA synthesis at the presumptive joint may also be related to the contribution of synovial fibroblast-like cells, and not macrophages, to the initial generation of such tissue separation which is vital to friction-free movement (Pitsillides *et al.*, 1995; Edwards *et al.*, 1994; Archer *et al.*, 1994). This possibility is also stressed by the fact that UDPGD activity in SLCs is markedly reduced in synovium from both RA joints and an antigen-induced rabbit model of chronic inflammation (Pitsillides *et al.*, 1993a; Pitsillides and Blake, 1992), where normal joint function becomes compromised. Thus, therapies aimed at re-establishing these particular SLC characteristics, may restore HA synthesis, where function has been disrupted by disease, and perhaps facilitate normal joint movement.

As outlined above, it appears that HA synthesis and turnover can be regulated by hyaladherin expression at the cell surface. However, although a role for aberrant expression of such molecules in the progression of joint diseases has been postulated (Haynes *et al.*, 1991; Sherman *et al.*, 1994; Lee *et al.*, 1992; Kohda *et al.*, 1996), their normal function within joints remains to be defined, and their potential regulatory function in the control of HA turnover in these tissues is still a central issue.

Nevertheless, it is unlikely that the regulation of a developmental process is related to a single change in cell behaviour (Adams and Watt, 1993). Indeed, as alluded to, changes in the synthesis and expression of a number of cellular components, as well as differential local growth rates may also be instrumental factors. Another contributory factor may be the mechanical strain, or shear, environment at the joint line, and many, including ourselves, have shown that movement is essential for both the generation and subsequent preservation of diarthrodial joint spaces. Interestingly, changes induced by immobilisation appeared to decrease UDPGD activity at the joint line. This observation is consistent with the elaboration of a stiffer ECM.

This raises interesting questions regarding the ECM changes evident in diseased joints. We have found that the concentration of HA and its binding to synovial tissue components, as well as the expression of CD44, are decreased in RA synovial lining (Pitsillides *et al.*, 1994; Henderson *et al.*, 1993). Further, we have also shown that cells with high UDPGD activity appear in tissue lining a cavity containing a moving plastic implant, but that in contrast to the synovial lining, cells lining a subcutaneous air pouch in rats lack high UDPGD activity (Wilkinson *et al.*, 1993). This suggests that movement, or shear, may also be important in inducing the specialised behaviour of synovial lining cells. However, it remains possible that such ECM alterations in RA joints are a consequence of the lack of mobility which is associated with joint pathology, and are not necessarily a principal factor involved in disease etiology.

Therefore, it may be concluded that our studies in joint development may contribute to a mechanistic understanding of how synovial lining cells facilitate friction-free movement. In terms of defining how these mechanisms fail in joints functionally compromised by disease, it may be considered that we have made relatively little progress. However, several studies suggest that synovial lining cells in both RA joints and in experimental immune-induced arthritic joints show early evidence of joint pathology (Fassbender, 1982; Chayen and Bitensky, 1982; Henderson and Pettipher, 1985).

Using quantitative cytochemical analyses of tissue removed from human rheumatoid arthritic joints, Chayen and co-workers had showed that the disturbance of three associated biochemical systems was characteristic of the disease. These were four-fold increases in glucose 6-phosphate dehydrogenase (G6PD) activity which generates NADPH; a elevated reductive balance in cellular -SH: -S-S- balance, and markedly labilised lysosomal membranes in synovial lining cells (Butcher *et al.*, 1973; Chayen *et al.*, 1969; Chayen *et al.*, 1973; Pitsillides *et al.*, 1991). These workers have also shown that human non-rheumatoid synovium could be maintained *in vitro* in organ culture at pH 7.8, but that it was not maintained at pH 7.4. In contrast, human rheumatoid synovium did not survive at pH values above 7.4 (Poulter *et al.*, 1970).

Together, these findings indicate that in the chronically inflamed joints, there is a more reductive balance and a pH approaching neutrality. As discussed earlier, both UDPGD activity and the ability of cell surface-associated hyaladherins to actively bind HA are sensitive to such changes. Thus, it is possible that these early redox-related changes in synovial lining cells, which occur in RA, alter the biosynthesis of HA by a mechanism dependent to some extent on the interaction of HA with its cell surface-associated hyaladherins, such as CD44. This is manifest as an alteration in HA's molecular weight and concentration in inflamed joints, and as a consequence the joint's HA-related functional competence becomes compromised. Thus, it is evident that by combining studies of normal developmental mechanisms with a knowledge of how these fail in disease, novel therapeutic strategies for the restoration of friction-free movement in diarthrodial joints will be established.

SUMMARY

Synovial joints are susceptible to many disorders, including rheumatoid arthritis (RA), which result in loss of joint mobility. Synovium's facilitation of efficient, pain-free, joint and tendon movement has been recognised for some time. However, despite the fact that synovial lining cells show primary evidence of joint pathology, their cellular biology remains ill-defined. By establishing the mechanisms which control initial formation and subsequent maintenance of joint cavities during development, we aim to formulate rational approaches for the maintenance, or restoration, of synovium's functional competence where it is compromised by disease.

During development, joint cavities form by a process involving the separation of opposed cartilaginous elements, producing non-adherent articular surfaces and associated synovial structures. In adults, these surfaces are associated with synovial fluid containing high hyaluronan (HA) concentrations. It was hypothesised that differential HA synthesis and its association with hyaladherins at the forming joint line, produce the loss of tensile strength which is required to facilitate movement.

HA synthesis involves the transfer of UDP-glucuronate and UDP-N-acetyl glucosamine to nascent chains of HA by HA synthase, and UDPglucose dehydrogenase

(UDPGD) activity is essential for UDP-glucuronate production. Using *in situ* biochemistry for UDPGD activity and its microspectrophotometric assessment, we showed that cells immediately adjacent to forming cavities contained increased UDPGD activity when compared to neighbouring epiphyseal chondrocytes, and that this differential was maintained after cavitation. We also confirmed the presence of free HA at these sites, and its co-localisation with high levels of HA-synthase expression, suggesting that the specialised differentiation of these cells involves alterations specifically associated with increased differential HA synthesis. We have shown that hyaladherins (RHAMM, IVD4 receptors and most markedly CD44) are expressed at sites of cavitation, and that CD44 co-localises with labelling for ERM actin-capping proteins, as well as with the specific alignment of filamentous actin, suggesting that CD44 is expressed in a form capable of binding HA (confirmed using biotinylated HA). Finally, we have found that the lack of cavitation and 'fusion' induced by in ovo immobilisation is associated with marked decreases in UDPGD activity at sites of presumptive cavitation. These findings indicate that HA-hyaladherin interactions may be pivotal in initial joint tissue separation, and suggest that with a knowledge of how these processes fail in disease, novel approaches for restoring friction-free movement in diarthrodial joints may be possible.

ACKNOWLEDGEMENTS

Recent work described in this article was supported by a grant (P0504) from the Arthritis and Rheumatism Council. I would like to thank both Dr Gary Dowthwaite (ARC funded) for his major contributions to this work, and Anne C. Ward (PhD Studentship from The Royal Veterinary College) for her recent work on the effects of in ovo immobilisation. Thanks are due to Professors Charles Archer, Bruce Caterson and Dr Jim Ralphs for allowing us to use their confocal microscope facility. I would also like to thank Drs Sachiko Tsukita and Mike Bayliss, and Professors Bryan Toole, Eva Turley, Shoichiro Tsukita and Peter Prehm for supplying antibodies. In addition the helpful discussions with Professor Jo C.W. Edwards are warmly acknowledged.

REFERENCES

Adams, J.C. and Watt, F.M. (1993) Regulation of development and differentiation by the extracellular matrix. *Development*, **117**, 1183–1198.

Andersen, H. (1962) Histochemical studies on the development of the human hip joint. *Acta Anatomical*, **48**, 258–276.

Andersen, H. (1963) Development, morphology and histochemistry of the early synovial tissue in human fetuses. *Acta Anatomica*, **58**, 90–115.

Andersen, H. and BroRasmussen, F. (1961) Histochemical studies on the histogenesis of the joints in human fetuses with special reference to the development of the joint cavities in the hand and foot. *Am. J. Anat.*, **108**, 111–122.

Archer, C.W., Morrison, H. and Pitsillides, A.A. (1994) Cellular aspects of the development of diarthrodial joints and articular cartilage. *J. Anat.*, **184**, 447–456.

Aruffo, A., Stamenkovic, I., Melnick, M., Underhill, C.B. and Seed, B. (1990) CD44 is the principal cell surface receptor for hyaluronate. *Cell*, **61**, 1303–1308.

Balazs, E.A. (1974) The physical properties of synovial fluid and the special role of hyaluronic acid. In: *Disorders of the knee*. pp. 63–75 (A. Helfet, ed.). Lippincott, Philadelphia, USA.

Balazs, E.A., Watson, D., Duff, I.F. and Roseman, S. (1967) Hyaluronic acid in synovial fluid: 1. Molecular parameters of hyaluronic acid in normal and arthritic human fluids. *Arth. Rheum.*, **10**, 357–375.

Banerjee, S.D. and Toole, B.P. (1991) Monoclonal antibody to chick embryo hyaluronan-binding protein: changes in the distribution of binding during early brain development. *Dev. Biol.*, **146**, 186–197.

Banerjee, S.D. and Toole, B.P. (1992) Hyaluronan-binding protein in endothelial cell morh[hogenesis. *J. Cell Biol.*, **146**, 186–197.

Bernays, A. (1878) Die entwicklungsgeschichte des kniegelenkes des menschen, mit bemerkungen Ÿber die gelenke im allgemeinen. *Morphol. Jahrb.*, **4**, 403–446.

Blumberg, B.S. and Ogston, A.G. (1958) Physicochemical studies on hyaluronic acid. In: *Chemistry and Biology of mucopolysaccharides*. pp. 22–37. Churchill, London (Ciba Foundation Symposium).

Brecht, M., Mayer, U., Schlosser, E. and Prehm, P. (1986) Increased hyaluronate synthesis is required for fibroblast detachment and mitosis. *Biochem. J.*, **239**, 445–450.

Butcher, R.G., Bitensky, L., Cashman, B. and Chayen, J. (1973) Differences in the redox balance in human rheumatoid and non-rheumatoid synovial lining cells. *Beitr. Path*, **148**, 265–274.

Chayen, J., Bitensky, L., Butcher, R.G. and Poulter, L.W. (1969) Redox control of lysososomes in human synovia. *Nature*, **222**, 281–282.

Chayen, J., Bitensky, L., Butcher, R.G. and Cashman, B. (1973) The effect of experimentally induced redox changes on humanrheumatoid and non-rheumatoid synovial tissue *in vitro*. *Beitr. Path*, **149**, 127–144.

Chayen, J. and Bitensky, L. (1982) The effects of pharmacologically active agents on cytosolic reducing equivalents. *Rev. Pure and Appl. Pharm. Sci.*, **3**, 271–317.

Chayen, J. (1984) Quantitative cytochemistry: a precise form of cellular biochemistry. *Biochem. Soc. Trans.*, **12**, 887–898.

Chayen, J. and Bitensky, L. (1992) *Practical Histochemistry*. London, Wiley and Sons.

Craig, F.M., Bentley, G. and Archer, C.W. (1987) The temporal and spatial patterns of collagen I and III and keratan sulphate in developing chick MTP joint. *Development*, **99**, 383–391.

Craig, F.M., Bayliss, M.T., Bentley, G. and Archer, C.W. (1990) A role for hyaluronan in joint development. *J. Anat.*, **171**, 17–23.

DeLuca, G., Speziale, P., Balduini, C. and Castellani, A.A. (1975) Biosynthesis of glycosaminoglycans: uridine diphosphate 4-epimerase from cornea and epiphysial-plate cartilage. *Conn. Tiss. Res.*, **3**, 39–47.

DeLuca, G., Speziale, P., Rindi, S., Balduini, C. and Castellani, A.A. (1976) Effects of some nucleotides on regulation of glycosaminoglycan biosynthesis. *Conn. Tiss. Res.*, **4**, 247–254.

DeLuca, G. and Castellani, A.A. (1984) Regulatory aspects of glycosaminoglycan biosynthesis. *Acta Biol. Hung.*, **35**, 109–121.

Dougherty, B.A. and van de Rijn, I. (1993) Molecular characterisation of hasB from an operon required for hyaluronic acid synthesis in Group A Streptococci. *J. Biol. Chem.*, **268**, 7118–7124.

Dowthwaite, G.P., Edwards, J.C.W. and Pitsillides, A.A. (1997) The role of hyaluronan binding proteins during joint development. *Transactions ORS*, **22**, 59.

Dowthwaite, G.P., Edwards, J.C.W. and Pitsillides, A.A. (1998) An essential role for the interaction between hyaluronan and hyaluronan-binding proteins during joint development. *J. Histochem. Cytochem.*, **465**, 1–11.

Drachmann, D.B. and Sokoloff, L. (1966) The role of movement in embryonic joint development. *Dev. Biol.*, **14**, 401–420.

Duprez, D.M., Kostakopoulou, K., Francis-West, P.H., Tickle, C. and Brickell, P.M. (1996) Activation of Fgf-4 and HoxD gene expression by BMP-2 expressing cells in the developing chick limb. *Development*, **122**, 1821–1828.

Edwards, J.C.W., Wilkinson, L.S., Jones, H.M., Soothill, P., Henderson, K.J., Worrall, J.G. and Pitsillides, A.A. (1994) The formation of human synovial joint cavities: a possible role for hyaluronan and CD44 in altered interzone cohesion. *J. Anat.*, **185**, 355–367.

Edwards, J.C.W., Wilkinson, L.S., Soothill, P., Hembry, R.M., Murphy, G. and Reynolds, J.J. (1996) Matrix metalloproteinases in the formation of human synovial joint cavities. *J. Anat.*, **188**, 355–360.

Fassbender, H.G. (1982) Potential agressiveness of the synovial tissue in rheumatiod arthritis. In: *Articular synovium*. (P. Franchimont, ed.). Karger, Basel, pp. 34–44.

Fell, H.B. and Canti, R.B. (1934) Experiments on the development *in vitro* of the avian knee joint. *Proc. R. Soc. B.*, **116**, 316–351.

Fessler, J.H. and Fessler, L.I. (1966) Electron microscopic visualisation of the polysaccharide hyaluronic acid. *Proc. Natl. Acad. Sci. USA*, **56**, 141–147.

Fisher, M. and Solursh, M. (1977) Glycosaminoglycan localisation and role in maintenance of tissue spaces in early chick embryos. *J. Embryol. Exp. Morph.*, **42**, 195–207.

Gardner, E. and Gray, D.J. (1950) Prenatal development of the human hip joint. *Am. J. Anat.*, **87**, 163–212.

Ginsburg, V. (1964) Sugar nucleotides and the synthesis of carbohydrates. *Adv. Enzymol. Relat. Subj. Biochem.*, **26**, 35–88.

Haddon, C.M. and Lewis, J.H. (1991) Hyaluronan as a propellant for epithelial movement: the development of semi-circular canals in the inner ear of Xenopus. *Development*, **112**, 541–549.

Hamburger, V. and Waugh, M. (1940) The primary development of the skeleton in nerveless and poorly innervated limb transplants of chick embryos. *Physiol. Zool.*, **13**, 367–380.

Handly, C.J. and Phelps, C.F. (1972) The biosynthesis *in vitro* of chondroitin sulphate in neonatal rat epiphyseal cartilage. *Biochem. J.*, **126**, 417–432.

Hardingham, T.E., Ewins, R.J.F. and Muir, H. (1976) Cartilage proteoglycans: structure and heterogeneity of the core protein and the effects of specific protein modification on the binding to hyaluronate. *Biochem. J.*, **157**, 127–143.

Hardingham, T.E. and Fosang, A.J. (1992) Proteoglycans: many forms and functions. *FASEB. J.*, **6**, 861–870.

Hardwick, C., Hoare, K., Owens, R., Hohn, H.P., Hook, M., Moore, D., Cripps, V., Austen, L., Nance, D.M. and Turley, E.A. (1992) Molecular cloning of a novel hyaluronan receptor that mediates tumour cell motility. *J. Cell. Biol.*, **117**, 1343–1350.

Hascall, V.C., Heinegard, D.K. and Wight, T.N. (1991) Proteoglycans: metabolism and pathology. pp. 149–172. In: *Cell Biology of Extracellular matrix.* 2nd edition (Hay, E.D., ed.). Plenum Press, New York and London.

Haynes, B.F., Liao, H-X. and Patton, K.L. (1991) The transmembrane hyaluronate receptor (CD44): multiple functions, multiple forms. *Cancer Cells*, 3(9), 347–350.

Heatley, F. and Scott, J.E. (1988) A water molecule participates in the secondary structure of hyaluronan. *Biochem. J.*, **254**, 489–493.

Henderson, B. and Pettipher, E.R. (1985) The synovial lining cell: biology and pathobiology. *Seminars in Arth. and Rhuem.*, **15**, 1–32.

Henderson, K.J., Pitsillides, A.A., Edwards, J.C.W. and Worrall, J.G. (1993) Reduced expression of CD44 in rheumatoid synovial lining cells. *Brit. J. Rheum.*, **32**(1), 25.

Hickery, M., Pitsillides, A.A., Edwards, J.C.W. and Bayliss, M.T. (1993) Measurement of glycosaminoglycan chain synthesis and UDP-glucose dehydrogenase activity in the presence of rhTGFb and rhIL-1a in human articular cartilage. *Trans. Orth. Res. Soc.*, **18**, 2.

Hinchcliffe, J.R. (1977) The chondrogenic pattern in chick limb morphogenesis. In: *Vertebrate limb and somite morphogenesis* (D.A. Ede, J.R. Hinchcliffe and M. Balls, eds), pp. 293–309. Cambridge University Press, London, New York and Melbourne.

Hronowski, L. and Anastassiades, T.P. (1980) The effect of cell density on net rates of glycosaminoglycan synthesis and secretion by cultures rat fibroblasts. *J. Biol. Chem.*, **255**, 10091–10099.

Isacke, C.M. (1994) The role of the cytoplasmic domain in regulating CD44 function. *J. Cell Sci.*, **107**, 2353–2359.

Izpisua-Belmonte, J-C. and Duboule, D. (1992) Homeobox genes and pattern information in the vertebrate limb. *Dev. Biol.*, **152**, 26–36.

Kendall, F.E., Heidelberger, M. and Dawson, M.H. (1937) A seriologically inactive polysaccharide elaborated by mucoid strains of Group A hemolytiv streptococcus. *J. Biol. Chem.*, **118**, 61–69.

Klewes, L., Turley, E.A. and Prehm, P. (1993) The hyaluronate synthase from a eukaryotic cell line. *Biochem. J.*, **290**, 791–795.

Knudson, C.B. and Knudson, W. (1993) Hyaluronan-binding proteins in development, tissue homeostasis and disease. *FASEB J.*, **7**, 1233–1241.

Knudson, C.B. and Toole, B.P. (1985) Changes in the pericellular matrix during differentiation of limb bud mesoderm. *Dev. Biol.*, **112**, 308–318.

Kohda, D., Morton, C.J., Parkar, A.A., Hatanaka, H., Inagaki, F.M., Campbell, I.D. and Day, A.J. (1996) Solution structure of the link module: a hyaluronan-binding domain involved in extracellular matrix stability and cell migration. *Cell*, **86**, 767–775.

Kulyk, W.M. and Kosher, R.A. (1987) Temporal and spatial analysis of hyaluronidase activity during development of embryonic chick limb bud. *Dev. Biol.*, **120**, 535–542.

Lacy, B.E. and Underhill, C.B. (1987) The hyaluronate receptor is associated with actin filaments. *J. Cell Biol.*, **105**, 1395–1404.

Laurent, T.C. (1989) Introduction. In: *The Biology of Hyaluronan* (D. Evered and J. Whelan, eds), pp. 1–5. Ciba Foundation Symposium, 143. J. Wiley and Sons, Chichester, UK.

Laurent, T.C. and Fraser, J.R.E. (1986) The properties and turnover of hyaluronan. In: *Functions of proteoglycans*. Ciba Foundation Symposium 124, pp. 9–29. Wiley, Chichester, England.

Laurent, T.C. and Fraser, J.R.E. (1992) Hyaluronan. *FASEB J.*, **6**, 2397–2404.

Lee, T., Wisniewski, H-G. and Vilcek, J. (1992) A novel secretory tumour necrosis factor-inducible protein (TSG-6) is a member of the family of hyaluronan binding proteins, closely related to the adhesion receptor CD44. *J. Cell Biol.*, **116**, 545–557.

Lelkes, G. (1958) Experiments *in vitro* on the role of movement in the development of joints. *J. Embryol. Exp. Morph.*, **6**, 183–186.

Lesley, J., Hyman, R. and Kinkade, P.W. (1993) CD44 and its interaction with the cellular matrix. *Adv. Immunol.*, **54**, 271–335.

Lewis, J.H. (1977) Growth and determination in the developing limb. In Ede, D.A., Hinchcliffe, J.R. and Balls, M., eds., *Vertebrate limb and somite morphogenesis*. Cambridge, London, New York and Melbourne, Cambridge University Press, 215.

Liao, H-X., Levesque, M.C., Patton, K., Bergamo, B., Jones, D., Moody, M., Telon, M.J. and Haynes, B.F. (1993) Regulation of human CD44H and CD44E isoform binding to hyaluronan by phorbol myristate acetate and anti-CD44 monoclonal and polyclonal antibodies. *J. Immunol.*, **151**, 6490–6499.

Mason, R.M., Crossman, M.V. and Sweeney, C. (1989) Hyaluronan and hyaluronan-binding proteins in cartilagenous tissues. In: *The Biology of Hyaluronan* (D. Evered and J. Whelan, eds), pp. 107–120. Ciba Foundation Symposium, 143. J. Wiley and Sons, Chichester, UK.

Mehdizadeh, S., Bitensky, L. and Chayen, J. (1991) The assay of uridine diphosphoglucose dehydrogenase activity. *Cell Biochem. Funct.*, **9**, 103–110.

Meyer, K. (1947) The biological significance of hyaluronic acid and hyaluronidase. *Physiol. Rev.*, **27**, 335–359.

Meyer, K. and Palmer, J.W. (1934) The polysaccharide of the vitrous humour. *J. Biol. Chem.*, **107**, 629–634.

McGarry, A. and Gahan, P.B. (1985) A quantitative cytochemical study of UDP-D glucose: NAD-oxidoreductase (E.C.1.1.1.22.) activity during stelar differentiation in Pisum sativum L.cv Meteor. *Histochemistry*, **83**, 551–554.

Mian, N. (1986) Characterisation of a high-Mr plasma-membrane bound protein and its role as a constituent of hyaluronan synthase complex. *Biochem. J.*, **237**, 333–342.

Milaire, J. (1947) In: *Normal and abnormal embryological development* (C.H. Frantz, ed.), pp. 61. Washington DC, National Research Council.

Mitrovic, D.R. (1971) La nécrose physiologique dans le mésenchyme articulaire des embryons de rat et poulet. *Comptes Rendus Hebdoinaires Séancces Rendu Academie de Science Paris*, **273**, 642–645.

Mitrovic, D.R. (1974) Vaisseaux sanguins au cours de l'arthrogénése et leur participation éventuelle a la cavatation articulaire. *Zeitschrift Für Anatomie und Entwick*, **144**, 39–60.

Mitrovic, D. (1977) Development of the metatarsophalangeal joint of the chick embryo. Morphological, ultrastructural and histochemical studies. *Am. J. Anat.*, **150**, 333–348.

Mitrovic, D. (1978) Development of the diarthrodial joint in the rat embryo. *Am. J. Anat.*, **151**, 474–486.

Mitrovic, D. (1982) Development of the articular cavity in peralysed chick embryos and in chick embryo limbs cultured on chorioallantoic membranes. *Acta. Anat.*, **113**, 313–324.

Molz, R.J. and Danishefsky, I. (1971) Uridine diphosphate glucose dehydrogenase in rat tissue. *Biochim. Biophys. Acta*, **250**, 6–13.

Munaron, G. (1954) Osservasione istofisiche ed istochimiche sul mesenchimima intermedio delle articolazioni embryonali e suio derivati. *Bolletino dell Societa di Biologia Spermentale*, **30**, 919–922.

Murakami, S., Shimabukuru, Y., Miki, Y., Saho, T., Hino, E., Kasai, D., Nozaki, T., Kusumoto, Y. and Okada, H. (1994) Inducible binding of human lymphocytes to hyaluronate via CD44 does not require cytoskeleton association but does require new protein synthesis. *J. Immunol.*, **152**, 467–477.

Murphy, G. and Reynolds, J.J. (1993) Extracellular matrix degradation. In: *Connective tissue and its heritable disorders* (P.M. Royce and B. Steinmann, eds), pp. 287–316. Wiley-Liss, New York.

Murray, P.D.F. and Drachmann, D.B. (1969) The role of movement in the development of joints and related structures: the head and neck in the chick embryo. *J. Embryol. Exp. Morph.*, **22**, 349–371.

Nalin, A.M., Greenlee, Jr. T.K. and Sandell, L.J. (1995) Collagen gene expression during development of avian synovial joints: transient expression of types II and XI collagen genes in the joint capsule. *Dev. Dynamics*, **203**, 352–362.

Neame, P.J. and Barry, F.P. (1993) The link proteins. *Experimentia*, **49**, 393–402.

Nomina Anatomica (1950) Revised by the International Anatomical Nomenclature Committee appointed the 5th International Congress of Anatomists, Oxford.

Ogston, A.G. and Stanier, J.E. (1953) The physiological functions of hyaluronic acid in synovial fluid; viscous, elastic and lubricant properties. *J. Physiol. (London)* **199**, 244–252.

O'Rahilly, R. and Gardner, E. (1978) The embryology of moveable joints. In: *The joints and synovial fluid* (L. Sokoloff, ed.). Vol. 1, pp. 49–97. Academic Press, New York.

Oster, G.F., Murray, J.D. and Maini, P.K. (1985) A model for chondrogenic condensations in the developing limb: role of extracellular matrix and cell intertractions. *J. Emb. Exp. Morph.*, **89**, 93–112.

Perkins, S.J., Nealis, A.S., Dudhia, J. and Hardingham, T.E. (1989) Immunoglobulin fold and tandem repeat structures in proteoglycan N-terminal domains and Link protein. *J. Mol. Biol.*, **206**, 737–753.

Perschl, A., Lesley, J., English, N., Trowbridge, I. and Hyman, R. (1995) Role of CD44 cytoplasmic domain in hyaluronan binding. *Eur. J. Immunol.*, **25**, 495–501.

Phelps, C.F. (1973) The biosynthesis of glycosaminoglycans. *Biochem. Soc. Trans.*, **1**, 814–819.

Pitsillides, A.A., Blake, S.M., Glynn, L.E., Frost, G.T.B., Bitensky, L. and Chayen, J. (1991) The effect of menadione epoxide on the experimental immune arthritis in the rabbit. *Int. J. Exp. Path.*, **72**, 301–309.

Pitsillides, A.A. and Blake, S.M. (1992) Uridine diphosphoglucose dehydrogenase activity in synovial lining cells in the experimental antigen induced model of rheumatoid arthritis: an indication of synovial lining cell function. *Ann. Rheum. Dis.*, **51**, 992–995.

Pitsillides, A.A., Wilkinson, L.S., Mehdizadeh, S., Bayliss, M.T. and Edwards, J.C.W. (1993a) Uridine diphos-phoglucose dehdrogenase activity in normal and rheumatoid synovium: the description of a specialized synovial lining cell. *Int. J. Exp. Path*, **74**, 27–34.

Pitsillides, A.A., Hickery, M., Bayliss, M.T. and Edwards, J.C.W. (1993b) The effect of rhIL-1 and rhTGFb on glycosaminoglycan chain synthesis and UDP-glucose dehydrogenase activity in human articular cartilage. *Brit. J. Rheumatol.*, **32**(1), 120.

Pitsillides, A.A., Will, R.K., Bayliss, M.T. and Edwards, J.C.W. (1994) Circulating and synovial fluid hyaluronan levels: effects of intraarticualr corticosteroid on the concentration and the rate of turnover. *Arth. Rheum.*, **37**, 1030–1038.

Pitsillides, A.A., Archer, C.W., Prehm, P., Bayliss, M.T. and Edwards, J.C.W. (1995) Alterations in hyaluronan synthesis during developing joint cavitation. *J. Histochem. Cytochem.*, **43**(3), 263–273.

Poulter, L.W., Bitensky, L., Cashman, B. and Chayen, J. (1970) The maintenance of human synovial tissue *in vitro*. *Virchows Arch (Zellpath)*, **4**, 303–309.

Pratt, R.M., Larsen, M.A. and Johnston, M.C. (1975) Migration of cranial neural crest cells in a cell-free hyaluronate-rich matrix. *Dev. Biol.*, **44**, 298–305.

Prehm, P. (1980) Induction of hyaluronic acid synthesis in teratocarcinoma stem cells by retinoic acid. *FEBS Lett.*, **111**, 295–298.

Prehm, P. (1983) Synthesis of hyaluronan in differentiated teratocarcinoma cells. II. Mechanisms of chain growth. *Biochem. J.*, **211**, 191–198.

Prehm, P. (1984) Hyaluronate is synthesised at the plasma membrane. *Biochem. J.*, **220**, 597–600.

Prehm, P. (1989) Identification and regulation of the eukaryote hyaluronate synthase. In: *The Biology of Hyaluronan* (D. Evered and J. Whelan, eds), pp. 21–40. Ciba Foundation Symposium, 143. J. Wiley and Sons, Chichester.

Prehm, P. and Mausolf, A. (1986) Isolation of streptococcal hyaluronan synthase. *Biochem. J.*, **235**, 887–889.

Preston, B.N., Davies, M. and Ogston, A.G. (1965) The composition and physicochemical properties of hyaluronic acid prepared from ox synovial fluid and froma case of mesothelioma. *Biochem. J.*, **96**, 449–471.

Rapport, M.M., Weissman, B., Linker, A. and Meyer, K. (1951) Isolation of a crystalline disaccharide, hyoalobiuronic acid, from hyaluronic acid. *Nature (London)* **168**, 996–997.

Roden, L. (1980) Structure and metabolism of connective tissue proteoglycans. In: *The biochemistry of glycoproteins and proteoglycans* (W.J. Lennarz, ed.), pp. 267–371. Plenum Press, New York and London.

Ruano-Gil, D., Nardi-Vilardaga, J. and Teixidor-Johe, A. (1980) Embryonic mobility and joint development. *Folia Morphologica.*, **28**, 221–223.

Sato, N., Funayama, N., Nagafuchi, A., Yonemura, S., Tsukita, S.A. and Tsukita, S.H. (1992) A gene family consisting of ezrin, radixin, and moesin: its specific localisation at actin filament/plasma membrane associated sites. *J. Cell Sci.*, **103**, 131–143.

Saunders, J.W. (1948) The proximo-distal sequence of the origin of the parts of the chick wing and the role of the ectoderm. *J. Exp. Zool.*, **108**, 363–404.

Scott, J.E. (1989) Secondary structure in hyaluronan solutions: chemical and biological implications. In: *The Biology of Hyaluronan* (D. Evered and J. Whelan, eds), pp. 6–20. Ciba Foundation Symposium, 143. J. Wiley and Sons, Chichester, UK.

Scott, J.E., Cummings, C., Brass, A. and Chen, Y. (1991) Secondar and tertiary structures of hyaluronan in aque-ous solution, investigated by rotary shadowing-electron microscopy and comuter simulation. *Biochem. J.*, **274**, 699–705.

Scott, J.E. and Dorling, J. (1965) Differential staining of acid glycosaminoglycans (mucopolysaccharides) by alcian blue in salt solutions. *Histochemie.*, **5**, 277–285.

Sherman, L., Sleeman, J., Herrlich, P. and Ponta, H. (1994) Hyaluronate receptors: key players in growth, differentiation and tumour progression. *Curr. Op. Cell Biol.*, **6**, 726–733.

Storm, E.E., Huynh, T.V., Copeland, N.G., Jenkins, N.A., Kingsley, D.M. and Lee, S-J. (1994) Limb altera-tions in brachypodism mice due to mutations in a new member of the TGFb-superfamily. *Nature*, **368**, 639–643.

Summerbell, D. (1977) Reduction of the rate of outgrowth, cell density, and cell division following removal of the apical ectodermal ridge of the chick limb-bud. *J. Embryol. Exp. Morph.*, **40**, 1–21.

Sundbland, L. (1953) Studies on hyaluronic acid in synovial fluids. *Acta. Soc. Med. Ups.*, **58**, 113–119.

Tickle, C. (1995) *Current opinion in Genetics and Development*, **5**, 478–484.

Toole, B.P. (1981) Glycosaminoglycans in morphogenesis. In: *Cell biology of the extracellular matrix* (E.D. Hay, ed.), pp. 259–294. Plenum Press, New York.

Toole, B.P. (1982) Developmental role of hyaluronate. *Connective Tiss. Res.*, **10**, 93–100.

Toole, B.P., Munaim, S.I., Welles, S. and Knudson, C.B. (1989) Hyaluronate-cell interactions and growth factor regulation of hyaluronate synthesis during limb development. In: *The Biology of Hyaluronan* (D. Evered and J. Whelan, eds), pp. 138–149. Ciba Foundation Symposium, 143. J. Wiley and Sons, Chichester, UK.

Toole, B.P. (1990) Hyaluronan and its binding proteins, the hyaladherins. *Current Op. Cell Biol.*, **2**, 839–844.

Toole, B.P., Biswas, C. and Gross, J. (1979) Hyaluronate and invasiveness of the rabbit V2 carcinoma. *Proc. Natl. Acad. Sci. USA*, **76**, 6299–6303.

Toole, B.P. and Trelstad, R.L. (1971) Hyaluronate production and removal during corneal development and virus-transformed cell lines – Binding and aggregation studies. *Exp. Cell Res.*, **131**, 419–427.

Tsukita, S.A., Oishi, K., Sato, N., Sagara, J., Kawai, A. and Tsukita, S.H. (1994) ERM family members as molecular linkers between the cell surface glycoprotein CD44 and actin-based cytoskeletons. *J. Cell Biol.*, **126**, 391–401.

Turley, E.A. (1989) The role of cell associated hyaluronan-binding protein in fibroblast behaviour. In: *The Biology of Hyaluronan* (D. Evered and J. Whelan, eds), pp. 121–137. Ciba Foundation Symposium, 143. J. Wiley and Sons, Chichester, UK.

Turley, E.A., Austen, L., Vandeligt, K. and Clary, C. (1991) Hyaluronan and cell-associated hyaluronan binding protein regulate the locmotion of ras-transformed cells. *J. Cell Biol.*, **112**, 1041–1047.

Underhill, C.B. (1989) The interaction of hyaluronate with the cell surface. In: *The Biology of Hyaluronan* (D. Evered and J. Whelan, eds), pp. 87–106. Ciba Foundation Symposium, 143. J. Wiley and Sons, Chichester, UK.

Underhill, C. (1992) CD44: The hyaluronan receptor. *J. Cell. Science*, **103**, 293–298.

Ward, A.C. and Pitsillides, A.A. (1998) Developmental immobilisation induces failure of joint cavity formation by a process involving selective local changes in glycosaminoglycan metabolism. *Trans. ORS.*, **23**, 199(34).

Wayner, E.A., Carter, W.G. (1987) Identification of multiple cell adhesion receptors for collagen and fibronectin in human fibrosarcoma cells possessing unique alpha and common beta sub-units. *J. Cell Biol.*, **105**, 1873–1884.

Weigel, P.H., Hascall, V.C. and Tammi, M. (1997) Hyaluronan synthases. *J. Biol. Chem.*, **272**(22), 13997–14000.

Wilkinson, L.S., Pitsillides, A.A., Worrall, J.G. and Edwards, J.C.W. (1992) Light microscopic characterisation of the fibroblast-like synovial intimal cell (synoviocyte). *Arth. Rheum.*, **35**(10), 1179–1184.

Wilkinson, L.S., Moore, A.R., Pitsillides, A.A., Willoughby, D.A. and Edwards, J.C.W. (1993) Comparison of surface fibroblastic cells in subcutaneous air pouch and synovial lining: differences in UDP-glucose dehydrogenase activity. *Int. J. Exp. Path*, **74**, 113–115.

Wolpert, L. (1989) Positional information revisited. *Development*, **107**, 3–12.

Yasuda, Y. (1973) Differentiation of human limb buds *in vitro*. *Anat. Rec.*, **175**, 561–578.

Yu, Q., Banerjee, S.D. and Toole, B.P. (1992) The role of hyaluronan-binding proteins in assembly of pericellular matrices. *Dev. Dynam.*, **193**, 145–152.

NOTE ADDED IN PROOF

Recent studies have suggested that the antibodies raised putatively to hyaluronan synthase and used in our experiments (Klewes *et al.*, 1993) may not necessarily recognise hyaluronan synthase and therefore should be considered with caution (see Wiegel *et al.*, 1997).

5 Growth and Differentiation Factors/ Morphogens in Joint Development and Tissue Specification

Frank P. Luyten*

Bone Research Branch, National Institute of Dental Research, National Institutes of Health, Bethesda, MD 20892, USA

INTRODUCTION

Joint diseases are a major health issue. They can be divided into inflammatory joint diseases (e.g. rheumatoid arthritis), infectious and degenerative or osteoarthritic diseases. Regardless of the type of arthritis, in most cases the joint disease process results in irreversible damage of the joint and joint associated tissues ultimately leading to an increasing amount of therapeutic surgical procedures including total joint replacement. The restoration of joint tissues using tissue engineering approaches appears to become a valid alternative to the existing more invasive surgical treatments.

Increasing evidence indicates that tissue regeneration recapitulates a cascade of molecular events taking place in embryonic tissue formation. Therefore, the study and understanding of the molecular mechanisms underlying skeletal tissue formation is of critical importance in order to device new approaches in skeletal repair protocols.

Tissue formation and repair is a cascade of events involving cell proliferation and angiogenesis, induction or initiation of tissue specification or differentiation, cell maturation and matrix synthesis, and tissue remodelling. All these stages are coupled to specific signalling molecules, matrix molecules and progenitor cell populations.

We have been focusing on the signalling molecules involved in the formation of skeletal tissues especially cartilage and bone. One of the major advances in this field has been the discovery of the Bone Morphogenetic Proteins (BMPs), a group of morphogens structurally

*Current address: Lab. for Skeletal Development & Joint Disorders, Onderwijs & Navorsing, Herestraat 49, B 3000 Leuven, Belgium.

belonging to the TGFβ superfamily. Bone inductive activity was originally described in demineralized bone matrix (Urist, 1965) and was further characterized and purified from extracts of demineralized bone using an *in vivo* ectopic bone induction assay (Reddi and Huggins, 1972; for review Reddi, 1992). Peptide sequences were obtained from highly purified osteogenic protein preparations (Wang *et al.*, 1988; Luyten *et al.*, 1989; Sampath *et al.*, 1990) and allowed the cloning of a number of BMPs (Wozney *et al.*, 1988; Celeste *et al.*, 1990; Özkaynak *et al.*, 1990). Subsequently, it has been demonstrated that BMPs are involved in many developmental processes, especially as mediators in epithelial-mesenchymal interactions. In addition, recombinantly expressed BMPs in combination with a variety of carriers have been shown to successfully heal craniofacial and periodontal lesions in non-human primates (Ripamonti *et al.*, 1992, 1995). These data are good examples of the use of developmentally crucial signalling molecules in postnatal tissue repair. Successful tissue repair with minimal scar tissue formation also involves other critical parameters such as the delivery vehicle, and the availability of responding cells. It is very likely that the ultimate repair protocol will be a combination of any of these components and will depend on the clinical indication, the individual patient and the underlying disease processes.

This manuscript will focus on our recent efforts to further elucidate and characterize the role of members of the Bone Morphogenetic Protein family in skeletal tissue formation and joint morphogenesis and explore the potential impact on joint tissue regeneration.

CARTILAGE-DERIVED CHONDROGENIC/ OSTEOGENIC ACTIVITIES

We decided to explore the possible presence of chondrogenic/osteogenic factors in cartilaginous tissues in order to determine if there are cartilage-specific morphogens controlling cartilage differentiation and maturation, and if so, are they distinct from bone derived osteogenic proteins (Luyten and Reddi, 1992). The same *in vivo* bioassay for ectopic subcutaneous cartilage and bone induction was used to characterize potential activities. Crude extracts from articular cartilage and epiphyseal cartilage using the same chaotropic conditions as described for bone extraction (e.g. 4 M GuHCl or 6 M urea) did not reveal any biological activity. On the contrary, the implants displayed substantial inflammatory infiltrations possibly preventing to uncover chondrogenic or osteogenic activities. Therefore procedures were designed to remove the bulk of the proteoglycan material by applying the extracts on an ion exchange column. Indeed, when implanted *in vivo*, the 0.15 M NaCl eluate of articular cartilage and epiphyseal cartilage extracts after DEAE Sephadex chromatography revealed the formation of several islands of chondrocytes, prompting us to further characterize the potential chondrogenic factors in cartilaginous tissues. We focused on the articular cartilage since this unique tissue is not replaced by bone postnatally and can be readily dissected free from bone tissue. A significant improvement was the development of a 1.2 M GuHCl, 0.5% CHAPS extraction procedure resulting in the recovery of substantial chondrogenic activity and leaving behind the majority of the cartilage matrix, thereby facilitating protein purification with much less viscous samples.

Further purification of the activity was essentially based on the protocols developed for bone derived osteogenic activity (Luyten *et al.*, 1989). The purification steps with yields, activities and protein content are shown in Table 5.1. Batches of 200–400 gram wet weight articular cartilage collected from 20 to 30 pairs of newborn calf hoofs (metatarsophalangeal and ankle joints) were processed. The tissues were finely minced and washed twice in ice cold phosphate buffer (PBS). Extraction was performed overnight in extraction buffer (1.2 M GuHCl, 0.5% CHAPS, 50 mM Tris.HCl pH 7.2 with enzyme inhibitors; 1 l extraction buffer/100–150 grams tissue) in the cold after brief homogenization of the tissues using a Polytron. The extract was centrifuged at $3,000 \times g$ for 30 min and the supernatant was subsequently equilibrated in 6 M urea/50 mM Tris.HCl pH 7.4 with 0.15 M NaCl by diafiltration (Ultrasette™, Filtron Technologies). The solution was subsequently mixed in batch for 2 h at room temperature with 500 ml Heparin-Sepharose (Pharmacia Biotech) previously equilibrated in the same buffer. The slurry was then loaded on a column, and washed with 10 volumes of 6 M urea/50 mM Tris.HCl pH 7.4 containing 0.15 M NaCl. Although some biological activity was eluted with 0.5 M NaCl, the majority of the activity was recovered between 0.5 and 1 M NaCl. Therefore, stepwise elution with 2 column volumes 1M NaCl was routinely used. Heparin-Sepharose affinity chromatography was a critical step because in most batches chondrogenic activity was not detectable in the crude extracts even using the modified extraction procedure in low GuHCl as described above. The 1 M NaCl eluate was concentrated by diafiltration, and 10 ml aliquots (2 to 5 aliquots) loaded on a Sepharose S-200 molecular sieve column (XK 50/100, Pharmacia Biotech) equilibrated in 4 M GdnHCl, 50 mM Tris.HCl pH 7.4. The bioactive fractions were then pooled and subjected to an additional molecular sieve step on Superose 12 (Pharmacia Biotech) under the same conditions. Molecular sieve chromatography, as shown in Table 5.1, resulted in a significant increase in total activity as measured by units alkaline phosphatase per mg implanted protein, suggesting the presence of specific or non-specific inhibitors. Indeed, reconstitution of higher molecular weight fractions with active samples inhibits the chondrogenic activity (unpublished). Highly purified fractions were obtained after Concanavalin A-Sepharose chromatography using conditions as described before (Chang *et al.*, 1994), and preparative SDS polyacrylamide gel electrophoresis followed by gel elution (Luyten *et al.*, 1989), indicating that the activity resided in the area between 35–40 kDa. As shown in Table 5.1, the specific activity of the highly

TABLE 5.1
Purification of cartilage derived chondrogenic/osteogenic activity.

	Total activity (units Alk. Phos.)	Protein (mg)	Specific activity (U/mg)	Purification-fold
Crude Extract	not detectable	4,063	—	—
Heparin Sepharose	121	760	0.16	1
Sephacryl S-200HR	1,008	48	21	132
Superose 12	382	3.5	112	703
Concanavalin A	84	0.175	480	3,015
SDS PAGE/elution	15	0.007	2,143	13,459

Abbreviations: Alk. Phos., Alkaline Phosphatase.

purified fractions was more than 2,000 Units of alkaline phosphatase/mg implanted protein the same order of magnitude as for the bone derived purified samples. However, the limited amount of protein available did not allow further purification. Therefore, we decided to obtain primary sequencing data at this point of the purification. Samples were subjected to enzymatic digestion (including trypsin) and the peptides were separated by reverse phase HPLC. Primary sequencing data of about 30 peptides of 3 different batches were obtained and surprisingly no sequences were found corresponding to any of the known BMPS. Several peptides suggested the possibility of BMP-like proteins. These data, together with the loss of activity after reduction and alkylation, suggested the possibility of the existence of other BMP members in cartilage extracts.

In parallel, we decided to pursue the further characterization of BMP-like genes in cartilage using molecular biology approaches. Based on the high degree of conservation of the C-terminal domain of the BMPs and TGF-β superfamily members, a large number of degenerate primer sets were designed and used in RT-PCR, a strategy previously successfully used to identify TGF-β superfamily members in Drosophila (Wharton *et al.*, 1991). Using mRNA prepared from newborn articular cartilage, we identified 2 novel members of the BMP family, designated Cartilage-derived Morphogenetic Proteins-1 and -2 (CDMP-1, CDMP-2) (Chang *et al.*, 1994). Based on the high percentage identity of their carboxyl-terminal domain (about 80%), they can be classified as members of a novel subfamily.

Using antibodies against specific BMPs we have analyzed the presence of BMPs/CDMPs in the Concanavalin A-Sepharose bound biologically active purified protein preparations of cartilage obtained as described above. Preliminary data indicate that BMP-2, BMP-3 and CDMP-2, and possibly CDMP-1, are immunodetectable in these highly purified protein preparations. Since recombinant BMP-2 (Wozney *et al.*, 1988), BMP-3 (A.H. Reddi, personal communication) and the CDMPs appear to display *in vivo* chondrogenic/osteogenic activities (unpublished data), it is very likely that a combination of BMPs/CDMPs in the highly purified protein preparations are responsible for the biological activity. However, the presence of other BMPs such as BMPs 4, 5, 6 and 7 has not yet been tested and therefore, cannot be excluded.

BONE MORPHOGENETIC PROTEINS/ CARTILAGE-DERIVED MORPHOGENETIC PROTEINS IN MOUSE SKELETAL DEVELOPMENT

The potential role of several BMPs in skeletal and joint tissue formation was supported by their expression pattern during skeletal morphogenesis (Lyons *et al.*, 1989, 1990; Vukicevic *et al.*, 1994a,b).

The first evidence that at least some BMPs are key physiological regulators in the formation of skeletal structures, was provided by the defects in many small bone and cartilage structures in *short ear* mice, caused by a nonsense mutation in the middle of the *Bmp5* coding region (Kingsley *et al.*, 1992). Additional data have emerged through homologous recombination approaches supporting a discrete role for OP-1/BMP-7 in skeletal development (Dudley *et al.*, 1995; Luo *et al.*, 1995).

The role of CDMP-1, the human homologue of *Gdf-5*, as a regulator of skeletal growth has now been well documented. Storm *et al.* (1994) and Chang *et al.* (1994) established independently that *Gdf-5/Cdmp-1* mapped close to the brachypodism *(bp)* locus on chromosome 2 in mice. This disorder is characterized by the shortening of the limbs. Owens and Solursh (1982), as a result of careful in-depth *in vitro* studies, suggested that the underlying molecular defect in *bp* mice might be the result of the lack of a chondrogenic signal normally produced by mesenchymal cells at the time of cartilage condensation and chondrogenesis. These data were very suggestive of the possibility of the involvement of a BMP-like gene such as *Gdf-5/Cdmp-1* in this brachypodism phenotype. Storm *et al.*, subsequently established that null mutations in the *Gdf-5* gene, resulting in the loss of function of the protein product, are indeed associated with several *bp* mice strains and are most likely directly responsible for the skeletal phenotype (Storm *et al.*, 1994).

BONE MORPHOGENETIC PROTEINS/ CARTILAGE-DERIVED MORPHOGENITIC PROTEINS IN HUMAN SKELETAL DEVELOPMENT

A distinct role for the CDMPs in human skeletal development is suggested by their expression patterns (Chang *et al.*, 1994). CDMP-1 is predominantly expressed in the pre-cartilage condensations of the developing limbs, and subsequently in the joint interzone, and the epiphyseal cartilage of the cartilaginous cores. The expression levels were the highest in the more distal parts of the limbs. No hybridization was detected in the cranio-facial nor axial skeleton. CDMP-2 is mainly expressed in the hypertrophic chondrocytes, the primary ossification center and is also associated with the periosteal layer at the primary ossification centers of the developing long bones. These localisation patterns suggests an important role for these genes in the development of the appendicular skeleton and joint morphogenesis.

Taking a candidate disorder approach, we established the role of CDMP-1 in human skeletal development and joint morphogenesis (Thomas *et al.*, 1996). The main criteria we selected to identify a candidate human disorder where the presence of short limbs, preferentially in a proximal-distal fashion, the distal parts of the limbs more severly affected than the proximal parts. We subsequently excluded those chondrodysplasias displaying abnormalities in the craniofacial and/or axial skeleton. The inheritance pattern should be autosomal recessive. This analysis suggested the acromesomelic chondrodysplastic diseases as the most likely candidate subgroup. Several distinct phenotypes have been described in this group of acromesomelic diseases including the Hunter-Thompson and Grebe types.

The Hunter-Thompson chondrodysplasia is an autosomal recessive disorder characterized by short limbs. The distal parts of the limbs are especially poorly developed. We identified a 22 bp frameshift mutation (tandem duplication) in the mature region of CDMP-1 resulting in a complete loss of function of the growth factor (Thomas *et al.*, 1996). The corresponding clinical characteristics of the affected individuals not only present short limbs but also a joint phenotype with hypoplastic condyles and dislocations which may be associated with ligament laxity, although it is difficult to establish if this is a primary or a secondary feature. In addition, several joints are missing as is the case for the fifth digit in the hands and feet. Mapping experiments show that the gene is located on human chromosome 20q11.2 which in a region on mouse chromosome 2 is syntactic with the locus described for Gdf-5 (Lin *et al.*, 1996).

These data have been expanded to include new mutations found in the CDMP-1 gene in other acromesomelic chondrodysplasias (Grebe type) (Thomas *et al.*, 1997). Interestingly, in these human phenotypes we could not see any major abnormalities in the sternoclavicular, acromioclavicular and temporomandibular joints! This suggests that the molecular signals guiding the formation of these joints may be quite distinct from the ones involved in appendicular joint morphogenesis. This is not really surprising since it is known that jaws and their accompanying jaw joints preceded all other joint evolution. Their developmental sequence was established before the appendicular joints and is, therefore, expected to be distinct. This is certainly a fertile area for further investigation.

BONE MORPHOGENETIC PROTEINS/CARTILAGE-DERIVED MORPHOGENETIC PROTEINS: ROLE IN THE SPECIFICATION OF JOINT TISSUE FORMATION

There is accumulating evidence that several BMPs/osteogenic proteins (OPs) are important regulators of discrete stages during cartilage and bone formation. Examples include the promotion of chemotaxis and proliferation of mesenchymal cells (Postlethwaite *et al.*, 1994), inhibition of myogenesis and conversion into osteoblast-like cells (Katagiri *et al.*, 1994), cartilage differentiation and chondrocyte maturation (Vukicevic *et al.*, 1989; Carrington *et al.*, 1991; Chen, P. *et al.*, 1991, 1993, 1995; Harrison *et al.*, 1991, 1992; Luyten *et al.*, 1992, 1994) and growth and differentiation of osteoprogenitor cells and mature osteoblasts (Vukicevic *et al.*, 1990; Yamaguchi *et al.*, 1991; Thies *et al.*, 1992; Chen, T. *et al.*, 1991; Hiraki *et al.*, 1991; Sampath *et al.*, 1992; Ripamonti *et al.*, 1992). This list is far from complete but it underlines the concept that the biological response to BMPs appears to be dependent on the stage of differentiation of the cells. For instance, osteogenic protein-1 (OP-1) can promote proliferation, differentiation and/or maturation in the same cell lineage (Chen, P. *et al.*, 1995).

Preliminary studies using recombinantly expressed protein indicate that CDMP-1 protein promotes chondrogenesis and osteogenesis *in vitro* and *in vivo*. These biological traits confirm the BMP-like nature of the protein and confirm the potential of CDMP-1 as an agent promoting cartilage and bone differentiation. Our data indicate that CDMP-2, the second member of this family and expressed at high levels in postnatal cartilage tissues, has also some chondrogenic potential *in vitro* and *in vivo* in certain models but appears not to support osteogenic differentiation *in vitro*. In addition, the biological effects in *in vitro* models of the CDMPs seem to be more restricted when compared with other BMPs such as BMP-2 and OP-1, indicating that the CDMPs may also act through distinct receptors and signalling pathways.

CHALLENGES FOR THE FUTURE

The BMP family of signalling molecules has provided the scientific community with a set of tools to further define the mechanisms involved in skeletal development and patterning as well chondrogenesis, chondrocyte maturation and osteogenesis. Their discovery has, therefore, been a major contribution to make substantial progress in the field of skeletal development and the biological regeneration of skeletal tissues especially bone.

It is obvious that the CDMPs might provide new opportunities to understand more about the mechanisms involved in skeletal development and joint formation. The data suggest that the soluble signals and cascade of events involved in the development of the appendicular skeleton are distinct from the ones determining the morphogenesis of the axial and craniofacial skeleton. The genetic data indicate that a subset of BMP-like genes including CDMP-1 are critical mediators in the joint formation process. However, there are several indications that some joints such as the temporomandibular joint have distinct signalling cascades. The precise function of CDMP-1 in skeletal development and joint morphogenesis in particular is still unclear. Both the genetic data and the *in vivo* and *in vitro* studies with recombinantly expressed protein indicate that CDMP-1 may certainly be involved in the initiation and promotion of chondrogenesis, chondrocyte maturation and promotion of bone formation. Its role in the early skeletal pattern formation and joint cavitation processes is still unknown but is probably linked to the maintenance and progression of the joint tissues. Ongoing studies seek to define the possible role of other BMP-like genes in joint morphogenesis.

Another opportunity with far-reaching consequences in the field of skeletal tissue repair and engineering is the possibility that depending on the signal one might be able to commit precursor cells into specific cell lineages. This suggests the possibility of directing *ex vivo* or *in vivo* cell and tissue specific differentiation. From here one can devise a number of tissue engineering applications including joint resurfacing protocols. This will be in association with appropriate delivery systems and/or enriched with the proper precursor cells. Recent studies using autologous articular chondrocytes, expanded *in vitro*, for the repair of local cartilage defects in the human knee joint surface support the concept of this tissue engineering approach (Brittberg *et al.*, 1994). The relative success of this study might be at least partially attributed to the use of the proper articular chondrocyte to repair the articular cartilage defects. Therefore, it is important to further identify molecular markers associated with specific cell types which would allow the scientist and clinician to repair tissue damage with the appropriate cells and avoid scar formation to the greatest extent possible.

REFERENCES

Brittberg, M., Lindahl, A., Nilsson, A., Ohlson, C., Isaksson, O. and Peterson, L. (1994) Treatment of deep cartilage defects in the knee with autologous chondrocyte transplantation. *N. Engl. J. Medicine*, **331**, 889–895.
Carrington, J.L., Chen, P., Yanagishita, M. and Reddi, A.H. (1991) Osteogenin (Bone morphogenetic protein-3) stimulates cartilage formation by chick limb bud cells *in vitro*. *Dev. Biol.*, **146**, 406–415.

Celeste, A.J., Ianazzi, J.A., Taylor, R.C., Hewick, R.M., Rosen, V., Wang, E.A. and Wozney, J.M. (1990) Identification of transforming growth factor β family members in bone inductive protein purified from bone. *Proc. Natl. Acad. Sci. USA*, **87**, 9843–9850.

Chang, S., Hoang, B., Thomas, J.T., Vukicevic, S., Luyten, F.P., Ryba, N.J.P., Kozak, C.A., Reddi, A.H. and Moos, M. Jr. (1994) Cartilage-derived morphogenetic proteins: new members of the TGF-β superfamily, predominantly expressed in long bones during human embryonic development. *J. Biol. Chem.*, **269**, 28227–28234.

Chen, T.L., Bates, R.L., Dudley, A., Hammonds, R.G. and Amento, E.P. Jr. (1991) Bone morphogenetic protein-2b stimulation of growth and osteogenic phenotypes in rat osteoblast-like cells: comparison with TGF-β_1. *J. Bone Miner. Res.*, **6**, 1387–1393.

Chen, P., Carrington, J.L., Hammonds, R.G. and Reddi, A.H. (1991) Stimulation of chondrogenesis in limb bud mesoderm cells by recombinant human bone morphogenetic protein 2B (BMP-2B) and modulation by transforming growth factor β_1 and β_2. *Exp. Cell Res.*, **195**, 509–515.

Chen, P., Vukicevic, S., Sampath, T.K. and Luyten, F.P. (1993) Bovine articular chondrocytes do not undergo hypertrophy when cultured in the presence of serum and osteogenic protein-1. *Biochem. Biophys. Res. Commun.*, **197**, 1253–1259.

Chen, P., Vukicevic, S., Sampath, T.K. and Luyten, F.P. (1995) Osteogenic Protein-1 promotes growth and maturation of chich\k sternal chondrocytes in serum-free cultures. *J. Cell Science*, **108**, 105–114.

Dudley, A.T., Lyons, K.M. and Robertson, E.J. (1995) A requirement for BMP-7 during development of the mammalian kidney and eye. *Genes Dev.*, **9**, 2795–2807.

Harrison, E.T. Jr., Luyten, F.P. and Reddi, A.H. (1991) Osteogenin promotes reexpression of cartilage phenotype by dedifferentiated articular chondrocytes in serum-free medium. *Exp. Cell Res.*, **192**, 340–345.

Harrison, E.T. Jr., Luyten, F.P. and Reddi, A.H. (1992) Transforming growth factor-beta: its effect on phenotype reexpression by dedifferentiated chondrocytes in the presence and absence of osteogenin. *In Vitro Cell Dev. Biol.*, **28A**, 445–448.

Hiraki, Y., Inoue, H., Shigeno, C., Sanma, Y., Bentz, H., Rosen, D.M., Asada, A. and Suzuki, F. (1991) Bone morphogenetic proteins (BMP-2 and BMP-3) promote growth and expression of the differentiated phenotype of rabbit chondrocytes and osteoblastic MC3T3-E1 *in vitro. J. Bone. Miner. Res.*, **6**, 1373–1385.

Katagiri, T., Yamaguchi, A., Komaki, M., Abe, E., Takahashi, N., Ikeda, T., Rosen, V., Wozney, J.M., Fujisawa-Sehara, A. and Suda, T. (1994) BMP-2 converts the differentiation pathway of C2C12 myoblasts into the osteoblast lineage. *J. Cell Biol.*, **127**, 1755–1766.

Kingsley, D.M., Bland, A.E., Grubber, J.M., Marker, P.C., Russell, L.B., Copeland, N.G. and Jenkins, N.A. (1992) The mouse short ear skeletal morphogenesis locus is associated with defects in a bone morphogenetic member of the TGF beta superfamily. *Cell*, **71**, 399–410.

Lin, K., Thomas, J.T., Mc Bride, O.W. and Luyten, F.P. (1996) Assignment of a new TGFβ superfamily member, human cartilage-derived Morphogenetic Protein-1, to chromosome 20q11.2 *Genomics*, **34**, 150–151.

Luo, G., Hoffman, C., Bronckers, A.L.J.J., Sohocki, M., Bradley, A. and Karsenty, G., (1995) BMP-7 is an inducer of nephrogenesis and is also required for eye development and skeletal patterning. *Genes Dev.*, **9**, 2808–2820.

Luyten, F.P., Cunningham, N.S., Ma, S., Muthukumaran, N., Hammonds, R.G., Nevins, W.B., Wood, W.I. and Reddi, A.H. (1989) Purification and partial amino acid sequence of osteogenin, a protein initiating bone differentiation. *J. Biol. Chem.*, **264**, 13377–13380.

Luyten, F.P., Yu, Y.M., Yanagishita, M., Vukicevic, S., Hammonds, R.G. and Reddi, A.H. (1992) Natural bovine osteogenin and recombinant human bone morphogenetic protein-2B are equipotent in the maintenance of proteoglycans in bovine articular cartilage explant cultures. *J. Biol. Chem.*, **267**, 3691–3695.

Luyten, F.P., Chen, P., Paralkar, V. and Reddi, A.H. (1994) Recombinant bone morphogenetic protein-4, transforming growth factor-beta 1, and activin A enhance the cartilage phenotype of articular chondrocytes *in vitro. Exp. Cell Res.*, **210**, 224–229.

Luyten, F.P. and Reddi, A.H. (1992) Articular Cartilage Repair: Potential Role of Growth and Differentiation Factors. In: M. Adolphe (ed.) *Biological Regulation of the Chondrocyte*, CRC Press, **9**, 227–236.

Lyons, K.M., Pelton, R.W. and Hogan, B.L.M. (1990) Organogenesis and pattern formation in the mouse: RNA distribution patterns suggest a role for bone morphogenetic protein-2A (BMP-2A). *Development*, **109**, 833–844.

Lyons, K.M., Pelton, R.W. and Hogan, B.L.M. (1989) Patterns of expression of murine Vgr-1 and BMP-2a RNA suggest that transforming growth factor-β-like genes coordinately regulate aspects of embryonic development. *Genes Dev.*, **3**, 1657–1668.

Owens, E.M. and Solursh, M. (1982) Cell–cell interaction by mouse limb cells during *in vitro* chondrogenesis: analysis of the brachypod mutation. *Dev. Biol.*, **91**, 376–388.

Özkaynak, E., Rueger, D.C., Drie, E.A., Corbett, C., Ridge, R.J., Sampath, T.K. and Opperman, H. (1990) OP-1 cDNA encodes an osteogenic protein in the TGF-β family. *EMBO J.*, **9**, 2085–2093.

Postlethwaite, A.J., Raghou, R., Stricklin, G., Ballou, L. and Sampath, T.K. (1994) Osteogenic Protein-1, a bone morphogenic protein member of the TGF-β superfamily, shares chemotactic but not fibrogenic properties with TGF-β. *J. Cell Physiol.*, **161**, 562–570.

Reddi, A.H. (1992) Regulation of cartilage and bone differentiation by bone morphogenetic proteins. *Curr. Opin. Cell Biol.*, **4**, 850–855.

Reddi, A.H. and Huggins, C.B. (1972) Biochemical sequences in the transformation of normal fibroblast in adolescent rat. *Proc. Natl. Acad. Sci. USA*, **69**, 1601–1605.

Ripamonti, U., Ma, S.S., van den Heever, B. and Reddi, A.H. (1992) Osteogenin, a bone morphogenetic protein, adsorbed on porous hydroxyapatite substrata, induces rapid bone differentiation in calvarial defects of adult primates. *Plast. Reconstr. Surg.*, **90**, 382–393.

Ripamonti, U. and Reddi, A.H. (1995) Bone Morphogenetic Proteins: Applications in Plastic and Reconstructive Surgery. *Plast. Reconstr. Surg.*, **11**, 47–74.

Sampath, T.K., Coughlin, J.E., Whetstone, R.M., Banach, D., Corbett, C., Ridge, R.J., Özkaynak, E., Opperman, H. and Rueger, D.C. (1990) Bovine osteogenic protein is composed of dimers of OP-1 and BMP-2A, two members of the transforming growth factor-β superfamily. *J. Biol. Chem.*, **265**, 13198–13205.

Sampath, T.K., Maliakal, J.C., Hauschka, P.V., Jones, W.K., Sasak, H., Tucker, R.F., White, K.H., Coughlin, J.E., Tucker, M.M., Pang, R.H.L., Corbett, C., Özkaynak, E., Oppermann, H. and Rueger, D.C. (1992) Recombinant human osteogenic protein (hOP-1) induces new bone formation *in vivo* with specific activity comparable to natural bovine osteogenic protein and stimulates osteoblast proliferation and differentiation *in vitro*. *J. Biol. Chem.*, **267**, 20352–20362.

Storm, E.E., Huynh, T.V., Copeland, N.G., Jenkins, N.A., Kingsley, D.M. and Lee, S.J. (1994) Limb alterations in brachypodism mice due to mutations in a new member of the TGF beta-superfamily. *Nature*, **368**, 639–43.

Thies, R.S., Bauduy, M., Ashton, B.A., Kurtzberg, L., Wozney, J.M. and Rosen, V. (1992) Recombinant human BMP-2 induces osteoblastic differentiation in W-20-17 stromal cells. *Endocrinology*, **130**, 1318–1324.

Thomas, J.T., Lin, K., Nandedkar, M., Camargo, M., Cervenka, J. and Luyten, F.P. (1996) A Human Chondrodysplasia due to a Mutation in a TGF-β Superfamily Member. *Nature Genetics*, **12**, 315–7.

Thomas, J.T., Kilpatrick, M.W., Lin, K., Eiracher, L., Lembessis, P., Costa, T., Tsipouras, P. and Luyten, F.P. (1997) Disruption of human limb morphogenesis by a dominant negative mutation in CDMP1. *Nature Genetics*, **17**, 58–64.

Urist, M.R. (1965) Bone: Formation by autoinduction. *Science*, **159**, 893–899.

Vukicevic, S., Luyten, F.P. and Reddi, A.H. (1989) Stimulation of the expression of osteogenic and chondro-genic phenotypes *in vitro* by osteogenin. *Proc. Natl. Acad. Sci. USA*, **86**, 8793–8797.

Vukicevic, S., Luyten, F.P. and Reddi, A.H. (1990) Osteogenin inhibits proliferation and stimulates differentia-tion in mouse osteoblast like cells (MC3T3-E1). *Biochem. Bioph. Res. Commun.*, **166**, 750–756.

Vukicevic, S., Latin, V., Chen, P., Batorsky, R., Reddi, A.H. and Sampath, T.K. (1994a) Localisation of OP-1 during human embryonic development: high affinity binding to basement membranes. *Biochem. Biophys. Res. Commun.*, **198**, 693–700.

Vukicevic, S., Helder, M.N. and Luyten, F.P. (1994b) Developing human lung and kidney are major sites for synthesis of Bone Morphogenetic Protein-3/Osteogenin. *J. Histochem. & Cytochem.*, **42**, 869–875.

Wang, E., Rosen, V., Cordes, P., Hewick, R.M., Kriz, M.J., Luxenberg, D.P., Sibley, B.S. and Wozney, J.M. (1988) Purification and characterization of other distinct bone-inducing factors. *Proc. Natl Acad. Sci. USA*, **85**, 9484–8488.

Wharton, K.A., Thomsen, G.H. and Gelbart, W.M. (1991) Drosophila 60A gene, another transforming growth factor beta family member, is closely related to human bone morphogenetic proteins. *Proc. Natl. Acad. Sci. USA*, **88**, 9214–9218.

Wozney, J.M., Rosen, V., Celeste, A.J., Mitsock, L.M., Whitters, M.J., Kriz, R.W., Hewick, R.M. and Wang, E.A. (1988) Novel regulators of bone formation: Molecular clones and activities. *Science*, **242**, 1528–1533.

Yamaguchi, A., Katagiri, T., Ikeda, T., Wozney, J.M., Rosen, V., Wang, E.A., Kahn, A.J., Suda, T. and Yoshiki, S. (1991) Recombinant human bone morphogenetic protein-2 stimulates osteoblastic maturation and inhibits myogenic differentiation *in vitro*. *J. Cell Biol*, **113**, 681–687.

Section 2
Articular Cartilage

6 Articular Cartilage Morphology and Biology

J.A. Buckwalter[1,*] and E.B. Hunziker[2]

[1]*University of Iowa, Department of Orthopaedics, Iowa City, Iowa;*
[2]*Muller Institute, Bern, Switzerland*

The remarkable mobility and dexterity of vertebrates depend on synovial joints. These complex structures consist of multiple tissues including synovium, bone, ligament, joint capsule and cartilage. They vary considerably in size, shape and range of motion; but for all synovial joints normal function depends on the smooth low friction gliding and load bearing surface provided by articular cartilage. Articular cartilage differs in thickness and cell density, and varies slightly in matrix composition and mechanical properties among species (Athanasiou *et al.*, 1991) and among joints of the same individual. Yet, in all synovial joints it consists of the same components, has the same general structure and performs the same functions. Although at most only a few millimeters thick, it has surprising stiffness to compression and resilience, and exceptional ability to distribute loads (Mow and Rosenwasser, 1988), thereby minimising peak stresses on subchondral bone. Perhaps most important, it has great durability – in many people it provides normal joint function for 80 years or more.

Grossly and microscopically, adult articular cartilage appears to be a simple inactive tissue. When examined from inside a synovial joint, normal articular cartilage appears as a slick firm surface that resists deformation. Light microscopic examination shows that it consists primarily of extracellular matrix, it has only one type of cell, the chondrocyte, and it lacks blood vessels, lymphatic vessels and nerves (Buckwalter *et al.*, 1988, 1990). Compared with tissues like muscle or bone, cartilage has a low level of metabolic activity and is less responsive to changes in loading, and it cannot repair significant structural damage caused by injury or disease (Buckwalter *et al.*, 1988, 1990, 1996; Buckwalter and Mow, 1992). Yet, despite its unimpressive appearance, low level of metabolic activity and limited ability to repair itself, detailed study of the morphology and biology of adult articular cartilage shows that it has an elaborate highly ordered structure and that

* Corresponding author. 01013 Pappajohn Pavilion, Department of Orthopaedics, University of Iowa, College of Medicine, Iowa City 52242.

a variety of complex interactions between the chondrocytes and the matrix actively maintain the tissue.

This chapter provides an overview of the morphology and biology of normal adult articular cartilage stressing the interdependence of articular cartilage composition, structure and function. The first section summarises the individual components of the tissue: the chondrocytes, the matrix water and the matrix macromolecules and the second section describes how the cells and matrix macromolecules are organised to form adult articular cartilage. The next section discusses the interdependence of the chondrocytes and the matrix and, in particular, the interactions between the chondrocytes and the matrix that maintain the tissue, and the last section reviews current understanding of the morphologic and biologic changes in articular cartilage with age.

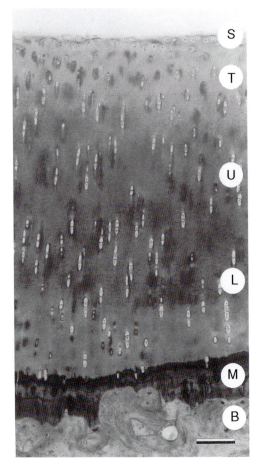

FIGURE 6.1   Light micrograph of vertically-sectioned adult human articular cartilage (femoral condyle), showing the superficial S, transitional T, upper U and lower L radial and calicified cartilage zones M; the latter abuts on the suchondral bone plate B. Notice that the radial zone forms most of the thickness of human articular cartilage and that in this zone the cells arrange themselves in columns. Magnification × 135; bar = 100 μm.

ARTICULAR CARTILAGE COMPONENTS

Articular cartilage consists of cells, matrix water and a matrix macromolecular framework organised to form the bearing surfaces of synovial joints (Figure 6.1). The cells contribute little to the volume of the tissue, about one percent in adult human articular cartilage (in other species, especially small animals like mice, rats and rabbits with thin articular cartilages, the cell density is many times greater than in humans) (Stockwell, 1967, 1978).

CHONDROCYTES

Only one type of cell exists within normal articular cartilage: the highly specialised chondrocyte (Buckwalter *et al.*, 1990) surrounded by extracellular matrix (Figure 6.2).

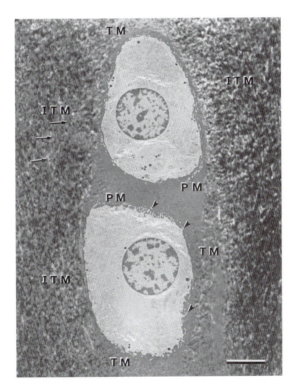

FIGURE 6.2   Electron micrograph of a pair of chondrocytes (a chondrone) from the lower radial zone of adult human articular cartilage processed by high pressure freezing, freeze-substitution and Epon embedding. At this relatively low magnification, the pericellular matrix compartment PM appears as a homeogeneously stained mantel around each chondrocyte; in contrast, the territorial matrix compartment TM forms a fibrillar coat around the chondrone. These matrix compartments vary considerably in width. The interterritorial matrix compartment or interterritorium ITM is distinguished from the other matrix compartments by the high concentration of parallel oriented collagen fibrils (arrows). Notice the fine cellular process extending from the chondrocytes into the pericellular matrix (arrow heads). Magnification × 4,000; bar = 4 μm.

Chondrocytes from different cartilage zones differ in size, shape and probably metabolic activity (Aydelotte *et al.*, 1996, 1992; Schumacher *et al.*, 1994; Wong *et al.*, 1996), but all of these cells have a complex relationship with their extracellular matrix (Figures 6.3 and 6.4) and contain the organelles necessary for matrix synthesis, including endoplasmic reticulum and Golgi complexes. Also, they frequently contain intracytoplasmic filaments, lipid, glycogen and secretory vesicles; and at least some chondrocytes have short processes or

(A)

(B)

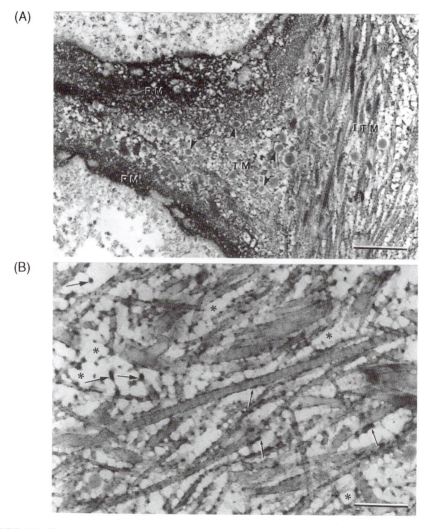

FIGURE 6.3   Electron micrographs of upper radial zone human articular cartilage fixed in the prescence of RHT. (A) shows the relationship of chondrocytes to the matrix: pericellular compartment PM, territorial compartment TM and interterritorial compartment ITM. (B) shows the interterritorial matrix at a higher magnification. RHT precipitates proteoglycans to form matrix granules (large solid arrows in (B)) which frequently condense along the surfaces of collagen fibrils (small arrows in (B)). The precipitation process forms 'empty' spaces (asterisks in (B)) between collagen fibrils and the granules and leads to a general shrinkage of this matrix compartment. Notice the abundant membrane bound vesicles (arrowheads) in the matrix. (A) magnification × 25,000; bar = 1 μm. (B) magnification × 50,000; bar = 0.5 μm.

microvilli extending from the cell into the matrix (Figure 6.4). These structures may have a role in sensing mechanical changes in the matrix. Chondrocytes surround themselves with their extracellular matrix and do not form cell to cell contacts (Figures 6.2, 6.3 and 6.4). A spheroidal shape, synthesis of type II collagen, large aggregating proteoglycans and specific non-collagenous proteins, and formation of these molecules into

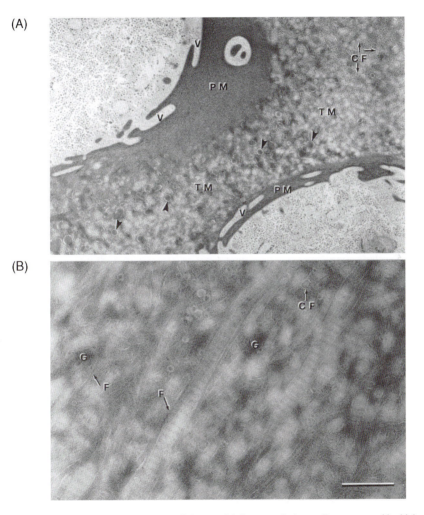

FIGURE 6.4 Electron micrographs of upper radial zone adult human articular cartilage processed by high pressure freezing, freeze substitiution and embedding in Epon. (A) Portions of two chondrocytes forming a chondrone with the intervening matrix. Small microvilli V that vary in width project from the cell surfaces into the pericellular matrix PM. The pericellular matrix is clearly demarcated from the territorial matrix TM, which is rich in membrane-bound vesicles (arrowheads) and, in this location, contains predominately cross-sectioned collagen fibrils CF. Notice how much more clearly structures can be seen in this section than in the chemically processed tissue shown in Figure 6.3A. Magnification × 25,000; bar = 1 μm. (B) The interterritorial matrix compartment from the same zone as (A). Notice the isotropic arrangement of the collagen fibrils (indicated by the presence of both cross- and longitudinally-sectioned fibrils). The interfibrillar proteoglycan-rich space is completely filled with a fine granular material G. Compare this appearance with Figure 6.3B in which 'empty' spaces are apparent. CF: cross-sectioned collagen fibrils; F: longitudinally-sectioned fibrils. Magnification × 50,000; bar = 0.5 μm.

a cartilaginous matrix that covers and binds to the cell membranes distinguish mature chondrocytes from other cells.

At first glance articular cartilage chondrocytes seem to be inactive. They appear to remain unchanged in location, appearance and activity for decades. Although the mechanical properties of articular cartilage depend on the matrix, i.e., the types of macromolecules that form the framework of the matrix and the concentrations of water and macromolecules, a matrix formed by mixing appropriate concentrations of water and the cartilage macromolecules (collagens, proteoglycans and non-collagenous proteins) will not duplicate the properties of articular cartilage. To produce a tissue that can provide normal synovial joint function the chondrocytes must first synthesise appropriate types and amounts of macromolecules and then assemble and organise them into a highly ordered macromolecular framework. Maintenance of the articular surface requires turnover of the matrix macromolecules, that is continual replacement of degraded matrix components; and probably alteration in the matrix macromolecular framework in response to joint use. To accomplish these activities, the cells must sense changes in the matrix composition due to degradation of macromolecules and in the demands placed on the articular surface, and then respond by synthesising appropriate types and amounts of macromolecules.

In adult animals, nutrients must pass from synovial capillaries through the synovial membrane and synovial fluid and then through the cartilage matrix to reach the chondrocytes. These multiple barriers limit the types and concentrations of nutrients available to the cells, and in particular the matrix is not only restrictive as to the size of the materials but also to their charge and other features such as molecular configuration. The nature of this system leaves chondrocytes with a low oxygen concentration relative to most other tissues, and, therefore, they depend primarily on anaerobic metabolism.

Articular cartilage chondrocytes differ in activity and function during skeletal development and growth and after completion of growth. In growing individuals they produce new tissue to expand and remodel the articular surface; in skeletally mature individuals they do not significantly change the volume of the tissue, but they replace degraded matrix macromolecules and they may remodel the articular surface (Buckwalter, 1995a; Buckwalter and Lane, 1996). Articular cartilage first forms from undifferentiated mesenchymal cells that form condensed cell clusters. They then begin to synthesise cartilage collagens, proteoglycans and non-collagneous proteins. The tissue becomes recognisable as cartilage by light microscopy when accumulation of matrix separates the cells and they assume a spherical shape. Recent investigations suggest that expression of the non-collagenous matrix protein tenascin is associated with the early stages of chondrogenesis and the formation and development of articular cartilage (Gluhak *et al.*, 1996; Mackie and Ramsey, 1996; Pacifici, 1995). During formation and growth of articular cartilage, the cell density is high and the cells reach their highest level of metabolic activity, as the chondrocytes proliferate rapidly and synthesise large volumes of matrix. With skeletal maturation, the rates of cell metabolic activity, matrix synthesis and cell division decline. After completion of skeletal growth, most chondrocytes probably never divide, but continue to synthesise collagens, proteoglycans and non-collagenous proteins.

The continued synthetic activity suggests that maintenance of articular cartilage requires substantial ongoing internal remodelling of the matrix macromolecular framework. Enzymes produced by chondrocytes presumably are responsible for degradation of the matrix macromolecules, and chondrocytes probably respond to the presence of fragmented matrix molecules by increasing their synthetic activity to replace the degraded components of the macromolecular framework. Other mechanisms must also influence the balance between synthetic and degradative activity. For example, the frequency and intensity of joint loading influences chondrocyte metabolism. Joint immobilisation or marked decreased joint loading alters chondrocyte activity so that degradation exceeds synthesis of at least the proteoglycan component of the matrix (Buckwalter, 1995a,b). Persistent increased joint use may also alter the composition and organisation of the matrix, but this has not been clearly demonstrated in skeletally mature individuals (Buckwalter, 1995a,b).

EXTRACELLULAR MATRIX

The articular cartilage matrix consists of two components: the tissue fluid and the framework of structural macromolecules that give the tissue its form and stability and maintain the tissue fluid within the matrix. The interaction of the tissue fluid and the macromolecular framework make possible mechanical properties of stiffness and resilience (Buckwalter and Mow, 1992; Mow and Rosenwasser, 1988).

TISSUE FLUID

Water contributes up to 80% of the wet weight of articular cartilage and the interaction of water with the matrix macromolecules significantly influences the mechanical properties of the tissue (Buckwalter *et al.*, 1990; Lai *et al.*, 1981; Linn and Sokoloff, 1965; Loeser, 1993; Mankin, 1978; Maroudas and Schneiderman, 1987; Mow and Rosenwasser, 1988). This tissue fluid contains gasses, small proteins, metabolites, and a high concentration of cations to balance the negatively charged proteoglycans. At least some of the water can move freely in and out of the tissue. Its volume, concentration and behaviour within the tissue depends primarily on its interaction with the structural macromolecules: in particular, the large aggregated proteoglycans that help maintain the fluid within the matrix and the fluid electrolyte concentrations. Because these macromolecules have large numbers of negative charges that attract positively charged ions and repel negatively charged ions they increase the concentration of positive ions like sodium and decrease the concentration of negative ions like chloride. The increase in total inorganic ion concentration increases the tissue osmolarity, that is, creates a Donnan effect. The collagen network resists the Donnan osmotic pressure caused by the inorganic ions associated with the proteoglycans (Buckwalter and Mow, 1992; Mow and Rosenwasser, 1988).

STRUCTURAL MACROMOLECULES

The cartilage structural macromolecules, collagens, proteoglycans, and non-collagenous proteins contribute 20% to 40% of the wet weight of the tissue (Buckwalter *et al.*, 1990).

The three classes of macromolecules differ in their concentrations within the tissue and in their contributions to the tissue properties. Collagens contribute about 60% of the dry weight of cartilage, proteoglycans contribute 25% to 35%, and the non-collagenous proteins and glycoproteins contribute 15% to 20%. The collagen fibrillar meshwork gives cartilage its form and tensile strength (Buckwalter and Mow, 1992). Proteoglycans and non-collagenous proteins bind to the collagenous meshwork or become mechanically entrapped within it, and water fills this molecular framework. Some non-collagenous proteins help organise and stabilise the matrix macromolecular framework while others help chondrocytes bind to the macromolecules of the matrix.

COLLAGENS

Articular cartilage, like most tissues, contains multiple genetically distinct collagen types: specifically collagen types II, VI, IX, X and XI (Eyre, 1995; Eyre *et al.*, 1992; Sandell, 1995). Collagen types II, IX and XI form the large cross-banded fibrils seen by electron microscopy (Figure 6.5). A network of finer cross-banded filaments, between 10 and 15 nm in diameter, also exists throughout the matrix (Figure 6.5). The composition of these structures has not been determined but their periodicity suggests that they may be a form of collagen. The organisation of fibrils and filaments into a tight meshwork that extends through out the tissue (Figures 6.6, 6.7 and 6.8) provides the tensile stiffness and strength of articular cartilage and contributes to the cohesiveness of the tissue by mechanically entrapping the large proteoglycans. The principal articular cartilage collagen, type II,

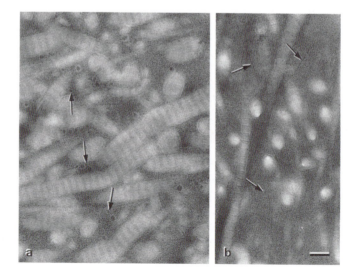

FIGURE 6.5   High magnification electron micrographs of mature bovine articular cartilage matrix (lower radial zone) after high pressure freezing, freeze-substitution and Epon-embedding. The matrix consists of fibrillar and non-fibrillar components. Aggregating proteoglycans lie between and surround the fibrillar components. The large cross-banded collagen fibrils form the most prominent fibrillar component of the matrix, but a network of fine banded filaments [cross-sections (a) and longitudinally-sections (b)] 10–15 nm in diameter is apparent between collagen fibrils. Bar = 200 nm.

(A)

(B)

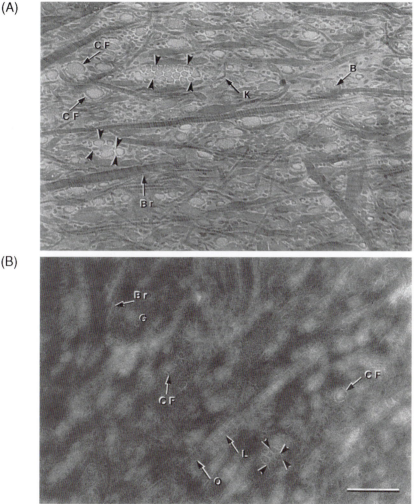

FIGURE 6.6   Electron micrographs showing the interterritorial matrix from the lower radial zone of adult human articular cartilage processed by high pressure freezing. (A) Unstained ultrathin cryosection. Cross-sectioned collagen fibrils CF vary in size and shape. Their profile areas manifest a characteristic 'staining' pattern: a pale central region, a narrow dark boundary and a perifibrillar electron-lucent halo. These features are more apparent in fibril bundles (arrowheads) and in freeze-substituted/metal-stained tissue. Longitudinally-sectioned fibrils with a repeating banding pattern of about 67 nm and a subbanding pattern of about 22.5 nm sometimes exhibit brushing Br, that is a splinting into finer elements. Single fibrils sometimes abruptly change their course or form 'kinks' K. Notice the bubbling B cause by prolonged exposure of the section to the electron beam. (B) Ultrathin section of freeze-substituted tissue embedded in Epon and stained with uranyl acetate and lead citrate. The proteoglycan-rich interfibrillar space is completely filled with a fine granular material G, which does not have the reticular network typically formed in the presence of ice crystals. Cross-sectioned collagen fibrils CF have a variety of shapes and the characteristic staining pattern shown in (A). Individual longitudinally sectioned fibrils may also have regional differences in profile staining, according to whether they are transected centrally or peripherally, when they will appear light L or dark O, respectively. Notice that in (A) and (B), collagen fibrils and fibril bundles are isotopically organised. Magnification × 50,000; bar = 0.5 μm.

(A)

(B)

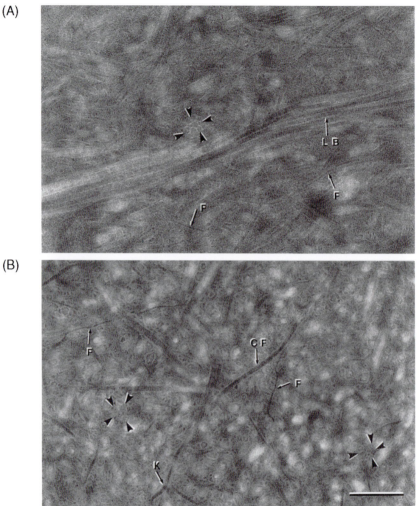

FIGURE 6.7   Electron micrographs of adult human articular cartilage processed by high pressure freezing/ freeze substitution and embedded in Epon. (A) Interterritorial matrix from the lower radial zone showing part of a large longitudinally-sectioned fibril bundle LB, crossing diagonally from the lower left-hand edge of the micrograph to the upper right-hand edge. The fibrils forming the bundle vary in diameter and spiral around the central axis of the bundle. The banding of each fibril is aligned in register with that of its neighbours. A number of fine cross-banded filaments F, with a diameter of 10–15 nm, can be seen dispersed throughout the matrix. Both filaments and collagen fibrils are mantled by an electron-lucent zone; this is most apparent in cross-sectioned elements where it appears as a halo, particularly in fibril bundles (arrowheads). (B) Interterritorial matrix from the upper radial zone showing both cross- and longitudinally-sectioned filaments F and collagen fibrils CF, as well as several cross-sectioned fibril bundles (arrowheads). Notice the random course followed by fibrils and the abrupt changes in direction or kinking K. The coarser appearance of the proteoglycan rich inter-fibrillar space together with the increased breadth of the electron-lucent perifibrillar halos, compared to the lower radial zone (A), indicate that the tissue water was not truly vitrified in this region. Magnification × 50,000; bar = 0.5 μm.

(A)

(B)

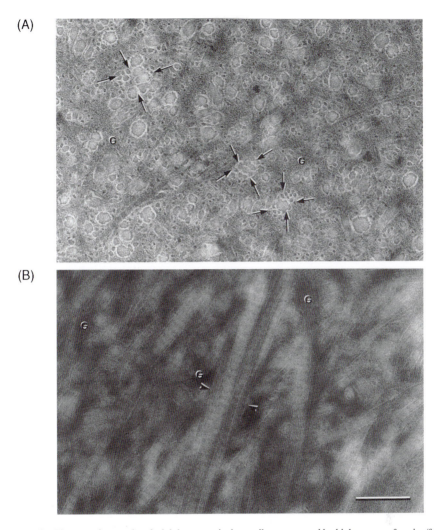

FIGURE 6.8   Electron micrographs of adult human articular cartilage processed by high pressure freezing/freeze substitution and embedding in Epon. (A) Interterritorial matrix from the upper radial zone. Notice the broad range of fibril diameters, even within an individual fibril bundle (arrowheads); and the staining profile of these acetone freeze-substituted collagen fibrils, that is a pale central region surrounded by a narrow dark boarder. The broad perifibrillar halo and the coarse granular appearance of the proteoglycan-rich interfibrillar space G indicate the tissue water was not optimally frozen. (B) Interterritorial matrix from the lower radial zone. Notice the finer granularity of the interfibrillar space G and the narrower breadth of the perifibrillar halos compared with (A). In this section the tissue water has been vitrified. Individual collagen fibrils within the longitudinally-sectioned fibril bundle (arrowheads) show in register alignment of their banding patterns. Magnification × 50,000; bar = 0.5 μm.

accounts for 90% to 95% of the cartilage collagen. Polymerised type II molecules form the primary component of the large cross-banded fibrils. Type XI collagen molecules bind covalently to type II collagen molecules and probably form part of the interior structure of the cross-banded fibrils. Type IX collagen molecules bind covalently to the superficial layers of the cross-banded fibrils and project into the matrix where they also can bind covalently to other type IX collagen molecules. The functions of type IX and type XI collagens remain uncertain, but, presumably, they help form and stabilise the collagen fibrils assembled primarily from type II collagen. The projecting portions of type IX collagen molecules may also help bind together the collagen fibril meshwork and connect the collagen meshwork with proteoglycans (Roughley and Lee, 1994). Recent work has suggested that a water rich layer or halo (Figures 6.6, 6.7 and 6.8) surrounds the collagen fibrils and that type IX collagen may have a role in creating this layer (Hunziker et al., 1996; Studer et al., 1996). The thin layer of water may reduce friction between the fibrils and the surrounding matrix macromolecules during compression and decompression of articular cartilage. Type VI collagen appears to form an important part of the matrix immediately surrounding chondrocytes and help chondrocytes attach to the matrix (Hagiwara et al., 1993; Marcelino and McDevitt, 1995). The presence of Type X collagen near the cells of the calcified cartilage zone of articular cartilage and the hypertrophic zone of growth plate (where the longitudinal cartilage septa begin to mineralise) suggests that it may have a role in cartilage mineralisation.

PROTEOGLYCANS (AGGRECANS AND SMALL PROTEOGLYCANS)

Proteoglycans consist of a protein core and one or more glycosaminoglycan chains (long unbranched polysaccharide chains consisting of repeating dissacharides that contain an amino sugar) (Hardingham et al., 1992; Rosenberg, 1992; Rosenberg and Buckwalter, 1986; Roughley and Lee, 1994). Each disaccharide unit has at least one negatively charged carboxylate or sulphate group so the glycosaminoglycans form long strings of negative charges that repel other and other negatively charged molecules, and attract cations. Glycosaminoglycans found in cartilage include hyaluronan (hyaluronic acid), chondroitin sulphate, keratan sulphate and dermatan sulphate. The concentrations of these molecules varies among sites within articular cartilage and also with age, cartilage injury and disease.

Articular cartilage contains two major classes of proteoglycans: large aggregating proteoglycans or aggrecans and small proteoglycans including decorin, biglycan, and fibromodulin. Because it may have a glycosaminoglycan component, type IX collagen is also considered a proteoglycan (Roughley and Lee, 1994). Aggrecans have large numbers of chondroitin sulphate and keratan sulphate chains attached to a protein core filament. Cartilage also contains large non-aggregating proteoglycans that resemble aggrecans in structure and composition and may represent degraded aggrecans (Buckwalter et al., 1994; Rosenberg and Buckwalter, 1986). Decorin has one dermatan sulphate chain, biglycan has two dermatan sulphate chains and fibromodulin has several keratan sulphate chains (Roughley and Lee, 1994). The tissue probably also contains other small proteoglycans that have not been identified. Aggrecan molecules fill most of the interfibrillar space of the cartilage matrix. They contribute about 90% of the total cartilage matrix proteoglycan mass, while large non-aggregating proteoglycans contribute 10% or less and small non-aggregating proteoglycans contribute about 3%. Although the small proteoglycans contribute relatively little to the total mass of proteoglycans compared with the aggrecans, because of their small size, they may be present in equal or higher molar amounts.

In the articular cartilage matrix, most aggrecans non-covalently associate with hyaluronan and link proteins, small non-collagenous proteins, to form proteoglycan aggregates (Buckwalter *et al.*, 1993a; Buckwalter and Rosenberg, 1982, 1983) that occupy the space between collagen fibrils (Figure 6.5). These large molecules have a central hyaluronan backbone that can vary in length from several hundred nanometers to more than ten thousand nanometers (Buckwalter and Rosenberg, 1982, 1983). Large aggregates may have more than 300 associated aggrecan molecules (Buckwalter and Rosenberg, 1983). Link proteins stabilise the association between monomers and hyaluronic acid and appear to have a role in directing the assembly of aggregates (Buckwalter *et al.*, 1984; Neame and Barry, 1993; Tang *et al.*, 1996). Aggregate formation helps anchor proteoglycans within the matrix, preventing their displacement during deformation of the tissue, and helps organise and stabilise the relationship between proteoglycans and the collagen meshwork.

Centrifugation, biochemical and electron microscopic studies show that two populations of proteoglycan aggregates exist within articular cartilage: a slow sedimenting population of aggregates with a low chondroitin sulphate to hyaluronate ratio and few monomers per aggregate and a faster sedimenting population of aggregates with a higher chondroitin sulphate to hyaluronate ratio and more monomers per aggregate (Buckwalter *et al.*, 1993a; Muller *et al.*, 1989; Pita *et al.*, 1990, 1992). The superficial regions of articular cartilage contain primarily the smaller slow sedimenting aggregates and the deeper regions contain both types of aggregates. Loss of the larger aggregates appears to be one of the earliest changes in osteoarthritis and joint immobilisation. Increasing age is also associated with a loss of large proteoglycan aggregates from articular cartilage (Buckwalter *et al.*, 1985, 1994).

The small non-aggregating proteoglycans have shorter protein cores than aggrecan molecules and unlike aggrecans they do not fill a large volume of the tissue or contribute directly to the mechanical behaviour of the tissue. Instead they bind to other macromolecules and probably influence cell function. Decorin and fibromodulin bind with type II collagen and may have a role in organising and stabilising the type II collagen meshwork (Roughley and Lee, 1994). Biglycan is concentrated in the pericellular matrix and may interact with type VI collagen (Miosge *et al.*, 1994; Roughley and Lee, 1994). The small proteoglycans also can bind transforming growth factor beta and may influence the activity of this cytokine in cartilage (Hildebrand *et al.*, 1994). At the articular surface, or on a cut surface of articular cartilage, they may prevent cell adhesion to the matrix (Noyori and Jasin, 1994).

NON-COLLAGENOUS PROTEINS AND GLYCOPROTEINS

The non-collagenous proteins and glycoproteins are not as well understood as the collagens and proteoglycans. A wide variety of these molecules exist within normal articular cartilage and thus far only a few of them have been studied. In general, they consist primarily of protein and have a few attached monosaccharides and oligosaccharides (Heinegard *et al.*, 1992, 1995). At least some of these molecules appear to help organise and maintain the macromolecular structure of the matrix. Cartilage oligomeric protein (COMP), an acidic protein, is concentrated primarily within the chondrocyte territorial matrix and appears to be present only within cartilage and have the capacity to bind to chondrocytes (DeCesare *et al.*, 1994; Hedbom *et al.*, 1992). This molecule may have value as a marker of cartilage turnover and of the progression of cartilage degeneration in patients with osteoarthritis (Lohmander *et al.*, 1994; Saxne and Heinegard, 1992; Sharif *et al.*, 1995). Fibronectin and tenascin, non-collagenous matrix proteins that are found in a variety of tissues, have also been identified within cartilage (Chevalier *et al.*, 1992, 1994; Gluhak *et al.*, 1996; Hayashi *et al.*, 1996; Mackie and Ramsey, 1996; Nishida *et al.*, 1995; Pacifici, 1995; Savarese *et al.*, 1996). Their functions in articular cartilage remain poorly understood, but they may have roles in matrix organisation, cell matrix interactions and in the responses of the tissue in inflammatory arthritis and osteoarthritis.

ARTICULAR CARTILAGE MORPHOLOGY

To form articular cartilage, chondrocytes organise the collagens, proteoglycans and non-collagenous proteins into a unique, highly ordered structure (Buckwalter *et al.*, 1990). The composition, organisation and mechanical properties of the matrix, cell morphology and, probably, cell function, vary with the depth from the articular surface (Figure 6.1). Matrix composition, organisation and function also vary with the distance from the cell.

ZONES

The morphologic changes in chondrocytes and matrix from the articular surface to the subchondral bone make it possible to identify four zones, or layers: the superficial zone, the transitional zone, the radial zone and the zone of calcified cartilage (Figure 6.1) (Buckwalter *et al.*, 1988). The relative size and appearance of these zones varies among species and among joints within the same species; and although each zone has different morphologic features, the boundaries between zones cannot be sharply defined. Nonetheless, recent biological and mechanical studies have shown that the zonal organisation has functional significance. The matrices differ in water, proteoglycan and collagen concentrations and in the size of the aggregates (Buckwalter *et al.*, 1990). Cells in different zones not only differ in shape, size and orientation relative to the articular surface (Figure 6.1), they also differ numerical density and in metabolic activity (Aydelotte *et al.*, 1992; Wong *et al.*, 1996). For example, a recent study of bovine articular cartilage showed that the cell numerical density was 54,000 cells/mm^3 in the superficial zone compared with 30,000 cells/mm^3 in the deeper zones, that chondrocytes in the superficial zone had about half the cell volume and surface area of chondrocytes in the radial zone and that chondrocytes in the superficial zone demonstrated about one tenth the synthetic activity of chondrocytes in the radial zone (Wong *et al.*, 1996). In addition to these differences, chondrocytes in different articular cartilage zones may respond differently to mechanical loading, suggesting that development and maintenance of normal articular cartilage depend in part on differentiation of phenotypically distinct populations of chondrocytes.

SUPERFICIAL ZONE

The unique structure and composition of the thinnest articular cartilage zone, the superficial zone, give it specialised mechanical and possibly biological properties. It typically consists of two layers: an acellular layer and a deeper cellular layer. The acellular layer consists of a thin covering of amorphous material (Jurvelin *et al.*, 1996) overlying a deeper sheet of fine fibrils with little polysaccharide (Buckwalter *et al.*, 1988, 1990). The acellular portion of the superficial zone presumably corresponds to the clear film, often identified as the 'lamina splendens', that can be stripped from the articular surface in some regions. Deep to the acellular sheet of fine fibrils, flattened ellipsoid shaped chondrocytes in a collagenous matrix arrange themselves so that their major axes are parallel to the articular surface (Figure 6.1). They synthesise a matrix that has a high collagen concentration and a low proteoglycan concentration relative to the other cartilage zones, and studies of superficial zone cells in culture shows that they degrade proteoglycans more rapidly and synthesise less collagen and proteoglycans than cells from the deeper zones (Aydelotte *et al.*, 1992; Wong *et al.*, 1996). Fibronectin and water concentrations are also highest in this zone.

The dense mat of collagen fibrils lying parallel to the joint surface in the superficial zone helps determine the mechanical properties of the tissue and affects the movement of molecules in and out of cartilage. It gives this cartilage zone greater tensile stiffness and strength than the deeper zones and it may resist shear forces generated during joint use (Buckwalter *et al.*, 1988; Mow and Rosenwasser, 1988). *In vitro* experiments show that the superficial zone also makes an important contribution to the compressive behaviour of articular cartilage (Setton *et al.*, 1993). Removal of this zone increases tissue permeability and probably increases loading of the macromolecular framework during compression; and disruption or remodelling of the dense collagenous matrix of the superficial zone is one of the first detectable structural changes in experimentally induced articular cartilage degeneration (Guilak *et al.*, 1994), suggesting that alterations in this zone may contribute to the development of osteoarthritis by altering the mechanical behaviour of the tissue. The densely packed collagen fibrils of the superficial zone also create a barrier for the articular cartilage that may limit ingress of large molecules such as antibodies or other proteins and the egress of large cartilage molecules.

TRANSITIONAL ZONE

As the name 'transitional zone' implies, the morphology and matrix composition of the transitional zone is intermediate between the superficial zone and the radial zone. It usually has several times the volume of the superficial zone. The cells have a higher concentration of synthetic organelles, endoplasmic reticulum and Golgi complex membranes, than superficial zone cells. Transitional zone cells assume a spheroidal shape and synthesise a matrix that has larger diameter collagen fibrils, a higher proteoglycan concentration, but lower concentrations of water and collagen than the superficial zone matrix.

RADIAL (MIDDLE) ZONE

The chondrocytes in the radial or middle zone are spheroidal in shape, and they tend to align themselves in columns perpendicular to the joint surface (Figure 6.1). This zone contains the largest diameter collagen fibrils, the highest concentration of proteoglycans and the lowest concentration of water. The collagen fibers of this zone and pass into the 'tidemark', a thin basophilic line seen on light microscopic sections of decalcified articular cartilage that roughly corresponds to the boundary between calcified and uncalcified cartilage. The nature of the 'tidemark' remains uncertain (Oegema and Thompson, 1995). It may result from concentration of basophilic calcified material at the interface between calcified and uncalcified matrix, possibly accentuated by the tissue processing, and thus represent a 'high water mark' for calcification. Alternatively, one study identified a band of fine fibrils corresponding to the tidemark (Redler et al., 1975) suggesting that it represents a well-defined matrix structure.

CALCIFIED CARTILAGE ZONE

A thin zone of calcified cartilage separates the radial zone (uncalcified cartilage) and the subchondral bone. The cells of the calcified cartilage zone have a smaller volume than the cells of the radial zone and contain only small amounts of endoplasmic reticulum and Golgi complex membranes. In some regions these cells appear to be completely surrounded by calcified cartilage. This appearance suggests that they have an extremely low level of metabolic activity. However, recent work suggests that they may have a role in the development and progression of osteoarthritis (Oegema and Thompson, 1995).

MATRIX REGIONS

Variations in the matrix within zones distinguish three regions or compartments: the pericellular region, the territorial region and the interterritorial region (Buckwalter et al., 1990) (Figure 6.9). The pericellular and territorial regions appear to serve the needs of chondrocytes, that is, binding the cell membranes to the matrix macromolecules and protecting the cells from damage during loading and deformation of the tissue. They may also help transmit mechanical signals to the chondrocytes when the matrix deforms during joint loading. The primary function of the interterritorial matrix (Figures 6.6, 6.7 and 6.8) is to provide the mechanical properties of the tissue.

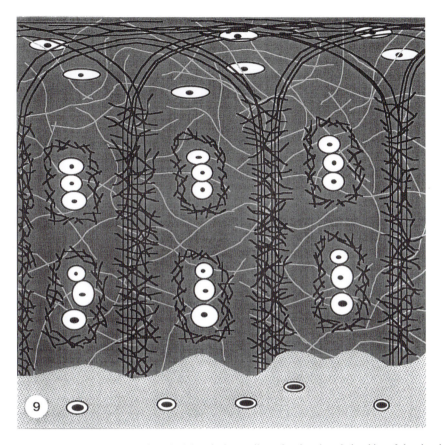

FIGURE 6.9 Schematic representation of adult articular cartilage showing the relationships of the chondrocytes to the fibrillar components of the matrix and the organisation of these components. The pericellular matrix compartment surrounds individual chondrocytes and varies in width; it is free of fibrillar components but contains an abundance of isotropically arranged cross-banded filaments which extend throughout all matrix compartments. The territorial matrix contains a basket-like arrangement of collagen fibrils and makes chondrones distinct morphologic entities. The interterritorial matrix forms the bulk of the tissue and contains two populations of fibrils and fibril bundles. The first population consists of fibrils with a highly oriented parallel arrangement that form the arcade-like structures. The second population consists of more randomly oriented fibrils.

PERICELLULAR MATRIX

Chondrocyte cell membranes appear to attach to the thin rim of the pericellular matrix that covers the cell surface (Figures 6.2, 6.3 and 6.4). This matrix region is rich in proteoglycans and also contains non-collagenous matrix proteins and non-fibrillar collagens including type VI collagen (Hagiwara *et al.*, 1993; Lee *et al.*, 1993; Marcelino and McDevitt, 1995; Poole *et al.*, 1992). It has little or no fibrillar collagen. Cytoplasmic extensions from the chondrocytes project into and through the pericellular matrix to the territorial matrix.

TERRITORIAL MATRIX

An envelope of territorial matrix surrounds the pericellular matrix of individual chondrocytes and, in some locations, pairs or clusters of chondrocytes and their pericellular matrices (Figures 6.2, 6.3 and 6.4). In the radial zone, a territorial matrix surrounds each chondrocyte column. The thin collagen fibrils of the territorial matrix nearest to the cell appear to adhere to the pericellular matrix. At a distance from the cell they decussate and intersect at various angles, forming a fibrillar basket around the cells. This collagenous basket may provide mechanical protection for the chondrocytes during loading and deformation of the tissue. An abrupt increase in collagen fibril diameter and a transition from the basket-like orientation of the collagen fibrils to a more parallel arrangement marks the boundary between the territorial and interterritorial matrices. However, many collagen fibrils connect the two regions, making it difficult to precisely identify the boundary between these regions.

INTERTERRITORIAL MATRIX

The interterritorial matrix makes up most of the volume of mature articular cartilage (Figure 6.9). It contains the largest diameter collagen fibrils. Unlike the collagen fibrils of the territorial matrix, these fibrils are not organised to surround the chondrocytes and many of them change their orientation relative to the joint surface 90 degrees from the superficial zone to the deep zone. In the superficial zone, the fibril diameters are relatively small and the fibrils generally lie parallel to the articular surface. In the transition zone, interterritorial matrix collagen fibrils assume more oblique angles relative to the articular surface and in the radial zone many of them form bundles that lie perpendicular (or radial) to the joint surface (Figure 6.9).

CHONDROCYTE–MATRIX INTERACTIONS

The relationship between the chondrocytes and the matrix does not end when the cells secrete the matrix macromolecules: instead the continued interactions of chondrocytes and the matrix makes possible the maintenance of the tissue throughout life. The cells bind to the matrix macromolecules through specialised cell surface receptors including a variety of integrins (Durr et al., 1993; Loeser, 1993; Salter et al., 1992, 1995). The matrix protects the chondrocytes from mechanical damage during normal joint use, it helps maintain their shape and their phenotype. Nutrients, substrates for synthesis of matrix molecules, newly synthesised molecules, degraded matrix molecules, metabolic waste products and molecules that help regulate cell function, like cytokines and growth factors, all pass through the matrix, and in some instances may be stored in the matrix. The types of molecules that can pass through the matrix and the rate at which they can pass depend on the composition and organisation of the matrix – primarily the concentration, composition and organisation of the large proteoglycans.

Throughout life, chondrocytes degrade and synthesise matrix macromolecules. The mechanisms that control the balance between these activities remain poorly understood, but cytokines with catabolic and anabolic effects appear to have important roles. For example, Interleukin 1 (IL-1) induces expression of matrix metalloproteases that can degrade the matrix macromolecules and interferes with synthesis of matrix proteoglycans at the transcriptional level. Other cytokines such as insulin-like growth factor I (IGF-I) and transforming growth factor β (TGF-β) oppose these catabolic activities by stimulating matrix synthesis and cell proliferation. In response to a variety of stimuli, chondrocytes synthesise and release these cytokines into the matrix where they may bind to receptors on the cell surfaces (stimulating cell activity either by autocrine or paracrine mechanisms) or become trapped within the matrix. The anabolic activities appear in large measure to be responses to matrix structural needs or other stimuli possibly including mechanical loading of the tissue detected by the chondrocytes. The degradative response on the other hand appears to be the result of a complex cascade that includes interleukin-1, stromelysin, aggrecanase, plasmin and collagenase being activated or inhibited by factors such as prostaglandins, transforming growth factors beta, tumor necrosis factor (TNF), tissue inhibitors of metalloproteases (TIMPs), tissue plasminogen activator, plasminogen activator inhibitor and other molecules.

The matrix also acts as a signal transducer for the chondrocytes. It transmits signals that result from mechanical loading of the articular surface to the chondrocytes and the chondrocytes respond to these signals by altering the matrix, possibly through expression of cytokines that act through autocrine or paracrine mechanisms. Experimental studies show that persistent abnormally decreased loading of a joint, or immobilisation of a joint, decreases the articular cartilage proteoglycan concentration, the degree of proteoglycan aggregation and alters cartilage mechanical properties (Buckwalter, 1995a,b; Buckwalter et al., 1995). Resumption of joint use restores matrix composition and mechanical properties toward normal, thus maintenance of normal articular cartilage composition requires a minimal level of joint loading and motion (Buckwalter, 1995b; Buckwalter and Lane, 1996). Repetitive joint loading and motion above normal levels may increase chondrocyte synthetic activity, but the chondrocytes have limited, if any, ability to expand the tissue volume in adults.

The details of how mechanical loading of joints influences chondrocyte function remain unknown, but matrix deformation produces mechanical, electrical and physicochemical signals that may have significant roles in stimulating chondrocytes (Buckwalter, 1995c; Buckwalter and Lane, 1996; Buschmann et al., 1995; Gray et al., 1988; Grodzinsky, 1993; Grodzinsky et al., (in press); Kim et al., 1994). Compression of the articular surface deforms the matrix and may directly deform chondrocytes. Matrix deformation also produces electrical and physicochemical effects that may influence chondrocytes. It causes flow of the tissue fluid and counterions relative to the fixed charged groups of the matrix macromolecules. This flow alters the charge density around the cells and produces a streaming potential. Changes in charge density within the matrix will alter the Donnan osmotic pressure and osmotic pressure gradients. Mechanically-induced matrix fluid flow may also accelerate flow of nutrients and metabolites through the matrix. Loading may also cause persistent changes in matrix molecular organisation that alter chondrocyte responses to subsequent loading. Thus, the matrix may not only transduce and transmit signals, it may 'record' the loading history of the tissue and alter the response of the cells based on the recorded loading history.

AGING OF CHONDROCYTES AND MATRIX

Because of the strong association between increasing prevalence of osteoarthritis or degenerative joint disease and increasing age, many patients, and some physicians, attribute the development of osteoarthritis to aging of articular cartilage. Despite this association, comparison of the age related morphologic and biologic changes in articular cartilage with the changes that occur in osteoarthritis shows that aging alone cannot explain the development of osteoarthritis (Buckwalter and Lane, 1996; Buckwalter and Mankin, 1997b; Buckwalter *et al.*, 1993b; Bullough and Brauer, 1993; Martin and Buckwalter, 1996a). However, aging changes may increase the risk of articular cartilage degeneration (Buckwalter and Lane, 1996; Buckwalter and Mankin, 1997b; Buckwalter *et al.*, 1993b).

The most apparent age-related morphologic change in articular cartilage is superficial fibrillation. Shallow fissures or clefts in the articular surface first appear near skeletal maturity (Buckwalter and Lane, 1996; Buckwalter and Mankin, 1997b; Bullough and Brauer, 1993; Martin and Buckwalter, 1996a). Longitudinal studies of articular cartilage fibrillation have not been done and are not currently feasible; but arthroscopic and autopsy examination of human joints strongly suggests that asymptomatic superficial fibrillation of at least some joint surfaces in middle age and older individuals is almost universal whereas these changes are rare in adolescents and young adults. It may not be possible in a specific joint to distinguish age-related superficial fibrillation from the early stage of osteoarthritis, but, the available evidence suggests that in many, if not most, individuals localised fibrillation of the articular surface does not progress into the deeper layers of the articular cartilage leading to loss of the articular cartilage surface even over a period of many decades.

With increasing age, chondrocyte morphology and synthetic function change (Buckwalter and Lane, 1996; Buckwalter and Mankin, 1997b; Buckwalter *et al.*, 1993b; Martin and Buckwalter, 1996a). The cells accumulate intracytoplasmic filaments and may lose some of their endoplasmic reticulum. They change their synthetic patterns to produce smaller more variable proteoglycans that may adversely alter the stability and mechanical properties of the macromolecular framework (Buckwalter *et al.*, 1993b; Martin and Buckwalter, 1996a). In addition, they become less responsive to growth factors that stimulate matrix synthesis (Buckwalter *et al.*, 1993b; Guerne *et al.*, 1995; Martin and Buckwalter, 1996a,b). These changes may make the cells less effective in maintaining the tissue and in repairing the matrix following injury.

Studies of the mechanical properties of cartilage have not found significant age-related changes in compressive properties, but they have shown significant decreases in tensile stiffness, fatigue resistance and strength (Kempson, 1991, 1980, 1982, Roberts *et al.*, 1986) that could make the tissue more vulnerable to injury from single or repetitive impact or torsional loads (Buckwalter and Lane, 1996). The underlying matrix alterations responsible for the age-related changes in matrix tensile properties have not been identified, but the water content generally decreases with age and both the proteoglycans and collagens that form the primary components of the articular cartilage matrix macromolecular framework undergo age-related changes (Buckwalter et al., 1993b; Roughley, 1993).

Aggregating proteoglycans and small proteoglycans both change with age. With skeletal maturation aggrecans they become much smaller and more variable in size, their keratan sulphate content increases, their chondroitin sulphate content decreases and the proportion of these molecules that form large aggregates declines (Buckwalter et al., 1994, 1993b; Roughley, 1993). As these changes in aggrecans occur, the size of proteoglycan aggregates decreases because of the decrease in aggrecan size and in the number of aggrecan molecules per aggregate. The decline in aggregation and aggregate size probably results from several changes in the molecules and in the matrix. Proteolytic degradation leaves molecular fragments in the matrix that occupy space and that may bind to hyaluronan where they can inhibit aggregation of fully functional molecules. Link proteins, the protein molecules responsible for stabilising and organising large proteoglycan aggregates, also undergo increasing proteolytic modification with age and the altered molecules accumulate in the matrix. Although the altered link proteins bind to hyaluronan and aggrecan they may be less effective in stabilising aggregates. Hyaluronan, the glycosaminoglycan that forms the central filament of proteoglycan aggregates, decreases in size and increases in concentration with maturation (Thonar et al., 1986, 1978). It is not certain if the increased concentration of hyaluronan results from increased synthesis or accumulation of degraded molecules. Since aggregation helps organise and stabilise proteoglycans within the matrix, the decline in aggregation and in aggregate size may alter the stability and mechanical properties of the matrix. Age-related changes may also occur in the small proteoglycans. The concentration of biglycan remains relatively constant while the concentration of decorin increases from about half the concentration of biglycan in newborns to twice the concentration of biglycan in adults (Poole et al., 1991; Roughley, 1993). The increasing concentration of decorin may affect matrix turnover and inhibit repair.

Cartilage collagens also undergo age-related changes that may alter the tissue properties (Martin and Buckwalter, 1996a; Roughley, 1993) During aging, cross-linking of collagen molecules may increase through non-enzymic glycation reactions. The matrix collagen fibrils increase in diameter with age and in their variability in diameter, changes thought to be related at least in part to the decreased content of type XI collagen relative to type II collagen. Larger diameter collagen fibrils with a greater degree of cross-linking may be less flexible and make the cartilage matrix more rigid. The increased rigidity combined with decreased water content could limit the ability of the macromolecular framework to deform repetitively when loaded without damaging its structure.

SUMMARY

The ability of articular cartilage to provide low friction joint motion for 80 years or more depends on its unique morphologic and biologic features including the interactions between chondrocytes and the matrix. Chondrocytes form the tissue matrix macromolecular framework from three classes of molecules: collagens, proteoglycans and non-collagenous proteins. Type II, type IX and type XI collagens form a fibrillar meshwork that gives the tissue its form and tensile stiffness and strength. Type VI collagen forms part of the matrix immediately surrounding chondrocytes and may help them attach to the matrix macromolecular framework. Large aggregating proteoglycans, aggrecans, give the tissue its stiffness to compression, resilience and contribute to its durability. Small proteo-glycans, including decorin, biglycan and fibromodulin, bind to other matrix macromole-cules and thereby help stabilise the matrix. They may also influence chondrocyte function and bind growth factors. Cartilage oligomeric protein (COMP) may have value as a marker of cartilage turnover and degeneration, and other non-collagenous proteins including tenascin and fibronectin can influence chondrocyte matrix interactions. The matrix protects the cells from injury due to normal joint use, it determines the types and concentrations of molecules that reach the cells and it helps maintain the chondrocyte phenotype. Throughout life, the tissue undergoes continual internal remodelling as the cells replace matrix macromolecules lost through degradation. The available evidence indicates that normal matrix turnover depends on the ability of chondrocytes to detect alterations in matrix macromolecular composition and organisation, including the pres-ence of degraded molecules, and respond by synthesising appropriate types and amounts of new molecules. In addition, the matrix acts as a signal transducer for the cells. Loading of the tissue due to joint use creates mechanical, electrical and physicochemical signals that help direct chondrocyte synthetic and degradative activity. Prolonged severely decreased joint use leads to alterations in matrix composition and eventually loss of tissue structure and mechanical properties, whereas joint use stimulates chondrocyte synthetic activity and possibly internal tissue remodelling. Aging leads to alterations in matrix composition and in chondrocyte activity including the ability of the cells to respond to a variety of stimuli including growth factors. These alterations may increase the probability of cartilage degeneration.

ACKNOWLEDGEMENT

Many of the concepts presented in this chapter were revised and updated from previous publications (Buckwalter et al., 1988; Buckwalter and Mankin, 1997a).

REFERENCES

Athanasiou, K.A., Rosenwasser, M.P., Buckwalter, J.A., Malinin, T.I. and Mow, V.C. (1991) Interspecies com-parisons of in situ intrinsic mechanical properties of distal femoral cartilage. J. Ortho. Res., 9, 330–340.
Aydelotte, M.B., Michal, L.E., Reid, D.R. and Schumacher, B.L. (1996) Chondrocytes from the articular surface and deep zones express different, but stable phenotypes in alginate gel culture. Trans. Ortho. Res. Soc., 21, 317.
Aydelotte, M.B., Schumacher, B.L. and Kuettner, K.E. (1992) Heterogeneity of articular chondrocytes. In: Kuettner, K.E., Schleyerbach, R., Peyron, J.G. and Hascall, V.C. (Editors) Articular Cartilage and Osteoarthritis, pp. 237–249. New York: Raven Press.
Buckwalter, J.A. (1995a) Activity vs. rest in the treatment of bone, soft tissue and joint injuries. Iowa Orthop. J., 15, 29–42.

Buckwalter, J.A. (1995b) Osteoarthritis and articular cartilage use, disuse and abuse: experimental studies. *J. Rheumatol.*, (suppl 43), **22**, 13–15.
Buckwalter, J.A. (1995c) Should bone, soft-tissue and joint injuries be treated with rest or activity? *J. Orthop. Res.*, **13**, 155–156.
Buckwalter, J.A., Einhorn, T.A., Bolander, M.E. and Cruess, R.L. (1996) Healing of musculoskeletal tissues. In: Rockwood, C.A. and Green, D. (Editors) *Fractures*, pp. 261–304. Lippincott.
Buckwalter, J.A., Hunziker, E.B., Rosenberg, L.C., Coutts, R.D., Adams, M.E. and Eyre, D.R. (1988) Articular cartilage: composition and structure. In: Woo, S.L. and Buckwalter, J.A. (Editors) *Injury and Repair of the Musculoskeletal Soft Tissues*, pp. 405–425. Park Ridge, IL: American Academy of Orthopaedic Surgeons.
Buckwalter, J.A., Kuettner, K.E. and Thonar, E.J-M. (1985) Age-related changes in articular cartilage proteo-glycans: electron microscopic studies. *J. Orthop. Res.*, **3**, 251–257.
Buckwalter, J.A. and Lane, N.E. (1996) Aging, sports and osteoarthritis. *Sports Med. Arth. Rev.*, **4**, 276–287.
Buckwalter, J.A., Lane, N.E. and Gordon, S.L. (1995) Exercise as a cause of osteoarthritis. In: Kuettner, K.E. and Goldberg, V.M. (Editors) *Osteoarthritic Disorders*, pp. 405–417. Rosemont, IL: American Academy of Orthopaedic Surgeons.
Buckwalter, J.A. and Mankin, H.J. (1997a) Articular cartilage I. Tissue design and chondrocyte-matrix interac-tions. *J. Bone Joint Surg.*, **79A**, (In Press).
Buckwalter, J.A. and Mankin, H.J. (1997b) Articular cartilage II. Degeneration and osteoarthrosis, repair, regen-eration and transplantation. *J. Bone Joint Surg.*, **79A**, 612–632.
Buckwalter, J.A. and Mow, V.C. (1992) Cartilage repair in osteoarthritis. In: Moskowitz, R.W., Howell, D.S., Goldberg, V.M. and Mankin, H.J. (Editors) *Osteoarthritis Diagnosis and Management*, 2nd edition, pp. 71–107. Philadelphia: Saunders.
Buckwalter, J.A., Pita, J.C., Muller, F.J. and Nessler, J. (1993a) Structural differences between two populations of articular cartilage proteoglycan aggregates. *J. Orthop. Res.*, **12**, 144–148.
Buckwalter, J.A., Rosenberg, L.A. and Hunziker, E.B. (1990) Articular cartilage: composition, structure, response to injury, and methods of facilitation repair. In: Ewing, J.W. (Editor) *Articular Cartilage and Knee Joint Function Basic Science and Arthroscopy*, pp. 19–56. New York: Raven Press.
Buckwalter, J.A. and Rosenberg, L.C. (1982) Electron microscopic studies of cartilage proteoglycans: Direct evidence for the variable length of the chondroitin sulphate rich region of the proteoglycan subunit core protein. *J. Biol. Chem.*, **257**, 9830–9839.
Buckwalter, J.A. and Rosenberg, L.C. (1983) Structural changes during development in bovine fetal epiphyseal cartilage. *Collagen Rel. Res.*, **3**, 489–504.
Buckwalter, J.A., Rosenberg, L.C., Coutts, R., Hunziker, E., Reddi, A.H. and Mow, V.C. (1988) Articular carti-lage: injury and repair. In: Woo, S.L. and Buckwalter, J.A. (Editors) *Injury and Repair of the Musculoskeletal Soft Tissues*, pp. 465–482. Park Ridge, IL: American Academy of Orthopaedic Surgeons.
Buckwalter, J.A., Rosenberg, L.C. and Tang, L.H. (1984) The effect of link protein on proteoglycan aggregate structure. *J. Biol. Chem.*, **259**(9), 5361–5363.
Buckwalter, J.A., Roughley, P.J. and Rosenberg, L.C. (1994) Age-related changes in cartilage proteoglycans: quantitative electron microscopic studies. *Micros. Res. Tech.*, **28**, 398–408.
Buckwalter, J.A., Woo, S.L.-Y., Goldberg, V.M., Hadley, E.C., Booth, F., Oegema, T.R. and Eyre, D.R. (1993b) Soft tissue aging and musculoskeletal function. *J. Bone Joint Surg.*, **75A**, 1533–1548.
Bullough, P.G. and Brauer, F.U. (1993) Age-related changes in articular cartilage. In: Buckwalter, J.A., Goldberg, V.M. and Woo, S.L.-Y. (Editors) *Soft Tissue Aging: Impact on Musculoskeletal Function and Mobility*, pp. 117–135. Rosemont, IL: American Academy of Orthopaedic Surgeons.
Buschmann, M.D., Gluzband, Y.A., Grodzinsky, A.J. and Hunziker, E.B. (1995) Mechanical compression mod-ulates matrix biosynthesis in chondrocyte/agarose culture. *J. Cell Sci.*, **108**, 1497–1508.
Chevalier, X., Groult, N. and Labat-Robert, J. (1992) Biosynthesis and distribution of fibronectin in normal and osteoarthritic human cartilage. *Clin. Phys. Biochem.*, **9**(1), 1–6.
Chevalier, X., Groult, N., Larget-Piet, B., Zardi, L. and Hornebeck, W. (1994) Tenascin distribution in articular cartilage from normal subjects and from patients with osteoarthritis and rheumatoid arthritis. *Arth. Rheum.*, **37**, 1013–1022.
DeCesare, P.E., Morgelin, M., Mann, K. and Paulsson, M. (1994) Cartilage oligomeric protein and thrombo-spondin 1. Purification from articular cartilage, electron microscopic structure, and chondrocyte binding. *European J. Biochem.*, **223**, 927–937.
Durr, J., Goodman, S., Potocnik, A., Mark, Hvd. and Mark, Kvd. (1993) Localization of beta 1-integrins in human cartilage and their role in chondrocyte adhesion to collagen and fibronectin. *Exp. Cell Res.*, **207**(2), 235–244.
Eyre, D.R. (1995) Collagen structure and function in articular cartilage: metabolic changes in the development of osteoarthritis. In: Kuettner, K.E. and Goldberg, V.M. (Editors) *Osteoarthritic Disorders*, pp. 219–227. Rosemont, IL: American Academy of Orthopaedic Surgeons.

Eyre, D.R., Wu, J.J. and Woods, P. (1992) Cartilage-specific collagens: structural studies. In: Kuettner, K.E., Schleyerbach, R., Peyron, J.G. and Hascall, V.C. (Editors) *Articular Cartilage and Osteoarthritis*, pp. 119–131. New York: Raven Press.

Gluhak, J., Mais, A. and Mina, M. (1996) Tenascin-C is associated with early stages of chondrogenesis by chick mandibular ectomesenchymal cells *in vivo* and *in vitro*. *Developmental Dynamics*, **205**(1), 24–40.

Gray, M.L., Pizzanelli, A.M., Grodzinski, A.J. and Lee, R.C. (1988) Mechanical and physicochemical determinants of chondrocyte biosynthesis response. *J. Orthop. Res.*, **6**, 788–792.

Grodzinsky, A.J. (1993) Age-related changes in cartilage: physical properties and cellular response to loading. In: Buckwalter, J.A., Goldberg, V. and Woo, S.-L.Y. (Editors) *Musculo-skeletal Soft Tissue Aging: Impact on Mobility*, pp. 137–149. Rosemont, IL: American Academy of Orthopaedic Surgeons.

Grodzinsky, A.J., Kim, Y.J., Bucschmann, M.D., Garcia, M.L. and Hunziker, E.B. Response of the chondrocyte to mechanical stimuli. In: Lohmander, S. and Brandt, K. (Editors) *Osteoarthritis*. Oxford Medical Publications, Oxford, UK.

Guerne, P.A., Blanco, F., Kaelin, A., Desgeorges, A. and Lotz, M. (1995) Growth factor responsiveness of human articular chondrocytes in aging and development. *Arth. Rheum.*, **38**, 960–968.

Guilak, F., Ratcliffe, A., Lane, N., Rosenwasser, M.P. and Mow, V.C. (1994) Mechanical and biochemical changes in the superficial zone of articular cartilage in canine experimental osteoarthritis. *J. Orthop. Res.*, **12**, 474–484.

Hagiwara, H., Schroter-Kermani, C. and Merker, H.J. (1993) Localization of collagen type VI in articular cartilage of young and adult mice. *Cell Tiss. Res.*, **272**(1), 155–160.

Hardingham, T.E., Fosang, A.J. and Dudhia, J. (1992) Aggrecan, the chondroitin/keratan sulphate proteoglycan from cartilage. In: Kuettner, K.E., Schleyerbach, R., Peyron, J.G. and Hascall, V.C. (Editors) *Articular Cartilage and Osteoarthritis*, pp. 5–20. New York: Raven Press.

Hayashi, T., Abe, E. and Jasin, H.E. (1996) Fibronectin synthesis in superficial and deep layers of normal articular cartilage. *Arth. Rheum.*, **39**, 567–573.

Hedbom, E., Antonsson, P., Hjerpe, A., Aeschlimann, D., Paulsson, M., Rosa-Pimentel, E., Sommarin, Y., Wendel, M., Oldberg, A. and Heinegard, D. (1992) Cartilage matrix proteins. An acidic oligomeric protein (COMP) detected only in cartilage. *J. Biol. Chem.*, **267**, 6132–6136.

Heinegard, D., Lorenzo, P. and Sommarin, Y. (1995) Articular cartilage matrix proteins. In: Kuettner, K.E. and Goldberg, V.M. (Editors) *Osteoarthritic Disorders*, pp. 229–237. Rosemont, IL: American Academy of Orthopaedic Surgeons.

Heinegard, D.K. and Pimentel, E.R. (1992) Cartilage matrix proteins. In: Kuettner, K.E., Schleyerbach, R., Peyron, J.G. and Hascall, V.C. (Editors) *Articular Cartilage and Osteoarthritis*, pp. 95–111. New York: Raven Press.

Hildebrand, A., Romaris, M., Rasmussen, L.M., Heinegard, D., Twardzik, D.R., Border, W.A. and Ruslahti, E. (1994) Interaction of the small interstitial proteoglycans biglycan, decorin and fibromodulin with transforming growth factor beta. *Biochem. J.*, **302**, 527–534.

Hunziker, E.B., Wagner, J. and Studer, D. (1996) Vitrified articular cartilage reveals novel ultra-structural features respecting extracellular matrix architecture. *Histochem. Cell Biol.*, **106**, 375–382.

Jurvelin, J.S., Muller, D.J., Wong, M., Studer, D., Engel, A. and Hunziker, E.B. (1996) Surface and subsurface morphology of bovine humeral articular cartilage as assessed by atomic force and transmission electron microscopy. *J. Struct. Biol.*, **117**, 45–54.

Kempson, G.E. (1991) Age-related changes in the tensile properties of human articular cartilage: a comparitive study between the femoral head of the hip joint and the talus of the ankle joint. *Biochim. Biophys. Acta*, **1075**, 223–230.

Kempson, G.E. (1980) The mechanical properties of articular cartilage. In: Sokoloff, L. (Editor) *The Mechanical properties of Articular Cartilage*, pp. 177–238. New York: Academic Press.

Kempson, G.E. (1982) Relationship between the tensile properties of articular cartilage from the human knee and age. *Ann. Rheum. Dis.*, **41**, 508–511.

Kim, Y.J., Sah, R.L., Grodzinsky, A.J., Plaas, A.H. and Sandy, J.D. (1994) Mechanical regulation of cartilage biosynthetic behaviour: physical stimuli. *Arch. Biochem. Biophys.*, **311**(1), 1–12.

Lai, W.M., Mow, V.C. and Roth, V. (1981) Effects of nonlinear strain-dependent permeability and rate of compression on the stress behaviour of articular cartilage. *J. Biomech. Eng.*, **103**, 61–66.

Lee, G.M., Johnstone, B., Jacobsen, K. and Caterson, B. (1993) The dynamic structure of the pericellular matrix on living cells. *J. Cell. Biol.*, **123**, 1899–1907.

Linn, F.C. and Sokoloff, L. (1965) Movement and composition of interstitial fluid of cartilage. *Arth. Rheum.*, **8**, 481–494.

Loeser, R.F. (1993) Integrin-mediated attachment of articular chondrocytes to extracellular matrix proteins. *Arth. Rheum.*, **36**(8), 1103–1110.

Lohmander, L.S., Saxne, T. and Heinegard, D.K. (1994) Release of cartilage oligomeric protein (COMP) into joint fluid after knee injury and in osteoarthritis. *Ann. Rheum. Dis.*, **53**, 8–13.

Mackie, E.J. and Ramsey, S. (1996) Expression of tenascin in joint-associated tissues during development and postnatal growth. *J. Anat.*, **188**, 157–165.

Mankin, H.J. (1978) The water of articular cartilage. In: Simon, W.H. (Editor) *The Human Joint in Health and Disease*, pp. 37–42. Philadelphia: University of Pennsylvannia Press.

Marcelino, J. and McDevitt, C.A. (1995) Attachment of articular cartilage chondrocytes to the tissue form of type VI collagen. *Biochem. Biophys. Acta*, **1249**(2), 180–188.

Maroudas, A. and Schneiderman, R. (1987) "Free" and "exchangeable" or "trapped" and "non-exchangeable" water in cartilage. *J. Orthop. Res.*, **5**, 133–138.

Martin, J.A. and Buckwalter, J.A. (1996a) Articular cartilage aging and degeneration. *Sports Med. Arth. Rev.*, **4**, 263–275.

Martin, J.A. and Buckwalter, J.A. (1996b) Fibronectin and cell shape affect age related decline in chondrocyte synthetic response to IGF-I. *Trans. Ortho. Res. Soc.*, **21**, 306.

Miosge, N., Flachsbart, K., Goetz, W., Schultz, W., Kresse, H. and Herken, R. (1994) Light and electron microscopical immunohistochemical localization of the small proteoglycan core proteins decorin and biglycan in human knee joint cartilage. *Histochemical J.*, **26**(12), 939–945.

Mow, V.C. and Rosenwasser, M.P. (1988) Articular cartilage: Biomechanics. In: Woo, S.L. and Buckwalter, J.A. (Editors) *Injury and Repair of the Musculoskeletal Soft Tissues*, pp. 427–463. Park Ridge, IL: American Academy of Orthopaedic Surgeons.

Muller, F.J., Pita, J.C., Manicourt, D.H., Malinin, T.I., Schoonbeck, J.M. and Mow, V.C. (1989) Centrifugal characterization of proteoglycans from various depth players and weight-bearing areas of normal and abnormal human articular cartilage. *J. Ortho. Res.*, **7**, 326–334.

Neame, P.J. and Barry, F.P. (1993) The link proteins. *Experientia*, **49**(5), 393–402.

Nishida, K., Inoue, H. and Murakami, T. (1995) Immunohistochemical demonstration of fibronectin in the most superfical layer of normal rabbit articular cartilage. *Ann. Rheum. Dis.*, **54**, 995–998.

Noyori, K. and Jasin, H.E. (1994) Inhibition of human fibroblast adhesion by cartilage surface proteoglycans. *Arth. Rheum.*, **37**(11), 1656–1663.

Oegema, T.R. and Thompson, R.C. (1995) Histopathology and pathobiochemistry of the cartilage-bone interface in osteoarthritis. In: Kuettner, K.E. and Goldberg, V.M. (Editors) *Osteoarthritic Disorders*, pp. 205–217. Rosemont, IL: American Academy of Orthopaedic Surgeons.

Pacifici, M. (1995) Tenascin-C and the development of articular cartilage. *Matrix Biology*, **14**(9), 689–698.

Pita, J.C., Manicourt, D.H. and Muller, F.J. (1990) Centrifugal and biochemical comparison of two populations of proteoglycan aggregates from articular cartilage of immobilized dog joints. *Trans. 33rd Meeting Ortho. Res. Soc.*, **15**, 17.

Pita, J.C., Muller, F.J., Manicourt, D.H., Buckwalter, J.A. and Ratcliff, A. (1992) Early matrix changes in experimental osteoarthritis and joint disuse atrophy. In: Kuettner, K.E., Schleyerbach, R., Peyron, J.G. and Hascall, V.C. (Editors) *Articular Cartilage and Osteoarthritis*, pp. 455–469. New York: Raven Press.

Poole, A.R., Reiner, A., Inonescu, M. *et al.* (1991) Immunochemical analyses of the small proteoglycans decorin and biglycan in normal and osteoarthritic human cartilages. *Trans. Combined Ortho. Res. Soc. USA, Japan, Canada*, **1**, 80.

Poole, C.A., Ayad, S. and Gilbert, R.T. (1992) Chondrons from articular cartilage. V Immunohistochemical evaluation of type VI collagen organization in isolated chondrons by light, confocal and electron microscopy. *J. Cell Sci.*, **103**, 1101–1110.

Redler, I., Mow, V.C., Zimny, M.L. and Mansell, J. (1975) The ultrastructure and biomechanical significance of the tidemark of articular cartilage. *Clin. Ortho. Rel. Res.*, **112**, 357–362.

Roberts, S., Weightman, B., Urban, J. and Chappell, D. (1986) Mechanical and biochemical properties of human articular cartilage in osteoarthritic femoral heads and in autopsy specimens. *J. Bone Joint Surg.*, **68B**, 278–288.

Rosenberg, L.C. (1992) Structure and function of dermatan sulphate proteoglycans in articular cartilage. In: Kuettner, K.E., Schleyerbach, R., Peyron, J.G. and Hascall, V.C. (Editors) *Articular Cartilage and Osteoarthritis*, pp. 45–63. New York: Raven Press.

Rosenberg, L.C. and Buckwalter, J.A. (1986) Cartilage proteoglycans. In: Kuettner, K.E., Schleyerbach, R. and Hascall, V.C. (Editors) *Articular Cartilage Biochemistry*, pp. 39–57. New York: Raven Press.

Roughley, P.J. (1993) Articular cartilage: matrix changes with aging. In: Buckwalter, J.A., Goldberg, V.M. and Woo, S.L.-Y. (Editors) *Soft Tissue Aging: Impact on Musculoskeletal Function and Mobility*, pp. 151–164. Rosemont, IL: American Academy of Orthopaedic Surgeons.

Roughley, P.J. and Lee, E.R. (1994) Cartilage proteoglycans: structure and potential functions. *Micros. Res. Tech.*, **28**, 385–397.

Salter, D.M., Godolphin, J.L. and Gourlay, M.S. (1995) Chondrocyte heterogeneity: immunohistologically defined variation in integrin expression at different sites in human fetal knees. *J. Histochemistry Cytochemistry*, **43**(4), 447–457.

Salter, D.M., Hughes, D.E., Simpson, R. and Gardner, D.L. (1992) Integrin expression by human articular chondrocytes. *Brit. J. Rheum.*, **31**(4), 231–234.

Sandell, L.J. (1995) Molecular biology of collagens in normal and osteoarthritic cartilage. In: Kuettner, K.E. and Goldberg, V.M. (Editors) *Osteoarthritic Disorders*, pp. 131–146. Rosemont, IL: American Academy of Orthopaedic Surgeons.

Savarese, J.J., Erickson, H. and Scully, S.P. (1996) Articular chondrocyte tenascin-C production and assembly into de novo extracellular matrix. *J. Ortho. Res.*, **14**, 273–281.

Saxne, T. and Heinegard, D. (1992) Cartilage oligomeric matrix protein: a novel marker of cartilage turnover detectable in synovial fluid and blood. *Brit. J. Rheum.*, **31**, 583–591.

Schumacher, B.L., Block, J.A., Schmid, T.M., Aydelotte, M.B. and Kuettner K.E. (1994) A novel proteoglycan synthesized and secreted by chondrocytes of the superficial zone of articular cartilage. *Arch. Biochem. Biophys.*, **311**(1), 144–152.

Setton, L.A., Zhu, W. and Mow, V.C. (1993) The biphasic poroviscoelastic behaviour of articular cartilage: role of the surface zone in governing the compressive behaviour. *J. Biomech.*, **26**, 581–592.

Sharif, M., Saxne, T., Shepstone, L., Kirwan, J.R., Elson, C.J., Heinegard, D. and Dieppe, P.A. (1995) Relationship between serum cartilage oligomeric matrix protein levels and disease progression in osteoarthritis of the knee joint. *Brit. J. Rheum.*, **34**(4), 306–310.

Stockwell, R.A. (1967) The cell density of human articular and costal cartilage. *J. Anat.*, **101**, 753–763.

Stockwell, R.A. (1978) Chondrocytes. *J. Clin. Pathol.* (suppl), 7–13.

Studer, D., Chiquet, M. and Hunziker, E.B. (1996) Evidence for a distinct water-rich layer surrounding collagen fibrils in articular cartilage extracellular matrix. *J. Structural Biol.*, **117**, 81–85.

Tang, L.H., Buckwalter, J.A. and Rosenberg, L.C. (1996) The effect of link protein concentration on articular cartilage proteoglycan aggregation. *J. Orthop. Res.*, **14**, 334–339.

Thonar, E-M., Bjornsson, S. and Kuettner, K.E. (1986) Age-related changes in cartilage proteoglycans. In: Kuettner, K.E., Schleyerbach, R. and Hascall, V.C. (Editors) *Articular Cartilage Biochemistry*, pp. 273–287. New York: Raven Press.

Thonar, E.J.-M. and Sweet, M.B.E., Immelman, A.R. and Lyons, G. (1978) Hyaluronate in articular cartilage: age-related changes. *Calcif. Tiss. Res.*, **26**, 19–22.

Wong, M., Wuethrich, P., Eggli, P. and Hunziker, E. (1996) Zone-specific cell biosynthetic activity in mature bovine articular cartilage: a new method using confocal microscopic stereology and quantitative autoradiography. *J. Ortho. Res.*, **14**(3), 424–432.

7 Regulation of Proteoglycan Metabolism in Articular Cartilage

Vincent C. Hascall*, John D. Sandy[1] and Christopher J. Handley[2]

*Department of Biomedical Engineering,
WB3 Cleveland Clinic Foundation, Cleveland, OH 44195, USA*

KEY WORDS aggrecan, aggrecanase, cartilage, articular; explant culture; hyaluronan, link protein, metabolism, proteoglycan; hyaluronan; steady state

INTRODUCTION

In normal cartilage, chondrocytes are surrounded by an extracellular matrix which gives the tissue its mechanical properties while providing the cells with an environment that sustains their metabolic activities. Under these circumstances, each chondrocyte ideally maintains the structure and function of its immediate matrix, or modifies it within a 'normal' range in response to biomechanical changes. In this sense a chondrocyte in a normal matrix operates to **maintain** its matrix. If the matrix is removed or damaged sufficiently, chondrocytes are confronted with a problem of matrix **repair**, and in the process of attempting repair, they can often undergo major changes in their phenotypic expression.

The proteoglycan aggrecan is the major structural macromolecule in the cartilage matrix responsible for tissue resilience and elasticity (Hascall, 1988; Wight *et al.*, 1991). This molecule consists of a core protein of ~220,000 molecular weight with distinct regions (Figure 7.1): the globular 1 (G1) domain at the N-terminus which has a binding site for hyaluronan (hyaluronic acid) that is critical for proteoglycan aggregate formation; an interglobular domain; a globular 2 (G2) domain; a region enriched in keratan sulfate chains; two regions enriched in chondroitin sulphate chains; and a globular 3 (G3) domain at the C-terminus. Chondrocytes actively metabolise aggrecan throughout the lifetime of the tissue.

* Corresponding author.
Current address: [1] Shriners Hospital for Crippled Children, Tampa Unit, 12502 North Pine Drive, Tampa, FL 33612-9499; [2] School of Human Biosciences, La Trobe University, Bundoora, Victoria 3083, Australia.

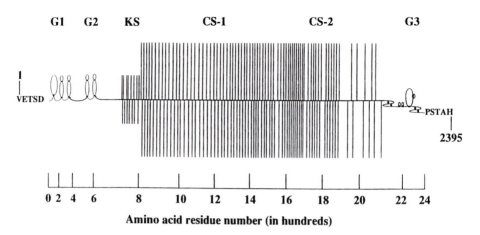

FIGURE 7.1 *Schematic model of aggrecan.* The determined amino terminus (residue 1) and the predicted carboxyl terminus (residue 2395) are indicated. The domain structure is discussed in the text and more thoroughly in Chapter 12. The long lines denote locations of -serine-glycine- in the sequences each of which may contain a chondroitin sulphate chain. They also denote the limits of the chondroitin sulphate-rich domain which was initially subdivided into two regions (CS-1 and CS-2) based upon different internal repetitive sequence motifs (Doege *et al.*, 1991). The short lines indicate serine and theonine sites in the keratan sulfate-rich domain each of which may contain either an O-linked oligosaccharide or a keratan sulfate chain. For simplicity the locations of the numerous other serine and threonine sites for substitution in other regions of the core are not indicated.

The purpose of this chapter is to describe how chondrocytes regulate proteoglycan metabolism when they are in a normal 'maintenance' mode. Most of the experimental studies pertaining to this problem have used articular cartilage explants *in vitro* as a model for investigating chondrocyte metabolism under conditions where they are surrounded by a 'normal' extracellular matrix. Under appropriate medium conditions, such cultures balance proteoglycan synthesis with proteoglycan catabolism and thereby keep the proteoglycan concentration in their local environment constant over long periods of time. This condition is referred to as *steady state metabolism* of proteoglycans. Because the cultures are a closed system, they offer a unique opportunity to define factors which modulate both the biosynthetic and catabolic responses, to characterise the catabolic products released from the tissue in order to define boundary conditions for the catabolic mechanisms, and to assess the consequences of controlled matrix damage on proteoglycan metabolic parameters.

STEADY STATE METABOLISM OF PROTEOGLYCANS

In the presence of sufficient amounts of foetal bovine serum, chondrocytes in explant cultures of young bovine articular cartilage from metacarpalphalangeal joints can maintain steady state metabolism of proteoglycans in the *metabolically active pool* for several weeks (Hascall *et al.*, 1983a). The major factor in serum responsible for achieving steady state conditions was shown to be insulin-like growth factor-I (IGF-I) (McQuillan *et al.*, 1986). Subsequent work showed that IGF-I at physiological concentrations (~10 ng/ml) is sufficient, as the sole medium supplement, to maintain steady state parameters for at least 5 weeks (Luyten *et al.*, 1988). Unlike serum, which can stimulate cell division and outgrowth in the cultures (Tian *et al.*, 1989), the cell number in cultures with IGF-I does not change with time. Transforming growth factor $\beta 1$ (Morales and Roberts, 1988) and osteogenin (bone morphogenic protein 3) (Luyten *et al.*, 1992) can also sustain steady state metabolism of proteoglycans in such cultures.

Figure 7.2 shows experimental data for 3 culture medium conditions: basal medium with either 0, 5 or 20 ng/ml IGF-I (Luyten *et al.*, 1988). Panel *a* shows the proteoglycan

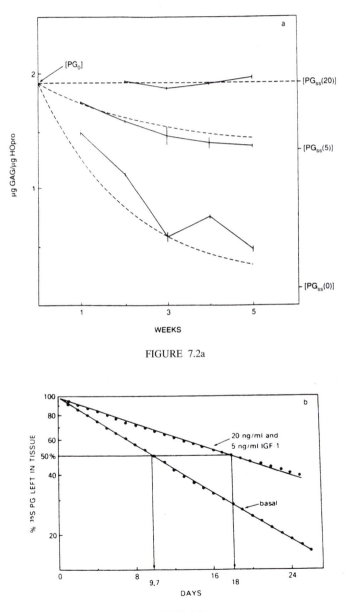

FIGURE 7.2a

FIGURE 7.2b

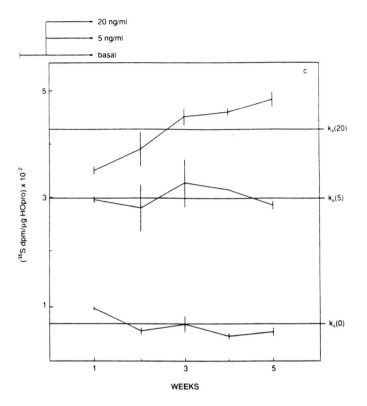

FIGURE 7.2c

FIGURE 7.2   *Metabolic responses of cartilage explant cultures to time in culture with basal medium alone or supplemented with 5 ng/ml or 20 ng/ml of IGF-1.* Panel *a* shows the glycosaminoglycan (GAG) concentrations in cultures isolated at different times of culture. The dashed lines are curves derived from the equations in the text for cultures in basal medium alone or with 5 ng/ml IGF-I. The values at the right indicate the concentrations predicted when steady state conditions are reached. The value [PG$_0$] is assumed to be the concentration in the metabolically active pool as described in the text. Panel *b* shows the catabolic loss of radiolabelled proteoglycans from cultures treated with basal medium alone or with 20 ng/ml IGF-I. The decay curve for cultures with 5 ng/ml IGF-I was identical to that for 20 ng/ml IGF-I and is not shown. The half lives of 9.7 days (basal) and 18 days (IGF-I supplemented) are indicated as the times when 50% of the labelled proteoglycans are lost from the matrix compartment. Panel *c* shows the rates of proteoglycan synthesis in the same cultures analysed in panel *a*. The values at the right indicate the levels used to estimate the zero-order rate constants for each medium condition as described in the text. The data are taken from reference Luyten *et al.* (1992) with permission.

concentrations for these cultures during the 5 weeks of the experiment. The proteoglycan concentration remained constant in the cultures with 20 ng/ml IGF-I whereas it declined with time for cultures in the other two medium conditions. Thus, cultures with 20 ng/ml IGF-I were in steady state proteoglycan metabolism while the others were not.

Proteoglycan catabolism was measured for each medium condition by radiolabelling cultures with ^{35}S-sulphate on day minus 2 and then determining the proportion of total counts remaining in the tissue with time, setting day 0 as 100%. When plotted on a semi-logarithmic scale (panel *b*), the curves were linear with time. Those for the 5 ng/ml (data not shown) and the 20 ng/ml IGF-I conditions were indistinguishable from each other, and their loss rate was less rapid than for basal conditions without IGF-I. The linearity of the curves indicates that the catabolic mechanism for the radiolabelled proteoglycans in all culture conditions exhibited *first order kinetics*. This means that the rate of catabolism of the *radiolabelled proteoglycans* in any culture condition is proportional to their concentration in the *metabolically active pool*. Therefore, catabolism in the total metabolic pool can be defined with a catabolic rate constant, k_c, which will be characteristic for each medium condition; i.e. the catabolic rate equals $k_c \times [\mathrm{PG}(t)]$, where $[\mathrm{PG}(t)]$ is the total proteoglycan concentration in the metabolic pool as a function of time (t).

The rates of proteoglycan synthesis in this experiment remained constant (0 and 5 ng/ml IGF-I) or nearly constant (20 ng/ml IGF-I) with time (panel c). Thus, the proteoglycan synthetic rates exhibit *zero order kinetics*, i.e. they are independent of proteoglycan concentration, with synthetic rate constants, k_s, that are characteristic for each medium condition.

MATHEMATICAL MODELLING OF CARTILAGE PROTEOGLYCAN METABOLISM

These data can be treated mathematically as follows (Hascall *et al.*, 1990):

When the system is not in steady state, the change in proteoglycan concentration in the metabolically active pool with time will be equal to the difference in the synthetic and catabolic rates:

$$d[\mathrm{PG}(t)]/dt = k_s - k_c \times [\mathrm{PG}(t)] \qquad [1]$$

Once steady state is achieved the proteoglycan concentration will not change, and $d[\mathrm{PG}(t)]/dt = 0$. In this case:

$$[\mathrm{PG_{ss}}] = k_s/k_c \qquad [2]$$

Where $[\mathrm{PG_{ss}}]$ is the steady state proteoglycan concentration for the particular k_s and k_c values that characterise a particular medium condition. The differential equation 1 can then be solved:

$$[\mathrm{PG}(t)] = [\mathrm{PG_{ss}}] \times (1 - A \times e^{-(k_c t)}) \qquad [3]$$

At $t = 0$, $[\mathrm{PG}(t=0)]$ will be the initial proteoglycan concentration, $[\mathrm{PG_0}]$, in the metabolically active pool, and the constant A becomes:

$$A = ([\mathrm{PG_{ss}}] - [\mathrm{PG_0}])/[\mathrm{PG_{ss}}] \qquad [4]$$

Equation 3 then becomes:

$$[\mathrm{PG}(t)] = [\mathrm{PG_{ss}}] - ([\mathrm{PG_{ss}}] - [\mathrm{PG_0}]) \times e^{-(k_c t)} \qquad [5]$$

These equations can now be used to evaluate the data in Figure 7.2. If it is assumed that all of the proteoglycans in the tissue are in the metabolically active pool, then $[\mathrm{PG_0}]$ in this experiment is ~1.9 mg/mg when measured as glycosaminoglycan per hydroxyproline, or the equivalent of ~2.2 mg proteoglycan per mg hydroxyproline (see Figure 7.2a). For the cultures with 20 ng/ml IGF-I, one half of the radiolabelled proteoglycans have been catabolised by day 18 (Figure 7.2b). This defines $k_c(20)$, the catabolic rate constant for the radiolabelled proteoglycans, $[PG^{\#}(t)]$, in the 20 ng/ml cultures:

$$[PG^{\#}(t=18)]/PG^{\#}(t=0)]=0.5=e^{-(k_c(20) \times 18)} \qquad [6]$$

and

$$k_c(20)=0.693/18=0.039/\text{day}$$

Because the cultures for 20 ng/ml were in steady state, equation 2 gives the synthetic rate constant, $k_s(20)$:

$$k_s(20)=k_c(20) \times [PG_{ss}]$$

$$=k_c(20) \times [PG_0]$$

$$=0.085 \text{ mg PG per mg hydroxyproline per day}$$

This rate is sufficient to replace ~3.9% of the total proteoglycans in the tissue per day. The DNA content per mg hydroxyproline was constant for all culture conditions, ~35 µg per mg hydroxyproline (Luyten et al., 1988). Assuming that each cell contains an average of about 9 pg DNA (Kimura et al., 1981), the proteoglycan synthetic rate in the cultures with 20 ng/ml IGF-I was approximately 22 pg per cell per day.

The parameters for the other culture conditions can now be determined. For cultures with 5 ng/ml IGF-I, $k_c(5)=k_c(20)$ since the catabolic curves were the same, and from Figure 7.2c, the synthetic rate constant, $k_s(5)$ is calculated as*:

$$k_s(5)=0.7 \times k_s(20)$$

Therefore, from equation 2, the proteoglycan concentration at steady state would be:

$$[PG_{ss}(5)]=k_s(5)/k_c(5)=0.7 \times k_s(20)/k_c(20)$$

$$=0.7 \times [PG_{ss}(20)]=0.7 \times [PG_0]$$

The closed solution to equation 5 with these parameters gives the dashed curve (Figure 7.2a) for the predicted change in proteoglycan concentration with time in the cultures with 5 ng/ml IGF-I.

Similarly, for basal medium, $k_s(0)=0.15 \times k_s(20)$, (Figure 7.2c), and the $k_c(0)$ can be calculated to be ~0.0714 per day from the half life value of ~9.7 days (Figure 7.2b) as shown in equation 6 for the 20 ng/ml cultures. Equation 5 with these parameters gives the dashed curve (Figure 7.2a) for the predicted change in proteoglycan concentration with time in cultures in basal medium.

As can be seen, the theoretical curves (dashed lines, Figure 7.2a) for the proteoglycan concentrations in the cultures with 0 or 5 ng/ml IGF-I agree rather well with the data, and both of these culture conditions appeared to be approaching the expected steady state

---

* Although in this experiment the rate of synthesis for the cultures with 20 ng/ml IGF-I increased somewhat with time, for the purpose of these analyses the indicated average $k_s(20)$ was used.

concentrations after 5 weeks. This suggests that the single assumption stated above, namely that $[PG_0]$ for the metabolically active pool is nearly equivalent to the entire population of proteoglycans in the tissue, is reasonable for these cultures with cartilage from young animals. Direct measurements of the amounts of glycosaminoglycan released into the culture medium for similar cultures in steady state support this conclusion (Morales and Hascall, 1988). The metabolically active proteoglycan pool in cultures of articular cartilage from older animals, however, is much smaller than the total proteoglycan content (see below).

Another important result in this experiment is that the concentration of IGF-I required to affect catabolic parameters is less than that which affects synthetic rates. Thus, 5 ng/ml IGF-I has a maximum effect on slowing the catabolic rates, but only stimulates synthesis to ~70% of maximum. When dose curves for both parameters were done, the IGF-I concentrations for half maximal effects were ~1.5 and ~4.5 ng/ml for catabolic and synthetic rates respectively (Luyten et al., 1988). Thus, the mechanisms for regulating synthetic and catabolic rates can be uncoupled experimentally.

PROTEOGLYCAN METABOLISM IN CARTILAGE FROM OLDER ANIMALS

Experiments such as those in Figure 7.2 can be used to measure k_s and k_c under a variety of conditions. If steady state criteria are satisfied, these values provide a direct estimate of the size of the metabolically active pool of proteoglycans (equation 2). As noted above, for explant cultures from young animals, the metabolic pool can represent most of the proteoglycans in the tissue. While this approach has not been rigorously applied to study the effect of animal age on these parameters, other lines of investigation indicate that it is likely that the metabolic pool will be considerably less than the total proteoglycan pool in cartilage from older individuals. For example, bovine cartilage explants from young (~1-week-old) and mature (~5-year-old) animals were pulse-labelled with ^{35}S-sulphate and chased for times up to 18 days (Handley, unpublished). Tissue for each animal was processed and sectioned for radioautography at different chase times. The incorporated radioactivity rapidly distributed throughout the matrix in the tissue from the young animal, a result similar to that reported earlier (Hardingham and Muir, 1972). However, in the tissue from the older animal the radioactivity remained more localised near the cells, most probably limited primarily to the territorial matrix. In both cases, there was a gradual loss with time of total radioactivity in tissue from young and old animals (half lives of ~28 and ~7 days, respectively) reflecting active catabolism of proteoglycans in the metabolically active pool.

Similar experiments with tissue from human articular cartilage show the same general results (Bayliss, 1992). In this case, explants of normal cartilage from a 9-year-old and a 60-year-old were radiolabelled with ^{35}S-sulphate for 4 h and either prepared for radioautography at the end of radiolabelling or after a 20 h chase. For both tissues, the radioactivity was closely associated with the cells after the radiolabelling period. For the tissue from the 60-year-old, the radiolabel remained close to the cells after the chase, while in the tissue from the 9-year-old it became widely dispersed into the matrix.

The simplest hypothesis to explain this age-related difference is to assume that the proteoglycans in the older individuals are divided into two distinct pools, a metabolically active pool and a metabolically inert pool. If the former constitutes the proteoglycans primarily in the territorial, and the latter those in the interterritorial regions, then it is likely that only a minority of the total proteoglycans are actively being turned over since the territorial matrix constitutes a small proportion of the total matrix (Hunziker, 1992). Experiments (Maroudas et al., 1992) measuring the rate of racemization of aspartic acid in proteoglycans isolated from articular cartilage of humans of different ages also suggest that a large proportion of the proteoglycans reside in a pool with a very low rate of turnover.

One consequence of a two-pool model is that structural damage to the proteoglycans in the territorial matrix could be repaired by metabolic replacement processes over relatively short time spans whereas structural damage to proteoglycans in the interterritorial matrix would be cumulative over long time periods. Such damage to proteoglycan monomers in aggregates in the metabolically inert pool would lead to foreshortening of the core protein, with the cleaved C-terminal portion being released from the tissue while the N-terminal portion with the HA-binding domain remains bound to HA in the matrix. This is consistent with early models for proteoglycan structure in which it was proposed that the proteoglycan monomers isolated from hyaline cartilages exhibited a continuous distribution of core protein sizes to account for the enrichment of chondroitin sulphate in larger proteoglycans and keratan sulphate in smaller proteoglycans (Hascall and Sajdera, 1970; Rosenberg et al., 1976). The two-pool model also poses a difficult problem for experimental strategies based upon promoting repair of damaged, or matrix depleted cartilage by endogenous chondrocytes. The proportion of matrix repaired may be limited if the metabolic control of the cells extends only through the territorial matrix.

CATABOLISM OF PROTEOGLYCANS IN ARTICULAR CARTILAGE

The explant cultures of articular cartilage provide a closed system such that products of catabolism released into the culture medium can be quantitated and analysed, as can the molecules retained in the matrix. The quantitative data for radiolabel-chase experiments can be used to measure kinetic parameters as discussed in the previous section, and structural data can be used to determine constraints on proposed mechanisms. Such an experimental approach involves metabolic radiolabelling of cultures in steady state with ^{35}S-sulphate to label proteoglycans and with a ^{3}H precursor such as ^{3}H-glucosamine or ^{3}H-acetate to label hyaluronan as well as proteoglycans. The cultures are washed to remove precursors and chased for 2 days to remove a small, rapid turnover pool of proteoglycans (perhaps cell surface proteoglycans) (Campbell et al., 1984; Hascall et al., 1983b). Culture medium samples are collected daily, and tissue samples are analysed after various times in culture.

Molecular sieve analyses of dissociative extracts of tissue shortly after radiolabelling revealed (Campbell et al., 1984) a major peak with large hydrodynamic size for aggrecan and a minor peak (~10% of the ^{35}S) for the smaller interstitial proteoglycans, decorin and biglycan. The rate of loss of these smaller proteoglycans from the tissue is significantly slower than that for aggrecan (Campbell *et al.*, 1984) indicating that their catabolic mechanism differs from that for aggrecan. This probably reflects the distinctly different organisations of these two different classes of proteoglycan in the cartilage matrix. Aggrecan is present in aggregate structures with hyaluronan and link protein, while the small proteoglycans appear to be primarily associated with collagen fibrils (Scott, 1988). Further, the size distribution of the radiolabelled aggrecan extracted from the tissue does not change after long chase times, even when more than 50% of the labelled aggrecan molecules have been lost from the tissue (Hascall *et al.*, 1983b). These data and other analyses indicate that the catabolic mechanism for aggrecan is *conservative*, i.e. entire proteoglycan molecules are catabolised while those left in the matrix remain intact.

Between 90–95% of the radiolabel present in the medium any day during the chase period elutes as a broad, high molecular weight peak, but with smaller average hydrodynamic size than for intact aggrecan in tissue extracts. The remaining 5–10% of the radioactivity elutes as free radiosulphate in the total column volume (Campbell *et al.*, 1984; Hascall *et al.*, 1983b). The free radiosulphate reflects that proportion of the catabolised proteoglycans which were endocytosed by the chondrocytes and totally degraded in lysosomes. Re-utilisation of radiosulphate by the cells is negligible (Hascall *et al.*, 1983a; Campbell *et al.*, 1984). The average sizes of the individual glycosaminoglycan chains after release from the protein core are the same in both medium and extract proteoglycan species indicating that endoglycosidic cleavage of the glycosaminoglycans is not part of the catabolic mechanism. Only a small proportion of the released proteoglycans will aggregate with hyaluronan in contrast with intact aggrecan molecules. Thus, most of the catabolised aggrecan molecules are recovered in the culture medium as macromolecules which have been partially degraded by the proteolytic mechanism described below.

Inhibition of cellular and peptidase activity by the inclusion of cycloheximide or cytocidal proteinase inhibitors in the medium of cartilage explants markedly decreases the rate of loss (to less than ~50% of normal) of aggrecan from the extracellular matrix of cartilage explant cultures (Bolis *et al.*, 1989). A large proportion of the aggrecan macromolecules appearing in the medium of such cultures are able to aggregate with hyaluronan, indicating that they contain functional G1 domains and hence the N-terminal region of the core protein (Bolis *et al.*, 1989). Thus, cellular activity is necessary to generate the aggrecan fragments observed in metabolically viable explants. The results also show that small amounts of functional aggrecan molecules can be lost from the extracellular matrix by passive means, probably as proteoglycan aggregates, and this probably accounts for the small amount of functional aggrecan molecules recovered in the medium from metabolically inactive explant cultures.

PROTEASES THAT CATABOLISE AGGRECAN

N-Terminal amino acid sequence data of the aggrecan macromolecules lost to the medium of bovine cartilage explant cultures from both immature and mature animals revealed a number of specific proteolytic cleavage sites within the core protein. A major cleavage site occurs between a glutamate–alanine bond in the interglobular region between the G1 and G2 domains (Sandy *et al.*, 1991; Ilic *et al.*, 1992; Loulakis *et al.*, 1992) (Figure 7.3). This bond occurs at Glu^{373}–Ala^{374} assuming human aggrecan sequence enumeration and a N-terminus at valine 20 (Doege *et al.*, 1991). This site has also been implicated in the catabolism of human and bovine aggrecan *in vivo* since aggrecan core protein fragments with similar mobility on SDS-PAGE (Ilic *et al.*, 1992; Sandy *et al.*, 1992) and with the corresponding N-terminal amino-acid sequences (Sandy *et al.*, 1992) have been isolated from the synovial fluid from these species. Two other predominant cleavage sites in the core protein of aggrecan have been identified (Sandy *et al.*, 1991, 1992; Ilic *et al.*, 1992; Loulakis *et al.*, 1992) (see Figure 7.3). These are located in the chondroitin sulphate attachment domain between glutamate and alanine (residues 1819–1820) and glutamate and leucine (residues 1919–1920 of human aggrecan). A third possible site in this region (between glutamate and glycine, residues 1714–1715) has also

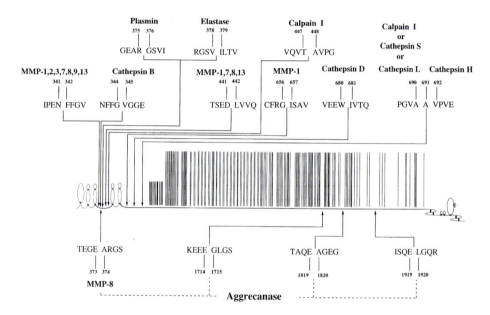

FIGURE 7.3 *Summary of the known cleavage points for "aggrecanase" and purified proteinases on aggrecan core protein.* Data on the cleavage points shown was obtained from the following references: "Aggrecanase" (Sandy *et al.*, 1991; Ilic *et al.*, 1992; Loulakis *et al.*, 1992); MMP-1 (Flannery and Sandy, 1993); MMP-2 (Flannery *et al.*, 1992a; Fosang *et al.*, 1992); MMP-3 (Flannery *et al.*, 1992a; Flannery and Sandy, 1993); MMP-7 (Flannery *et al.*, 1992a); MMP-8 (Fosang *et al.*, 1994; Arner *et al.*, 1997); MMP-9 (Flannery *et al.*, 1992a; Flannery and Sandy, 1993); MMP-13 (Flannery and Sandy, 1995; Fosang *et al.*, 1996); Cathepsin B (Flannery *et al.*, 1992a; Fosang *et al.*, 1992; Flannery and Sandy, 1993); Cathepsins D, L, H and S and Plasmin (Flannery and Sandy, 1993); Calpain 1 (Suzuki *et al.*, 1994, 1995); Elastase (Mok *et al.*, 1992). The residue numbers were calculated assuming that residue 1 corresponds to valine-20 in the original sequence analysis (Doege *et al.*, 1991). The figure shows each proteinase adjacent to the residue numbers and sequence of the bond cleaved. For example, MMPs 1, 2, 3, 7, 8, 9,13 (top left) cleave the bond between asparagine (N)-341 and phenylalanine (F)-342. The lines denoting potential keratan sulphate and chondroitin sulphate substitution sites (as shown in Figure 7.1) in this case are projected from only one side to illustrate "aggrecanase" sites of cleavage more clearly.

been identified (Loulakis *et al.*, 1992). The similarity in amino acid sequences around these sites (TEGE-ARGS, KEEE-GLGS, TAQE-AGEG and ISQE-LGQR) suggests that there may be only one endopeptidase involved in this critical step in the catabolic mechanism, and this protease has been given the name 'aggrecanase' (Figure 7.3). The same activity, leading to the generation of fragments with the above mentioned N-terminals of ARGS, AGEG and LGQR, has now also been described in all zones of fetal bovine growth plate explants treated with retinoic acid to promote aggrecan catabolism (Plaas and Sandy, 1993).

Digestion of aggrecan with physiologic concentrations of MMPs 1, 2, 3, 7, 8, 9 and 13 and a range of cathepsins, serine proteinases and calpain 1 has so far failed to produce products with the N-terminal sequences generated by aggrecanase (see Figure 7.3 legend for references). However, digestion of aggrecan with high concentrations of MMP-8 has been shown to generate a minor product with the N-terminal of Ala 374 (Fosang *et al.*, 1994). This finding suggests that aggrecanase may share some properties in common with MMP-8. However, potent inhibitors of the MMP-8 cleavage of aggrecan at the aggrecanase site do not prevent this cleavage by aggrecanase in IL-1 treated cartilage (Arner *et al.*, 1997), suggesting that MMP-8 is not the cartilage aggrecanase. Nonetheless, support for the involvement of an MMP in the IL-1 response in bovine explants has come from the finding (Bonassar *et al.*, 1997) that the release from the tissue of aggrecanase-generated G1 domain can be markedly inhibited by the inclusion of 4 µm TIMP-1 in the medium. In addition, a study of the effects of a range of potent low molecular weight MMP inhibitors on cytokine induced proteoglycan release from bovine explants has suggested that a collagenase-like MMP rather than a gelatinase-like MMP is involved (Brown *et al.*, 1996). On the other hand, a lipophilic inhibitor of cysteine endopeptidases (E64d) can also reduce aggrecan degradation in IL-1 treated explants whereas the inhibitor is ineffective without the lipophilic group (Buttle *et al.*, 1992). These results suggest that aggrecanase, or an activator of aggrecanase, may be a cysteine proteinase located in or close to the cell membrane.

Two predominant radiolabelled aggrecan core protein species (observed after chondroitinase digestion) are recovered in the extracts from cultures of bovine articular cartilage from mature animals (Figure 7.4) (Ilic *et al.*, 1992). Both have N-terminal amino acid sequences from the N-terminus of the G1 domain. The larger represents intact aggrecan core protein and the smaller the same macromolecule, but most likely without the C-terminal G3 globular region (Ilic *et al.*, 1992). No radiolabelled aggrecan molecules were observed in the *tissue extracts* that correspond to any of the catabolic cleavage sites discussed above (Figure 7.3). However, additional, smaller core protein fragments without radiolabel, but with functional G1 domains were observed in matrix extracts. The results suggest that proteolytic cleavage of the metabolically active aggrecan pool occurs at all three (or four) of the sites discussed above (see Figure 7.3). However, aggrecan molecules residing in the metabolically slower (or inactive) pool within the inter-territorial matrix of the tissue appear to undergo some additional proteolytic cleavage within the chondroitin sulphate attachment domain, and presumably accumulate over a much longer time of residence in the tissue. These data support the hypothesis that catabolism of aggrecan in the metabolically active pool is conservative (i.e. all or nothing), and that there are two metabolic pools in articular cartilage from older (mature) animals.

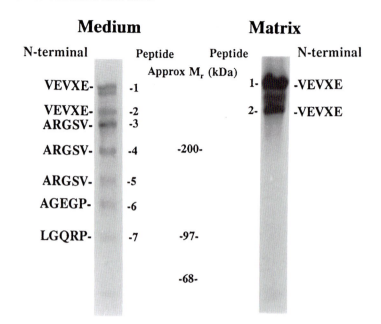

FIGURE 7.4   *Resolution of chondroitinase digested, metabolically radiolabelled proteoglycans isolated from the tissue (Matrix) or from the culture medium (Medium) of explant cultures.* The indicated bands were sequenced, yielding the N-terminal sequences noted beside each band. Band 1 represents intact core proteins; band 2, core proteins with intact N-terminus, but most likely lacking the G3 globular domain; band 3 the product of cleavage by 'aggrecanase' at residues 373–374; band 4, the product of cleavage at both 373–374 and probably 1919–1920; band 5, the product of cleavage at both 373–374 and probably 1819–1820; band 6, cleavage at 1819–1820; and band 7, cleavage at 1919–1920 (modified from data in reference Ilic *et al.* (1992) with permission).

CATABOLISM OF HYALURONAN IN AGGREGATES

Hyaluronan does not contain sulphate esters and is therefore not labelled with radio-sulphate. Thus, precursors which radiolabel hyaluronan, ^{3}H-glucosamine (Morales and Hascall, 1988) and ^{3}H-acetate (Ng *et al.*, 1992), have been used to study metabolism of this glycosaminoglycan in cartilage explants. Both of these precursors radiolabel the UDP-N-acetylhexosamine in the metabolic precursor pool for glycosaminoglycan synthesis. Because UDP-glcNAc (precursor for hyaluronan) and UDP-galNAc (precursor for chondroitin sulphate) are equilibrated by an epimerase, the specific radioactivity of the hexosamines in the chondroitin sulphate and hyaluronan incorporated during the labelling period are the same. Therefore, the ratio of radiolabel in the two glycosaminoglycans is equal to the ratio of their masses synthesised.

A label-chase experiment was done with ^{35}S-sulphate and ^{3}H-glucosamine, and tissue was isolated at different times during the chase (Morales and Hascall, 1988). Procedures using highly purified collagenase and associative extraction, followed by velocity and equilibrium density gradient centrifugation were used to purify native aggregates. The final preparations contained nearly 40% of the total aggregate originally in the tissue and were therefore considered representative. The chemical ratio of hyaluronan to chondroitin sulphate in the aggregates was ~1:32. The ^{3}H-labelling ratio was the same at all chase times and equivalent to the chemical ratio. Further, the ^{3}H half lives for both hyaluronan and proteoglycan in the aggregates were ~18 days, the same as for the ^{35}S-activity in proteoglycans. These data indicate that those newly synthesised hyaluronan and aggrecan molecules that are organised into aggregates are synthesised at rates proportional to their mass ratios in aggregates, and subsequently they are catabolised with identical kinetics. There is, however, a second, rapid turnover pool of hyaluronan in the tissue (Ng et al., 1989). Approximately 30–40% of the newly synthesised hyaluronan in explants is released into the medium within a few hours after synthesis. Little is yet known about this metabolic pool of hyaluronan, although it is possible that some of this may be synthesised by chondrocytes originally in the superficial layers and could contribute to the hyaluronan normally present in synovial fluid.

Later experiments using ^{3}H-acetate as a precursor also showed that catabolic rates of hyaluronan and aggrecan were the same under steady state conditions (Ng et al., 1992). Importantly, both studies (Morales and Hascall, 1988; Ng et al., 1992) showed that the culture medium compartment did not contain significant amounts of radiolabelled hyaluronan fragments for chase times greater than 2 days. Thus, unlike aggrecan, where ~95% of the molecules appear in the medium in a degraded, but macromolecular form, essentially none of the radiolabelled hyaluronan molecules in aggregates which are catabolised leave the tissue. This indicates that the catabolism of hyaluronan involves internalisation by the cells and eventually complete degradation in lysosomes.

The hyaluronan that is synthesised and organised into aggregates has a molecular weight distribution that is higher than that of the unlabelled hyaluronan in the tissue (Ng et al., 1992). In the explant matrix, the newly radiolabelled hyaluronan undergoes partial, random depolymerisation such that the high molecular weight hyaluronan species (excluded on Sephacryl 1000) disappears with a half life that is somewhat faster (~7 days) than the half lives for aggrecan and hyaluronan in the matrix. This depolymerisation process depends upon cellular viability. This suggests that scission of hyaluronan may be involved in the catabolic mechanism.

MODEL FOR CATABOLISM OF PROTEOGLYCAN AGGREGATES

The results described above suggest that catabolism of proteoglycan aggregates in the metabolically active pool is normally controlled by the chondrocyte at sites on or near the cell surface. The catabolic unit would contain a hyaluronan-binding component which can bind to an open region of hyaluronan in an accessible aggregate (Figure 7.5). The hyaluronan could be cleaved as part of a process which eventually leads to complete degradation of the aggregate in one direction or the other along the cleaved hyaluronan strand depending on the polarity of the mechanism. This would contribute to the observed depolymerisation of the initially high molecular weight of hyaluronan in newly synthesised aggregates. As part of the mechanism, the hyaluronan would be internalised,

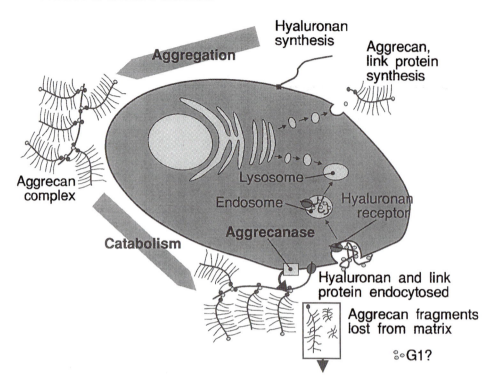

FIGURE 7.5   *Schematic model for aggrecan and hyaluronan (hyaluronan) synthesis and catabolism in cartilage.* See text for discussion.

perhaps partially depolymerised by endoglycosidases, and eventually completely degraded in lysosomes. The catabolic unit must also contain an endopeptidase ('aggrecanase') with specificity for the cleavages observed on the aggrecan degradation fragments. This protease could be anchored to the plasma membrane or localised near the cell surface. Whatever the mechanism, its activity must be restricted to aggrecan molecules on aggregates actively being catabolised since loss of aggrecan from the tissue and internalisation of hyaluronan for degradation are stoichiometric. The frequency that a catabolic unit would encounter an aggregate would depend upon the concentration of aggregate in the accessible matrix and thereby be consistent with the observed first-order kinetics of catabolism (see Figure 7.2). If the catabolic unit were located on a cell process, then the range of matrix susceptible to catabolism could extend throughout the territorial matrix in older animals (Hunziker, 1992) and even further in younger animals.

   In support of this model, a mechanism for degrading hyaluronan similar to that proposed above has been identified for cells with one of the isoforms of the cell surface receptor CD44 (Culty *et al.*, 1992). This receptor binds hyaluronan so that it can be internalised and degraded. Recent work with cultures of chondrocytes from bovine articular cartilage revealed that these cells can also endocytose and degrade hyaluronan by the same mechanism (Hua *et al.*, 1993; Chow *et al.*, 1995).

There are two other pieces of the puzzle, namely the hyaluran-binding proteins (G1 domain of aggrecan and the link protein). Recent work (Tester *et al.*, submitted) has shown that newly synthesised link protein is turned over within the extracellular matrix of explant cultures of articular cartilage at a similar rate to the newly synthesised pool of aggrecan. Furthermore, virtually no radiolabelled link protein was observed to be present in the medium of the cultures which strongly points to the internalisation of this matrix protein by chondrocytes, possibly associated with hyaluronan. This work is further evidence that the catabolism of newly synthesised aggrecan complexes occurs in a coordinated manner. To date nothing is known about the fate of the G1 domain within the newly synthesised pool of aggrecan, but in the light of the studies on link protein it is likely also to be internalised by chondrocytes.

Immunological studies of pig laryngeal cartilage explants indicate that a proportion of both the G1 and link protein can be recovered in the culture medium (Fosang *et al.*, 1991). It is possible that these molecules originate from action of aggrecanase on the pool of aggrecan complexes within the inter-territorial region of the matrix and thus are not able to be internalised because of their physical distance from the chondrocytes (see also the section 'Non steady state proteoglycan metabolism' below).

Degradation of aggregates in the metabolically inert pool also occurs over long time periods, perhaps time frames approaching the mature lifetime of the individual. This can occur by a number of mechanisms; from proteases released as a result of cell death or injury responses, free radical reactions, mechanical damage, activation of latent enzymes such as stromelysin bound to matrix components, etc. Any cleavage in the glycosaminoglycan-attachment region would release the C-terminal fragment from the aggregate allowing it to diffuse from the tissue. The N-terminal fragment, remaining bound to hyaluronan, would be retained. The consequence of this process would be the accumulation of a polydisperse population of aggrecan molecules with the G1 binding domain (minimally) and varying lengths of the G2 and the glycosaminoglycan attachment regions (Hascall and Sajdera, 1970; Rosenberg *et al.*, 1976; Flannery *et al.*, 1992a; Roughley *et al.*, 1992). Chemical evidence for such polydisperse populations led to the early models of aggrecan which incorporated this foreshortening (Hascall and Sajdera, 1970; Rosenberg *et al.*, 1976). Consistent with this, the quantitation of G3 domain on aggrecan from immature and mature bovine articular cartilage has indicated a marked aged-dependent reduction in the G3 content of G1-bearing molecules (Flannery *et al.*, 1992b).

Evidence has also been obtained on the structure of the accumulated G1 domain (Flannery *et al.*, 1992a) and partially degraded link protein (Roughley *et al.*, 1992; Hughes *et al.*, 1992) in tissue from older individuals. Analyses by C-terminal identification and peptide quantitation (Flannery *et al.*, 1992a) have indicated that a small proportion of the accumulated G1 domain is a product of the action of one or more of the matrix metalloproteinases, all of which (MMP-1, 2, 3, 7, 9, 9 and 13) cleave the same asparagine–phenylalanine bond (residues 341–342 of human aggrecan) in the interglobular domain (Figure 7.3). The C-terminal sequences for all of the accumulated G1 domain populations remain to be determined. In a similar way, characterisation of the degraded form of link protein (LP3) in adult cartilage (Hughes *et al.*, 1992) has suggested that the MMP-3-generated product is quantitatively minor, and that other as yet unidentified proteolytic agents appear to be responsible for link protein degradation in the long-lived, metabolically inactive pool.

Analyses of 'reporter' peptides (Flannery *et al.*, 1992b) in tryptic digests of aggrecan from calf chondrocyte cultures have shown that the newly synthesised molecules have a markedly higher G3 domain content than the aggrecan present in the matrix of calf cartilage, which in turn was higher than that in steer cartilage. In addition, analyses of the two sub-populations of aggrecan present in steer cartilage, and separable by agarose gel electrophoresis, showed that the faster migrating band has a lower content of G3 domain. Taken together, these results are consistent with the slow accumulation of truncated proteoglycans in the metabolically inactive pool.

CLINICAL IMPLICATIONS

Aggrecan degradation products are released from articular cartilage into synovial fluid (Ilic *et al.*, 1992; Sandy *et al.*, 1992). Analyses of these products indicate that the processes described for the explant cultures operate *in vivo* in a range of joint diseases (Lohmander *et al.*, 1993). N-terminal sequence analyses of aggrecan fragments present in the synovial fluid of patients with joint injury, osteoarthritis, acute pyrophosphate arthritis, reactive arthritis, psoriatic arthritis, and juvenile rheumatoid arthritis show that a sizeable proportion were generated by the 'aggrecanase' involved in catabolism of the metabolically active pool. If the half life of the metabolically active pool is similar *in vivo* to that measured *in vitro*, then most of the released fragments in synovial fluid represent aggrecan molecules which have resided in the tissue for only a few weeks. It is important to note that the chemistry of these fragments, then, will not be representative of the chemistry of the bulk of the aggrecan molecules in the tissue, which in general have much longer residence times. These fragments can, however, provide valuable information about metabolic changes that can occur in cartilage as a consequence of pathobiological changes, and several laboratories are studying them to identify markers for early osteoarthritic events (Lohmander, 1992; Thonar *et al.*, 1992; Shinmei *et al.*, 1992).

NON STEADY STATE PROTEOGLYCAN METABOLISM

The metabolism of aggrecan can be altered away from steady state in explant cultures by various procedures that may mimic pathological mechanisms. For example, when basal medium is used, aggrecan synthesis is decreased and catabolism increased as was analysed in detail above. The addition of lipopolysaccharide (Morales *et al.*, 1984; Morales and Hascall, 1989), interleukin-1 (Tyler, 1989; Morales and Hascall, 1989; Fosang *et al.*, 1991) or retinoic acid (Campbell and Handley, 1987a,b; Morales and Roberts, 1992) to culture medium which would otherwise maintain steady state likewise suppresses synthesis and accelerates catabolism of aggrecan. All these conditions appear to have a relatively selective effect on aggrecan metabolism. For example, synthesis of the small proteoglycans is not altered by retinoic acid treatment (Campbell and Handley, 1987a), and general protein synthesis is minimally affected by either interleukin-1, lipopoly-saccharides or retinoic acid. In all cases aggrecan synthesis increases and catabolism decreases when the culture medium is restored to steady state conditions, provided that the treatment was not prolonged for more than 1–2 weeks. Usually the tissue does not return to the original levels of proteoglycan metabolism, however.

Non-steady state degradation of aggrecan in bovine explants by addition of interleukin-1 or retinoic acid results in an increased release of the aggrecan G1 domain and hyaluronan as well as chondroitin sulphate bearing fragments into the medium (Bonassar *et al.*, 1997). Under these conditions it would appear that the aggrecanase activity is uncoupled from the control of the cell associated catabolic unit described in the model (Figure 7.5) and that products can diffuse directly out of the tissue. The degradative events induced by IL-1 and retinoic acid appear to be similar with respect to the aggrecan matrix. However, IL-1 treatment alone induces rapid swelling of the collagen network (Bonassar *et al.*, 1997). This swelling can also be induced by MMP-3 cleavage of the telopeptide region of Type II collagen in explants (Bonassar *et al.*, 1995). In addition, MMP-1 dependent cleavage and "unwinding" of the triple helical region also appears to occur in IL-1 treated explants as determined by the appearance of epitopes reactive with an antibody (COL2-3/4m) to a sequence which is normally hidden in native collagen (Hollander *et al.*, 1994).

It is interesting that the collagen network appears to remain intact in these experimental conditions for at least 1–2 weeks as monitored by loss of collagen peptides (hydroxyproline) into the medium. After this time there is less ability for the aggrecan metabolic responses to recover when the reagent is removed. This suggests that integrity of the collagen network may be a key element for regulating chondrocyte metabolism of proteoglycans. This is also suggested by experiments in which highly purified collagenase was used to disrupt the collagen network of explants to a limited extent. Chondrocytes in such cultures became mitogenic when exposed to growth factors (basic fibroblast growth factor, epidermal growth factor) whereas in other cultures treated with trypsin to remove proteoglycans while leaving the collagen intact, they did not (Scully, S., Hascall, V. and Bolander, M., unpublished). Further, trypsin treated cultures maintain high steady state levels of proteoglycan synthesis and decrease their catabolic rate, as would be expected for a first order process, leading to net increase of proteoglycan in the tissue with time (Hascall *et al.*, 1983b). Thus, chondrocytes respond to losses of proteoglycans in their matrix by different processes (maintenance) than they do to damage of the collagen network (repair, mitosis).

CONCLUDING REMARKS

The purpose of this chapter, in part, is to present a provocative model for a normal catabolic unit located in or near the plasma membrane of the chondrocyte (Figure 7.5). This model does satisfy the constraints imposed upon it by the experimental data, but like most models it only deserves considerable scepticism until additional experimental constraints confirm or deny various of its aspects. Since the model treats the tissue as if it were isotropic, it clearly represents an over-simplification, and detailed information for different regions, from the superficial to deep zones of the articular cartilage, will be needed to evaluate the validity of the concepts at each level. We hope, however, that this chapter does demonstrate the utility of the explant model and of the steady state approach to the analysis of the experimental data.

REFERENCES

Arner, E.C., Decicco, C.P., Cherney, R. and Tortorella, M.D. (1997). Cleavage of native cartilage aggrecan by neutrophil collagenase (MMP-8) is distinct from endogenous cleavage by aggrecanase. *J. Biol. Chem.*, **272**, 9294–9299.

Bayliss, M.T. (1992) Metabolism of animal and human osteoarthritic cartilage. In: *Articular Cartilage and Osteoarthritis*, (Kuettner, K., Schleyerbach, R., Peyron, J.G. and Hascall, V.C., eds), pp. 487–500. New York: Raven Press.

Bolis, S., Handley, C.J. and Comper, W.D. (1989) Passive loss of proteoglycan from articular cartilage explants. *Biochem. Biophys. Acta*, **993**, 157–167.

Bonassar, L.J., Frank, E.H., Murray, J.C., Paguio, C.G., Moore, V.L., Lark, M.W., Sandy, J.D., Wu, J.J., Eyre, D.R. and Grodzinsky, A.J. (1995) Changes in cartilage composition and physical properties due to stromelysin degradation. *Arth. Rheum.*, **38**, 173–183.

Bonassar, L.J., Sandy, J.D., Lark, M.W., Plaas, A.H.K., Frank, E.H. and Grodzinsky, A.J. (1997) Inhibition of cartilage degradation and changes in physical properties induced by IL-1b and retinoic acid using matrix metalloproteinase inhibitors. *Arch. Biochem. Biophys.*, **344**, 404–412.

Brown, C.J., Rahman, S., Morton, A., Beauchamp, C.L., Bramwell, H. and Buttle, D.J. (1996) Inhibitors of collagenase but not of gelatinase reduce cartilage explant proteoglycan breakdown despite only low levels of MMP activity. *J. Clin. Pathol.: Mol. Pathol.*, **49**, M331–339.

Buttle, D.J., Saklatvala, J., Tamai, M. and Barrett, A.J. (1992) Inhibition of interleukin 1-stimulated cartilage proteoglycan degradation by lipophilic inactivator of cysteine endopeptidases. *Biochem. J.*, **281**, 175–177.

Campbell, M.A. and Handley, C.J. (1987a) The effect of retinoic acid on proteoglycan biosynthesis in bovine articular cartilage cultures. *Arch. Biochem. Biophys.*, **253**, 462–474.

Campbell, M.A. and Handley, C.J. (1987b) The effect of retinoic acid on the turnover of proteoglycans in cultured articular cartilage. *Arch. Biochem. Biophys.*, **258**, 143–155.

Campbell, M.A., Handley, C.J., Hascall, V.C., Campbell, R.A. and Lowther, D.A. (1984) Turnover of proteoglycans in cultures of bovine articular cartilage. *Arch. Biochem. Biophys.*, **234**, 275–281.

Chow, G., Knudson, C.B., Homandberg, G. and Knudson, W. (1995) Increased expression of CD44 in bovine articular chondrocytes by catabolic cellular mediators. *J. Biol. Chem.*, **270**, 27734–27741.

Culty, M., Nguyen, N.A. and Underhill, C.B. (1992) The hyaluronan receptor (CD44) participates in the uptake and degradation of hyaluronan. *J. Cell Biol.*, **116**, 1055–1062.

Doege, K., Sasaki, M., Kimura, T. and Yamada, Y. (1991) Complete coding sequence and deduced primary structure of the human cartilage large aggregating proteoglycan, aggrecan. *J. Biol. Chem.*, **266**, 894–902.

Flannery, C.R., Lark, M.W. and Sandy, J.D. (1992a) Identification of a stromelysin cleavage site within the interglobular domain of human aggrecan: Evidence for proteolysis at this site *in vivo* in human articular cartilage. *J. Biol. Chem.*, **267**, 1008–1014.

Flannery, C.R. and Sandy, J.D. (1995) Identification of MMP-13 (collagenase-3) as the major matrix metalloproteinase expressed by chondrocytes during retinoic acid-induced matrix catabolism. *Trans. Orthop. Res. Soc.*, **20**, 102.

Flannery, C.R. and Sandy, J.D. (1993) Aggrecan catabolism in cartilage: studies on the nature of a novel proteinase ("Aggrecanase") which cleaves the Glu373-Ala374 bond of the interglobular domain. *Trans. Orthop. Res. Soc.*, **17**, 677.

Flannery, C.R., Stanescu, V., Morgelin, M., Boynton, R., Gordy, J. and Sandy, J. (1992b) Variability in the G3 domain content of bovine aggrecan from cartilage extracts and chondrocyte cultures. *Arch. Biochem. Biophy.*, **297**, 52–60.

Fosang, A.J., Last, K., Neame, P.J., Murphy, G., Knauper, V., Tschesche, H., Hughes, C., Caterson, B. and Hardingham, T.E. (1994) Neutrophil collagenase (MMP-8) cleaves at the aggrecanase site (E373-A374) in the interglobular domain of cartilage aggrecan. *Biochem. J.*, **304**, 347–351.

Fosang, A.J., Last, K., Knauper, V., Murphy, G. and Neame, P.J. (1996) Degradation of cartilage aggrecan by collagenase-3 (MMP-13). *FEBS Lett.*, **380**, 17–20.

Fosang, A.J., Neame, P.J., Last, K., Hardingham, T.E., Murphy, G. and Hamilton, J.A. (1992) The inter-globular domain of cartilage aggrecan is cleaved by PUMP, gelatinases and cathepsin B. *J. Biol. Chem.*, **267**, 19470–19474.

Fosang, A.J., Tyler, J.A. and Hardingham, T.E. (1991) Effect of interleukin-1 and insulin-like growth factor-I on the release of proteoglycan components and hyaluronan from pig articular cartilage in explant culture. *Matrix*, **11**, 17–24.

Hardingham, T.E. and Muir, H. (1972) Biosynthesis of proteoglycans in slices: fractionation by gel chromatography and equilibrium density gradient centrifugation. *Biochem. J.*, **126**, 791–803.

Hascall, V.C. (1988) Proteoglycans: the chondroitin sulfate/keratan sulfate proteoglycan of cartilage. *ISI Atlas of Science: Biochemistry*, **1**, 189–198.

Hascall, V.C., Handley, C.J., McQuillan, D.J., Robinson, H.C. and Lowther, D.A. (1983a) The effect of serum on biosynthesis of proteoglycans by bovine articular cartilage in culture. *Arch. Biochem. Biophys.*, **224**, 206–223.

Hascall, V.C., Luyten, F.P., Plaas, A.H.K. and Sandy, J.D. (1990) Steady state metabolism of proteoglycans in bovine articular cartilage explants. In: *Methods in Cartilage Research*, (Maroudas, A. and Kuettner, K., eds), pp. 108–112. NY: Academic Press.

Hascall, V.C., Morales, T.I., Hascall, G.K., Handley, C.J. and McQuillan, D.J. (1983b) Biosynthesis and turnover of proteoglycans in organ culture of bovine articular cartilage. *J. Rheum.*, **11**, 45–52.

Hascall, V.C. and Sajdera, S.W. (1970) Physical properties and polydispersity of proteoglycans from bovine nasal cartilage. *J. Biol. Chem.*, **245**, 4920–4930.

Hollander, A.P., Heathfield, T.F., Webber, C., Iwata, Y., Bourne, R., Rorabeck, C. and Poole, A.R. (1994) Increased damage to Type II collagen in osteoarthritic articular cartilage detected by a new immunoassay. *J. Clin. Invest.*, **93**, 1722–1732.

Hua, Q., Knudson, C.B. and Knudson, W. (1993) Internalization of hyaluronan by chondrocytes occurs via receptor-mediated endocytosis. *J. Cell. Sci.*, **106**, 365–375.

Hughes, C.E., Caterson, B., White, R.J., Roughley, P.J. and Mort, J.S. (1992) Monoclonal antibodies recognizing protease-generated neoepitopes from cartilage proteoglycan degradation. *J. Biol. Chem.*, **267**, 16011–16014.

Hunziker, E.B. (1992) *Articular Cartilage and Osteoarthritis* (Kuettner, K.E., Schleyerbach, R., Peyron, J.G. and Hascall, V.C., eds), pp. 183–199. New York: Raven Press.

Ilic, M.Z., Handley, C.J., Robinson, H.C. and Mok, M.T. (1992) Mechanism of catabolism of aggrecan by articular cartilage. *Arch. Biochem. Biophys.*, **294**, 115–122.

Kimura, J.H., Thonar, E.J.-M.A., Hascall, V.C., Reiner, A. and Poole, A.R. (1981) Identification of core protein, an intermediate in proteoglycan biosynthesis in cultured chondrocytes from the Swarm rat chondosarcoma. *J. Biol. Chem.*, **256**, 7890–7897.

Lohmander, L.S. (1992) Molecular markers of cartilage turnover. A role in monitoring and diagnosis of osteoarthritis. In: *Articular Cartilage and Osteoarthritis* (Kuettner, K.E., Schleyerbach, R., Peyron, J.G. and Hascall, V.C., eds), pp. 653–667. New York: Raven Press.

Lohmander, L.S., Neame, P.J. and Sandy, J.D. (1993) The structure of aggrecan fragments in human synovial fluid: evidence that 'aggrecanase' mediates cartilage degradation in inflammatory joint disease, joint injury and osteoarthritis. *Arth. Rheum.*, **36**, 1214–1222.

Loulakis, P., Shrikhande, A., Davis, G. and Maniglia, C.A. (1992) N-terminal sequence of proteoglycan fragments isolated from medium of interleukin-1-treated articular cartilage cultures. Putative site(s) of enzymatic cleavage. *Biochem. J.*, **284**, 589–593.

Luyten, F.P., Hascall, V.C., Nissley, S.P., Morales, T.I. and Reddi, A.H. (1988) Insulin-growth factors maintain steady state metabolism of proteoglycans in bovine articular cartilage explants. *Arch. Biochem. Biophys.*, **267**, 416–425.

Luyten, F.P., Yu, Y.M., Yanagishita, M., Vukicevic, S., Hammonds, R.G. and Reddi, A.H. (1992) Natural bovine osteogenin and recombinant human bone morphogenetic protein-2B are equipotent in the maintenance of proteoglycans in bovine articular cartilage explant cultures. *J. Biol. Chem.*, **267**, 3691–3695.

Maroudas, A., Palla, G. and Gilav, E. (1992) Racemization of aspartic acid in human articular cartilage. *Conn. Tiss. Res.*, **27**, 1–8.

McQuillan, D.J., Handley, C.J., Campbell, M.A., Bollis, S., Milway, V.E. and Herington, A.C. (1986) Stimulation of proteoglycan synthesis by serum and insulin-like growth factor-I in cultured bovine articular cartilage. *Biochem. J.*, **240**, 423–430.

Mok, M.T., Ilic, M.Z., Handley, C.J. and Robinson, H.C. (1992) Cleavage of proteoglycan aggregate by leukocyte elastase. *Arch. Biochem. Biophys.*, **292**, 442–447.

Morales, T.I. and Hascall, V.C. (1988) Correlated metabolism of proteoglycans and hyaluronan in bovine articular cartilage organ cultures. *J. Biol. Chem.*, **263**, 3632–3638.

Morales, T.I. and Hascall, V.C. (1989) Effects of interleukin-1 and lipopolysaccharides on protein and carbohydrate metabolism in bovine articular cartilage organ tissues. *Conn. Tiss. Res.*, **19**, 255–275.

Morales, T.I. and Roberts, A.B. (1992) The interactions between retinoic acid and the transforming growth factor-ß in calf articular cartilage organ cultures. *Arch. Biochem. Biophys.*, **293**, 79–84.

Morales, T.I. and Roberts, A.B. (1988) TGF-ß regulates proteoglycan metabolism in bovine articular cartilage organ cultures. *J. Biol. Chem.*, **263**, 12828–12831.

Morales, T.I., Wahl, L.M. and Hascall, V.C. (1984) The effect of bacterial polysaccharides on the biosynthesis and release of proteoglycans in bovine cartilage organ cultures. *J. Biol. Chem.*, **259**, 6720–6729.

Ng, C.K., Handley, C.J., Mason, R.M. and Robinson, H.C. (1989) Synthesis of hyaluronate in cultured bovine cartilage. *Biochem. J.*, **263**, 761–767.

Ng, C.K., Handley, C.J., Preston, B.P. and Robinson, H.C. (1992) The extracellular processing and catabolism of hyaluronan in cultured adult articular cartilage explants. *Arch. Biochem. Biophys.*, **298**, 70–79.

Plaas, A.K. and Sandy, J.D. (1993) A cartilage explant system for studies on aggrecan structure, biosynthesis and catabolism in discrete zones of the mammalian growth plate. *Matrix*, **13**, 135–147.

Rosenberg, L., Wolfenstein-Todel, C., Margolis, R., Pal, S. and Strider, W. (1976) Structural basis for the polydispersity of proteoglycan sub-unit. *J. Biol. Chem.*, **251**, 6439–6444.

Roughley, P.J., Nguyen, Q. and Mort, J.S. (1992) The role of proteinases and oxygen radicals in the degradation of human articular cartilage. In: *Articular Cartilage and Osteoarthritis* (Kuettner, K.E., Schleyerbach, R., Peyron, J.G. and Hascall, V.C., eds), pp. 305–316. New York: Raven Press.

Sandy, J.D., Flannery, C.R., Neame, P.J. and Lohmander, L.S. (1992) The structure of aggrecan fragments in human synovial fluid. Evidence for the involvement in osteoarthritis of a novel proteinase which cleaves the glu 373-Ala 374 bond of the interglobular domain. *J. Clin. Invest.*, **89**, 1512–1516.

Sandy, J.D., Neame, P.J., Boynton, R.E. and Flannery, C.R. (1991) Catabolism of aggrecan in cartilage explants. Identification of a major cleavage site within the interglobular domain. *J. Biol. Chem.*, **266**, 8683–8685.

Scott, J.E. (1988) Proteoglycan-fibrillar collagen interactions. *Biochem. J.*, **252**, 313–323.

Shinmei, M., Inamori, Y., Yoshihara, Y., Kikuchi, T. and Hyakawa, T. (1992) The potential of cartilage markers in joint fluid for drug evaluation. In: *Articular Cartilage and Osteoarthritis* (Kuettner, K.E., Schleyerbach, R., Peyron, J.G. and Hascall, V.C., eds), pp. 597–608. New York: Raven Press.

Suzuki, K., Shimizu, K. and Sandy, J.D. (1994) Aggrecan degradation by calpain. *Trans. Orthop. Res. Soc.*, **19**, 319.

Suzuki, K., Neame, P.J. and Sandy, J.D. (1995) Bovine aggrecan G2 domain. Isolation and structural analysis. *Trans. Orthop. Res. Soc.*, **20**, 425.

Tester, A.M., Ilic, M.Z., Robinson, H.C. and Handley, C.J. (submitted) Turnover and metabolic processing of link protein in bovine articular cartilage.

Thonar, E.J.-A., Manicourt, D.H., Williams, J.A., Fukuda, K., Campion, G., Sweet, B.M.E., Lenz, M.E., Schnitzer, T.J. and Kuettner K.E. (1992) Serum keratan sulfate, a measure of cartilage proteoglycan metabolism. In: *Articular Cartilage and Osteoarthritis* (Kuettner, K.E., Schleyerbach, R., Peyron, J.G. and Hascall, V.C., eds), pp. 429–445. New York: Raven Press.

Tian, X., Chen, S., Morales, T.I. and Hascall, V.C. (1989) Biochemical and morphological studies of steady state and lipopolysaccharide treated bovine articular cartilage explant cultures. *Conn. Tiss. Res.*, **19**, 195–218.

Tyler, J.A. (1989) Insulin-like growth factor-I can decrease the degradation and promote synthesis of proteoglycan in cartilage exposed to cytokines. *Biochem. J.*, **260**, 543–548.

Wight, T.N., Heinegard, D.K. and Hascall, V.C. (1991) Proteoglycans: structure and function. In: *Cell Biology of the Extracellular Matrix*, 2nd Edition (Hay, E., ed), pp. 45–78. NY: Plenum Press.

8 Collagens in Joint Tissue

Linda J. Sandell[1,2,3,*], Andrew M. Nalin[1,3] and Yong Zhu[1,3]

[1]*Departments of Orthopaedics,*
[2]*Biochemistry, University of Washington,*
[3]*Seattle Veterans Affairs Medical Center, Seattle, WA 98108, USA*

COLLAGENS IN JOINT TISSUE

COLLAGENS

The extracellular matrix molecules present in connective tissues of the joint reflect the structure and function of individual tissues. Mature collagen fibers provide the capacity to withstand tensile and shear forces (Kempson *et al.*, 1970; Kempson, 1974), while proteoglycans are generally responsible for solute flow and deformation of the tissue. The predominant collagens in the mature tissue are: type II in cartilage, type I in tendon, types I and III in ligament, and types I and III in synovium. Collagens in the joint capsule of adult interphalangeal joints include types I and III in the central slip, volar plate and collateral ligament while the attachment zones additionally contain type II in the regions that are fibrocartilaginous (Ralphs and Benjamin, 1994).

The collagen gene family has grown greatly over the last few years. To qualify as a collagen, a molecule must contain a stretch of at least 20 or so amino acids of the sequence Gly-X-Y where X and Y are often proline and hydroxyproline. This coding sequence forms the characteristic collagen triple helical structure when three chains are wound around each other during biosynthesis. There are now 19 collagen molecular "types" made of up more than 30 different gene products (see Table 8.1).

"MINOR" COLLAGENS IN JOINT TISSUES

During development and later in the articular joint, cartilages also contain various forms of collagens present in less abundance, usually not more than 10% of the total collagen

---

* Corresponding author. University of Washington, Department of Orthopaedics ORT 112, VA Puget Sound Health Care Systems, 1660 S, Columbian Way, Seattle, WA 98108, USA.

TABLE 8.1
Collagen superfamily.

Class	Type	Molecules	mature-chain $Mr. \times 10^{-3}$	Tissue distribution
Fibrillar	I	$[\alpha1(I)]_2\ \alpha2(I)$	95	Most connective tissues, except cartilage and basement membrane
	II	$[\alpha1(II)]_3$	95	Cartilage, vitreous humor
	III	$[\alpha1(III)]_3$	95	Synovium, Tendon, Ligament, some in cartilage
	V/XI	$[\alpha1(V)]_2\ \alpha2(V)$ $[\alpha1(V)\ \alpha2(V)\ \alpha3(V)]$ $[\alpha1(XI)\ \alpha2(XI)\ \alpha3(XI)]$ mixed molecules of V and XI	120–145	Heterotypic fibrils of V with I and XI with II, but mixed molecules of V/XI with I and/or II possible
Microfibrillar	VI	$[\alpha1(VI)\ \alpha2(VI)\ \alpha3(VI)]$	$\alpha1/\alpha2=140$ $\alpha3=200–280$	Skin, cartilage, blood vessels
Fibril-associated (FACITs)	IX	$[\alpha1(IX)\ \alpha2(IX)\ \alpha3(IX)]$	$\alpha1=66$ (short form) or 84 (long form), $\alpha2=66$ (non-glycanated) or 66–115 (glycanated) $\alpha3=72$	cartilage, vitreous humor
	XII	$[\alpha1(XII)]_3$	220 (short form) 340 (long form) long form can be glycanated	fetal tendon and skin
	XIV	$[\alpha1(XIV)]_3$	220 can be glycanated	fetal tendon and skin
	XVI	$[\alpha1(XVI)]_3$	160	fibroblasts, keratinocytes
Short-chain Non-fibrillar	X	$[\alpha1(X)]_3$	59	growth plate
	IV	$[\alpha1(IV)]_2\ \alpha2(IV)$	150	basement membrane
	VII	$[\alpha1(VII)]_3$	270	Anchoring fibrils in epithelial basement membrane
	VIII	$[\alpha1(VIII)]_2\alpha2(VIII)]$	70	Descemet's membrane
	XIII	$[\alpha1(XIII)]_3$	60	Many tissues
	XV	$[\alpha1(XV)]_3$	140	Fibroblasts
	XVII	$[\alpha1(XVII)]_3$	140	Epithelial hemidesmosomes
	XVIII	$[\alpha1(XVIII]3$	130	Liver, lung
	XIX	$[\alpha1(XIX)]_3$	115	Rhabdosarcoma

Ayad S. and Sandell L.J. (1996) Collagens of the intervertebral disc: structure, function and changes during aging and disease. Weinstein, J.N. and Gordon, S.L. (eds), AAOS Press, Rosemont, IL, in press.

present. However, these collagens may be important functional components of the tissue. Two of these minor collagens, types IX and XI, are thought to be involved in assembly of collagen fibers. For example, if one chain of the collagen type XI molecule is missing, the fibril diameter on the major type II collagen fibril will be altered (Li *et al.*, 1995). Type IX collagen is also thought to be involved in the packing and overall diameter of the type II collagen fibril (Mendler *et al.*, 1989). In tissues containing type I collagen, minor collagen types XII and XIV are associated with fibrils.

TABLE 8.2.
Collagen fibril diameters in cartilage.

Zone/Region	Diameter (nm)	
	mean ± SD	(n)
Superficial zone		
1. Pericellular	15.4 ± 8.3	(18)
2. Territorial	29.2 ± 5.4	(22)
Middle zone		
3. Pericellular	21.5 ± 12.7	(18)
4. Territorial	31.8 ± 5.0	(23)
Deep zone		
5. Pericellular	19.0 ± 4.4	(23)
6. Territorial	48.5 ± 7.0	(23)
7. Interterritorial	57.5 ± 7.6	(25)

From Poole A.R. *et al.* (1982) *J. Cell Biol.*, **93**, 921–937. All measurements were made from one experiment (BC14). Student's *t* test analyses revealed that the following were significantly different from each other (P < 0.001): 1 and 2, 3 and 4, 5 and 6, 6 and 7, 4 and 6, 4 and 7.

In articular cartilage of mammals, the content of predominant and minor collagens as well as other collagen-binding molecules contributes to the differences in collagen fibril diameters observed in different zones of the tissue. Collagen fibril diameters are listed in Table 8.2. Many of the differences are related to depth in the tissue because heterogeneity plays a role in determining the biomechanical properties of normal articular cartilage essential for tissue function. The articular cartilage can be divided into three zones based on the type of matrix synthesized, the arrangement of cells and the collagen fibril diameter (Figure 8.1) (Poole *et al.*, 1982). In pericellular areas collagen fibril diameters are much less than in territorial and interterritorial areas. Type II collagen represents 85–90 per cent of the total tissue collagen. Type V collagen is primarily found in the pericellular region near the chondrocytes (Poole *et al.*, 1982).

Articular cartilage of the chicken differs from that of the mammal by containing a significant proportion of type I collagen in addition to type II (Seyer *et al.*, 1974). Eyre and colleagues (Eyre *et al.*, 1978) investigated the changes with age and with depth from the articular surface in the proportions of types I and II collagens in chicken knee cartilage. They found that the total content of type I increased after hatching, becoming the major collagen component at maturity. At all ages, type I was essentially the only collagen type at the articular surface and it gradually interchanged with type II with increasing depth. We have examined the origin of the articular chondrocytes and the development of the chicken joint during the embryonic and fetal periods by following collagen gene expression (discussed in the next section).

There are other collagen types not related to the predominant fibrillar collagens, such as type IV and type VI collagens. Cartilage contains the type VI collagen which has many functional domains and very little triple helical domain. Type IV is observed wherever basement membranes occur and is present in the synovium (Schneider *et al.*, 1994).

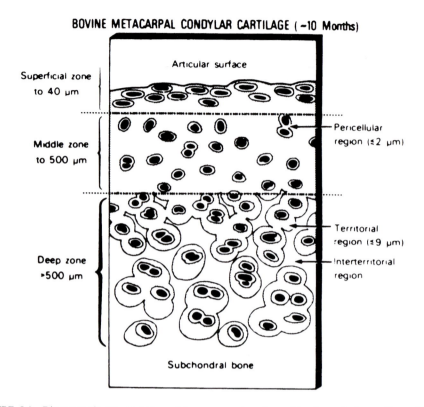

BOVINE METACARPAL CONDYLAR CARTILAGE (~10 Months)

FIGURE 8.1   Diagrammatic representation of the zones and regions of bovine articular cartilage. (From Poole, A.R. *et al.*, *J. Cell Biol.*, **93**: 921–937, 1982.)

COLLAGEN EXPRESSION DURING JOINT DEVELOPMENT

Collagen gene products can be used as biochemical markers to describe the differentiation state of connective tissues. Simply, mesenchymal and undifferentiated cells express type I collagen while chondrocytes express type II. Upon differentiation of osteoblasts, these bone-forming cells characteristically produce abundant type I collagen. The joint develops from the primitive avascular, densely packed cellular mesenchyme called the skeletal blastema (shown diagrammatically in Figure 8.2). The cartilaginous skeletal nodules appear in the middle of the blastema surrounded by perichondrium. The cartilage anlagen grow by cell division and apposition of extracellular matrix and by apposition of chondroblasts proliferating from the inner, chondrogenic layer of the perichondrium. In the region of the future joint, a narrow band of densely packed cellular blastema remains and forms the interzone between the nodules. The interzone differentiates into three morphologically identifiable layers: two chondrogenic, perichondrium-like layers that cover the cartilaginous articulating surfaces and one intermediate layer composed of a loose cellular tissue. Blood vessels appear at the periphery of the joint in the capsulo-synovial blastemal mesenchyme prior to the separation of the adjacent articulating surfaces (Mitrovic, 1977, 1978).

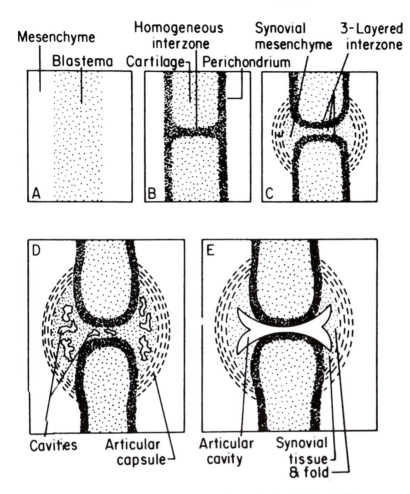

FIGURE 8.2   Diagram of the development of a synovial joint. Joints develop from the blastema, not surrounding the mesenchyme. The interzone remains avascular and highly cellular. The synovial mesenchyme develops from the periphery of the interzone (C) and becomes vascularized. Following shortly after differentiation of synovial membrane is cavitation, which may begin centrally in the interzone or peripherally (D) and merge to form the joint cavity (E). (From O'Rahilly, R. and Gardner, E. In: *The Joints and Synovial Fluid*, Sokoloff, L. (ed), vol. 1, New York, Academic Press, 1978.)

The distribution of collagen types and keratin sulfate proteoglycan has been studied immunohistochemically in the developing joint (von der Mark *et al.*, 1976; Craig *et al.*, 1987). Using antibodies that specifically react with type I or type II collagen, in the chicken, von der Mark and colleagues (1976) were able to identify collagen types at the cellular level in these areas of rapid collagen transition. Type II collagen was found in all cartilaginous structures that showed metachromatic staining. Type I collagen appeared in the perichondrium of the tibia at stage 28 and was also found in osteoid, periosteal and enchondral bone after decalcification, in periosteum, and in tendons, ligaments and the joint capsule. In addition, they proposed that during enchondral ossification type I collagen is deposited onto the surface of cartilage, where it partially diffuses into the cartilage matrix forming a "hybrid" anlagen matrix with type II collagen. During appositional growth of the diaphyseal cartilage and differentiation of epiphyseal perichondrium into articular cartilage, perichondrial cells switch from type I to type II collagen synthesis when differentiating into chondroblasts. In the transition zones, chondroblasts are imbedded in a "hybrid" matrix consisting of a mixture of type I and type II collagens. The development of the mammalian joint is apparently similar to the chick with two differences. First, after the joint space is formed, the exposed epiphyseal cartilage lacks a chondrogenic perichondrial layer on its surface, and it can continue to expand only by interstitial growth. Second, the articular surface does not contain the fibrocartilaginous layer and type I collagen.

ANALYSIS OF TYPE II PROCOLLAGEN SPLICE FORMS REVEALS A NEW CELL POPULATION

The studies described above have provided a good understanding of the morphology of joint development and have defined certain domains of the tissue; however, the cellular origin of the matrix molecules remains unknown. Since the 1970s, when most of the morphological studies were conducted, additional collagen gene products and splice forms have been discovered that may play important roles in joint development. Of particular interest in chondrogenesis is the expression of alternative splice forms of type II procollagen (Ryan and Sandell, 1990; Sandell et al., 1991; Nah and Upholt, 1991) and the expression of type XI collagen (Li et al., 1995). Expression of type II collagen splice forms, IIA and IIB, is developmentally regulated with the expression of IIA preceding IIB. Type IIA procollagen is synthesized by chondroprogenitor cells that are fibroblastic in appearance, while type IIB is synthesized once the cells become chondroblasts (Sandell et al., 1994). The difference between the two forms is that the type IIA procollagen is a longer form containing a cysteine-rich amino propeptide. This domain is removed from the type IIB procollagen by alternative splicing of the mRNA.

The expression of the two procollagen splice forms was studied by in situ hybridization to mRNA during development of the chicken interphalangeal joint (Nalin et al., 1995). Early in development of the limb, type IIA procollagen expression predominates in the early condensation of the cartilage primordium and may play a role in morphogenesis of the primitive limb structure. As the cells differentiate into chondrocytes, the synthesis of type IIB procollagen mRNA is dominant and the characteristic morphology of cartilage with abundant synthesis of extracellular matrix is observed. Figure 8.3 shows in situ hybridization of an 8 day gestation chicken embryo (stage 33). Type IIA procollagen mRNA is expressed primarily by the chondroprogenitor cells, while in the center of each cartilaginous precursor, cells are beginning to synthesize type IIB (panels B and C). It can be seen that in the central region of the large precartilaginous domain, less type IIA message is being made while more type IIB is present. The expression of type IIB procollagen mRNA is coincident with the metachromatic staining of the extracellular matrix. As development proceeds, the cartilage anlagen synthesize only type IIB procollagen mRNA while the periosteum synthesizes type IIA mRNA (Figure 8.4). These type IIA-synthesizing cells are the progenitors for appositional cartilage development. As formation

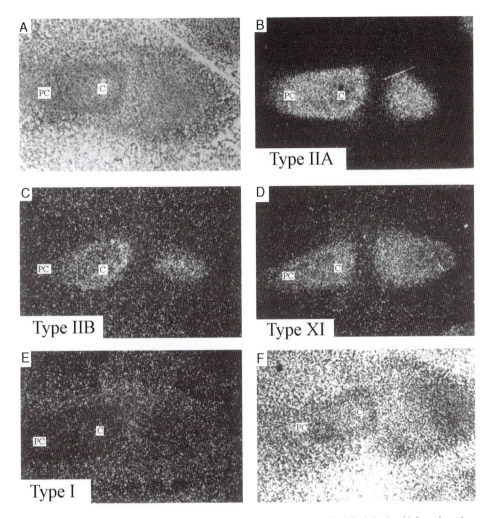

FIGURE 8.3 *In situ* hybridization of 8 day (stage 33) chicken embryo hind limb bud, mid-frontal sections. A: Brightfield image of B showing newly formed chondrocytes (C) and pre-chondrocytes (PC). B: Expression of type IIA message in both populations of cells. C: Expression of type IIB only in chondrocytes. D: Type XI mRNA is present in both chondrocytes and pre-chondrocytes. E: Type I message is expressed in surrounding mesenchyme F: Brightfield image of D. Bar = 100 microns. (From Nalin *et al.*, *Dev. Dynamics*, **203**, 352–362, 1995.)

of the joint cavity occurs, the type I-synthesizing cells of the interzone observed in Figure 8.4, Panel F, form a layer over the cartilage and become part of the fibrocartilage. These cells then synthesize type I collagen in the young chick.

The cells that synthesize type I, type IIA and type IIB procollagens do not overlap. At birth, the cartilage is covered by the type IIA-synthesizing cells, then a layer of type I synthesizing cells. The dense cell layer previously identified as perichondrium actually contains a different cell type that synthesizes type IIA procollagen (see diagram in Figure 8.5).

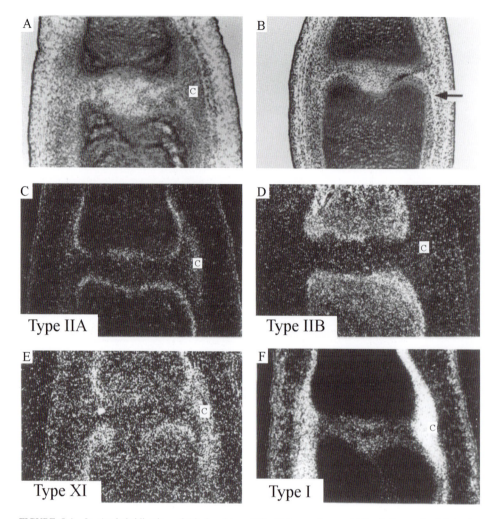

FIGURE 8.4   *In situ* hybridization of 13 day (stage 39) chicken embryo middle digit, proximal interphalangeal joint, mid-frontal sections. A: Brightfield image showing developing joint and capsule (C).
B: Equivalent paraffin section of opposite limb of same animal, clearly showing onset of cavitation laterally
(arrow). C: Expression of type IIA in articular surface cells, perichondrium, and capsule. D: Type IIB message
is expressed only in chondrocytes of the anlagen. E: Type XI mRNA is expressed in the surface cells, perichondrium, capsule, and lower levels in chondrocytes. F: Type I message is present in cells of the interzone and capsule. Panels C–F are darkfield, Bar = 100 m. (From Nalin *et al.*, *Dev. Dynamics*, **203**, 352–362, 1995.)

FUNCTION OF TYPE IIA PROCOLLAGEN IN JOINT DEVELOPMENT

Recent studies in human tissue have revealed a similar distribution of type II procollagen
mRNAs. We have developed an antibody specific for the type IIA procollagen amino
propeptide (Oganesian *et al.*, 1997). With this reagent, we have been able to show that the
type IIA procollagen is indeed present in the extracellular matrix. This observation is
important as it shows that the cysteine-rich domain of the procollagen can be functional

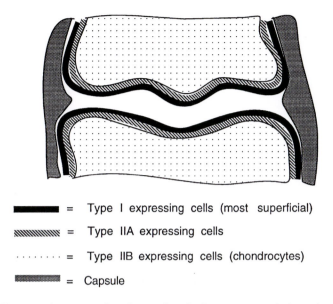

■■■■■   =   Type I expressing cells (most superficial)

▨▨▨▨▨   =   Type IIA expressing cells

· · · · · · ·   =   Type IIB expressing cells (chondrocytes)

▓▓▓▓▓   =   Capsule

FIGURE 8.5   Diagrammatic representation of expression of collagen types at articular surface in morphologically mature interphalangeal joint. Type I mRNA is expressed by the most superficial, flattened cells of the surface, followed deeper by a layer of similar appearing cells producing type IIA message. Type IIB is expressed
by overt chondrocytes in the deepest layer. Type XI message (not shown) is found in all layers except the most
superficial, type I expressing cells. (From Nalin *et al.*, *Dev. Dynamics*, **203**, 352–362, 1995.)

in the extracellular matrix. Figure 8.6 shows the distribution of type IIA procollagen
in a human joint. Panel A shows *in situ* hybridization of exon 2 of the collagen type IIA
procollagen mRNA. mRNA is present primarily in the zone of chondroprogenitor cells
at the growing ends and in the perichondrium. Panels C and D show double-immunofluo-
rescence using an antibody to the NH_2-propeptide of type IIA (Panel C) and the fibrillar
domain of type II (Panel D). Type IIA remains in the matrix. In cartilage, where it is no
longer synthesized, it is forced into the interterritorial zone. The composite photograph
(Panel E) shows that only the fibrillar collagen (type IIB) surrounds the chondrocytes
(green) while type IIA is predominant in the growing tissue and perichondrium. Further
examination by electron microscopy reveals that the amino propeptide is retained on the
collagen molecule and incorporated into the fibril (Y. Zhu, A. Oganesian, D. Keene and
L. Sandell, unpublished data).

JOINT CAVITATION DURING DEVELOPMENT

In order for the joint cavity to form, a space in the interzone must be made. Cavitation
generally begins laterally and moves toward the center of the joint. There have been several theories to explain the mechanism of cavitation: programmed cell death in the interzone (Mitrovic, 1972), vascular ingression and enzymatic degradation of matrix of the
interzone (Mitrovic, 1974), mechanical disruption of cells of the interzone due to muscle
activity (Drachman and Sokoloff, 1966), forces produced by differential growth rates of

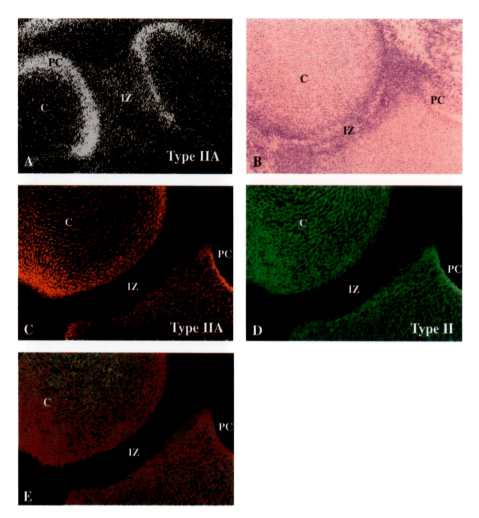

FIGURE 8.6 *In situ* hybridization and immunofluorescent staining of type II procollagen in human fetal joint at 50 days gestation. A: *In situ* hybridization with type IIA mRNA in knee joint, mainly in the perichondrium (PC), at low levels in the interzone (IZ), and absent in the cartilage (C). B: Brightfield image of panels C, D, and E. C–E: Immunolocalization of antibodies to type IIA procollagen (panel C) showing high staining in the perichondrium, type II fibrillar collagen (panel D) showing staining in the cartilage, and a composite of the two (panel E). Sections were visualized with confocal microscopy.

tissues (Lewis, 1977), and biochemical changes in the matrix at the site of cavity formation (Craig *et al.*, 1990; Edwards *et al.*, 1994; Pitsillides *et al.*, 1995). Much recent work has pointed to the latter explanation, although cavitation is a complex process and probably involves an interplay of the proposed mechanisms.

Just prior to cavitation, there is a turnover of matrix constituents in the interzone in the area where separation will occur. The cells lining the presumptive joint line synthesize a matrix rich in hyaluronan (HA) rather than collagen and other matrix components (Craig *et al.*, 1990; Edwards *et al.*, 1994; Pitsillides *et al.*, 1995), which represents

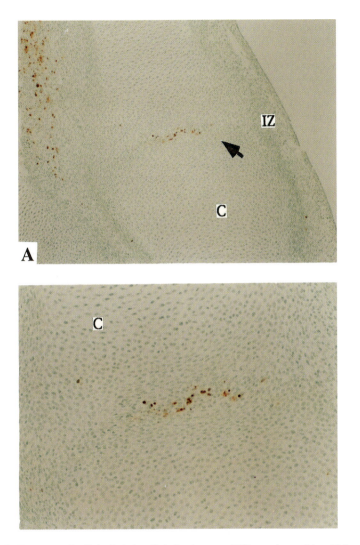

FIGURE 8.7   Programmed cell death during digit development. PCD was detected in mid-frontal sections of day 9 paraffin-embedded embryos by TUNEL. A: Digit showing cartilage anlage (C) and interzonal regions (IZ). Positive cells can be observed in the interzones (arrow) B: Higher magnification of A.

a change in the matrix from a cohesive solid to a more fluid state, similar to synovial fluid in the mature joint. This area potentially represents a region of low tensile strength, amenable to separation and maintenance of the joint space under mechanical stresses. This process may occur additionally due to hydraulic means, as the HA in the area of cavitation may realize its full swelling potential in the absence of the collagen network.

Nalin *et al.* (1995) showed that apoptosis does indeed occur in the interzone of developing chicken interphalangeal joints prior to cavitation (Figure 8.7). Cells in the interzone at stages 33 and 35 were positive for apoptosis using the TUNEL technique, with no apparent apoptosis at stages 38–41 when overt cavitation occurs. This implies that programmed cell death may contribute to the early part of the cavitation process, perhaps delineating the line where the joint space will form.

SUMMARY

A complex pattern of collagens is expressed in the mature joint tissues and differentially during development. Recent evidence indicates that in addition to the traditionally defined function of the collagen fibrils, components of minor fibrillar collagens contribute to the fibril diameter, thus microtuning the functional fibrils throughout different depths of the tissue. Furthermore, non-collagenous domains of collagen molecules such as the amino propeptide of type IIA collagen and the EGF repeats of type VI and XII collagens may play important regulatory and signaling roles in the joint tissues.

ACKNOWLEDGMENTS

The author thanks Margo Weiss for expert assistance in the preparation of the manuscript. The study was supported in part by National Institutes of Health Research Grant AR36994, the Department of Veterans Affairs, and the Department of Orthopaedics, University of Washington.

REFERENCES

Craig, F.M., Bentley, G. and Archer, C.W. (1987) The spatial and temporal pattern of collagens I and II and keratan sulphate in the developing chick metatarsophalangeal joint. *Develop.*, **99**, 383–391.

Craig, F.M., Bayliss, M.T., Bentley, G. and Archer, C.W. (1990) A role for hyaluronan in joint development. *J. Anat.*, **171**, 17–23.

Drachman, D.B. and Sokoloff, L. (1966) The role of movement in embryonic joint development. *Dev. Biol.*, **14**, 401–420.

Edwards, J.C.W., Wilkinson, L.S., Jones, H.M., Soothill, P., Henderson, K.J., Worrall, J.G. and Pitsillides, A.A. (1994) The formation of human synovial joint cavities: a possible role for hyaluronan and CD44 in altered interzone cohesion. *J. Anat.*, **185**, 355–367.

Eyre, D.R., Brickley-Parsons, D.M. and Glimcher, M.J. (1978) Pre-dominance of type I collagen at the surface of avian articular cartilage. *FEBS Lett.*, **85**, 259–263.

Kempson, G.E., Muir, H., Swanson, S.A.V. and Freeman, M.A. (1970) Correlations between stiffness and the chemical constituents of cartilage on the human femoral head. *Biochim. Biophy. Acta.*, **215**, 70–77.

Kempson, G.E. (1974) Mechanical properties of articular cartilage. In: *Adult Articular Cartilage*. Freeman, M.A.R. (ed): New York, Grune & Stratton, p. 196.

Lewis, J. (1977) Growth and determination in the developing limb. In: *Vertebrate Limb and Somite Morphogenesis*. Ede, D.A., Hinchcliffe, J.R. and Balls, M. (eds), pp. 215–228. Cambridge University Press, Cambridge.

Li, Y., Lacerda, D.A., Warman, M.L., Beier, D.R., Yoskioka, H., Ninomiya, Y., Oxford, J.T., Morris, N.P., Andrikopoulos, K., Ramirez, F. *et al.* (1995) A fibrillar collagen gene, COLIIa1 is essential for skeletal morphogenesis. *Cell*, **80**, 423–430.

Mendler, M., Eich-Bender, S.G., Vaughan, L., Winterhalter, K.H. and Bruckner, P. (1989) Cartilage contains mixed fibrils of collagen types II, IX, and XI. *J. Cell Biol.*, **108**, 191–197.

Mitrovic, D. (1972) Presence of degenerated cells in the developing articular cavity of the chick embryo. *CR Acad. Sci. Hebd. Seances. Acad. Sci. D.*, **275**, 2941–2944.

Mitrovic, D. (1974) Blood vessels and arthrogenesis. A possible relationship with the cavitation process. *Zeitschrift fur Anatomie und Entwicklungsgeschichte*, **144**, 39–60.

Mitrovic, D. (1977) Development of the metatarsophalangeal joint of the chick embryo: Morphological, ultrastructural and histochemical studies. *Am. J. Anat.*, **150**, 333–348.

Mitrovic, D. (1978) Development of the diarthroidal joints in the rat embryo. *Am. J. Anat.*, **151**, 475–486.

Nah, H.-D. and Upholt, W.B. (1991) Type II collagen mRNA containing an alternatively spliced exon predominates in the chick limb prior to chondrogenesis. *J. Biol. Chem.*, **266**, 23446–23452.

Nalin, A.M., Greenlee, Jr. T.K. and Sandell, L.J. (1995) Collagen gene expression during development of avian synovial joints: Transient expression of types II and XI collagen genes in the joint capsule. *Dev. Dynamics*, **203**, 352–362.

Oganesian, A., Yong, Z. and Sandell, L.J. (1997) Type IIA procollagen amino propeptide is localized in Human Embryonic Tissues. *J. Histochem. Cytochem.*, **45**(11), 1469–1480.

Pitsillides, A.A., Archer, C.W., Prehm, P., Bayliss, M.T. and Edwards, J.C.W. (1995) Alternations in hyaluronan synthesis during developing joint cavitation. *J. Histochem. Cytochem.*, **43**, 263–273.

Poole, A.R., Pidoux, I., Reiner, A. and Rosenberg, L. (1982) An immunoelectron microscope study of proteoglycan monomer, link protein, and the collagen in the matrix of articular cartilage. *J. Cell Biol.*, **93**, 921–937.

Ralphs, J.R. and Benjamin, M. (1994) The joint capsule: structure, composition, aging and disease. *J. Anat.*, **184**, 503–509.

Ryan, M.C. and Sandell, L.J. (1990) Differential expression of a cysteine-rich domain in the amino-terminal propeptide of Type II (Cartilage) procollagen by alternative splicing of mRNA. *J. Biol. Chem.*, **265**, 10334–10339.

Sandell, L.J., Morris, N., Robbins, J.R. and Goldring, M.R. (1991) Alternatively spliced type II procollagen mRNAs define distinct populations of cells during vertebral development: differential expression of the amino-propeptide. *J. Cell Biol.*, **114**, 1307–1319.

Sandell, L.J., Nalin, A. and Reife, R. (1994) Alternative splice form of type II procollagen mRNA (IIA) is predominant in skeletal precursors and non-cartilaginous tissues during early mouse development. *Dev. Dynamics*, **199**, 129–140.

Schneider, M., Voss, B., Rauterberg, J., Menke, M. and Pauly, T. (1994) Basement membrane proteins in synovial membrane: distribution in rheumatoid arthritis and synthesis by fibroblast-like cells. *Clin. Rheumatol.*, **13**, 90–97.

Seyer, J.M., Brickley, D.M. and Glimcher, M.J. (1974) The identification of two types of collagen in the articular cartilage of postnatal chickens. *Calcif. Tiss. Res.*, **17**, 43–55.

von der Mark, H., von der Mark, K. and Gay, S. (1976) Study of differential collagen synthesis during development of the chick embryo by immunofluorescence. *Dev. Biol.*, **48**, 237–249.

9 The Collagens of Articular and Meniscal Cartilages

Victor C. Duance, Anne Vaughan-Thomas,
Robert J. Wardale and Sandra F. Wotton

*Connective Tissue Biology Labs, Cardiff School of Biosciences,
University of Wales Cardiff,
Museum Avenue, Cardiff CF1 3US, UK*

ARTICULAR CARTILAGE

The major macromolecular components of the extracellular matrix of articular cartilage are the collagens and large aggregating proteoglycans (Kuettner, 1992). The relative concentrations of these macromolecules change during development and ageing and may reflect the varying characteristics and functions of the different cartilages in specific locations. 50–60% of the organic dry weight of articular cartilage (10–20% of the wet weight) is collagen, and in the adult, 90% of this is the "fibril-forming" type II collagen (Kuettner, 1992). However, articular cartilage includes up to 10 genetically distinct collagens altogether; types II, VI, IX, X and XI have long been recognised as cartilage components (Thomas *et al.*, 1994; Bruckner and van der Rest, 1994) but there are reports of type I (Duance, 1983; Wardale and Duance, 1993) type III, (Wotton and Duance, 1994; Aigner *et al.*, 1993; Young *et al.*, 1995) type V, (Eyre and Wu, 1987) and types XII and XIV (Watt *et al.*, 1992) being present. It is clear that many if not all the fibrils of the collagen network in articular cartilage, are heterotypic, being comprised of collagen types II, IX and XI (Figure 9.1). Type XI collagen is thought to be partially buried within the fibril while type IX is found on the surface covalently bound to the type II collagen (Mendler *et al.*, 1989; Jacenko and Olsen, 1995; Olsen, 1997). These so called "minor collagens" appear to play pivotal roles in the normal functioning of articular cartilage. In this chapter we will review the detailed structure and current views on the function of the collagens of articular and meniscal cartilages with particular reference to types IX and XI collagen.

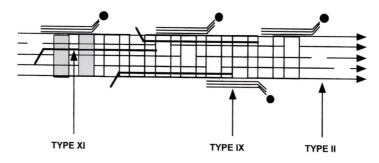

TYPE XI   TYPE IX   TYPE II

(Adapted from Jacenko and Olsen, 1995)

FIGURE 9.1   Diagram to show a heterotypic fibril consisting of types II, IX and XI collagen.

TYPE IX COLLAGEN

MOLECULAR STRUCTURE AND ORGANISATION

Type IX collagen is classified as a FACIT collagen (Fibril Associated Collagen with an Interrupted Triple-helix) forming heterotypic fibrils with types II and XI collagen. It is a heterotrimer $[\alpha1(IX)\alpha2(IX)\alpha3(IX)]$, the 3 chains being products of 3 distinct genes (Eyre and Wu, 1995). It can represent up to 10% of the total cartilage collagen in foetal or very young animals but decreases with age to between 1 and 5% in the adult (Duance and Wotton, 1991). The type IX molecule has a number of unusual characteristics. It has 3 triple-helical collagenous domains (COL 1, 2 and 3) and 4 non-collagenous domains (NC1, 2, 3 and 4). These non-collagenous regions are more susceptible to pro-teolysis than collagenous domains, thus type IX collagen is isolated from mature cartilage by standard pepsin extraction procedures as the 3 separate triple helical domains (COL1, COL 2 and COL3) (Shimokomaki *et al.*, 1980, 1981; Ayad *et al.*, 1981, 1982; Reese *et al.*, 1982; von der Mark *et al.*, 1982). Overall it is shorter than the fibrillar interstitial collagens and is stabilised by interchain disulphide bonds. There are long and short forms depending on the presence or absence of a large globular domain (NC4) at the amino-terminal of the $\alpha1$ chain. Most unusually for a collagen molecule it has a chondroitin sul-phate chain, leading to its additional classification as a proteoglycan. Thus the molecular weights of the α-chains differ, the $\alpha1$ chain including the NC4 domain being approxi-mately 84,000 kDa, the $\alpha2$ chain which bears the chondroitin sulphate chain varying between 65,000 and 115,000 kDa and the $\alpha3$ chain being approximately 68,000 kDa. A schematic representation of the type IX molecule is shown in Figure 9.2.

Long and short forms of type IX collagen

Rotary shadowing studies revealed a distinctive kink towards one end of the molecule and the presence of a globular domain or "knob" at the end of the kink (Irwin *et al.*, 1985; Duance *et al.*, 1984). DNA and amino acid sequencing of tryptic peptides from several species revealed that NC4 contains 245–266 amino acids including the signal peptide and 5 cysteine residues which form 2 disulphide bridges (Vasios *et al.*, 1988; Abe *et al.*,

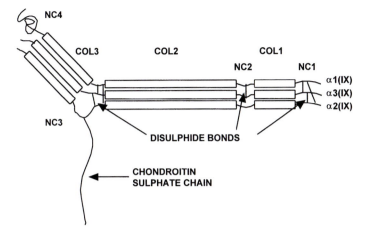

FIGURE 9.2   Diagram of the type IX collagen molecule.

1994; Kimura *et al.*, 1989). The domain is basic with a pl about 9.7. The short form of type IX collagen lacks NC4 on the $\alpha1(IX)$ chain which is present in the long form. This arises through the use of an alternative promoter between exons 6 and 7 of the col9a1 gene (Nishimura *et al.*, 1989). Thus in the short form exons 1–6 as well as exon 7 are not transcribed while the alternative exon 1 encodes a different, much shorter, NC4 peptide.

The expression of these forms of type IX collagen is tissue specific and developmentally regulated. In articular cartilage type IX is present mainly in the long form but in the hypertrophic cartilage of the growth plate the short form becomes dominant (Olsen, 1992). The mRNAs for the $\alpha2(IX)$ chain in cartilage and cornea are of similar size, whereas corneal $\alpha1(IX)$ mRNA is smaller by about 700 nucleotides than cartilage $\alpha1(IX)$ mRNA indicating only the short form is present (Svoboda *et al.*, 1988; Muragaki *et al.*, 1990a,b). In the notochord of chick embryos a transition from the early production of the short form to the appearance of the long form during stages 27 and 31 (Hayashi *et al.*, 1992). Swiderski and Solursh (1992) could not detect the long form of type IX in the notochord up to stage 28 but found both forms in the developing chondrogenic vertebrae, the chondrocranium and Meckle's cartilage, although expression of the short form was more restricted in these regions.

The proteoglycan form of type IX collagen

In 1983 Noro *et al.* isolated a proteoglycan (PG-Lt) which was subsequently identified as type IX collagen using ion-exchange chromatography and cross-reactivity with a polyclonal antibody to type IX collagen (Vaughan *et al.*, 1985). ^{35}S labelling and chondroitinase ABC treatment have revealed that the chondroitin sulphate chain is linked to the NC3 region of the $\alpha2(IX)$ chain (Bruckner *et al.*, 1985; Duance *et al.*, 1985; Huber *et al.*, 1986; Konomi *et al.*, 1986; Irwin and Mayne, 1986). This domain of the $\alpha2(IX)$ chain has the sequence, Val-Glu-Gly-Ser-Ala, containing the serine residue to which the glycosaminoglycan side chain is covalently linked (McCormick *et al.*, 1987). The usual attachment sequence is Ser-Gly but type IX collagen does have an acidic residue preceding the glycine which may be acceptable for the xylosyltransferase (Huber *et al.*, 1988). However, Chandrasekhar and Harvey (1987) found that β-xylosides, which inhibit the synthesis of both the large and small proteoglycans of cartilage, did not affect the synthesis of type IX collagen suggesting that a different metabolic pathway to that of the classical cartilage proteoglycans may be involved.

The proportion of type IX molecules which are substituted with a glycosaminoglycan side-chain varies and is tissue and species specific. In chick cartilage over 70% of the type IX is substituted (Huber *et al.*, 1988); in the vitreous of the eye (both chick and bovine) the substitution is 100% (Bishop *et al.*, 1994); while in human and bovine articular cartilage the proteoglycan form is only a minor component (Ayad *et al.*, 1989; Diab *et al.*, 1996). In mammalian cartilage both proteoglycan and non-proteoglycan forms of type IX collagen are synthesised as two discrete populations (Ayad *et al.*, 1991). The size and composition of the glycosaminoglycan side chain also varies. In chick vitreous the side chains are about 10 times larger (M_r 350 kDa) than those found in cartilage (Yada *et al.*, 1990) and consist predominantly of chondroitin-6-sulphate. However, type IX collagen in the bovine vitreous possesses a comparatively short glycosaminoglycan chain which is mainly 4-sulphated (Bishop *et al.*, 1994).

Type IX collagen cross-linking

Type IX collagen can only be isolated as a complete molecule from embryonic cartilage, chondrocyte cultures or tissues from animals fed a diet containing the lathyrogen β-aminoproprionitrile which inhibits lysyl oxidase mediated collagen cross-linking (Duance *et al.*, 1984). Tryptic peptide analysis and amino acid sequencing has revealed that type IX is covalently cross-linked to the telopeptide regions of the type II collagen molecules by the mature cross-links, hydroxylysyl pyridinoline and lysyl pyridinoline (Wu and Eyre, 1984). Type IX to type IX bonding was also discovered linking the $\alpha1(IX)$ and $\alpha3(IX)$ chains (Eyre *et al.*, 1987; van der Rest and Mayne, 1988; Shimokomaki *et al.*, 1990; Diab *et al.*, 1996). All three chains of type IX collagen contain a cross-linking site at the amino terminus of the COL2 triple helix which can attach to the $\alpha1(II)$ N-telopeptide while the $\alpha3(IX)$ COL2 domain has an additional attachment site for the $\alpha1(II)$ C-telopeptide (Wu *et al.*, 1992; Diab *et al.*, 1996). The distance between these two attachment sites is equal to the length of the gap zone of a type II collagen fibril (137 residues) suggesting that type IX collagen spans the gap region. In addition, the type IX molecules are arranged in an antiparallel direction to the type II molecules (Wu *et al.*, 1992) (see Figure 9.1).

TYPE IX COLLAGEN IMMUNOLOCALISATION

Immunolocalisation studies on articular cartilage have shown that while type II is present throughout the interterritorial matrix, type IX collagen is located in the pericellular environment in an area which had been shown in ultrastructural studies to contain fine non-banded collagen fibrils (Duance *et al.*, 1982; Evans *et al.*, 1983; Ricard-Blum *et al.*, 1982). Furthermore, the association of type IX collagen with the fine non-striated fibrils in the pericellular region was confirmed using immuno-electron microscopy (Hartmann *et al.*, 1983; Wotton *et al.*, 1988). In embryonic chick sternal and foetal calf articular cartilage, type IX collagen was reported to be distributed throughout the matrix (Irwin et al., 1985; Vilamitjana et al., 1989). These researchers suggested that incomplete removal of the proteoglycans and a greater accessibility of epitopes could result in type IX collagen appearing to be concentrated around the chondrocytes. More recent studies, using high resolution confocal microscopy, revealed these differences in distribution were age-related (Wotton et al., 1991; Duance et al., 1990). In older rats type IX collagen can be clearly localised to the pericellular areas of the articular cartilage but in young or foetal rats the labelling appears to be throughout the matrix. However, because young and foetal articular cartilage is much more cellular than the adult tissue this "matrix" labelling is still preferentially located around chondrocytes. In an ultrastructural study of juvenile rib growth plate cartilage type IX collagen was shown to be present on both fine and large banded fibrils (Keene et al., 1995), whether this distribution remains in adult human cartilage is unknown.

The pericellular labelling of type IX collagen is consistent with immunolocalisation studies conducted on isolated chondrons from articular cartilage or rat chondrosarcoma tissue. The chondron consists of the chondrocyte with its immediate pericellular matrix bounded by a "felt-like" capsule of fine fibrous material. Immunolocalisation revealed very strong type IX collagen labelling in the capsule of chondrons isolated from both porcine articular cartilage and rat chondrosarcoma (Poole et al., 1988a). Double labelling with antibodies to type IX and type II collagens demonstrated that they co-localised in the chondron capsule. Optical sectioning in the confocal microscope of rat chondrosarcoma chondrons labelled with antibody to type IX collagen demonstrated a complex concentric arrangement of capsules surrounding individual and clusters of chondrocytes, perhaps indicating how the capsular material may consolidate to form the felt-like structure as the cells divide and the matrix expands during development and growth (Wotton et al., 1991). It has been suggested that chondrons protect the chondrocytes from excessive loads and that their development may correlate with the amount and/or distribution of mechanical stress experienced within the cartilage (Poole et al., 1988a).

DEGRADATION OF TYPE IX COLLAGEN

Relatively few enzymes, MMP-1 (MMP-2, MMP-8 and MMP-13) are able to attack native collagen triple helices but a number of proteinases can degrade non-triple-helical regions of collagen molecules or denatured collagen. Type IX collagen is resistant to digestion by interstitial collagenase but is susceptible to stromelysin (MMP-3), neutrophil elastase and cathepsins B and L.

Stromelysin (MMP-3) is the only metalloproteinase which is known to degrade type IX collagen cleaving all three chains of type IX in the NC2 domain. It also "trims" off the large N-terminal globular NC4 domain from the $\alpha1(IX)$ chain and probably the smaller N-terminal peptides from the $\alpha2(IX)$ and $\alpha3(IX)$ chains (Okada et al., 1989; Wu et al., 1991).

Neutrophil elastase also degrades type IX collagen (Gadher et al., 1988, 1990). Interestingly, Jasin and Taurog (1991) found that incubation of articular cartilage with neutrophil elastase seemed to expose type II collagen epitopes and increase the binding of antibody to type II on the surface of the cartilage perhaps through the removal of type IX collagen.

There are a number of cysteine proteinases which can degrade various connective tissue proteins, of these, cathepsins B and L have been found to degrade both cartilage proteoglycans and collagens (Maciewicz *et al.*, 1990a,b). The cathepsins act primarily intracellularly within lysosomes and function optimally at acid pH (Murphy and Reynolds, 1993). However cathepsins B and L have been detected in active forms in human synovial fluids and the extracellular matrix of the rat chondrosarcoma (Maciewicz and Wotton, 1991) and can degrade types II, IX and XI collagen at pH values near neutrality (Maciewicz *et al.*, 1990b). Cleavage occurs only in the non-helical regions but degradation will progress further if the helix is destabilised. Type IX collagen is degraded principally by MMP-3 but cathepsins B and L may contribute as they are also capable of producing COL1, 2 and 3 fragments.

Loss of type IX collagen is likely to have profound effects on matrix integrity, through the loss of interactions with other matrix components and may affect the chondrocytes directly if there is a significant breakdown of the chondron structure. Furthermore the location of type IX collagen on the surface of type II fibrils and its susceptibility to number of proteases could result in it being degraded or removed as an early but significant event in arthritic diseases.

FUNCTION OF TYPE IX COLLAGEN

The exact function of type IX collagen is still not clear and although the concept of heterotypic fibrils consisting of types II, IX and XI collagens is now well accepted their precise arrangement within the fibrils is still the subject of some debate (Eikenberry *et al.*, 1992). Most researchers agree that type IX collagen plays a fundamental role in cartilage matrix integrity but despite several different approaches the nature of this important role has not been determined. Certainly the possession of a large globular N-terminal domain and a chondroitin sulphate chain are characteristics which suggest a potential to interact with other matrix components.

Localisation of type IX collagen to the capsule of the chondron where the fibrils were observed to be of much smaller diameters than those in the interterritorial matrix suggested that type IX collagen might have a role in regulating fibril diameter of type II collagen (Wotton *et al.*, 1987). Using *in vitro* fibrillogenesis with isolated type IX and type II collagens it was shown that the presence of type IX reduces the diameter of the heterotypic fibril aggregates. However, type IX collagen does not act by preventing fibrillogenesis since, in these experiments, it actually enhanced the proportion of type II which was incorporated into small diameter fibrils. Furthermore, using immunogold labelling, type IX collagen was demonstrated to be more associated with the fine fibrils which occur in greater concentrations close to the chondrocytes than further out into the matrix (Wotton *et al.*, 1988; Duance *et al.*, 1990).

Independently, Vaughan *et al.* (1988) visualised type IX collagen molecules decorating the surface of type II collagen heterotypic fibrils from chick embryonic sternal cartilage by rotary shadowing. They described a regular D-periodic arrangement of the type IX along these fibrils with the N-terminal domain projecting from the surface from the position of the kink. Subsequently a similar D-periodic pattern was found on mechanically extracted fibril fragments from human foetal cartilage (Bruckner *et al.*, 1988).

However they detected no difference in the degree of type IX association with fibrils whatever their diameter up to a size of 30 nm, although this is still a relatively small diameter compared to the fibrils found in adult human and pig cartilage where some diameters may exceed 150 nm. Their results support the concept that type IX collagen on the surface of the type II collagen fibrils could facilitate interactions with other matrix components limiting the formation of larger fibril aggregates. These interactions, along with the type IX–type II collagen interactions identified by the cross-linking studies (Wu *et al.*, 1992), provide a possible mechanism by which type IX could stabilise the fibrillar network.

The importance of type II collagen to normal cartilage function is well documented and is evident from the consequences of mutations in the COL2A1 gene which cause disorders ranging from death *in utero* as in achondrogenesis II to relatively mild spondyloarthropathies (reviewed in Eyre and Wu, 1995; Williams and Jimenez, 1995; Horton, 1996). It is now apparent that the other collagens of the heterotypic fibrils also have profound effects on cartilage integrity.

Transgenic mice have been produced with a defective col9a1 gene which express a truncated $\alpha1(IX)$ chain (Nakata *et al.*, 1993; Olsen, 1995). These animals developed pathological changes in the articular cartilage of the knee joints which resembled those seen in osteoarthritis. Furthermore mice which were homozygous for the mutation were found to have a mild chondrodysplasia. Another transgenic mouse has been generated which lacks the $\alpha1(IX)$ chain completely (Fassler *et al.*, 1994). Surprisingly, even the homozygous mutants appear normal at birth, but later they develop a severe degenerative joint disease with similarities to human osteoarthritis. These findings suggest that changes in or lack of type IX collagen chains do not directly affect the gross appearance of the cartilage or its overall development. However, they may affect the organisation of cartilage components at a molecular level leading to conditions such as chondrodysplasia or osteoarthritis, perhaps due to a loss of cartilage integrity which only becomes apparent when the cartilage is exposed to conditions of loading after birth.

In genetic linkage studies the $\alpha1(IX)$ collagen gene has been mapped to the human and mouse chromosome 6 (Yoshioko *et al.*, 1992; Warman *et al.*, 1993), the $\alpha3(IX)$ collagen gene to the human chromosome 20 (Brewton *et al.*, 1995) and the gene for the $\alpha2(IX)$ chain to human chromosome 1 or mouse chromosome 4 (Perala *et al.*, 1993; Warman *et al.*, 1994). In 1994 it was found that the locus for multiple epiphyseal dysplasia (EDM2) is on the short arm of chromosome 1, in the region of the type IX collagen gene, COL9A2, which encodes the $\alpha2$ chain (Briggs *et al.*, 1994). The major effect of EDM2 is early-onset osteoarthritis and the possible role of type IX collagen in determining the architecture of the cartilage extracellular matrix suggests that the COL9A2 gene could be involved in this disease. Subsequent studies have revealed a mutation predicted to cause a 12 amino acid deletion in the COL3 domain of the $\alpha2$ chain which associates with EDM2. It has been suggested that weak mutations in type IX collagen may represent genetic risk factors for late onset osteoarthritis (Olsen, 1997).

Most of the theories concerning the role of type IX collagen predict that events which result in a loss of type IX collagen eg by the action of proteolytic enzymes, will have a profound effect on matrix integrity and lead to cartilage degradation as occurs in osteo- and rheumatoid arthritis. Certainly the location of type IX on the surface of the type II fibrils and its non-collagenous domains would render it relatively susceptible to proteolytic digestion. Furthermore type IX collagen in articular cartilage is known to decrease with age (Duance and Wotton, 1991) which may predispose the cartilage to degenerative changes and if type IX collagen is not readily re-expressed the cartilage may be unable to repair itself effectively.

TYPE XI COLLAGEN

MOLECULAR STRUCTURE AND ORGANISATION

Type XI collagen was first isolated from human neonatal cartilage and was fractionated into three distinct polypeptide chains termed 1α, 2α, 3α (Burgeson and Hollister, 1979). Chemical cross-linking studies (Morris and Bachinger, 1987) showed that the chains, now known as $\alpha1(XI)$, $\alpha2(XI)$ and $\alpha3(XI)$, form predominantly heterotrimeric molecules containing one of each chain. The $\alpha1(XI)$ and $\alpha2(XI)$ chains are products of separate genes, COL11A1 and COL11A2 respectively, and the complete sequences of $pro\alpha1(XI)$ (Bernard et al., 1988; Yoshioka and Ramirez, 1990) and $pro\alpha2(XI)$ (Kimura et al., 1989; Zhidkova et al., 1993; Lui et al., 1996a) have been elucidated. The $pro\alpha3(XI)$ chain appears to be a product of the gene COL2A1, which codes for the $\alpha1(II)$ chain, differences between the two chains being due to post-translational hydroxylation and glycosylation (Burgeson et al., 1982). While type XI collagen is associated with type II collagen in cartilaginous matrices (Mendler et al., 1989) and type V collagen is usually associated with type I collagen, recent studies have shown that chains of collagen types V and XI coexist within tissues (Niyibizi and Eyre, 1989; Mayne et al., 1993; Kleman et al., 1992). It is probable that the α-chains of types V and XI can participate in the formation of heterotypic molecules of stoichiometries other than those previously assigned and therefore, are now considered as a single collagen type (see Fichard et al., 1994). For the purpose of this review however, our discussion will be limited to observations of the common $\alpha1(XI)$, $\alpha2(XI)$, $\alpha3(XI)$ molecules present in and isolated from cartilage and chondrocyte cultures. Type V collagen will be discussed briefly later.

In common with other fibrillar collagens, the α-chains of type XI collagen are synthesised as precursor procollagen chains consisting of a triple helical domain of more than 1000 amino acids, with globular extensions at the amino- and carboxy-termini (Figure 9.3). Type XI collagen has 5 major domains; NC1 (the non-collagenous C-propeptide), COL1 (the $\sim300\,nm$ triple helical region), NC2 (non-collagenous "hinge"-like region), COL2 (minor collagenous domain) and NC3 (N-terminal non-collagenous domain). Processing of type XI collagen has been studied in embryonic chick sterna in vitro (Thom and Morris, 1991). It is slower and more complex than that of collagen types I and II. All three chains of type XI collagen are initially processed at the C-terminal domains, which are linked through cysteines. $\alpha3(XI)$ undergoes one processing step at the N-terminal domain which results in the fully processed matrix form of this chain. $\alpha1(XI)$ and $\alpha2(XI)$ however, are processed at the N-terminal domain in two stages, involving the formation of intermediate forms with the matrix form retaining substantial N-terminal domains. By rotary shadowing electron microscopy (Morris et al., 1990;

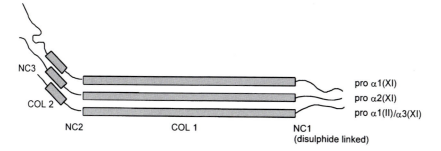

FIGURE 9.3   Diagram of the type XI collagen molecule.

Thom and Morris, 1991), the matrix form of type XI collagen appears as a molecule of approximately 315 nm in length.

NC1, the C-propeptide

The C-propeptide is highly conserved for all the fibrillar collagens and the cysteines present are believed to be involved in the initial recognition of procollagen chains and subsequent triple helix formation. On the basis of the NC1 sequences, it has been speculated (Kimura *et al.*, 1989) that the $\alpha2(XI)$ chains, like $\alpha3(XI)/\alpha1(II)$, can form homotrimers, the requirement being 8 cysteinyl residues in the C-propeptide. $\alpha1(XI)$ has 7 cysteine residues suggesting it can only form heterotrimeric molecules (Bernard *et al.*, 1988). Homotrimeric molecules of $\alpha2(XI)$ however have not been isolated.

COL1, the triple helical region

The triple helical region of $\alpha1(XI)$ is highly homologous to $\alpha2(XI)$ and $\alpha1(V)$. Likewise, $\alpha3(XI)$ and $\alpha2(V)$ show a high degree of homology. The domains consist of 338 or 339 uninterrupted Gly-X-Y repeats. As mentioned earlier, the $\alpha3(XI)$ is believed to be an overglycosylated $\alpha1(II)$ chain. $\alpha1(XI)$ and $\alpha2(XI)$ are also modified extensively by the intracellular activities of the procollagen glycosyl transferases and were found to contain 28 and 34 glycosylated hydroxylysines respectively, mostly glucosyl-galactosylhydroxylysines (Burgeson *et al.*, 1982). In contrast, $\alpha1(I)$ and $\alpha1(II)$ contain 5 and 10 glycosylated hydroxylysines respectively. Disaccharide modified hydroxylysine residues will increase the effective hydrated size of the type XI collagen helix, relative to type II, and may be important in determining the efficiency of molecular packing in the heterotypic fibril. The triple helix of type XI collagen also differs from that of collagen types I, II and III in its thermal stability. Type XI (and V) have thermal unfolding intermediates in the triple helix to coil transition (Morris *et al.*, 1990) with transitions occurring at around 38°C. The lower thermal stability of type XI collagen may lead to greater flexibility and also, increased susceptibility to gelatinase activities during matrix remodelling.

The COL1 domain has binding sites which may be involved in interacting with other extracellular matrix components. $\alpha1(XI)$ and $\alpha2(XI)$ triple helices both have heparin binding sites (Smith and Brandt, 1987). By comparison with the $\alpha1(V)$ sequence (Yaoi *et al.*, 1990), the heparin binding site of $\alpha1(XI)$ is probably in the highly conserved region of residues 342 to 374. It was found that the major cartilage proteoglycan aggrecan could bind to type XI collagen, presumably through the same sites and that this binding was reduced following proteolytic digestion, suggesting that the protein component of this proteoglycan stabilised the binding (Smith *et al.*, 1985). In a heparin binding assay, the only glycosaminoglycans found to compete for binding to native type XI collagen were heparin, heparan sulphate and dermatan sulphate (Vaughan-Thomas and Duance, 1994). It has been suggested that heparan sulphate-type XI collagen interactions may be of importance on the chondrocyte surface and Smith *et al.* (1989) demonstrated association of type XI collagen with the cell membrane. Preincubation of chondrocytes with heparin or with heparinase reduced attachment of the cells to type XI collagen coated substrates confirming the involvement of cell-surface heparan sulphate (unpublished observations). Along the COL1 domain of $\alpha2(XI)$ there are also three RGD motifs which could contribute to chondrocyte surface interaction. COL1 of $\alpha1(XI)$ however, has two inactive RGE sequences instead of the RGD motifs. It is interesting to note that $\alpha1(V)$, which Eyre and Wu (1987) have found replaces some of the $\alpha1(XI)$ chains with age, has two RGD motifs, suggesting that there may be additional chondrocyte–collagen interaction with increasing age.

NC2, the 'hinge region' and COL2, the 'minor helix'

NC2 is a non-collagenous region of around 36 amino acids. It is visualised by rotary shadowing as a flexible hinge or 'kink' which forms an angle between the COL1 and COL2 domains. Although all three chains of type XI collagen contain a putative N-proteinase cleavage site within this domain, there appears to be little or no utilisation of this site as all chains in the matrix retain the COL2 domain (Thom and Morris, 1991; Rousseau *et al.*, 1996; Wu and Eyre, 1995). COL2 is a 51 amino acid collagenous domain. As COL2 is retained on the constituent chains, the rod-like structure observed by rotary shadowing, corresponding to this domain, may be triple helical. Its retention on the type XI collagen molecule introduces another mechanism by which fibril diameter and packing could be affected by interfering with the accretion of further collagen molecules onto the surface of a heterotypic fibril by steric hindrance.

NC3, the non-collagenous, globular domain

The N-terminal domains of $pro\alpha1(XI)$ and $pro\alpha2(XI)$ (and $pro\alpha1(V)$) differ from those of collagen types I, II and III in length and structure. The NC3 domains of $pro\alpha1(XI)$ and $pro\alpha2(XI)$ may be divided into two main sub-domains (Figure 9.4). The most N-terminal of these is a module rich in basic residues, isolated originally from cartilage as a disulphide-bonded molecule called PARP (proline/arginine rich protein) (Neame *et al.*, 1990). Cloning and sequencing revealed that PARP is part of the $pro\alpha2(XI)$ chain (Zhidkova *et al.*, 1993). The $pro\alpha1(XI)$ chain contains a PARP-like module which has since been identified in several collagen chains, including the FACIT collagens.

C-terminal of PARP is a variable region (VR). The VR of rat $\alpha1(XI)$ contains exons V1a, V1b and V2, (Oxford *et al.*, 1995) and the human and chick VR contain exons IIA, IIB and IV, (Zhidkova *et al.*, 1995). Variation in the VR transcripts occurs as a result of alternative exon usage. There are three exons which may be differentially used; VIa

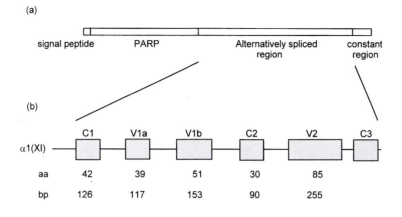

(a)

signal peptide   PARP   Alternatively spliced   constant
region   region

(b)

	C1	V1a	V1b	C2	V2	C3
α1(XI)						
aa	42	39	51	30	85	
bp	126	117	153	90	255	

Adapted from Oxford et al 1995.

FIGURE 9.4 (a) Diagram of NC3 subdomains and (b) organisation of exons coding for the alternatively spliced variable subdomain of NC3 of proα1(XI).

(or IIA) which is highly acidic, V1b (or IIB) which is very basic and V2 (or IV), which is also acidic. While it has been reported that transcripts of all these exons are found in cartilage there is a paucity of data on translated products. However, in their study of the processing of chick type XI collagen, Rousseau *et al.* (1996) suggested that the major cartilage form of α1(XI) is Vo which lacks exons IIA, IIB and IV. Their study showed that the fully processed form of α1(XI) in chondrocyte cultures begins at Gln-254, seven residues before the end of the PARP region, and was immediately followed by a sequence encoded by exon III.

In the α2(XI) gene, exon 7 (containing exons 7A, 7B and 7C) in human and exons 6 to 8 in mouse are also alternatively spliced (Lui *et al.*, 1996b; Tsumaki and Kimura, 1995). Tsumaki and Kimura (1995) found that most of the transcripts in mouse cartilage did not contain exons 6 to 8, but suggested that even transient expression of isoforms containing sequences derived from these exons may be important in cartilage interactions. α3(XI) is believed to be α1(IIB) (Wu and Eyre, 1995) which is the short spliced variant of COL2A1 (Sandell *et al.*, 1991, 1997).

The presence of isoforms of each chain of type XI collagen indicate functions and interactions which may be important at different stages of development and growth. Interactions with other basic or acidic molecules, rates and the extent of processing and fibril diameter regulation may all be mediated by these alternative transcripts.

Type XI collagen cross-linking

The major type XI collagen cross-links of foetal bovine cartilage are the divalent, borohydride-reducible ketoamines (Wu and Eyre, 1995). The cross-linking is chain specific and predominantly between N-telopeptides (NC2 domains) and the C-terminal region of the triple helix. This is consistent with a head to tail interaction between individual collagen molecules arranged in a 4D stagger within a fibrillar network. Type XI collagen molecules are mainly cross-linked to each other and it was concluded that a homopolymer is formed initially in the matrix. The cross-links identified were between the $\alpha1$(XI) N-telopeptide and $\alpha3$(XI) C-terminal helix, the $\alpha2$(XI) N-telopeptide and $\alpha1$(XI) C-terminal helix and the $\alpha3$(XI) N-telopeptide and $\alpha2$(XI) C-terminal helix. These cross-links are N-terminal of the putative N-telopeptide, defined by the predicted N-proteinase cleavage site. Also, a cross-link was identified between the amino-terminal site of the $\alpha1$(XI) triple helix and the $\alpha1$(II)/$\alpha3$(XI) C-telopeptide, forming potentially a lateral linkage of the type XI collagen homopolymer with type II collagen within the heterotypic fibril. The location of the cross-links amino-terminal to the putative N-proteinase cleavage site confirms that the N-terminal domains of the three chains of type XI collagen are retained in cartilage matrix. Wu and Eyre (1995) speculate that MMP-3, which is known to cleave C-terminal to the N-telopeptide cross-links of type XI collagen, may therefore allow for depolymerisation and remodelling of the collagenous components of matrix in cartilage.

Finally, type XI collagen may be a substrate for transglutaminase as reviewed by Fichard et al. (1994). However, expression of the enzyme is associated with terminal differentiation of chondrocytes and has not been detected in articular cartilage extracts (Aeschlimann et al., 1993).

IMMUNOLOCALISATION STUDIES

Type XI collagen is reported to be preferentially located in the pericellular regions of articular cartilage (Evans et al., 1983; Ricard-Blum et al., 1982). However, more generalised matrix labelling has also been described in chick embryo sternal cartilage (Mendler et al., 1989), rat articular cartilage (Duance and Wotton, 1991) and in porcine articular and growth plate cartilages (Wardale and Duance, 1993). Using electron microscopy Keene et al. (1995) found that both the amino terminal non-collagenous domain and the C-telopeptide of type XI collagen were readily accessible to specific antibody binding on the surface of fibrils. The labelled fibrils however, were less than 25 nm in diameter and thick fibrils did not label with the specific antibodies, even after treatment with chaotropic agents. In contrast, Mendler et al. (1989) found that the triple helical epitope of type XI collagen could only be detected in fibrils from chick embryo sternal cartilage partially disrupted by mechanical shear, indicating a homogeneous distribution of the molecule buried in the fibrils. Without disruption of the fibril, the type XI collagen was antigenically masked by type II collagen. Keene et al. (1995) suggested that the C-telopeptide may be accessible in the gap region of the fine cartilage fibril and that the amino terminal epitope may protrude from the surface. Therefore the inaccessibility of the triple helix due to masking by type II collagen is not contrary to their findings. Such an arrangement of type XI and II collagen would be in agreement with that hypothesised for type V and I collagen in corneal fibrils (Linsenmayer et al., 1993), with the triple helix of type XI collagen molecules being under the surface, and the N-terminal domains protruding onto the surface of the fibrils.

DEGRADATION OF TYPE XI COLLAGEN

The degradation of type XI collagen by enzymes known to have extracellular matrix degrading activities has been investigated. MMP-1 and MMP-13 are collagenases which are able to cleave the triple helices of the major collagen types I, II and III into specific 1/4 and 3/4 products. The triple helix of type XI collagen is not cleaved by MMP-1 or MMP-13 (Eyre *et al.*, 1984; Knauper *et al.*, 1997) at this site.

Of the other matrix degrading enymes, stromelysin (MMP-3) (Wu *et al.*, 1991), gelatinase (MMP-2) (Yu *et al.*, 1990), cathepsins B & L (Maciewicz *et al.*, 1990b) and neutrophil elastase (Gadher *et al.*, 1988) cleave type XI collagen. Gelatinase cleaves type XI collagen within the triple helix, and the initial products of this digest are similar to those obtained when using crude enzyme extracts from osteoarthritic cartilage. Cathepsins and stromelysin cleave type XI collagen at sites N-terminal of the triple helix, and therefore may act as telopeptidases.

FUNCTION OF TYPE XI COLLAGEN

Some potential interactions and biological functions of type XI collagen have already been discussed, mainly its role in fibril formation and interactions with components of cartilage proteoglycans and chondrocytes. In summary, there are several ways that incorporation of type XI collagen into the heterotypic fibril could limit its diameter. Firstly, the triple helix is heavily glycosylated resulting in a 'bulkier' molecule than type II collagen. The bulkiness of type XI collagen could alter intermolecular spacing in the fibril and therefore molecular packing. Secondly, the retained N-terminal domain could sterically hinder accretion of further molecules onto the fibril surface. Finally, alternative splicing of the N-terminal domains may allow interactions to occur with other matrix molecules which stabilise the fibrils at a certain diameter. It is interesting to note that type XI collagen molecules are cross-linked end to end, suggesting the formation initially of a homopolymer. The relationship between the homopolymer and the heterotypic fibril is unknown.

From immunolocalisation studies and the interaction of type XI collagen with glycosaminoglycan (including cell-surface species), it appears that type XI collagen is found in close proximity or bound to the chondrocyte membrane. Such a location suggests that type XI collagen may be important in cell-matrix interactions. The involvement of alternative exon usage in interactions with other molecules or chondrocytes remains to be elucidated.

Identification of mutations that cause specific chondrodysplasias have provided further evidence of the biological role of type XI collagen in cartilage and in skeletal morphogenesis. Mice homozygous for the autosomal recessive chondrodysplasia (*cho*) mutation have abnormalities in cartilage, notably larger collagen fibrils and loss of cohesion with increased ease of proteoglycan extraction, relative to the normal cartilage. Li *et al.* (1995) identified a deletion 570 nucleotides downstream of the translation initiation codon in COL11A1 causing a reading frame shift and introducing a premature stop codon. As a result of this mutation, $\alpha1(XI)$ chains could not be detected in the cartilage. Both the COL11A1 and COL11A2 genes have also been implicated in forms of Stickler syndrome (Vikkula *et al.*, 1995). Mutations in COL11A2 have been identified which result in forms of the syndrome in which there is no eye pathology as the vitreous hybrid type XI/V molecule contains no $\alpha2(XI)$ chain. However, a mutation identified in a family with Sticklers syndrome type 2 in which there are eye abnormalities, was recently found to be due to a mutation in the COL11A1 gene, encoding the $\alpha1(XI)$ chain of type XI/V collagen (Richards et al., 1996). Type XI collagen is now believed to be of central importance in regulating fibril morphology, matrix interactions and also, cell maturation and organisation in the growth plates of long bones.

In summary, type XI, or type V/XI collagen is a molecule which shows great diversity at several levels. First, there are at least six α-chains from which heterotrimers may be composed, four of which have been identified in cartilage. Second, it exists in cartilage as a triple helical molecule retaining non-triple helical domains and in tissue culture, this form has been shown to arise from complex processing events. Finally, different isoforms arise from the use of alternative splice sites within the gene sequences encoding the N-terminal domains. The functional significance of such structural diversity is yet to be elucidated, but along with type IX collagen, the constituent chains of type XI collagen potentially make the surface of cartilage collagen fibrils highly interactive.

OTHER MINOR COLLAGENOUS COMPONENTS OF ARTICULAR CARTILAGE

TYPE I COLLAGEN

Type I collagen is the major structural protein of the body and has been studied extensively in terms of its physical and chemical characteristics. It is present in the surface fibrocartilaginous layer of chicken articular cartilage (Eyre et al., 1978) but until recently it was thought to be absent from mammalian articular cartilage. However, Duance (1983) and Wardale and Duance (1993) demonstrated that type I collagen is present in porcine articular cartilage while Aigner et al. (1993) reported it in human articular cartilage. It is also predominant in the fibrocartilaginous repair tissue which is formed in response to articular cartilage destruction in equine arthritic diseases (Barr et al., 1994).

TYPE III COLLAGEN

Type III collagen exists mainly in association with type I collagen and is distributed widely throughout the body. Immunoelectron microscopy and cross-linking studies revealed that types I and III collagens coexist within individual fibres (Fleischmajer et al., 1990; Henkel and Glanville, 1982). This interaction is thought to regulate fibril formation and fibril growth. Recently type III was found in both normal and pathological human specimens of the cartilage end-plate, a hyaline cartilage (Roberts et al., 1991a,b). In all cases the type III collagen was localised to a pericellular region which appears to correspond to the outer margins of chondron-like structures and extending out slightly into the matrix. Biochemical and immunolocalisation studies have shown that type III collagen is also present in both normal (Wotton and Duance, 1994) and osteoarthritic human articular cartilage (Aigner et al., 1993). High resolution labelling studies using electron microscopy confirmed these findings and revealed the co-localisation of collagen types II and III within the same fibril (Young *et al.*, 1995; Lawrence *et al.*, 1995). The discovery of cross-links between types II and III collagens isolated from normal adult human articular cartilage (Wu *et al.*, 1996) provides further confirmation for the presence of type III and its colocalisation with type II collagen in cartilage. The function of type III in cartilage is unknown.

TYPE V COLLAGEN

As stated above there is high homology between type V and type XI collagen and tentative evidence suggests that hybrid molecules exist. The detailed composition and domain structure of type V collagen has been recently reviewed (Fichard *et al.*, 1994). Like type XI collagen the $\alpha 1$ and $\alpha 2$ chains undergo complex processing but both retain varying sized N-terminal non-triple helical domains. Analysis showed that the $\alpha 2$ chain retained all of the N-terminal domain whilst the $\alpha 1$ chain undergoes limited processing (Niyibizi and Eyre, 1993). Further analysis showed that 2 molecular forms existed, $\alpha 1(V)_2 \alpha 2(V)$ in which the chains retain N-terminal domains and $\alpha 1(V)_3$ in which the α-chains are fully processed (Moradiameli *et al.*, 1994). In cartilage, the $\alpha 1(V)$ chain increases while the $\alpha 1(XI)$ chain decreases with age (Eyre and Wu, 1987). Whether the $\alpha 1(V)$ chain is present as a separate molecule or as part of a hybrid molecule awaits further investigation.

In many tissues, type V collagen appears to be present in the form of heterotypic fibrils co-polymerised with type I collagen where it may control the diameter of the fibrils (Birk *et al.*, 1988). Studies on the cornea, where all the collagen fibrils are of a small uniform diameter, have demonstrated that type V collagen regulates the fibril diameter of the type I fibrils (Birk *et al.*, 1990; Linsenmayer *et al.*, 1993). A model of a collagen fibril was proposed with the amino terminal portion of type V collagen protruding through the surface preventing any further addition of type I molecules to the fibril by steric hindrance. This model has been further demonstrated with domain specific antibodies showing that the N-terminal tyrosine rich region of type V collagen is retained on the fibril surface (Peters *et al.*, 1996). Loss of antibody reactivity with age was shown to be due to masking rather than further processing of the type V collagen. Recent studies on matrix assembly using either cell culture or transgenic mice both demonstrate that type V collagen is a key component in type I collagen fibril assembly (Andrikopoulos *et al.*, 1995; Marchant *et al.*, 1996).

The importance of type V collagen in joint tissues has not been studied extensively. The precise role of type V collagen appearing in articular cartilage is unknown. Its presence in other tissue components of the joint such as the meniscus, joint capsule and subchondral bone suggest that alterations in type V collagen expression may have significant impact on the normal functioning of the joint.

TYPE VI COLLAGEN

Type VI collagen is a heterotrimer of three distinct chains, $\alpha 1(VI)$, $\alpha 2(VI)$ and $\alpha 3(VI)$, (Timpl and Engel, 1987). The triple-helical domain is short (105 nm) but the N- and C-terminal globular domains are very large and account for more than two-thirds of the mass of the molecule. All 3 α-chains have a multidomain structure; their globular domains containing modules homologous to von Willebrand factor A. The larger $\alpha3(VI)$ chain additionally contains modules with similarity to salivary proteins, to fibronectin type III repeats and to Kunitz type protease inhibitor (Chu *et al.*, 1990; Ayad *et al.*, 1994). The $\alpha2(VI)$ and $\alpha3(VI)$ chains exist in a number of different forms due to alternative splicing. In the $\alpha3(VI)$ chain splicing occurs in the N-terminal NC2 region and gives rise to four isoforms while in the $\alpha2(VI)$ three alternative forms are possible through splicing in the C-terminal region (Ayad *et al.*, 1994; Stokes *et al.*, 1991; Saitta *et al.*, 1990). The type VI molecules assemble into dimers in an antiparallel fashion which aggregate laterally to form disulphide bonded tetramers. These associate non-covalently to form networks of microfibrils. The type VI microfibrils have a beaded appearance and are found in most connective tissues including articular cartilage where they are stabilised by interaction of the large globular domain of the $\alpha3(VI)$ chain with hyaluronan (Kielty *et al.*, 1992; McDevitt *et al.*, 1991). Type VI collagen is rich in RGD sequences and has been shown to bind to the surface of many cells including chondrocytes (Marcelino and McDevitt, 1995).

Ayad *et al.* (1984) described the localisation of type VI collagen around the chondrocytes in bovine nasal cartilage and it was later found to be preferentially located in the pericellular capsule of chondrons (Poole *et al.*, 1988b). Type VI collagen has been shown to occur as concentric rings in isolated chondrons (Lee, 1995) similar to that observed for type IX collagen in the rat chondrosarcoma (Wotton *et al.*, 1991) and may indicate a role in matrix organisation. However, there was a suggestion that type VI collagen might have a wider distribution in the superficial layers of the cartilage particularly in young tissue (Duance and Wotton, 1991). Recent studies on cartilage development (Morrison *et al.*, 1996) have shown that type VI is widely distributed throughout the matrix in foetal cartilage but becomes restricted to the pericellular domain during growth. The increased expression of type VI collagen in osteoarthritis has been suggested to be an attempt at tissue repair (Arican *et al.*, 1996; Chang and Poole, 1996). In samples of all ages, labelling in close proximity to the chondrocytes throughout the full thickness of the cartilage was clearly seen which is consistent with a postulated cell binding function suggested by the presence of the cell binding motif, RGD, in the type VI sequence.

COLLAGEN TYPES XII AND XIV

These FACIT collagens have partial homology with type IX collagen (Gordon *et al.*, 1989; Keene *et al.*, 1991; Mazzorana, 1993). In collagen types IX, XII and XIV there is a highly conserved region of 100 amino acid residues/chain at the C-terminal of the triple helical COL1 domain and two cysteines separated by 4 amino acids at the junction of COL1 and NC1. It is likely this domain is involved in the interaction between the fibrillar and FACIT collagens. Types XII and XIV collagens are synthesised as disulphide bonded homotrimeric molecules, $[\alpha1(XII)]_3$ and $[\alpha1(XIV)]_3$ (Ayad *et al.*, 1994) and are structurally similar, having short interrupted triple-helical domains with 3 large globular domains (NC3) projecting from each α-chain. Types XII and XIV collagen both exist as two variants which arise by alternative splicing (Nishiyama *et al.*, 1994; Gerecke *et al.*, 1993). Types XII and XIV collagen are found mainly in tissues which are rich in type I collagen but recently they have also been reported in bovine articular cartilage

(Watt *et al.*, 1992) where they may exist in a proteoglycan form possessing an attached chondroitin sulphate chain. Although collagens XII and XIV occur together in many tissues they have distinct regional distributions. Nevertheless, at the ultrastructural level they have both been found to be associated with, but not cross-linked to banded collagen fibrils (Keene *et al.*, 1991; Nishiyama *et al.*, 1994). Fibril diameter does not seem to be affected and it has been suggested that these collagens may bridge adjacent fibrils or be involved in mediating matrix deformability through interaction of their NC3 domains with other tissue components.

MENISCAL CARTILAGE

The menisci of the mammalian knee joint are two semilunar, fibrous structures located between the articular surfaces of the tibial plateaux and the femoral condyles. The tissue is described historically as fibrocartilage as most species have a narrow inner region of hyaline cartilage which merges with the fibrous tissue that makes up the majority of the meniscus. Whilst this arrangement holds true for several studied species (eg canine, bovine, porcine and equine), some species such as human (Wardale *et al.*, 1996) appear never to have a hyaline region during any stages of development. As the human knee menisci develop by metaplasia from fibrous tissue (Clark and Ogden, 1983) rather than precartilage or hyaline cartilage as many of the other types of fibrocartilages do, it is perhaps not surprising that there is no area of hyaline cartilage. A recent study of developing rabbit meniscus (Bland and Ashhurst, 1997) has shown that the arrangement of collagen types is highly dynamic, starting with a type I collagen matrix, type II collagen not appearing until 3 weeks after birth and by 14 weeks only type II collagen mRNA is being expressed. The development of distinct fibrocartilage at tendon or ligament insertion sites and at boney pulleys where mechanical compression causes a change in fibrochondrocyte phenotype, results in a clearly defined area rich in type II and other hyaline cartilage collagens (Benjamin and Evans, 1990; Benjamin and Ralphs, 1997). This is clearly not the case in normal human knee menisci and it is debatable therefore, whether the term fibrocartilage should be applied to this tissue.

STRUCTURE

The menisci are characterised morphologically by thick collagen fibres that are predominantly circumferential in orientation. The compressive loads acting upon the wedge-shaped meniscal cartilage are converted to radially directed extrusive forces which are resisted by the strong anterior and posterior attachments of the menisci. These radial forces are balanced by the tensile stresses developed by the circumferentially orientated collagen bundles (Skaggs and Mow, 1990). The collagen fibres are prevented from separating by large radial tie fibres which run perpendicular to and are stiffer than the majority of the type I collagen fibrils (Skaggs *et al.*, 1994) (Figure 9.5). It is inevitable, therefore, that any alteration in the biochemical composition of the tissue will have a significant effect on the mechanical properties of the menisci.

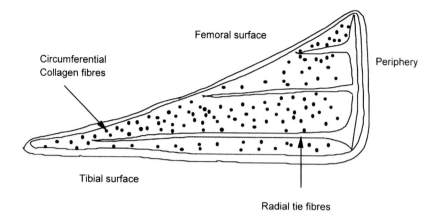

FIGURE 9.5   Diagrammatic representation of a transverse section of meniscus.

COLLAGENOUS COMPONENTS

Early work on lapine and bovine meniscus showed that collagen constitutes approximately 75% of the dry weight of total meniscal cartilage, the remainder being proteoglycan and noncollagenous proteins. The inner third (by weight) of bovine meniscus resembles hyaline cartilage and has been shown to contain a mixture of types I and II collagens while the outer two-thirds is fibrous in appearance and comprises predominantly type I collagen with traces of type V and type III collagen (Eyre and Wu, 1983; Cheung, 1987). Type VI collagen is present in extracts of whole meniscus and makes up 1–2% of the total (Wu *et al.*, 1987). Type I collagen from meniscus shows more post-translational modification than that from bone, skin or tendon, having higher levels of hydroxylysine and hydroxylysine glycoside (Eyre and Wu, 1983). Porcine and bovine menisci also contain high levels of the mature collagen cross-link hydroxylysylpyridinoline (Eyre and Oguchi, 1980; Nakano *et al.*, 1986).

CHANGES IN THE COLLAGENS WITH DISEASE

The menisci have a vital role in load-bearing and transmission of the load across the joint (Cox and Cordell, 1977) and therefore may contribute to the pathogenesis of osteoarthritis of the knee, one of the most affected joints (Cushnaghan and Dieppe, 1991). In most cases of osteoarthritis there are substantial degenerative changes in the meniscus and it is known that meniscectomy or any joint destabilisation predisposes the knee to develop osteoarthritis (Seedholm and Hargreaves, 1979; Cox *et al.*, 1975; Roos *et al.*, 1995) probably due to the subsequent exposure of the articular surfaces to abnormal forces.

To date very little information is available on the biochemical events associated with meniscal degeneration in patients with osteoarthritis. An increase in water content implying a compromise in the capacity of the collagenous fibrillar meshwork to resist the swelling pressure of the proteoglycans has been seen in the degenerating human meniscus (Herwig *et al.*, 1984). A decrease in collagen content has been shown in both osteoarthritic and rheumatoid arthritic meniscus when compared to normal, age-matched controls (Ghosh *et al.*, 1975). The maintenance of structural integrity during the extreme loads experienced by the meniscus must rely heavily on the interactions of collagen with the surrounding extracellular matrix.

Work on the biochemical composition of human meniscal cartilage has concentrated on studying an age range of normal and osteoarthritic tissue (Wardale *et al.*, 1996). Using SDS-PAGE of cyanogen bromide digested tissue and Western blotting, in combination with enhanced chemiluminescent detection and laser-scanning densitometry (Hills *et al.*, 1996), collagen types I, II, III, and VI have been quantified in meniscal samples. This work demonstrated a steady decline in total meniscal collagen with age from 75% (dry weight) at 5 years to 65% at 80 years. There is also a steady increase from 5 years to 65 years of levels of the mature collagen cross-link, hydroxylysyl-pyridinoline (HYL-PYR) in normal meniscus. There is a decrease in type I and an increase in type III collagen with age in normal menisci resulting in a steadily decreasing type I : type III ratio. Normal meniscal samples only rarely contain any detectable type II collagen and then only in minute quantities. Type VI collagen decreases in amount and becomes reorganised from a distribution throughout the matrix into a pericellular location with increasing age in normal samples.

However, if one compares normal with osteoarthritic (OA) meniscal samples there is a dramatic decrease in the levels of HYL-PYR with disease (Figure 9.6a). This loss of mature cross-links in OA menisci may contribute to the severity of the disease. There is reduced type I collagen in OA samples compared to normal samples (Figure 9.6b), and unchanged type III (Figure 9.6c) resulting in a lower than normal type I : type III ratio in the diseased tissue (Figure 9.6d). OA samples also contain higher levels of type VI collagen than in the normal samples (Figure 9.6e). The most interesting finding however, is that type II collagen is present in the majority of OA samples and comprises up to 8% of the total collagen (Figure 9.6f). A switch to type II collagen synthesis represents a radical event for the cell and it is likely that there is expression of other hyaline cartilage proteins altering the normal cell/matrix interactions known to be important for tissue homeostasis.

LOCALISATION OF COLLAGEN TYPES

Immunolocalisation studies showed that collagen types I and III are distributed throughout the matrix of the whole meniscus with very little variation with age or disease. As mentioned above, type II collagen is not usually detected in normal samples but is found in the majority of OA samples studied. The distribution is patchy and the expression is not in the inner area where any hyaline cartilage in other species of meniscus exists, but is distributed within the main body of the tissue (Figures 9.7a,b). The cells and matrix in the areas of new type II collagen expression do not resemble a hyaline cartilage and do not differ histologically from the surrounding tissue. Collagen types IX and XI were not detected with the type II expression either biochemically or immunohisto-chemically but it is possible that they are present below the detection limits of our techniques. Type VI collagen shows a distribution that is related to the age of the tissue. In young tissue the collagen is detected solely in the matrix of the meniscus (Figure 9.7c), whereas with increasing age the matrix staining is reduced with increasing concentrations

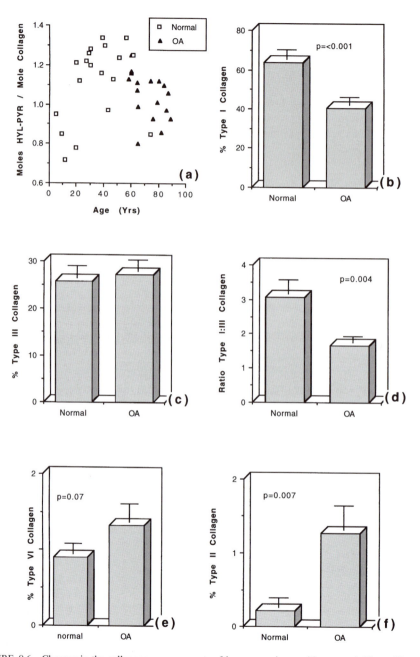

FIGURE 9.6   Changes in the collagenous components of human meniscus with osteoarthritis. a: Changes in the levels of the mature collagen cross-link hydroxylysyl-pyridinoline with age and OA. b and c: Changes in the percentage of collagen types I and III respectively with OA. d: Changes in the ratio of type I : type III collagen with OA. e and f: Changes in the percentage of collagen types VI and II respectively with OA. All percentages are with respect to total dry weight collagen.

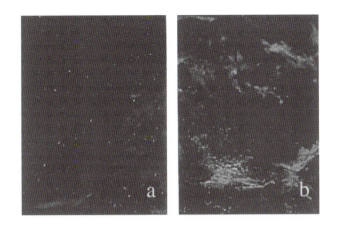

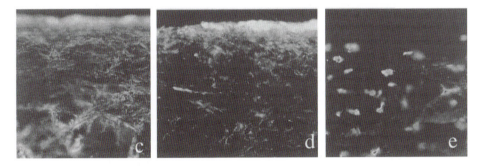

FIGURE 9.7   Immunolocalisation of collagen types in normal and OA human meniscus. a and b: Immunostaining for type II collagen, c–e: Immunostaining for type VI collagen. a: Normal tissue, 23 yrs, b: OA tissue, 82 yrs, c: Normal tissue, 5 yrs, d: Normal tissue, 20 yrs, e: OA tissue 81 yrs.

near the cells (Figure 9.7d). Finally, in old and particularly OA samples, the signal becomes totally pericellular with no staining of the surrounding matrix (Figure 9.7e).

In summary there is great variability in the composition, localisation, development and age-related changes in the collagens from different species of the mammalian meniscus. Until recently, few studies have been carried out on this tissue and little is known about the collagen fibril composition, collagenolytic enzyme composition and the response of meniscal cells to mechanical pressure and growth factors. As meniscal cartilage plays a vital role in maintaining the integrity of the articular cartilages of the knee joint and degeneration of the meniscus may be important in the development of osteoarthritis, it is a field that is worthy of more extensive research.

SUMMARY

Articular, growth plate and meniscal cartilages are 3 very distinct structures with different functions. To achieve this diversity of structure/function it is clear their compositions are required to be very different. Although all 3 cartilages have a major fibrillar collagen network, the matrix organisation and interactive properties are greatly influenced by the more minor collagenous and non-collagenous components. In this review, we have limited our discussions primarily to a few specific components in which there has been considerable interest in recent years. However, it is clear that these components function by interacting with other matrix constituents, which in most cases have yet to be defined. Knowledge of the role of these components in the function of the synovial joint will in the future help us devise new strategies for the treatment of many of the degenerative joint disorders.

REFERENCES

Abe, N., Yoshioka, H., Inoue, H. and Ninomiya, Y. (1994) The complete primary structure of the long form of mouse α1(IX) collagen chain and its expression during limb development. *Biochim. Biophys. Acta*, **1204**, 61–67.

Aeschlimann, D., Wetterwald, A., Fleisch, H. and Paulsson, M. (1993) Expression of tissue transglutaminase in skeletal tissue correlates with events of terminal differentiation of chondrocytes. *J. Cell Biol.*, **120**, 1461–1470.

Aigner, T., Bertlin, W., Stos, H., Wesoloh, G. and von der Mark, K. (1993) Independent expression of fibril-forming collagens I, II and III in chondrocytes of human osteoarthritic cartilage. *J. Clin. Invest.*, **91**, 829–837.

Andrikopoulos, K., Liu, X., Keene, D.R., Jaenisch, R. and Ramirez, F. (1995) Targeted mutation in the COL5A2 gene reveals a regulatory role for type V collagen during matrix assembly. *Nature Genetics*, **9**, 31–36.

Arican, M., Carter, S.D., Bennett, D., Ross, G. and Ayad, S. (1996) Increased metabolism of collagen VI in canine osteoarthritis. *J. Comp. Pathol.*, **114**, 249–256.

Ayad, S., Abedin, M.Z., Grundy, S.M. and Weiss, J.B. (1981) Isolation and characterisation of an unusual collagen from hyaline cartilage and intervertebral disc. *FEBS Lett.*, **123**, 195–199.

Ayad, S., Abedin, M.Z., Weiss, J.B. and Grundy, S.M. (1982) Characterisation of another short-chain disulphide bonded collagen from cartilage, vitreous and intervertebral disc. *FEBS Lett.*, **139**, 300–304.

Ayad, S., Evans, H., Weiss, J.B. and Holt, L. (1984) Type VI collagen but not type V collagen is present in cartilage. *Coll. Rel. Res.*, **4**, 165–168.

Ayad, S., Marriott, A., Morgan, K. and Grant, M.E. (1989) Bovine cartilage types VI and IX collagens. Characterisation of their forms *in vivo*. *Biochem. J.*, **262**, 753–761.

Ayad, S., Marriott, A., Brierley, V.H. and Grant, M.E. (1991) Mammalian cartilage synthesizes both proteo-glycan and non-proteoglycan forms of type IX collagen. *Biochem. J.*, **278**, 441–445.

Ayad, S., Boot-Handford, R.P., Humphries, M.J., Kadler, K.E. and Suttleworth, C.A. (1994) The Extracellular Matrix: Facts Book. Academic Press, London.

Barr, A.R.S., Duance, V.C., Wotton, S.F., Waterman, A.E. and Holt, P.E. (1994) Quantitative analysis of cyanogen bromide-cleaved peptides for the assessment of type I : type II collagen ratios in equine articular repair tissue. *Equine. Vet. J.*, **26**, 29–32.

Benjamin, M. and Evans, E.J. (1990) Fibrocartilage *J. Anat.*, **171**, 1–15.

Benjamin, M. and Ralphs, J.R. (1998) The attachment of tendons and ligaments to bone. Chapter 23 (this volume).

Bernard, M., Yoshioka, H., Rodriguez, E., van der Rest, M., Kimura, T., Ninomiya, Y., Olsen, B.R. and Ramirez, F. (1988) Cloning and sequencing of pro-alpha-1 (XI) collagen cDNA demonstrates that type XI belongs to the fibrillar class of collagens and reveals that the expression of the gene is not restricted to cartilagenous tissue. *J. Biol. Chem.*, **263**, 17159–17166.

Birk, D.E., Fitch, J.M., Babiarz, J.P. and Linsenmayer, T.F. (1988) Collagen type I and type V are present in the same fibril in the avian corneal stroma. *J. Cell Biol.*, **106**, 999–1008.

Birk, D.E., Fitch, J.M., Babiarz, J.P., Doane, K.J. and Linsenmayer, T.F. (1990) Collagen fibrillogenesis *in vitro*: interaction of types I and V collagen regulates fibril diameter. *J. Cell. Sci.*, **95**, 649–657.

Bishop, P.N., Crossman, M.V., Mcleod, D. and Ayad, S. (1994) Extraction and characterization of the tissue forms of collagen types II and IX from bovine vitreous. *Biochem. J.*, **299**, 497–505.

Bland, Y. and Ashhurst, D. (1997) Changes in the content of the fibrillar collagens and the expression of their mRNAs in the menisci of the rabbit knee joint during development and ageing. *Histochem. J.*, **28**, 265–274.

Brewton, R.G., Wood, B.M. *et al.* (1995) Molecular cloning of the alpha-3 chain of human type IX collagen – Linkage of the gene Col9α3 to chromosome 20q13.3. *Genomics*, **30**, 329–336.

Briggs, M.D., Choi, H., Warman, M.L., Loughlin, J.A., Wordsworth, P., Sykes, B.C., Irven, C.M.M., Smith, M., Wynne-Davies, R., Lipson, M.H., Biesecker, L.G., Garber, A.P., Lachman, R., Olsen, B.R., Rimoin, D.L. and Cohn, D.H. (1994) Genetic mapping of a locus for multiple epiphyseal dysplasia (EDM2) to a region of chromosome 1 containing a type IX collagen gene. *Am. J. Genet.*, **55**, 678–684.

Bruckner, P. and van der Rest, M. (1994) Structure and function of cartilage collagens. *Microscopy Research and Technique*, **28**, 378–384.

Bruckner, P., Vaughan, L. and Winterhalter, K.H. (1985) Type IX collagen from sternal cartilage of chicken embryo contains covalently bound glycosaminoglycans. *Proc. Natl. Acad. Sci. USA*, **82**, 2608–2612.

Bruckner, P., Mendler, M., Steinmann, B., Huber, S. and Winterhalter, K.H. (1988) The structure of human collagen type IX and its organisation in fetal and infant cartilage fibrils. *J. Biol. Chem.*, **263**, 16911–16917.

Burgeson, R.E. and Hollister, D.W. (1979) Collagen heterogeneity in human cartilage: identification of several new chains. *Biochem. Biophys. Res. Comm.*, **87**, 1124–1131.

Burgeson, R.E., Hebda, P.A., Morris, N.P. and Hollister, D.W. (1982) Human cartilage collagens – comparison of cartilage collagens with human type-V collagen. *J. Biol. Chem.*, **257**, 7852–7856.

Chandrasekhar, S. and Harvey, A.K. (1987) Synthesis of type IX collagen: Effect of b-xylosides. *Biochem. Biophys. Res. Comm.*, **146**, 1040–1046.

Chang, J. and Poole, C.A. (1996) Sequestration of type VI collagen in the pericellular microenvironment of adult chondrocytes cultured in agarose. *Osteoarthritis and Cartilage*, **4**, 275–285.

Cheung, H.S. (1987) Distribution of Type-I, Type-II, Type-III, and Type-V in the Pepsin Solubilized Collagens in Bovine Menisci. *Connect Tissue Res.*, **16**, 343–356.

Chu, M.L., Pan, T.C., Conway, D., Saitta, B., Stokes, D., Kuo, H.J., Glanville, R.W., Timpl, R., Mann, K. and Deutzmann, R. (1990) The structure of type VI collagen. *Ann. NY Acad. Sci.*, **580**, 55–63.

Clark, C.R. and Ogden, J.A. (1983) Development of the menisci of the human knee joint. *J. Bone Joint Surg.*, **65A**, 538–547.

Cox, J.S. and Cordell, L.D. (1977) The degenerative effects of medial meniscus tears in dogs knees. *Clin. Orthop. Rel. Res.*, **125**, 236–242.

Cox, J.S., Nye, D.E., Schaefer, W.W. and Woodstein, I.J. (1975) The degenerative effects of partial and total resection of the medial meniscus in dogs knees. *Clin. Orthop. Rel. Res.*, **109**, 175–183.

Cushnaghan, J. and Dieppe, P.A. (1991) A study of 500 patients with limb joint osteoarthritis. 1. Analysis by age, sex and distribution of sympomatic joint sites. *Annals Rheum. Dis.*, **50**, 8–13.

Diab, M., Wu, J.J. and Eyre, D.R. (1996) Collagen type IX from human cartilage: a structural profile of inter-molecular cross-linking sites. *Biochem. J.*, **314**, 327–332.

Duance, V.C. (1983) Surface of articular cartilage: Immunohistological studies. *Cell Biochemistry and Function*, **1**, 143–144.

Duance, V.C. and Wotton, S.F. (1991) Changes in the distribution of mammalian cartilage collagens with age. *Biochem. Soc. Trans.*, **19**, 376S.

Duance, V.C., Shimokomaki, M. and Bailey, A.J. (1982) Immunofluorescence localisation of type-M collagen in articular cartilage. *Biosci. Rep.*, **2**, 223–227.

Duance, V.C., Wotton, S.F., Voyle, C.A. and Bailey, A.J. (1984) Isolation and characterisation of the precursor of type M collagen. *Biochem. J.*, **221**, 885–889.

Duance, V.C., Wotton, S.F. and Bailey, A.J. (1985) Isolation and characterization of mammalian parent type M collagen. *Ann. NY Acad. Sci.*, **460**, 422–425.

Duance, V.C., Wotton, S.F. and Young, R.D. (1990) Type IX function in articular cartilage. *Ann. NY Acad. Sci.*, **580**, 480–483.

Eikenberry, E.F., Mendler, M., Burgin, R., Winterhalter, K.H. and Bruckner, P. (1992) Fibrillar organisation in cartilage. In: *Articular Cartilage and Osteoarthritis* (Eds Kuettner, K.E., Schleyerbach, R., Peyron, J.G. and Hascall, V.C.), pp. 133–149, Raven Press, New York.

Evans, H.B., Ayad, S., Abedin, M.Z., Hopkins, S., Morgan, K., Walton, K.W., Weiss, J.B. and Holt, P.J.L. (1983) Localisation of collagen types and fibronectin in cartilage by immunofluorescence. *Ann. Rheum. Dis.*, **42**, 575–581.

Eyre, D.R. and Oguchi, H. (1980) The hydroxypyridinium crosslinks of skeletal collagens: their measurement, properties and a proposed pathway of formation. *Biochem. Biophys. Res. Commun.*, **92**, 403–410.

Eyre, D.R. and Wu, J.J. (1983) Collagen of fibrocartilage: a distinctive molecular phenotype in bovine meniscus. *FEBS Lett.*, **158**, 265–270.

Eyre, D. and Wu, J.J. (1987) Type XI or $1\alpha 2\alpha 3\alpha$ collagen. In: *Structure and Function of the Collagen Types* (Eds R.E. Mayne and R. Burgeson), pp. 261–268, Academic Press, Orlando, Fl.

Eyre, D. and Wu, J.J. (1995) Collagen structure and cartilage matrix integrity. *J. Rheumatol.*, **22**, 82–85.

Eyre, D.R., Brinkley-Parsons, D.M. and Glimcher, M.J. (1978) Predominance of type I collagen at the surface of avian articular cartilage. *FEBS Lett.*, **85**, 259–263.

Eyre, D.R., Apon, S., Wu, J.J., Ericsson, L.H. and Walsh, K.A. (1987) Collagen type IX: evidence for covalent linkages to type II collagen in cartilage. *FEBS Lett.*, **220**, 337–341.

Eyre, D.R., Wu, J.J. and Woolley, D.E. (1984) All 3 chains of 1-alpha-2-alpha-3-alpha collagen from hyaline cartilage resist human collagenase. *Biochem. Biophys. Res. Comm.*, **118**, 724–729.

Fassler, R., Schnegelsberg, P.N.J., Dausman, J., Shinya, T., Muragaki, Y., McCarthy, M.T., Olsen, B.R. and Jaenisch, R. (1994) Mice lacking $\alpha 1(IX)$ collagen develop noninflammatory degenerative joint disease. *Proc. Natl. Acad. Sci. USA*, **91**, 5070–5074.

Fichard, A., Kleman, J.-P. and Ruggiero, F. (1994) Another look at collagen V and XI molecules. *Matrix Biology*, **14**, 515–531.

Fleischmajer, R., Perlish, J.S., Burgeson, R.E., Shaikh-Bahai, F. and Timpl, R. (1990) Type I and type III collagen interactions during fibrillogenesis. *Ann. NY Acad. Sci.*, **580**, 161–175.

Gadher, S.J., Eyre, D.R., Duance, V.C., Wotton, S.F., Heck, L.W., Schmid, T.M. and Woolley, D.E. (1988) Susceptibility of cartilage collagens type II, type IX, type X and type XI to human synovial collagenase and neutrophil elastase. *Eur. J. Biochem.*, **175**, 1–7.

Gadher, S.J., Eyre, D.R., Wotton, S.F., Schmid, T.M. and Woolley, D.E. (1990) Degradation of cartilage collagens type II, type IX, type X and type-XI by enzymes derived from human articular chondrocytes. *Matrix*, **10**, 154–163.

Gerecke, D.R. *et al.* (1993) Type XIV collagen is encoded by alternative transcripts with distinct 5' regions and is a multidomain protein with homologies to von Willebrand's factor, fibronectin, and other matrix proteins. *J. Biol. Chem.*, **268**, 12177–12184.

Ghosh, P., Ingman, A.M. and Taylor, T.K.F. (1975) Variations in collagen, non collagenous proteins and hexosamine in menisci derived from osteoarthritic and rheumatoid arthritis knee joints. *J. Rheumatol.*, **2**, 100–107.

Gordon, M.K., Gerecke, D.R., Dublet, B., van der Rest, M. and Olsen, B.R. (1989) Type XII collagen. A large multidomain molecule with partial homology to type IX collagen. *J. Biol. Chem.*, **264**, 19772–19778.

Hartmann, D.J., Magliore, H., Ricard-Blum, S., Joffre, A., Couble, M.L., Ville, G. and Herbage, D. (1983) Light and electron immunoperoxidase localization of minor disulphide bonded collagens in fetal calf epiphyseal cartilage. *Coll. Rel. Res.*, **3**, 349–357.

Hayashi, M., Hayashi, K., Iyama, K.I., Trelstad, R.L., Linsenmayer, T.F. and Mayne, R. (1992) Notochord of chick embryos secretes short-form type IX collagen prior to the onset of vertebral chondrogenesis. *Developmental Dynamics*, **194**, 169–176.

Henkel, W. and Glanville, R.W. (1982) Covalent crosslinking between molecules of type I and III collagen. *Eur. J. Biochem.*, **122**, 205–213.

Herwig, J., Egner, E. and Buddecke, E. (1984) Chemical changes of human knee joint menisci in various stages of degeneration. *Ann. Rheum. Dis.*, **43**, 635–640.

Hills, N.J., Barr, A.R.S., Duance, V.C., Wardale, R.J. and Wotton, S.F. (1996) Quantification of collagens in equine articular cartilage by western blotting. *Int. J. Expt. Pathol.*, **77**, 19.

Horton, W.A. (1996) Molecular and genetic basis of the human chondrodysplasias. *Endocrinology & Metabolic Clinics of N. America*, **25**, 683.

Huber, S., van der Rest, M., Bruckner, P., Rodriguez, E., Winterhalter, K.H. and Vaughan, L. (1986) Identification of the type IX collagen polypeptide chains. The $\alpha 2(IX)$ polypeptide carries the chondroitin sulfate chains. *J. Biol. Chem.*, **261**, 5965–5968.

Huber, S., Winterhalter, K.H. and Vaughan, L. (1988) Isolation and sequence analysis of the glycosaminoglycan attachment site of type IX collagen. *J. Biol. Chem.*, **263**, 752–756.

Irwin, M.H. and Mayne, R. (1986) Use of monoclonal antibodies to locate the chondroitin sulfate chain(s) in type IX collagen. *J. Biol. Chem.*, **261**, 16281–16283.

Irwin, M.H., Silvers, S.H. and Mayne, R. (1985) Monoclonal antibody against type IX collagen: Preparation, characterisation, and recognition of the intact form of type IX collagen secreted by chondrocytes. *J. Cell Biol.*, **101**, 814–823.

Jacenko, O. and Olsen, B.R. (1995) Transgenic mouse models in studies of skeletal disorders. *J. Rheumatol.*, **22**, (suppl 43) 39–41.

Jasin, H.E. and Taurog, J.D. (1991) Mechanisms of disruption of the articular cartilage surface in inflammation. Neutrophil elastase increases availability of collagen type II epitopes for binding with antibody on the surface of articular cartilage. *J. Clin. Invest.*, **87**, 1531–1536.

Keene, D.R., Lunstrum, G.P., Morris, N.P., Stoddard, D.W. and Burgeson, R.E. (1991) Two type XII-like collagens localise to the surface of banded collagen fibrils. *J. Cell Biol.*, **113**, 971–978.

Keene, D.R., Oxford, J.T. and Morris, N.P. (1995) Ultrastructural localization of collagen type II, type IX and type XI in the growth-plate of human rib and fetal bovine epiphyseal cartilage – type XI collagen is restricted to thin fibrils. *J. Histochem. Cytochem.*, **43**, 967–979.

Kielty, C.M., Whittaker, S.P., Grant, M.E. and Shuttleworth, C.A. (1992) Type VI collagen microfibrils: Evidence for a structural association with hyaluronan. *J. Cell Biol.*, **118**, 979–990.

Kimura, T., Cheah, K.S.E., Chan, S.D.H., Lui, V.C.H., Mattei, M.G., van der Rest, M., Ono, K., Solomon, E., Ninomiya, Y. and Olsen, B.R. (1989) The human alpha-2(XI) collagen (COL11α2) chain – molecular cloning of cDNA and genomic DNA reveals characteristics of a fibrillar collagen with differences in genomic organization. *J. Biol. Chem.*, **264**, 13910–13916.

Kleman, J.P., Hartmann, D.J., Ramirez, F. and van der Rest, M. (1992) The human rhabdomyosarcoma cell line A204 lays down a highly insoluble matrix composed mainly of α1 type XI and α2 type V collagen chains. *Eur. J. Biochem.*, **210**, 329–335.

Knauper, V., Cowell, S., Smith, B., Lopez Otin, C., O'Shea, M., Morris, H., Zardi, L. and Murphy, G. (1997) The role of the c-terminal domain of human collagenase-3 (MMP-13) in the activation of procollagenase-3, substrate specificity and tissue inhibitor of metalloproteinase interaction. *J. Biol. Chem.*, **272**, 7608–7616.

Konomi, H., Seyer, J.M., Ninomiya, Y. and Olsen, B.R. (1986) Peptide-specific antibodies identify the α2 chain as the proteoglycan subunit of type IX collagen. *J. Biol. Chem.*, **261**, 6742–6746.

Kuettner, K.E. (1992) Biochemistry of articular cartilage in health and disease. *Clin. Biochem.*, **25**, 155–163.

Lawrence, P.A., Young, R.D., Duance, V.C. and Monaghan, P. (1995) High pressure cryofixation for immuno-electron microscopy of human cartilage. *Biochem. Soc. Trans.*, **23**, 508S.

Lee, G.M. (1995) Type VI collagen is arranged in concentric rings in isolated chondrons. *Molecular Biology of the Cell*, **6**, 2223.

Li, Y., Lacerda, D.A., Warman, M.L., Beier, D.R., Yoshioka, H., Ninomiya, Y., Oxford, J.T., Morris, N.P., Andrikopoulos, K., Ramirez, F., Wardell, B.B., Lifferth, G.D., Teuscher, C., Woodward, S.R., Taylor, B.A., Seegmiller, R.E. and Olsen, B.R. (1995) A fibrillar collagen gene, Col11A1, is essential for skeletal morphogenesis. *Cell*, **80**, 423–430.

Linsenmayer, T.F., Gibney, E., Igoe, F., Gordon, M.K., Fitch, J.M., Fessler, L.I. and Birk, D.E. (1993) Type V collagen: molecular structure and fibrillar organisation of the chicken α1(V) NH2-terminal domain, a putative regulator of corneal fibrillogenesis. *J. Cell Biol.*, **121**, 1181–1189.

Lui, V.C.H., Ng, L.J., Sat, E.W.Y. and Cheah, K.S.E. (1996a) The human alpha-2(xi) collagen gene (COL11α2) – completion of coding information, identification of the promoter sequence, and precise localization within the major histocompatibility complex reveal overlap with the ke5 gene. *Genomics*, **32**, 401–412.

Lui, V.C.H., Ng, L.J., Sat, E.W.Y., Nicholls, J. and Cheah, K.S.E. (1996b) Extensive alternative splicing within the amino-propeptide coding domain of alpha-2(XI) procollagen messenger-RNAs – expression of transcripts encoding truncated pro-alpha chains. *J. Biol. Chem.*, **271**, 16945–16951.

Maciewicz, R.A. and Wotton, S.F. (1991) Degradation of cartilage matrix components by the cysteine proteinases, cathepsins B and L. *Biomed. Biochim. Acta*, **50**, 561–564.

Maciewicz, R.A., Wardale, R.J., Wotton, S.F. and Duance, V.C. (1990a) Mode of activation of the precursor to cathepsin L: Implication for matrix degradation in arthritis. *Biol. Chem. Hoppe-Seyler*, **371**, 223–228.

Maciewicz, R.A., Wotton, S.F., Etherington, D.J. and Duance, V.C. (1990b) Susceptibility of the cartilage collagens types II, IX, & XI to degradation by the cysteine proteinases cathepsins B and L. *FEBS Lett.*, **269**, 189–193.

Marcellino, J. and McDevitt, C.A. (1995) Attachment of articular cartilage chondrocytes to the tissue form of type VI collagen. *Biochim. Biophys. Acta*, **1249**, 180–188.

Marchant, J.K., Hahn, R.A., Linsenmayer, T.F. and Birk, D.E. (1996) Reduction of type V collagen using a dominant-negative stategy alters the regulation of fibrillogenesis and results in the loss of corneal specific fibril morphology. *J. Cell Biol.*, **135**, 1415–1426.

Mayne, R., Brewton, R.G., Mayne, P.M. and Baker, J.R. (1993) Isolation and characterisation of the chains of type V/type XI collagen present in bovine vitreous. *J. Biol. Chem.*, **268**, 9381–9386.

Mazzorana, M., Gruffat, H., Sergeant, A. and van der Rest, M. (1993) Mechanisms of collagen trimer formation. Construction and expression of a recombinant minigene in HeLa cells reveals a direct effect of prolyl hydroxylation on chain assembly of type XII collagen. *J. Biol. Chem.*, **268**, 3029–3032.

McCormick, D., van der Rest, M., Goodship, J., Lozano, G., Ninomiya, Y. and Olsen, B.R. (1987) Structure of the glycosaminoglycan domain in the type IX collagen-proteoglycan. *Proc. Natl. Acad. Sci. USA*, **84**, 4044–4048.

McDevitt, C.A., Marcellino, J. and Tucker, L. (1991) Interaction of intact type VI collagen with hyaluronan. *FEBS Lett.*, **294**, 167–170.

Mendler, M., Eich-Bender, S.G., Vaughan, L., Winterhalter, K.H. and Bruckner, P. (1989) Cartilage contains mixed fibrils of collagen types II, IX and XI. *J. Cell Biol.*, **108**, 191–197.

Moradiameli, M., Rousseau, J.C., Kleman, J.P., Champliaud, M.F., Boutillon, M.M., Bernillon, J., Wallach, J. and van der Rest, M. (1994) Diversity in the processing events at the N-terminus of type-V collagen. *Eur. J. Biochem.*, **221**, 987–995.

Morris, N.P. and Bachinger, H.P. (1987) Type-XI collagen is a heterotrimer with the composition $(1\alpha, 2\alpha, 3\alpha)$ retaining non-triple-helical domains. *J. Biol. Chem.*, **262**, 11345–11350.

Morris, N.P., Watt, S.L., Davis, J.M. and Bachinger, H.P. (1990) Unfolding intermediates in the triple helix to coil transition of bovine type-XI collagen and human type-V collagens $\alpha 1_2 \alpha 2$ and $\alpha 1 \alpha 2 \alpha 3$. *J. Biol. Chem.*, **265**, 17, 10081–10087.

Morrison, E.H., Ferguson, M.W.J., Bayliss, M.T. and Archer, C.W. (1996) The development of articular cartilage, 1. The spacial and temporal patterns of collagen types. *J. Anatomy*, **189**, 9–22.

Muragaki, Y., Kimura, T., Ninomiya, Y. and Olsen, B.R. (1990a) The complete primary structure of two distinct forms of human $\alpha 1$(IX) collagen chains. *Eur. J. Biochem.*, **192**, 703–708.

Muragaki, Y., Nishimura, I., Henney, A., Ninomiya, Y. and Olsen, B.R. (1990b) The $\alpha 1$(IX) collagen gene gives rise to two different transcripts in both mouse embryonic and human fetal RNA. *Proc. Natl. Acad. Sci. USA*, **87**, 2400–2404.

Murphy, G. and Reynolds, J.J. (1993) Extracellular matrix degeneration. In: *Connective Tissue and Its Heritable Disorders* (Eds P.M. Royce and B. Steinman), pp. 287–316, Wiley-Liss, Inc. New York.

Nakano, T., Thompson, J.R. and Aherne, F.X. (1986) Distribution of gycosaminoglycans and the non-reducible crosslink, pyridinoline in porcine menisci. *Can. J. Vet. Res.*, **50**, 532–536.

Nakata, K., Ono, K., Miyazaki, J.I., Olsen, B.R., Muragaki, Y., Adachi, E., Yamamura, K.I. and Kimura, T. (1993) Osteoarthritis associated with mild chondrodysplasia in transgenic mice expressing $\alpha 1$(IX) collagen chains with a central deletion. *Proc. Natl. Acad. Sci. USA*, **90**, 2870–2874.

Neame, P.J., Young, C.N. and Treep, J.T. (1990) Isolation and primary structure of PARP, a 24 kDa proline- and arginine-rich protein from bovine cartilage closely related to the NH2-terminal domain in collagen @1(XI). *J. Biol. Chem.*, **265**, 20401–20408.

Nishimura, I., Muragaki, Y. and Olsen, B.R. (1989) Tissue-specific forms of type IX collagen-proteoglycan arise from the use of two widely separated promoters. *J. Biol. Chem.*, **264**, 20033–20041.

Nishiyama, T., McDonough, A.M., Bruns, R.R. and Burgeson, R.E. (1994) Type XII and XIV collagens mediate interactions between banded collagen fibres in vitro and may modulate extracellular matrix deformability. *J. Biol. Chem.*, **269**, 28193–28199.

Niyibizi, C. and Eyre, D.R. (1989) Identification of the cartilage $\alpha 1$(XI) chain in type V from bovine bone. *FEBS Lett.*, **242**, 314–318.

Niyibizi, C. and Eyre, D.R. (1993) Structural analysis of the extension peptides on matrix forms of type V collagen in fetal calf bone and skin. *Biochim. Biophys. Acta*, **1203**, 304–309.

Noro, A., Kimata, K., Oike, Y., Shinomura, T., Maeda, N., Yano, S., Takahashi, N. and Suzuki, S. (1983) Isolation and characterization of a third proteoglycan (PG-Lt) from chick embryo cartilage which contains disulphide-bonded collagenous polypeptide. *J. Biol. Chem.*, **258**, 9323–9331.

Okada, Y., Konomi, H., Yada, T., Kimata, K. and Nagase, H. (1989) Degradation of type IX collagen by matrix metalloproteinase 3 (stromelysin) from human rheumatoid synovial cells. *FEBS Lett.*, **244**, 473–476.

Olsen, B.J. (1992) Molecular biology of cartilage collagens. In: *Articular Cartilage and Osteoarthritis* (Eds K.E. Kuettner, R. Schleyerbach, J.G. Peyron and V.C. Hascall), pp. 151–165, Raven Press, New York.

Olsen, B.R. (1995) New insights into the function of collagens from genetic analysis. *Current Opinion in Cell Biol.*, **7**, 720–727.

Olsen, B.R. (1997) Collagen IX. *Int. J. Biochem. Cell Biol.*, **29**, 555–558.

Oxford, J.T., Doege, K.J. and Morris, N.P. (1995) Alternative exon splicing within the amino-terminal nontriple-helical domain of the rat pro-alpha-1(XI) collagen chain generates multiple forms of the messenger-RNA transcript which exhibit tissue-dependent variation. *J. Biol. Chem.*, **270**, 9478–9485.

Perala, M., Hanninen, M., Hastbacka, J., Elima, K. and Vuorio, E. (1993) Molecular cloning of the human $\alpha 2$(IX) collagen cDNA and assignment of the human COL9A2 gene to chromosome 1. *FEBS Lett.*, **319**, 177–180.

Peters, D.M., Kintner, R.L., Steger, C., Bultmann, K. and Brandt, C.R. (1996) Maturation of collagen fibrils in the corneal stroma results in the masking of tyrosine-rich region of type V procollagen. *Invest. Ophthalmol. & Vis. Sci.*, **37**, 2047–2059.

Poole, C.A., Wotton, S.F. and Duance, V.C. (1988a) Localization of type IX collagen in chondrons isolated from porcine articular cartilage and rat chondrosarcoma. *Histochem. J.*, **20**, 567–574.

Poole, C.A., Ayad, S. and Schofield, J.R. (1988b) Chondrons from articular cartilage: 1. Immunolocalization of type VI collagen in the pericellular capsule of isolated canine tibial chondrons. *J. Cell. Sci.*, **90**, 635–643.

Reese, C.A., Wiedmann, H., Kuhn, K. and Mayne, R. (1982) Characterization of a highly soluble collagenous molecule isolated from chicken hyaline cartilage. *Biochemistry*, **21**, 826–830.

Ricard-Blum, S., Hartmann, D.J., Herbage, D., Payen-Meyran, C. and Ville, G. (1982) Biochemical properties and immunolocalization of minor collagens in foetal calf cartilage. *FEBS Lett.*, **146**, 343–347.

Richards, A.J., Yates, J.R.W., Williams, R., Payne, S.J., Pope, F.M., Scott, J.D. and Snead, M.P. (1996) A family with Stickler syndrome type-2 has a mutation in the COL11A1 gene resulting in the substitution of glycine-97 by valine in alpha-1(XI) collagen. *Human Molecular Genetics*, **5**, 1339–1343.

Roberts, S., Menage, J., Duance, V., Wotton, S. and Ayad, S. (1991a) Collagen types around the cells of the intervertebral disc and cartilage end plate: An immunolocalization study. *Spine*, **16**, 1030–1038.

Roberts, S., Menage, J., Duance, V. and Wotton, S. (1991b) Type III collagen in the intervertebral disc. *Histochem. J.*, **23**, 503–508.

Roos, H., Adalberth, T., Dahlberg, L. and Lohmander, L.S. (1995) Osteoarthritis of the knee after injury to the anterior cruciate ligament or meniscus – the influence of time and age. *Osteoarthritis and Cartilage*, **3**(4), 261–267.

Rousseau, J.C., Farjanel, J., Boutillon, M.M., Hartmann, D.J., van der Rest, M. and Moradi-Amli, M. (1996) Processing of type XI collagen. *J. Biol. Chem.*, **271**, 23743–23748.

Saitta, B., Stokes, D.G., Vissing, H., Timpl, R. and Chu, M.L. (1990) Alternative splicing of the human $\alpha 2$(VI) collagen gene generates multiple mRNA transcripts which predict three protein variants with distinct carboxy termini. *J. Biol. Chem.*, **265**, 6473–6480.

Sandell, L.J., Nalin, A.M. and Zhu, Y. (1997) Collagens in joint tissue. Chapter 8 (this volume).

Sandell, L.J., Morris, N., Robbins, J.R. and Goldring, M.R. (1991) Alternatively spliced type II procollagen mRNAs define distinct populations of cells during vertebral development: differential expression of the amino-propeptide. *J. Cell Biol.*, **114**, 1307–1319.

Seedholm, B.B. and Hargreaves, D.J. (1979) Transmission of the load in the knee joint with special reference to the role of the menisci. *Eng. Med.*, **8**, 220–228.

Shimokomaki, M., Duance, V.C. and Bailey, A.J. (1980) Identification of a new disulphide bonded collagen from cartilage. *FEBS Lett.*, **121**, 51–54.

Shimokomaki, M., Duance, V.C. and Bailey, A.J. (1981) Identification of two further collagenous fractions from articular cartilage. *Biosci. Rep.*, **1**, 561–570.

Shimokomaki, M., Wright, D.W., Irwin, M.H., van der Rest, M. and Mayne, R. (1990) The structure and macro-molecular organisation of type IX collagen in cartilage. *Ann. NY Acad. Sci.*, **460**, 1–7.

Skaggs, D.L. and Mow, V.C. (1990) Function of radial tie fibers in the meniscus. *Trans. Orthop. Res. Soc.*, **15**, 248.

Skaggs, D.L., Warden, W.H. and Mow, V.C. (1994) Radial tie fibers influence the tensile properties of the bovine medial meniscus. *J. Orthop. Res.*, **12**(2), 176–185.

Smith, G.N. and Brandt, K.D. (1987) Interaction of cartilage collagens with heparin. *Coll. Rel. Res.*, **7**, 315–321.

Smith, G.N., Williams, J.M. and Brandt, K.D. (1985) Interaction of proteoglycans with the pericellular $(1\alpha, 2\alpha, 3\alpha)$ collagens of cartilage. *J. Biol. Chem.*, **260**, 761–767.

Smith, G.N., Hasty, K.A. and Brandt, K.D. (1989) Type-XI collagen is associated with the chondrocyte surface in suspension-culture. *Matrix*, **9**, 186–192.

Stokes, D.G., Saitta, B., Timpl, R. and Chu, M.L. (1991) Human $\alpha 3$(VI) collagen gene. Characterization of exons coding for the amino-terminal globular domain and alternative splicing in normal and tumor cells. *J. Biol. Chem.*, **266**, 8626–8633.

Svoboda, K.K., Nishimura, I., Sugrue, S.P., Ninomiya, Y. and Olsen, B.R. (1988) Embryonic chicken cornea and cartilage synthesize type IX collagen molecules with different amino-terminal domains. *Proc. Natl. Acad. Sci. USA*, **85**, 7496–7500.

Swiderski, R.E. and Solursh, M. (1992) Localisation of type II collagen; long form $\alpha 1$(IX) collagen, and short form $\alpha 1$(IX) collagen transcripts in the developing chick notochord and axial skeleton. *Developmental Dynamics*, **194**, 118–127.

Thom, J.R. and Morris, N.P. (1991) Biosynthesis and proteolytic processing of type XI collagen in embryonic chick sterna. *J. Biol. Chem.*, **266**, 7262–7269.

Thomas, J.T., Ayad, S. and Grant, M.E. (1994) Cartilage collagens: strategies for the study of their organisation and expression in the extracellular matrix. *Ann. Rheum. Dis.*, **53**, 488–496.

Timpl, R. and Engel, J. (1987) Type VI collagen. In: *Structure and Function of the Collagen Types* (Eds R.E. Mayne and R. Burgeson), pp. 105–143, Academic Press, Orlando, FI.

Tsumaki, N. and Kimura, T. (1995) Differential expression of an acidic domain in the amino-terminal propeptide of mouse pro-$\alpha 2$(XI) collagen by complex alternative splicing. *J. Biol. Chem.*, **270**, 2372–2378.

van der Rest, M. and Mayne, R. (1988) Type IX collagen proteoglycan from cartilage is covalently cross-linked to type II collagen. *J. Biol. Chem.*, 1615–1618.

Vasios, G., Nishimura, I., Konomi, H., van der Rest, M., Ninomiya, Y. and Olsen, B.R. (1988) Cartilage type IX collagen-proteoglycan contains a large amino-terminal globular domain encoded by multiple exons. *J. Biol. Chem.*, **263**, 2324–2329.

Vaughan, L., Winterhalter, K.H. and Bruckner, P. (1985) Proteoglycan Lt from chicken embryo sternum identi-fied as type IX collagen. *J. Biol. Chem.*, **260**, 4758–4763.

Vaughan, L., Mendler, M., Huber, S., Bruckner, P., Winterhalter, K.H., Irwin, M.I. and Mayne, R. (1988) D-periodic distribution of collagen type IX along cartilage fibrils. *J. Cell Biol.*, **106**, 991–997.

Vaughan-Thomas, A. and Duance, V.C. (1994) Interactions of type XI collagen with other extracellular matrix comonents. *Int. J. Exp. Path.*, **75**, A41–A42.

Vikkula, M., Mariman, E.C.M., Lui, V.C.H., Zhidkova, N.I., Tiller, G.E., Goldring, M.B., van Beersum, S.E.C., de Waal Malefijt, M.C., van den Hoogen, F.H.J., Ropers, H.-H., Mayne, R., Cheah, K.S.E., Olsen, B.R., Warman, M.L. and Brunner, H.G. (1995) Autosomal dominant and recessive osteochondrodysplasias associated with the COL11A2 locus. *Cell*, **80**, 431–437.

Vilamitjana, J., Barge, A., Julliard, A.K., Herbage, D., Baltz, T., Garrone, R. and Harmond, M.F. (1989) Problems in the immunolocalization of type IX collagen in fetal calf cartilage using a monoclonal antibody. *Connect. Tiss. Res.*, **18**, 277–292.

von der Mark, K., van Menxel, M. and Wiedemann, H. (1982) Isolation and characterization of new collagens from chick cartilage. *Eur. J. Biochem.*, **124**, 57–62.

Wardale, R.J. and Duance, V.C. (1993) Quantification and immunolocalisation of porcine articular and growth plate cartilage collagens. *J. Cell Sci.*, **105**, 975–984.

Wardale, R.J., Vaughan-Thomas, A., Bayliss, M., Langkamer, G. and Duance, V.C. (1996) Expression of Collagen in Osteoarthritic Meniscal Cartilage. *Int. J. Exp. Pathol.*, **77**, 21.

Warman, M.L., Tiller, G.E., Polumbo, P.A., Seldin, M.F., Rochelle, J.M., Knoll, J.H.M., Cheng, S.D. and Olsen, B.R. (1993) Physical and linkage mapping of the human and murine genes for the $\alpha 1$ chain of type IX collagen (COL9A1). *Genomics*, **17**, 694–698.

Warman, M.L., McCarthy, M.T., Perala, M., Vuorio, E., Knoll, J.H.M., McDaniels, C.N., Mayne, R., Beier, D.R. and Olsen, B.R. (1994) The genes encoding $\alpha 2(IX)$ collagen (COL9A2) map to human chromosome 1p32.3-p33 and mouse chromosome 4. *Genomics*, **23**, 158–162.

Watt, S.L., Lunstrum, G.P., McDonough, A.M., Keene, D.R., Burgeson, R.E. and Morris, N.P. (1992) Characterisation of collagen types XII and XIV from foetal bovine cartilage. *J. Biol. Chem.*, **267**, 20093–20099.

Williams, C.J. and Jimenez, S.A. (1995) Heritable diseases of cartilage caused by mutations in collagen genes. *J. Rhematol.*, **22**, 28–33.

Wotton, S.F. and Duance, V.C. (1994) Type III collagen in normal articular cartilage. *Histochem. J.*, **26**, 412–416.

Wotton, S.F., Duance, V.C. and Fryer, P.R. (1988) Type IX collagen: a possible function in articular cartilage. *FEBS Lett.*, **234**, 79–82.

Wotton, S.F., Jeacocke, R.E., Maciewicz, R.A., Wardale, R.J. and Duance, V.C. (1991) The application of scanning confocal microscopy in cartilage research. *Histochem. J.*, **23**, 328–335.

Wotton, S.F., Duance, V.C. and Poole, C.A. (1987) A possible function for type IX collagen in articular cartilage. *Proceedings of the Strangeways Research Laboratories 75th Anniversary Symposium*, 25–29.

Wu, J.J. and Eyre, D.R. (1984) Cartilage type IX collagen is cross-linked by hydroxypyridinium residues. *Biochem. Biophys. Res. Comm.*, **123**, 1033–1039.

Wu, J.J. and Eyre, D.R. (1995) Structural analysis of cross-linking domains in cartilage type XI collagen. *J. Biol. Chem.*, **270**, 18865–18870.

Wu, J.J., Eyre, D.R. and Slayter, H.S. (1987) Type VI collagen of the intervertebral disc. Biochemical and elec-tron-microscopic characterization of the native protein. *Biochem. J.*, **248**, 373–338.

Wu, J.J., Lark, M.W., Chun, L.E. and Eyre, D.R. (1991) Sites of stromelysin cleavage in collagen types II, IX, X and XI of cartilage. *J. Biol. Chem.*, **266**, 5625–5628.

Wu, J.J., Woods, P.E. and Eyre, D.R. (1992) Identification of cross-linking sites in bovine cartilage type IX collagen reveals an antiparallel type II-Type IX molecular relationship and type IX to type IX bonding. *J. Biol. Chem.*, **267**, 23007–23014.

Wu, J.J., Murray, J. and Eyre, D.R. (1996) Evidence for copolymeric crosslinking between types II and III colla-gens in human articular cartilage. Abstract 42-7, *42nd Annual Meeting, Orthopaedic Research Society*, 1996.

Yada, T., Suzuki, S., Kobayashi, K., Kobayashi, M., Hoshino, T., Horie, K. and Kimata, K. (1990) Occurrence in chick embryo vitreous humor of a type IX collagen proteoglycan with an extraordinarily large chondroitin sulfate chain and short $\alpha 1$ polypeptide. *J. Biol. Chem.*, **265**, 6992–6999.

Yaoi, Y., Hashimoto, K., Koitabashi, H., Takahara, K., Ito, M. and Kato, I. (1990) Primary structure of the heparin-binding site of type V collagen. *Biochim. Biophys. Acta*, **1035**, 139–145.

Yoshioka, H. and Ramirez, F. (1990) Pro-alpha-1(XI) collagen – structure of the amino-terminal propeptide and expression of the gene in tumor-cell lines. *J. Biol. Chem.*, **265**, 6423–6426.

Yoshioka, H., Zhang, H., Ramirez, F., Mattei, M.G., Moradi-Ameli, M., van der Rest, M. and Gordon, M.K. (1992) Synteny between the loci for a novel FACIT-like collagen locus (D6S228E) and $\alpha 1(IX)$ collagen (COL9A1) on 6q12-q14 in humans. *Genomics*, **13**, 884–886.

Young, R.D., Lawrence, P.A., Duance, V.C., Aigner, T. and Monaghan, P. (1995) Immunolocalization of type III collagen in human articular cartilage prepared by high-pressure cryofixation, freeze-substitution, and low-temperature embedding. *J. Histochem. Cytochem.*, **43**, 421–427.

Yu, L.P., Smith, G.N., Brandt, K.D. and Capello, W. (1990) Type XI collagen degrading activity in human osteoarthritic cartilage. *Arth. Rheum.*, **33**, 1626–1633.

Zhidkova, N.I., Brewton, R.G. and Mayne, R. (1993) Molecular-cloning of PARP (proline arginine-rich protein) from human cartilage and subsequent demonstration that PARP is a fragment of the NH2-terminal domain of the collagen alpha-2(XI) chain. *FEBS Letters*, **326**, 25–28.

Zhidkova, N.I., Justice, S.K. and Mayne, R. (1995) Alternative messenger-RNA processing occurs in the variable region of the pro-alpha-1(XI) and pro-alpha-2(XI) collagen chains. *J. Biol. Chem.*, **270**, 9486–9493.

10 Type X Collagen

Alvin P.L. Kwan

Connective Tissue Biology Labs, Cardiff School of Biosciences,
University of Wales Cardiff,
Museum Avenue, Cardiff CF1 3US, UK

THE EPIPHYSEAL GROWTH PLATE

The growth plate is a highly specialized form of hyaline cartilage that is responsible for linear skeletal growth (Ogden and Rosenberg, 1988; Brighton, 1984, 1987). In a growing long bone, the growth plate is sandwiched between the distal end of the bone (the epiphysis) and the metaphysis. Chondrocytes within the growth plate follow a stringently controlled sequence of cell proliferation, maturation and hypertrophy, which culminates in mineralization of the extracellular matrix and the invasion of blood vessels and osteogenic cells from the bone marrow, thus giving rise to bone elongation (Hunziker and Schenk, 1989). The growth plate can be divided into three main zones characterized by their prevailing cellular activities.

THE RESERVE OR RESTING ZONE

This region lies just beneath the epiphysis containing sparsely distributed spherical chondrocytes which rarely replicate but appear to be active in protein synthesis. The matrix contains random fibrils of type II collagen, chondroitin-4-sulphate and keratan sulphate and the highest proportion of collagen of any of the growth plate regions (Horton and Machado, 1988).

THE PROLIFERATIVE ZONE

The chondrocytes in this zone are active in cell division resulting in the cells flattening out and aligning into columns. Collagen fibrils become orientated in parallel with the cell columns, but biochemically there is little change in the extracellular matrix.

THE HYPERTROPHIC ZONE

In this zone, chondrocytes mature, cease division, hypertrophy and are finally destroyed by the advancing zone of calcification and vascularization. Changes in the matrix occur in this region with the deposition of type X collagen, less-aggregated proteoglycans and higher levels of hyaluronan. These alterations to the chondrocytes and surrounding matrix prepare the cartilage for the processes of endochondral ossification.

The growth plate cartilage matrix shows a well-defined structural organization that is maintained throughout the various zones. Three compartments have been described (Eggli *et al.*, 1985). The pericellular compartment around each chondrocyte is an aggrecan-rich matrix containing extremely fine fibrils (Keene and McDonald, 1993). The adjacent territorial matrix is characterised by a network of fine fibrillar collagens of types II, IX and XI. The interterritorial matrix compartment, located between the columns of cells, consists principally of longitudinally oriented collagen fibrils which give rise to the longitudinal septa where small membrane-bound structures called matrix vesicles (100–200 nm in diameter) are found (Anderson, 1989; Eggli *et al.*, 1985). In the hypertrophic zone, the septa appear more compressed by the enlarging cells and the collagen fibrils of the transverse septa (composed of territorial matrix) are more tightly packed than the longitudinally aligned fibrils of the interterritorial matrix. Calcification occurs in the interterritorial matrix of the longitudinal septa but not in the pericellular matrix and transverse septa. Type I collagen and fibronectin have been localized intracellularly and in the pericellular region of cells in the lower hypertrophic zone (Horton and Machado, 1988). Alkaline phosphatase activity is associated with the cell membranes and matrix vesicles in the same region (Anderson, 1989). However, the principal collagen present in this zone is type X which will be described in detail below.

MOLECULAR STRUCTURE AND ORGANIZATION

Type X collagen is a homotrimer comprising of three identical $\alpha 1(X)$ chains (M_r 59 kDa) (Schmid and Conrad, 1982) each contains a triple-helical domain of 45 kDa flanked by two non-collagenous regions (Schmid and Linsenmayer, 1983) (Figure 10.1). Type X collagen was first isolated from chick sternal and tibial chondrocyte cultures (Capasso *et al.*, 1982; Gibson *et al.*, 1982; Schmid and Conrad, 1982), and the complete amino acid sequence of chick collagen X was first described by LuValle *et al.* (1988). The molecular structures from different species are essentially identical with the exceptions of the bovine and ovine molecules. The helical domain of the $\alpha 1(X)$ chains from bovine and ovine collagen X contain a cysteine residue which form interchain disulfide bonds (Remington *et al.*, 1984; Gibson *et al.*, 1991) within the triple helix. In human collagen X, the N-terminal region (NC2) consists of only 38 amino acids, but the C-terminal domain (NC1) is considerably larger (161 amino acids) (Thomas *et al.*, 1991). The greatest degree of interspecies sequence identity is seen in the NC1 domain (87% nucleotide similarity/94% amino acid similarity between mouse and human) with 13 tyrosine residues and 6 asparagine residues in conserved positions. The triple helix contains eight imperfections of the Gly-X-Y triplet structure (Apte *et al.*, 1992). There are five

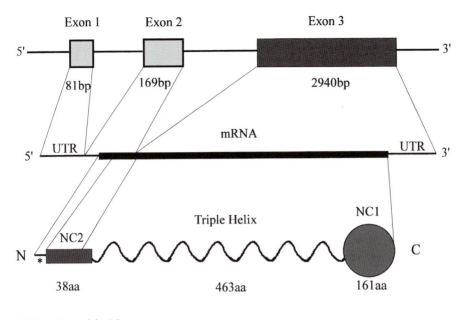

FIGURE 10.1   Structure of COL10A1 and Type X collagen. Diagrammatic representation of the condensed gene structure of COL10A1 which contains only three exons with exon 3 encoding the entire triple helical domain. The triple helical domain is flanked by a large globular C-terminal domain (NC1) and a smaller N-terminal non-collagenous domain (NC2).

imperfections of the type Gly-X-Gly and two Gly-X-Y-X-Y-Gly. Therefore, collagen X is cleaved at two sites by MMP-1 (Schmid *et al.*, 1986). In spite of the short helix with the eight imperfections, the melting temperature of collagen X is 47°C (Schmid and Linsenmayer, 1984) which is considerably greater than that of the fibrillar collagens. The large fragment (32 kDa) after MMP-1 cleavage remains triple helical at physiological temperatures and requires the action of Cathepsin B for complete degradation (Sires *et al.*, 1995). Denaturation–renaturation and site-directed mutagenesis studies have shown that the NC1 domain has a role in the assembly of the triple helix (Schmid and Linsenmayer, 1984; Chan *et al.*, 1996). It has been proposed that a highly conserved tyrosine-rich region within the NC1 acts as an aromatic zipper to align the three chains into a correct register before helix formation (Brass *et al.*, 1992).

Unlike the fibrillar collagens, the NC1 domain is not proteolytically removed in the extracellular matrix but is retained to form part of the supramolecular structure. Electron-microscopic studies have shown that collagen X molecules form an extended filamentous network in the cartilage matrix (Schmid and Linsenmayer, 1990). Rotary shadowing electronmicroscopy has shown that type X molecules aggregate via their NC1 domains forming an extended lattice structure with the aggregated NC1s arranged in a hexagonal array (Kwan *et al.*, 1991) (Figure 10.2). Partial characterization of the NC1 domain of chick collagen X showed potential covalent crosslinks that are non-reducible, non-lysine

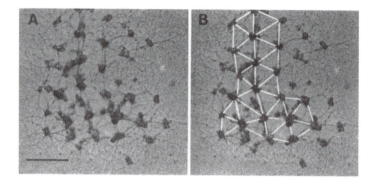

FIGURE 10.2 Rotary shadowing electron micrographs of the extended network of type X collagen aggregates. (A) Regularly spaced nodules of aggregated NC1 domains were interconnected with filamentous structures formed via interactions between adjacent triple helices. The nodules in this lattice were arranged into a regular hexagonal array. (B) The hexagonal nature of the type X collagen lattice is highlighted in this micrograph. Bar, 200 nm. (Courtesy of *J. Cell Biol.*)

derived and does not appear to be a γ-glutaminyl, ε-lysine crosslink (Barber and Kwan, 1996). The structure and role of this crosslink has yet to be defined but it is likely to increase the stability of the filamentous collagen X network. Within the helical region, several different forms of lysine-derived crosslinks have been identified (Rucklidge *et al.*, 1996a; Orth *et al.*, 1996). These crosslinks may be potential interactions between type X and other cartilage collagens.

TYPE X COLLAGEN GENE

The type X collagen gene, COL10A1, is distinct from the other large multi-exon fibrillar collagen genes in that its condensed gene structure contains only three exons (Thomas *et al.*, 1991; Elima *et al.*, 1993; Apte *et al.*, 1992; Reichenberger *et al.*, 1992). The human collagen X gene is approximately 7 kb and has been localized to the long arm of chromosome 6 at locus q21-22.3 (Thomas *et al.*, 1991). Exon 1 (81 bp), encodes most of the 5'-untranslated region, exon 2 (169 bp) codes for the signal peptide and the NC2 domain and exon 3 (2940 bp) contains the coding region for the entire triple-helical, the NC1 domain and part of the 3'-untranslated region (Figure 10.1). The exon sizes of COL10A1 are distinct from the fibrillar collagens' highly conserved exon sizes – multiples of 54 bp. This indicates that evolution of collagen X must, therefore, have taken a different path.

SPATIAL AND TEMPORAL EXPRESSION OF TYPE X COLLAGEN

The distribution of collagen X has been demonstrated by immunohistological techniques in chick (Schmid and Linsenmayer, 1985a,b; Gibson *et al.*, 1986; Kwan *et al.*, 1986), bovine (Kirsch and von der Mark, 1990; Marriott *et al.*, 1991), canine (Gannon *et al.*, 1991), porcine (Wardale and Duance, 1993) and human (Kirsch and von der Mark, 1991a) growth plates. These studies have concluded that collagen X is localised almost exclusively in the matrix of the hypertrophic zone and in the spicules of calcifying cartilage. *In situ* hybridisation has shown that collagen X mRNA appears at, or slightly before chondrocyte hypertrophy, and continues to be synthesised at a high level throughout the hypertrophic region (Oshima *et al.*, 1989; Linsenmayer *et al.*, 1991; Iyama *et al.*, 1991; Reichenberger *et al.*, 1991). The accumulation of collagen X mRNA and protein deposition in hypertrophic cartilage was found always to precede vascular invasion and mineralization of the matrix (Claassen and Kirsch, 1994). In chick sternal cartilage, collagen X is the major secreted product of this cell type, constituting approximately 45% of the total collagen produced (Reginato *et al.*, 1986). Chondrocytes from hypertrophic cartilage produce type X collagen when maintained in culture but chondrocytes from permanent cartilages do not (Gibson *et al.*, 1984; Reginato *et al.*, 1986; Gerstenfeld *et al.*, 1989). Furthermore, chondrocytes isolated from pre-hypertrophic embryonic tibia growth plate mature to a hypertrophic state and express collagen X mRNA when grown in a permissive culture environment (Castagnola *et al.*, 1986; O'keefe *et al.*, 1994). Therefore, it is generally accepted that type X collagen is a product of chondrocytes undergoing hypertrophy and collagen X expression is frequently used as a marker for chondrocyte hypertrophy (Kielty *et al.*, 1985; Gibson and Flint, 1985; Schmid and Linsenmayer, 1985b). However, recent observations have created questions to this widely accepted notion. Ekanayake and Hall (1994) demonstrated that chondrocytes derived from chick mandibular ectomesenchyme, a normally permanent cartilage, can be induced to undergo maturation in culture, but that chondrocyte hypertrophy is not a prerequisite for collagen X expression. Also, type X collagen has been immunolocalized in normal porcine, neonatal rat and human articular cartilage, and, in the mineralized fibrocartilage at the femoral insertion of the bovine medial collateral ligament where cell hypertrophy does not normally occur (Niyibizi *et al.*, 1996; Rucklidge *et al.*, 1996b).

Apart from the expression of type X collagen in normal bone development, histologic and biochemical studies on humeral fractures in chicks have identified type X collagen synthesis and endochondral ossification during fracture repair (Grant *et al.*, 1987). Expression of collagen X has also been demonstrated in regions of endochondral bone formation in pathologic condition of osteoarthritis (Hoyland *et al.*, 1991; Aigner *et al.*, 1993; Walker *et al.*, 1995; von der Mark *et al.*, 1995; Girkontaite *et al.*, 1996).

CONTROL OF TYPE X COLLAGEN EXPRESSION

The limited tissue distribution of type X collagen raises the question of how expression of this collagen is controlled. Earlier biochemical studies have shown the initiation of type X collagen synthesis when mesenchymal cells or non-hypertrophic chondrocytes were grown on or in a type I collagen gel. These experiments provided the earlier indications of the induction of collagen X synthesis during differentiation of mesenchymal cells to chondrocytes and subsequently to hypertrophic chondrocytes (Gibson *et al.*, 1982, 1984; Gibson and Flint, 1985; Solursh *et al.*, 1986; Schmid and Linsenmayer, 1983). Further experiments have shown that type X collagen synthesis in cultures can be inhibited by the addition of 5-bromodeoxyuridine; by transforming chick growth plate chondrocytes with Rous Sarcoma virus; treatment with sub-lethal doses of lead (Gionti *et al.*, 1983; Hicks *et al.*, 1996); or addition of the alkaline phosphatase inhibitor Levamisole (Thomas *et al.*, 1990). A recent report by Davies *et al.* (1996) has shown that the drug Doxycycline, a tetracycline derivative potentially useful in the treatment of osteoarthritis by reducing collagenase and gelatinase activity, also inhibits collagen X synthesis. Using rachitic chicks and shell-less chick embryos, it has been shown that calcium is a potential mediator of type X collagen synthesis (Kwan *et al.*, 1989; Reginato *et al.*, 1993). Studies by Bonen and Schmid (1991) also demonstrated an induction in collagen X synthesis when chondrocytes are cultured with increased concentrations of calcium. Thyroxine, retinoic acid, calcium β-glycerophosphate and recombinant human BMP-7 (osteogenic protein-1 OP-1) have all been shown to promote chondrocyte hypertrophy and hence up-regulate type X collagen production (Thomas *et al.*, 1990; Pacifici *et al.*, 1991; Böhme *et al.*, 1992; Chen *et al.*, 1995). Treatment of chick chondrocytes in high-density cultures with porcine TGFβ caused the appearance of collagen X mRNA 4 days earlier than cells not treated with TGFβ (Iwasaki *et al.*, 1995).

Measurements of type X mRNA levels and transcription rates in chondrocyte populations suggest that the restricted expression of collagen X mRNA to hypertrophic chondrocytes is controlled by transcriptional mechanisms both *in vivo* (LuValle *et al.*, 1989, 1992; Reginato *et al.*, 1995) and *in vitro* (Castagnola *et al.*, 1988). LuValle *et al.* (1993) have described the presence of multiple negative regulatory elements within a 4.2 kb fragment upstream of the promoter which can act in an additive manner to restrict transcription of the chick COL10A1 to hypertrophic chondrocytes. Transcriptional activation of COL10A1 in these chondrocytes is accompanied by decreases in the levels of both collagen IX and collagen II mRNAs (Oshima *et al.*, 1989; LuValle *et al.*, 1992). Analysis of the mammalian promoter regions revealed a single conserved TATAA box for trancription factor binding approximately 30 bp upstream of the transcription start site. Transfection studies also established that an enhancer element is presence in the region spanning 2400 and 900 bp upstream (Thomas *et al.*, 1995). *In vivo* footprinting experiments on the chick COL10A1 demonstrated use of the TATA binding region in hypertrophic chondrocytes, and use of other binding sites in non-hypertrophic chondrocytes and tendon fibroblasts (Long and Linsenmayer, 1995). In summary, these studies have identified several genetic factors enhancing COL10A1 transcription in hypertrophic chondrocytes whereas negative regulatory elements may be responsible for suppressing collagen X expression in non-hypertrophic chondrocytes. However, because recent studies have demonstrated the expression of collagen X in non-hypertrophic cells (Niyibizi *et al.*, 1996; Rucklidge *et al.*, 1996b), it is apparent that the identification of upstream elements is not sufficient to explain the tissue spatial and temporal expression of type X collagen.

ROLE OF TYPE X COLLAGEN

Earlier studies utilizing animal disease models have shown altered levels of type X collagen in association with certain skeletal abnormalities. Low levels of collagen X were found in both rachitic growth cartilage (Kwan *et al.*, 1989) and in chick tibial dyschon-droplasia (TD) (Bashey *et al.*, 1989) when the growth plate fails to ossify. These obser-vations, in addition to the reported spatial and temporal expression of collagen X at sites of new bone formation imply that this collagen is closely involved in the processes of endochondral ossification.

Direct evidence that collagen X is required for normal bone development has been obtained by the generation of transgenic mice expressing a truncated chicken and unstable chick/mouse hybrid collagen X (Jacenko *et al.*, 1993). These mice developed skeletal de-formities including compression of the hypertrophic zone and a decrease in newly formed trabecular bone. The skeletal and growth abnormalities resembled certain forms of human spondylometaphyseal dysplasias (SMD) and metaphyseal chondrodysplasia (MCD) sug-gesting that mutations in the human COL10A1 may be responsible for these diseases. In fact, several mutations of the human COL10A1 have been discovered to be linked to metaphyseal chondrodyplasia type Schmid (MCDS) (Warman *et al.*, 1993; Wallis *et al.*, 1994; Dharmavaram *et al.*, 1994). More recently, Kwan *et al.* (1997) reported the devel-opment of phenotypic changes in type X collagen-null mice including coxa vara, reduc-tion in thickness of growth plate resting zone and articular cartilage, altered bone content and atypical distribution of matrix components within the growth plate. However, investi-gations by Rosati *et al.* (1994) have produced conflicting results. These authors reported that mice without collagen X were viable and that they could detect no abnormalities in long bone growth and therefore proposed that this collagen has no function in long bone development.

Gordon and Olsen (1990) suggested that collagen X serves primarily as a structural element, either alone or in conjunction with other matrix components. The hypertrophic zone is structurally the weakest point within the growth plate by virtue of the increase in chondrocyte size and the decrease in the amount of type II collagen fibrils. It has been proposed that the hexagonal lattice structure of collagen X could provide considerable reinforcement of the hypertrophic matrix towards compressive stiffness (Aspden, 1994).

However, it is generally accepted that collagen X provides a permissive matrix for chondrocyte hypertrophy, mineralization and vascular invasion to occur during endo-chondral ossification. A correlation between collagen X deposition and matrix mineral-ization is supported by observations that collagen X gene expression is enhanced in the presence of calcium β-glycerophosphate and reduced in the presence of a mineralization inhibitor (levamisole) (Thomas *et al.*, 1990). Bonen and Schmid (1991) also demonstrated an induction in collagen X synthesis when chondrocytes are cultured with increased concentrations of calcium. Furthermore, type X collagen has been shown to have calcium binding properties (Kirsch and von der Mark, 1991b); to be associated with alkaline phosphatase (Habuchi *et al.*, 1985) and with matrix vesicles (Wu *et al.*, 1991a,b; Morris *et al.*, 1992), considered by some to be the initial site of mineral deposition in carti-lage (Anderson, 1989; Bonucci *et al.*, 1987), although conflicting evidence has also been put forward (Poole and Pidoux, 1989). A recent study by Tselepis *et al.* (1996) with chick chondrodysplastic (TD) growth plate cartilage has tentatively suggested that the absence of type X collagen in the matrix may be linked to the failure of chondrocyte hypertrophy in these lesions, contrary to currently accepted notion that type X collagen synthesis is a consequence of chondrocyte hypertrophy. Within the TD lesion, the levels of extracellular aggrecan and biglycan were also decreased suggesting that interactions between collagen X and these chondroitin sulphate proteoglycans are involved in maintaining tissue integrity which may be important in mediating cell differentiation.

DEGRADATION OF TYPE X COLLAGEN

The type X collagen triple helix is susceptible to cleavage by a variety of metalloproteinases because it contains two cleavage sites for vertebrate collagenase (Schmid and Conrad, 1982; Schmid et al., 1986) rather than one which is characteristic for the other collagens. It is also degraded more rapidly by collagenase than type II collagen (Schmid et al., 1986; Welgus et al., 1990). Collagen X is also cleaved by neutrophil elastase (Gahder et al., 1989), MMP-2 (Welgus et al., 1990), MMP-3 (Wu, J.-J. et al., 1991) and the 92 kDa gelatinase. Based on these observations, it has been speculated that collagen X provides a readily degradable matrix that can be easily resorbed and replaced by bone (Schmid and Linsenmayer, 1990). Growth plate cartilage also contains several metalloproteinases that are capable of degrading collagen X. Collagenase and stromelysin have been detected in the hypertrophic region of rat growth plates and the level of collagenase was shown to be elevated in the pericellular matrix of hypertrophic chondrocytes (Blair et al., 1989). Immunohistochemical methods (Brown et al., 1989) revealed the presence of MMP1, MMP2, MMP3 and TIMP-1 (tissue inhibitor of metalloproteinase-1) in rabbit growth plates. In the hypertrophic region, immunoreactivity for MMP1 and MMP3 were elevated whereas reactivity for TIMP-1 was diminished. The more degradable nature of a type X collagen-rich matrix may also promote invasion of blood vessels into the normally avascular cartilage.

CONCLUSION

Despite extensive investigations, the exact functional role of collagen X remains ill defined. It is important to consider that, the biomechanical and biochemical properties of cartilage are conferred by the composition of the extracellular matrix and spatial relationship or interactions between its molecular components. It is conceivable that the function of type X collagen may depend on the composition of the surrounding matrix. To date, little is known regarding interactions of type X collagen with cells and other matrix macromolecules although Gibson et al. (1996) have demonstrated the colocalization of proteoglycan epitope (7D4) with type X collagen in the longitudinal septum of bovine growth plate. Further experimental investigations into interactions of type X collagen with cells and other matrix components will no doubt provide more insight into the functional role of type X collagen in endochondral ossification.

ACKNOWLEDGEMENT

The financial support from the Arthritis and Rheumatism Council, Medical Research Council and Biotechnology and Biological Sciences Research Council are gratefully acknowledged.

REFERENCES

Aigner, T., Reichenberger, E., Bertling, W., Kirsch, T., Stob, H. and von der Mark, K. (1993) Type X collagen expression in osteoarthritic and rheumatoid articular cartilage. *Virchows Archiv. B Cell Pathol.*, **63**, 205–211.

Anderson, H.C. (1989) Mechanism of mineral formation in bone. *Lab. Invest.*, **60**, 320–330.

Apte, S.S., Seldin, M.F., Hayashi, M. and Olsen, B.R. (1992) Cloning of the human and mouse type X collagen genes and mapping of the mouse type X collagen gene to chromosome 10. *FEBS Lett.*, **206**, 217–224.

Aspden, R.M. (1994) Fibre reinforcing by collagen in cartilage and soft connective tissues. *Proceedings of the Royal Society of London*, **258**, 195–200.

Barber, R.E. and Kwan, A.P.L. (1996) Partial characterization of the C-terminal non-collagenous domain (NC1) of collagen type X. *Biochem. J.*, **320**, 479–485.

Bashey, R.I., Jimenez, S.A., Gay, C.V. and Leach, R.M. (1989) Type X collagen in avian tibial chondrodysplasia. *Lab. Invest.*, **60**, 106–112.

Blair, H.C., Dean, D.D., Howell, D.S., Teitelbaum, S.L. and Jeffrey, J.J. (1989) Hypertrophic chondrocytes produce immunoreactive collagenase *in vivo*. *Connect Tissue Res.*, **23**, 65–73.

Bohme, K., Conscience-Egli, M., Tschan, T., Winterhalter, K.H. and Bruckner, P. (1992) Induction of proliferation or hypertrophy of chondrocytes in serum-free culture: The role of insulin-like growth factor-I, insulin, or thyroxine. *J. Cell Biol.*, **116**, 1035–1042.

Bonen, D.K. and Schmid, T.M. (1991) Elevated extracellular calcium concentrations induce type X collagen synthesis in chondrocyte cultures. *J. Cell Biol.*, **115**, 1171–1178.

Bonucci, E. (1987) Fine structure of early cartilage calcification. *J. Ultrastruct. Res.*, **20**, 33–50.

Brass, A., Kadler, K.E., Thomas, J.T., Grant, M.E. and Boot-Handford, R.P. (1992) The fibrillar collagens, collagen VIII, collagen X and the C1q complement proteins share a similar domain in their C-terminal non-collagenous regions. *FEBS Lett.*, **303**, 126–128.

Brighton, C.T. (1984) The growth plate. *Orthop Clinics of North America*, **15**, 571–595.

Brighton, C.T. (1987) Morphology and biochemistry of the growth plate. *Rheum. Dis. Clin. North Am.*, **13**, 75–100.

Brown, C.C., Hembry, R.M. and Reynolds, J.J. (1989) Immunolocalisation of metalloproteinases and their inhibitor in the rabbit growth plate. *J. Bone Joint Surg.*, **71**, 580–593.

Capasso, O., Gionti, E., Pontarelli, G., Ambesi-Imprombato, F.S., Nitsch, L., Tajana, G. and Cancedda, R. (1982) The culture of chick embryo chondrocytes and the control of their differentiated functions *in vivo* 1. Characterisation of the chondrocyte-specific phenotypes. *Exp. Cell Res.*, **142**, 197–206.

Castagnola, P., Moro, G., Descalzi, F. and Cancedda, R. (1986) Type X collagen synthesis during *in vitro* development of chick embryo tibial chondrocytes. *J. Cell Biol.*, **102**, 2310–2317.

Castagnola, P., Dozin, B., Moro, G. and Cancedda, R. (1988) Changes in the expression of collagen genes show two stages in chondrocyte differentiation *in vitro*. *J. Cell Biol.*, **106**, 461–467.

Chan, D., Weng, Y.M., Hocking, A.M., Golub, S., McQuillan, D.J. and Bateman, J.F. (1996) Site-directed mutagenesis of human type X collagen. Expression of α1(X) NC1, NC2, and helical mutations *in vitro* and in transfected cells. *J. Biol. Chem.*, **271**, 13566–13572.

Chen, P., Vukicevic, S., Sampath, T.K. and Luyten, F.P. (1995) Osteogenic protein-1 promotes growth and maturation of chick sternal chondrocytes in serum-free cultures. *J. Cell Sci.*, **108**, 105–114.

Claassen, H. and Kirsch, T. (1994) Immunolocalization of type X collagen before and after mineralization of human thyroid cartilage. *Histo.*, **101**, 27–32.

Davies, S.R., Cole, A.A. and Schmid, T.M. (1996) Doxycycline inhibits type X collagen synthesis in avian hypertrophic chondrocyte cultures. *J. Biol. Chem.*, **271**, 25966–25970.

Dharmavaram, R.M., Elberson, M.A., Peng, M., Kirson, L.A., Kelley, T.E. and Jimenez, S.A. (1994) Identification of a mutation in type X collagen in a family with Schmid metaphyseal chondrodysplasia. *Hum. Mol. Genet.*, **3**, 507–509.

Eggli, P.S., Herrmann, W., Hunziker, E.B. and Schenk, R.K. (1985) Matrix compartments in the growth plate of the proximal tibia of rats. *Anat. Rec.*, **211**, 246–257.

Ekanayake, S. and Hall, B.K. (1994) Hypertrophy is not a prerequisite for type X collagen expression or mineralisation of chondrocytes derived from cultured chick mandibular ectomesenchyme. *Int. J. Dev. Biol.*, **38**, 683–694.

Elima, K., Eerola, I., Rosat, R., Metsäranta, M., Garofalo, S., Perälä, M., De Crombrugghe, B. and Vuorio, E. (1993) The mouse collagen X gene: complete nucleotide sequence, exon structure and expression pattern. *Biochem. J.*, **289**, 247–253.

Gahder, S.J., Schmid, T.M., Heck, L.W. and Wooley, D.E. (1989) Cleavage of collagen type X by human synovial collagenase and neutrophil elastase. *Matrix*, **9**, 109–115.

Gannon, J.M., Walker, G., Fischer, M., Carpenter, R., Thompson, R.C. and Oegema, T.R. Jr. (1991) Localization of type X collagen in canine growth plate and adult canine articular cartilage. *J. Ortho. Res.*, **9**, 485–494.

Gerstenfeld, L.C., Finer, M.H. and Boedtker, H. (1989) Quantitative analysis of collagen expression in embryonic chick chondrocytes having different developmental fates. *J. Biol. Chem.*, **264**, 5112–5120.

Gibson, G.J., Schor, S.L. and Grant, M.E. (1982) Effects of matrix molecules on chondrocyte gene expression: synthesis of a low molecular weight collagen species by cells cultured within collagen gels. *J. Cell Biol.*, **93**, 767–774.

Gibson, G.J., Beaumont, B.W. and Flint, M.H. (1984) Synthesis of a low molecular weight collagen by chondrocytes from the presumptive calcification region of the embryonic chick sterna. The influence of culture with collagen gels. *J. Cell Biol.*, **99**, 208–216.

Gibson, G.J., Francki, K.T., Hopwood, J.J. and Foster, B.K. (1991) Human and sheep growth-plate cartilage type X collagen synthesis and the influence of tissue storage. *Biochem. J.*, **277**, 513–520.

Gibson, G.J. and Flint, M.H. (1985) Type X collagen synthesis by chick sternal cartilage and its relationship to endochondral bone development. *J. Cell Biol.*, **101**, 277–284.

Gibson, G.J., Bearman, C.H. and Flint, M.H. (1986) The immunolocalisation of type X collagen in chick cartilage and lung. *Coll. Rel. Res.*, **6**, 163–184.

Gibson, G., Lin, D.L., Francki, K., Caterson, B. and Foster, B. (1996) Type X collagen is colocalized with a proteoglycan epitope to form distinct morphological structures in bovine growth cartilage. *Bone*, **19**, 307–315.

Gionti, E., Capasso, O. and Cancedda, R. (1983) The culture of chick embryo chondrocytes and the control of their differentiated functions *in vitro*. Transformation by Rous sarcoma virus induces a switch in the collagen type synthesis and enhances fibronectin expression. *J. Biol. Chem.*, **258**, 7190–7194.

Girkontaite, I., Frischholz, S., Lammi, P., Wagner, K., Swoboda, B., Aigner, T. and von der Mark, K. (1996) Immunolocalization of type X collagen in normal fetal and adult osteoarthritic cartilage with monoclonal antibodies. *Matrix Biol.*, **15**, 231–238.

Gordon, M.K. and Olsen, B.R. (1990) The contribution of collagenous proteins to tissue-specific matrix assemblies. *Curr. Opin. Cell Biol.*, **2**, 833–838.

Grant, W.T., Wang, G.J. and Balian, G. (1987) Type X collagen synthesis during endochondral ossification in fracture repair. *J. Biol. Chem.*, **262**, 9844–9849.

Habuchi, H., Conrad, H.E. and Glaser, J.H. (1985) Co-ordinate regulation of collagen and alkaline phosphatase levels in chick embryo chondrocytes. *J. Biol. Chem.*, **260**, 13029–13034.

Hicks, D.G., O'keefe, R.J., Reynolds, K.J., CorySlechta, D.A., Puzas, J.E., Judkins, A. and Rosier, R.N. (1996) Effects of lead on growth plate chondrocyte phenotype *Toxi. and App. Pharm.*, **140**, 164–172.

Horton, W.A. and Machado, M.M. (1988) Extracellular matrix alterations during endochondral ossification in humans. *J. Orthop. Res.*, **6**, 793–803.

Hoyland, J.A., Thomas, J.T., Donn, R., Marriott, A., Ayad, S., Boot-Handford, R.P., Grant, M.E. and Freemont, A.J. (1991) Distribution of type X collagen mRNA in normal and osteoarthritic human cartilage. *Bone Min.*, **15**, 151–164.

Hunziker, E.B. and Schenk, R.K. (1989) Physiological mechanisms adopted by chondrocytes in regulating longitudinal bone growth in rats. *J. Physiol. (Lond.)*, **414**, 55–71.

Iwasaki, M., Nakahara, H., Nakata, K., Nakase, T., Kimura, T. and Ono, K. (1995) Regulation of proliferation and osteochondrogenic differentiation of periosteum-derived cells by transforming growth factor-β and basic fibroblast growth factor. *J. Bone Joint Surg.*, **77A**, 543–554.

Iyama, K.I., Ninomiya, Y., Olsen, B.R., Linsenmayer, T.F., Trelstad, R.L. and Hayashi, M. (1991) Spatiotemporal pattern of type X collagen gene expression and collagen deposition in embryonic chick vertebrae undergoing endochondral ossification. *Anat. Rec.*, **229**, 462–472.

Jacenko, O., LuValle, P.A. and Olsen, B.R. (1993) Spondylometaphyseal dysplasia in mice carrying a dominant negative mutation in a matrix protein specific for cartilage-to-bone transition. *Nature*, **365**, 56–61.

Keene, D.R. and McDonald, K. (1993) The ultrastructure of the connective tissue matrix of skin and cartilage after high-pressure freezing and freeze substitution. *J. Histochem. Cytochem.*, **41**, 1141–1153.

Kielty, C.M., Kwan, A.P.L., Holmes, D.F., Schor, S.F. and Grant, M.E. (1985) Type X collagen, a product of hypertrophic chondrocytes. *Biochem. J.*, **227**, 545–554.

Kirsch, T. and von der Mark, K. (1990) Isolation of bovine type X collagen and immunolocalisation in growth plate cartilage. *Biochem. J.*, **265**, 453–459.

Kirsch, T. and von der Mark, K. (1991a) Isolation of human type X collagen and immunolocalisation in foetal cartilage. *Eur. J. Biochem.*, **196**, 575–580.

Kirsch, T. and von der Mark, K. (1991b) Ca^{2+} binding properties of type X collagen. *FEBS Lett.*, **294**, 149–152.

Kwan, A.P.L., Freemont, A.J. and Grant, M.E. (1986) Immunoperoxidase localisation of type X collagen in tibiae. *Biosci. Rep.*, **6**, 155–162.

Kwan, A.P.L., Dickson, I.R., Freemont, A.J. and Grant, M.E. (1989) Comparative studies of type X collagen expression in normal and rachitic chicken epiphyseal cartilage. *J. Cell Biol.*, **109**, 1849–1856.

Kwan, A.P.L., Cummings, C.E., Chapman, J.A. and Grant, M.E. (1991) Macromolecular organisation of chicken type X collagen *in vitro*. *J. Cell Biol.*, **114**, 597–604.

Kwan, K.M., Pang, M.K.M., Zhou, S., Cowan, S.K., Kong, R.Y.C., Pfordte, T., Olsen, B.R., Sillence, D.O., Tam, P.P.L. and Cheah, K.S.E. (1997) Abnormal compartmentalization of cartilage matrix components in mice lacking collagen X: Implications for function. *J. Cell Biol.*, **136**, 459–471.

Linsenmayer, T.F., Chen, Q., Gibney, E., Gordon, M.K., Marchant, J.K., Mayne, R. and Schmid, T.M. (1991) Collagen types IX and X in the developing chick tibiotarsus: analysis of mRNAs and proteins. *Development*, **111**, 191–196.

Long, F. and Linsenmayer, T.F. (1995) Tissue-specific regulation of the type X collagen gene. *J. Biol. Chem.*, **270**, 31310–31314.

LuValle, P., Hayashi, M. and Olsen, B.R. (1989) Transcriptional regulation of type X collagen during chondrocyte maturation. *Dev. Biol.*, **133**, 613–616.

Luvalle, P., Daniels, K., Hay, E.D. and Olsen, B.R. (1992) Type X collagen is transcriptionally activated and specifically localised during sternal cartilage maturation. *Matrix*, **12**, 404–413.

LuValle, P., Iwamoto, M., Fanning, P., Pacifici, M. and Olsen, B.R. (1993) Multiple negative elements in a gene that codes for an extracellular matrix protein, collagen X, restricts expression to hypertrophic chondrocytes. *J. Cell Biol.*, **121**, 1173–1179.

LuValle, P., Ninomiya, Y., Rosenblum, N.D. and Olsen, B.R. (1988) The type X collagen gene. *J. Biol. Chem.*, **263**, 18378–18385.

Marriott, A., Ayad, S. and Grant, M.E. (1991) The synthesis of type X collagen by bovine and human growth-plate chondrocytes. *J. Cell Sci.*, **99**, 641–649.

Morris, D.C., Moylan, P.E. and Anderson, H.C. (1992) Immunochemical and immunocytochemical identification of matrix vesicle proteins. *Bone Mineral*, **17**, 209–213.

Niyibizi, C., Visconti, C.S., Gibson, G. and Kavalkovich, K. (1996) Identification and immunolocalization of type X collagen at the ligament–bone interface. *BBRC*, **222**, 584–589.

Ogden, J.A. and Rosenberg, L.C. (1988) Defining the growth plate. In *Behaviour of the Growth Plate*. Uhthoff, H.K. and Wiley, J.J. (Eds), New York, Raven Press, pp. 1–16.

O'keefe, R.J., Puzas, J.E., Loveys, L., Hicks, D.G. and Rosier, R.N. (1994) Analysis of type II and type X collagen synthesis in cultured growth plate chondrocytes by *in situ* hybridization: Rapid induction of type X collagen in culture. *J. Bone Min. Res.*, **9**, 1713–1722.

Orth, M.W., Luchene, L.J. and Schmid, T.M. (1996) Type X collagen isolated from the hypertrophic cartilage of embryonic chick tibiae contains both hydroxylysyl- and lysylpyridinoline cross-links. *BBRC*, **219**, 301–305.

Oshima, O., Leboy, P.S., McDonald, S.A., Tuan, R.S. and Shapiro, I.M. (1989) Developmental expression of genes in chick growth plate cartilage detected by *in situ* hybridisation. *Calcif. Tissue Int.*, **45**, 182–192.

Pacifici, M., Golden, E.B., Iwamoto, M. and Adams, S.L. (1991) Retinoic acid treatment induces type X collagen gene expression in cultured chick chondrocytes. *Exp. Cell Res.*, **195**, 38–46.

Poole, A.R. and Pidoux, I. (1989) Immunoelectron microscopic studies of type X collagen in endochondral ossification. *J. Cell Biol.*, **109**, 2547–2554.

Reginato, A., Lash, J. and Jiminez, S. (1986) Biosynthetic expression of type X collagen in embryonic chick sternum cartilage during development. *J. Biol. Chem.*, **261**, 2897–2904.

Reginato, A.M., Tuan, R.S., Ono, T., Jimenez, S. and Jacenko, O. (1993) Effects of calcium deficiency on chondrocyte hypertrophy and type X collagen expression in chick embryonic sternum. *Dev. Dynam.*, **198**, 284–295.

Reginato, A.M., Sanz-Rodriguez, C. and Jimenez, S.A. (1995) Biosynthesis and characterization of type X collagen in human fetal epiphyseal growth plate cartilage. *Osteo. and Cart.*, **3**, 105–116.

Reichenberger, E., Aigner, T., von der Mark, K., Stöss, H. and Bertling, W. (1991) *In situ* hybridisation studies on the expression of type X collagen in fetal human cartilage. *Dev. Biol.*, **148**, 562–572.

Reichenberger, E., Beier, F., LuValle, P., Olsen, B.R., von der Mark, K. and Bertling, W.M. (1992) Genomic organisation and full-length cDNA sequence of human collagen X. *FEBS Lett.*, **311**, 305–310.

Remington, M.C., Bashey, R.I., Brighton, C.T. and Jimenez, S.A. (1984) Biosynthesis of a disulphide-bonded short-chain collagen by calf growth plate cartilage. *Biochem. J.*, **224**, 227–233.

Rosati, R., Horan, G.S.B., Pinero, G.J. Garofalo, S., Keene, D.R., Horton, W.A., Vuario, E., de Crombrugghe, B. and Behringer, R.R. (1994) Normal long bone growth and development in type X collagen-null mice. *Nature Genetics*, **8**, 129–135.

Rucklidge, G.J., Milne, G. and Robins, S.P. (1996a) Identification of lysine-derived crosslinks in porcine collagen type X from growth plate and newly mineralized bone. *Matrix Biol.*, **15**, 73–80.

Rucklidge, G.J., Milne, G. and Robins, S.P. (1996b) Collagen type X: a component of the surface of normal human, pig, and rat articular cartilage. *BBRC*, **224**, 297–302.

Schmid, T.M. and Conrad, H.E. (1982) A unique low molecular weight collagen secreted by cultured chick embryo chondrocytes. *J. Biol. Chem.*, **257**, 12444–12450.

Schmid, T.M. and Linsenmayer, T.F. (1983) A short-chain collagen from aged endochondral chondrocytes. *J. Biol. Chem.*, **258**, 9504–9509.

Schmid, T.M., Mayne, R., Bruns, R.R. and Linsenmayer, T.F. (1984) Molecular structure of short chain (SC) cartilage collagen by electron microscopy. *J. Ultrastruct. Res.*, **86**, 186–191.

Schmid, T.M. and Linsenmayer, T.F. (1985a) Immunohistochemical localization of short chain cartilage collagen (type X) in avian tissues. *J. Cell Biol.*, **100**, 598–605.

Schmid, T.M. and Linsenmayer, T.F. (1985b) Developmental acquisition of type X collagen in the embryonic chick tibiotarsus. *Dev. Biol.*, **107**, 373–381.

Schmid, T.M. and Linsenmayer, T.F. (1990) Immunoelectron microscopy of type X collagen: supramolecular forms within embryonic chick cartilage. *Dev. Biol.*, **138**, 53–62.

Schmid, T.M., Mayne, R., Jeffrey, J.J. and Linsenmayer, T.F. (1986) Type X collagen contains two cleavage sites for a vertebrate collagenase. *J. Biol. Chem.*, **261**, 4184–4189.

Sires, U.I., Schmid, T.M., Fliszar, C.J., Wang, Z.Q., Gluck, S.L. and Welgus, H.G. (1995) Complete degradation of type X collagen requires the combined action of interstitial collagenase and osteoclast-derived cathepsin-B. *J. Clin. Inv.*, **95**, 2089–2095.

Solursh, M., Jensen, K.L., Reiter, R.S., Schmid, T.M. and Linsenmayer, T.F. (1986) Environmental regulation of type X collagen production by cultures of limb mesenchyme, mesectoderm, and sternal chondrocytes. *Dev. Biol.*, **117**, 90–101.

Thomas, J.T., Boot-Handford, R.P. and Grant, M.E. (1990) Modulation of type X collagen gene expression by calcium β-glycerophosphate and levamisole: implications for a possible role for type X collagen in endochondral bone formation. *J. Cell Sci.*, **95**, 639–648.

Thomas, J.T., Cresswell, C.J., Rash, B., Nicolai, H., Jones, T., Solomon, E., Grant, M.E. and Boot-Handford, R.P. (1991) The human collagen X gene. *Biochem. J.*, **280**, 617–623.

Thomas, J.T., Sweetman, W.A., Cresswell, C.J., Wallis, G.A., Grant, M.E. and Boot-Handford, R.P. (1995) Sequence comparison of three mammalian type-X collagen promoters and preliminary functional analysis of the human promoter. *Gene*, **160**, 291–296.

Tselepis, C., Hoyland, J.A., Barber, R.E., Thorp, B.H. and Kwan, A.P.L. (1996) Expression and distribution of cartilage matrix macromolecules in avian tibial dyschondroplasia. *Avian Path*, **25**, 305–324.

von der Mark, K., Frischholz, S., Aigner, T., Beier, F., Belke, J., Erdmann, S. and Burkhardt, H. (1995) Upregulation of type X collagen expression in osteoarthritic cartilage. *Acta. Orthop. Scand. (Suppl. 266)*, **66**, 125–129.

Walker, G.D., Fischer, M., Gannon, J., Thompson, R.C. Jr. and Oegema, T.R. Jr. (1995) Expression of type-X collagen in osteoarthritis. *J. Ortho. Res.*, **13**, 4–12.

Wallis, G.A., Rash, B., Sweetman, W.A., Thomas, J.T., Super, M., Evans, G., Grant, M.E. and Boot-Handford, R.P. (1994) Amino acid substitutions of conserved residues in the carboxyl-terminal domain of the α1(X) chain of type X collagen occur in two unrelated families with metaphyseal chondrodysplasia type. *Schmid. Am. J. Hum. Genet.*, **54**, 169–178.

Warman, M.L., Abott, M., Apte, S.S., Hefferon, T., McIntosh, I., Cohn, D.H., Heicht, J.T., Olsen, B.R. and Francomano, C.A. (1993) A type X collagen mutation causes Schmid metaphyseal chondrodysplasia. *Nature Genet.*, **5**, 79–82.

Wardale, R.J. and Duance, V.C. (1993) Quantification and immunolocalisation of porcine articular and growth plate cartilage collagens. *J. Cell Sci.*, **105**, 975–984.

Welgus, H.G., Fliszar, C.J., Seltzer, J.L., Schmid, T.M. and Jeffrey, J.J. (1990) Differential susceptibility of type X collagen to cleavage by two mammalian interstitial collagenases and 72kDa type IV collagenase. *J. Biol. Chem.*, **265**, 13521–13527.

Wu, L.N.Y., Genge, B.R. and Wuthier, R.E. (1991a) Collagen binding proteins in collagenase-released matrix vesicles: specific binding of annexins, alkaline phosphatase, link and hyaluronic acid binding region proteins to native cartilage collagen. *J. Biol. Chem.*, **266**, 1195–1203.

Wu, L.N.Y., Genge, B.R. and Wuthier, R.E. (1991b) Evidence for specific interactions between matrix vesicle proteins and the connective tissue matrix. *Bone. Min.*, **17**, 247–252.

Wu, J.-J., Lark, M.W., Chun, L.E. and Eyre, D.R. (1991) Sites of stromelysin cleavage in collagen types II, IX, X and XI of cartilage. *J. Biol. Chem.*, **266**, 5625–5628.

11 Matrix Turnover in Joint Tissues: The Role of Metalloproteinases

Gillian Murphy[1,*], Vera Knäuper[1], Susan Cowell[2] and
Rosalind M. Hembry[2]

[1]*School of Biological Sciences, University of East Anglia,
Norwich, NR4 7TJ, UK*
[2]*Strangeways Research Laboratory, Worts' Causeway,
Cambridge CB1 4RN, UK*

METALLOPROTEINASES IN MORPHOGENESIS AND GROWTH

Embryonic development is a continuously and exquisitely regulated process involving reciprocal interactions between cells and their extracellular matrix. A key element of cellular differentiation and tissue morphogenesis and growth is the remodelling activity of proteinases. Matrix metalloproteinases (MMPs) have been shown to have a role in many developmental processes (reviewed by Matrisian and Hogan, 1990), although deletion of specific MMP gene products to date has failed to interfere with either reproductive or developmental events. Specific analyses of these proteinases in joint development have been undertaken in the anticipation that the data will promote the understanding of the precise role of individual MMPs in the turnover of extracellular matrix components and the subsequent modulation of cell–matrix interactions. Such knowledge should have implications for our interpretation of the excessive remodelling processes associated with degradative pathologies like the arthritides. Gelatinase B (MMP9) has hence been shown to be associated with bone development in the mouse embryo (Reponen *et al.*, 1994) and the regeneration of axolotl appendages (Yang and Bryant, 1994). Stromelysin-3 (MMP11) mRNA is specifically expressed at the interdigital regions of the developing limb buds in mice (Basset *et al.*, 1990) and during bone and spinal cord morphogenesis (Lefebvre *et al.*, 1995). Using both *in vitro* hybridization and immunohistochemistry MT.1MMP (MMP14)

* Corresponding author.

expression levels are high in the developing bones and the rib and femur primordia of the 9-day mouse embryo, together with gelatinase A and TIMP-2 (Kinoh *et al.*, 1996).

Studies of the growth plate in embryonic and post-partum animals have also demonstrated the association of MMP expression with endochondral ossification. Collagenase activity has been identified in growth plate cartilage from embryonic chick bone (Yasui *et al.*, 1981), collagenase and TIMP in normal and rachitic rat cartilage (Dean *et al.*, 1990), and proteoglycanase (probably stromelysin) activity in the bovine growth plate (Ehrlich *et al.*, 1985). Collagenase-1 (MMP1), gelatinases (MMP2, 9), stromelysin-1 (MMP3), and TIMP-1 have been detected by immunolocalisation studies in the distal femoral growth plate (Brown *et al.*, 1989) and mandibular condylar cartilage (Breckon *et al.*, 1994). Both cartilages showed unique patterns of synthesis and extracellular distribution of MMPs and TIMP-1 at specific stages of chondrocyte differentiation, which in the case of the mandibular condyle showed temporal variation during development. These observations suggest that extracellular matrix degradation within both primary and secondary cartilage is a carefully regulated event. Immunolocalisation in the mandibular condyle (Breckon *et al.*, 1994) has also shown extensive matrix staining for gelatinase in newly formed bone. A prominent role for MMPs, particularly gelatinase A has been suggested during studies of osteogenesis in the craniofacial region of the rabbit embryo (Breckon *et al.*, 1995).

A histochemical study of human fetal limbs was undertaken to assess the presence, and consequently the possible role, of MMPs and TIMP-1 in synovial joint cavity formation. Cryostat sections of fetal limbs from 7 to 14 week gestation were stained with specific antibodies to collagenase-1, gelatinases A and B, stromelysin-1 and TIMP-1. Immunoreactive collagenase-1, gelatinase A and stromelysin-1 were seen chiefly in chondrocytes, but in all cases in zones distant from the joint line before cavity formation. Collagenase-1 and gelatinase A were also localised both in synovium and on the articular surfaces of joints after cavity formation. In addition gelatinase A was seen in a 'collar' of perichondrium alongside the hypertrophic zone of chondrocytes and weakly in bone marrow spaces. Gelatinase B was seen in neutrophil leucocytes and in bone marrow spaces. TIMP-1 was generally distributed in connective tissue cells. No MMPs were seen along potential joint lines before or at the time of cavity formation, nor was there a specific decrease in TIMP-1 at this site. These findings confirm a role for metalloproteinases in developmental processes such as cartilage remodelling and bone marrow space formation. Collagenase-1 and gelatinase A may be involved in the remodelling of developing synovial tissue and the articular surfaces subsequent to cavity formation. However, no evidence was obtained to indicate that the loss of tissue strength at the joint line which allows synovial joint cavity formation relates to high local levels of MMPs (Edwards *et al.*, 1996). It can be concluded at this stage that the expression of a number of MMPs is related particularly to bone development, and at some stages to cartilage development, but that no clear indication of their precise function has emerged to date.

METALLOPROTEINASES AND ARTHRITIS

The irreversible destruction of the extracellular matrix of bone and cartilage tissues in diarthrodial joints is a major feature of arthritic diseases and causes permanent loss of joint function. It is known that proteinases of all mechanistic classes have the potential to contribute to the degradation (reviewed by Poole *et al.*, 1995). Because of their key role in the physiological maintenance and remodelling of connective tissues, the matrix metallo-proteinases (MMPs) have been particularly implicated in pathological degradative processes. There is now significant evidence of the over-expression of MMPs in tissues derived from patients with arthritic disease. Cultures of cells derived from rheumatoid synovia secreted collagenase (Dayer *et al.*, 1976) and stromelysin-1 (Sirum and Brinckerhoff, 1989) into the culture media and collagenase could be detected at sites of cartilage erosion in rheumatoid joints by immunolocalisation (Woolley *et al.*, 1977). Stromelysin-1 and collagenase-1 have also been demonstrated by immunolocalisation in lining cells of synovia, and their respective mRNAs detected by *in vitro* hybridisation (Okada *et al.*, 1990, 1992; Wolfe *et al.*, 1993; McCachren, 1991). This was confirmed by a recent immunolocalisation study of MMPs and TIMPs in synovial samples from joints with rheumatoid arthritis or osteoarthritis (Hembry *et al.*, 1995). The finding of stromelysin-1 in all synovial samples from 10 patients with disparate clinical diagnoses and histories, in contrast to its absence from normal synovia (Firestein *et al.*, 1991; McCachren, 1991), clearly implicates this enzyme in the arthritic process. It was also shown that collagenase-1, gelatinase A and matrilysin may have a role in the synovitis associated with rheumatoid arthritis, but are not a significant feature in osteoarthritic joints. However, marked regional variations were found in the synthesis of these MMPs, indicating that these diseases are episodic and that the control of enzyme synthesis is focal. This indicates the need for further work to co-localise MMP synthesis with cytokine and matrix expression in synovia from diseased joints, in order to further explore the mechanisms which control the synthesis and degradation of extracellular matrix components of articular cartilage. A better understanding of the control of these processes may indicate ways to down regulate MMP overproduction without compromis-ing normal tissue remodelling. Stromelysin-1 and collagenase-1 have also been measured in the synovial fluids from rheumatoid and osteoarthritic knee joints (Walakovits *et al.*, 1992; Lohmander *et al.*, 1993). The majority of the stromelysin-1 in the joint fluid is inactive, either as the proenzyme form or complexed to TIMP-1 or a_2 macroglobulin. Collagenase-1 levels in the fluids were an order of magnitude less than those of stromelysin. Analysis of TIMP-1 levels showed an excess of TIMP relative to stromelysin-1 in the control population, with the balance shifting to one of excess stromelysin-1 in the patients with joint disease. These observations are consistent with a previous study of extracts of human osteoarthritic cartilage which showed that there was an imbalance in favour of enzyme activity relative to normal tissue (Dean *et al.*, 1989).

Other studies of MMP expression in normal and diseased cartilage have documented the presence of stromelysin-1 (Okada *et al.*, 1992; Wolfe *et al.*, 1993) with lower levels of collagenase-1 (Wolfe *et al.*, 1993). Gelatinase B is expressed as both protein and mRNA in osteoarthritic cartilage but not in normal tissue (Mohtai *et al.*, 1993). The presence of low levels of collagenase-2 (MMPs) have been described (Cole *et al.*, 1996) and of MT1 MMP mRNA (Büttner *et al.*, 1996).

MMP expression has also been evaluated in animal models of arthritis, including rat streptococcal cell wall (Case *et al.*, 1989) and CIA models (Hasty *et al.*, 1990), both of which have elevated levels of MMPs at the cartilage–synovial interface. Injection of rabbit knee joints with IL-1 causes a 100 fold elevation in stromelysin levels (McDonnell *et al.*, 1992) and a rabbit meniscectomy model also showed elevated MMP mRNA levels in both the cartilage and synovium (Mehraban *et al.*, 1994). It is evident that MMPs are significantly raised in many animal models of arthritic disease. We have investigated the distribution of collagenase-1, stromelysin-1, gelatinases A and B, and TIMP-1 in cartilage and synovium removed from rabbits up to 27 days after induction of two models of arthritis by immunolocalisation (Hembry *et al.*, 1993). Following intra-articular injection of a poly-D-lysine/hyaluronic acid coacervate, collagenase and stromelysin were found bound to cartilage matrix, but there was little increase in chondrocyte synthesis of these enzymes. The synovium underwent a complex wound healing response involving invagination and encapsulation of the coacervate and inflammatory cell debris, during which all four metalloproteinases and tissue inhibitor of metalloproteinase could be immunolocalised. The second model, intra-articular injection of ovalbumin into sensitised rabbits, caused considerable chondrocyte necrosis; collagenase was found bound to cartilage matrix on day 13, although again there was little evidence of synthesis by chondrocytes. The data suggest that there are considerable differences between rheumatoid arthritis and these models and their use must therefore be carefully defined.

Immunochemical methods have also been developed to monitor the degradation and denaturation of type II collagen in cartilage (Hollander *et al.*, 1995). These measure the generation of a chain epitopes exposed after cleavage by collagenases. In ageing and osteoarthritis such cleavages are first detected around the chondrocytes, particularly at or just under the articular surface, from where it extends progressively deeper into the cartilage according to the Mankin grade (Hollander *et al.*, 1995). In contrast damage to the collagen can be detected throughout the matrix in rheumatoid arthritis.

A focus of attention in the study of matrix turnover in joint tissues has been the catabolism of aggrecan. This is a major component of cartilage conferring osmotic activity and hence the ability to resist compressive loads. Early studies showed that aggrecan turnover involved cleavage by metal-dependent proteolysis of the protein core at multiple sites, including cleavage close to the G1 domain, to release large GAG-containing fragments that no longer bind to hyaluronan. An understanding of the structures of these products and the development of assay procedures for individual components is now emerging. When aggrecan fragments from both culture models of cartilage breakdown and joint fluid from patients were sequenced, a specific reproducible cleavage at Glu 373–Ala 374 was identified (Sandy *et al.*, 1991; Lohmander *et al.*, 1993) and a new 'aggrecanase' proteinase was proposed (Figure 11.1). MMPs have been shown to cleave aggrecan at one major site between Asn 341 and Phe 342, although low activity can be shown at other sites (Fosang *et al.*, 1991, 1993; Flannery *et al.*, 1992, Figure 11.1). The recently described collagenase-3 (MMP13), which is discussed below, has been shown to cleave at the same site (Fosang *et al.*, 1996, Figure 11.1). The only MMP with activity against aggrecan at the Glu 373–Ala 374 bond is collagenase-2, but this enzyme still cleaves predominantly at the MMP site (Fosang *et al.*, 1994, Figure 11.1). The levels in cartilage are generally extremely low (Cole *et al.*, 1996) and are unlikely to be sufficient to account for the potentially large scale of aggrecan turnover. Aggrecan fragments from osteoarthritic cartilage provides evidence for both the Phe 342 and Ala 374 cleavage i.e. both MMP and 'aggrecanase' activities (Flannery *et al.*, 1992). Lark *et al.* (1995) recently produced

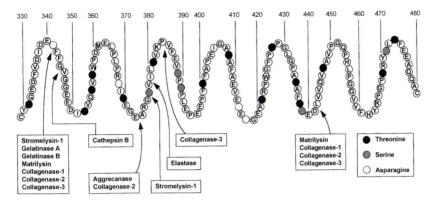

FIGURE 11.1   Cleavage of G1–G2 interglobular domain of aggrecan.

evidence that aggrecan cleavage at Glu 373 is the primary event in models of cartilage breakdown, but the use of specific antibodies to the C termini of the cleavage sites showed that 10% of cleaved aggrecan in normal and osteoarthritic cartilage and 20% in rheumatoid cartilage represented putative MMP cleavages. Upon immunohistochemical analysis both C termini appeared to be most abundant towards the surface of osteo-arthritic and rheumatoid cartilage and were most intense in areas of greatest damage, with significant but not exclusive co-distribution of both neo epitopes (Bayne *et al.*, 1995). The use of cleavage site-specific antisera can therefore provide useful data on the extent of activity of different proteinases. This approach will form an important basis for the ongoing development of synovial fluid analyses in monitoring disease progression.

CHARACTERISATION OF NOVEL MATRIX METALLOPROTEINASES

The recent cloning of a new sub group of membrane-associated MMPs (MT-MMPs; MMP14–17) as well as collagenase-3 (MMP13) led to the question of their potential role in extracellular matrix turnover, their expression in relation to joint tissues and their regulation. Somewhat unexpectedly MMP13; collagenase-3 mRNA was found to be expressed in osteoarthritic cartilage (Mitchell *et al.*, 1994; Reboul *et al.*, 1996) and in both rheumatoid and osteoarthritic synovium (Wernicke *et al.*, 1996). We have demon-strated the presence of collagenase-3 protein by immunolocalisation of cartilage from osteoarthritic patients (Cowell, Hembry, Murphy and Bayliss, unpublished).

Analysis of normal cartilage *ex vivo*, in which low levels of stromelysin-1 and gelatinase A could be found in scattered locations, showed no evidence for collagenase-1, collagenase-2 or collagenase-3. However, after 48 h exposure to IL-1b *in vitro*, collagenase-3 became detectable, particularly in chondrocytes at the articular surface. In agreement with data of Mitchell *et al.* (1994) and Reboul *et al.* (1996), inflammatory cytokines similarly upregulated collagenase-3 expression in both human chondrocytes and the chondrosarcoma cell line SW 1353 in culture (Cowell, Knäuper and Murphy, unpublished). A number of other MMPs were also upregulated including collagenase-1, stromelysin-1 and gelatinase B, but we could not detect collagenase-2 protein.

We have expressed procollagenase-3 from a myeloma cell line and purified it for biochemical characterisation (Knäuper et al., 1996a). The enzyme showed a high degree of N-linked glycosylation and was completely inactive in the proform. Collagenase-3 can be assigned to the collagenase subfamily of matrix metalloproteinases, according to substrate specificity analysis, hydrolysing the interstitial collagens I–III into 3/4 and 1/4 fragments and preferentially cleaving type II collagen over type I and III. In contrast, fibroblast collagenase preferentially cleaves type III and neutrophil collagenase type I collagen (Welgus et al., 1981; Hasty et al., 1987). Thus the three collagenases show distinct collagen substrate specificities, which implies that they may have evolved as specialised enzymes in order to degrade different connective tissues, depending on the collagen composition. Collagenase-3 may be especially important in the turnover of articular cartilage, which is rich in type II collagen. The specific activities of the three collagenases against type I collagen were in the range of 100–120 μg/min/nmol enzyme with the exception of 'superactive' collagenase-2, which cleaved 338 μg/min/nmol. By comparison of the ratios of collagenolytic/gelatinolytic activity or collagenolytic/peptidolytic activity of the three enzymes, it is clear that collagenase-1 is the most specific collagenase within this group, (Knäuper et al., 1996a). Collagenase-3 cleaved gelatin and the two synthetic peptide substrates with highly improved efficiency when compared with fibroblast or neutrophil collagenase. Thus, it appears that collagenase-3 not only efficiently degrades type I collagen, but it might also act as a gelatinase to further degrade the initial cleavage products of collagenolysis to small peptides suitable for further metabolism. This is in agreement with results obtained earlier for rat collagenase, which shows relatively high levels of gelatinolytic activity (Welgus et al., 1985) and shares the highest degree of homology with human collagenase-3, as does mouse collagenase (Henriet et al., 1992; Quinn et al., 1990). According to the high degree of functional and sequence homology between human collagenase-3 and the rodent collagenases, these enzymes belong to the collagenase-3 subfamily (MMP13) of matrix metalloproteinases and are distinct from human fibroblast collagenase (MMP-1).

Comparison of the ratios of gelatinolytic over peptidolytic activity of collagenase-3 with those values obtained for human gelatinase A revealed that collagenase-3 is 10 times less efficient than wild-type gelatinase A (Murphy et al., 1994). The high efficiency of wild-type gelatinase A against gelatin as a substrate can be attributed to the fibronectin-like type II repeats, since a gelatinase A deletion mutant ($D_{V191-Q364}$gelatinase A) lacking these sequence motifs has a similar ratio of gelatinolytic over peptidolytic activity to collagenase-3 (Murphy et al., 1994). Thus collagenase-3 shares some proteolytic characteristics with the gelatinase subfamily of matrix metalloproteinases, which is reflected in common structural elements shared by collagenase-3 and the gelatinases being localised within the active site cleft.

Analysis of the inhibition profile of collagenase-3 by the three homologous TIMPs revealed that all react with 1 : 1 stoichiometry by forming noncovalent tight-binding complexes, which is in agreement with earlier published data on other matrix metalloproteinases (for review, see Murphy and Willenbrock, 1995). Comparison of the efficacy of two synthetic peptide hydroxamate inhibitors against collagenase-3 confirmed the structural similarity to the gelatinases. CT1399, which has a K_i of less than 10 pM for gelatinase A and 16 pM for gelatinase B, had an approximate K_i of ~4 pM for collagenase-3 and a K_i of 385 nM for MMP-1. Similarly, CT1847, which has a K_i of 1.55 nM against gelatinase A and 2.1 nM against gelatinase B had K_i values of 0.54 nM against collagenase-3 and of 2.9 nM against MMP-1. It may be concluded that inhibitors directed against gelatinases will also be efficient in the control of collagenase-3.

Extracellular activation of the latent proform of many of the MMP family seems to be an important level of regulation and is effected by proteolytic removal of the N-terminal propeptide. Procollagenase-3 can be activated *in vitro* by stromelysin-1 or plasmin, but the latter rapidly destroys the active enzyme by further cleavages (Knäuper *et al.*, 1996b). We have found that procollagenase-3 is also processed to the active form by a cell-membrane associated mechanism involving MT.1-MMP (Knäuper *et al.*, 1996b) which was previously thought to be specific for progelatinase A (Atkinson *et al.*, 1995). Cell surface MT.1-MMP itself is probably activated intracellularly within the constitutive secretory pathway, since it contains the RXRXR/KR furin recognition site (Sato *et al.*, 1994). Active gelatinase A can also process procollagenase-3 to the active form and active collagenase-3 can generate active gelatinase A from the MT.1-MMP cleaved propeptide intermediate (Will *et al.*, 1996; Knäuper *et al.*, 1996b). Our data suggest that a cell surface associated activation cascade centred on MT-MMPs may exist (Figure 11.2). This may be compared with the plasmin cascade proposed earlier (Murphy *et al.*, 1992), centred on the urokinase-type plasminogen activator (uPA) receptor. Plasmin generated by plasminogen cleavage can be shown to mediate the activation of MMPs such as stromelysin-1, collagenase-1 and gelatinase B (Figure 11.2).

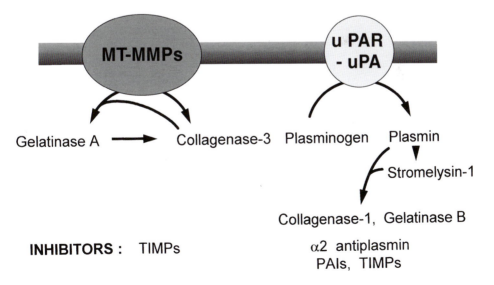

FIGURE 11.2 Cell Surface associated activation cascades for matrix metalloproteinases.

Our studies have indicated that human collagenase-3 is a potent proteinase with a broad spectrum of activity against extracellular matrix proteins as well as collagenolytic activity. The regulation and location of its expression in joint tissues relative to the other collagenases will be a matter of great importance for future study.

ACKNOWLEDGEMENTS

Our work is funded by the Arthritis and Rheumatism Council and the Medical Research Council. We thank Dr M. Bayliss and colleagues, Dr C. Lopez-Otin and colleagues and Dr J. Edwards and colleagues for their collaborations. We are grateful to Linda Thrift, Chris Green and Julie Parsison for preparing the manuscript.

REFERENCES

Atkinson, S.J., Crabbe, T., Cowell, S., Ward, R.V., Butler, M.J., Sato, H., Seiki, M., Reynolds, J.J. and Murphy, G. (1995) Intermolecular autolytic cleavage can contribute to the activation of progelatinase-A by cell-membranes. *J. Biol. Chem.*, **270**, 30479–30485.

Bayne, E.K., Donatelli, S.A., Sargeant, S., Singer, I.I., Lark, M.W., Hoerrner, L.A., Weidner, J.R., Williams, H.R., Mumford, R.A. and Lohmander, L.S. (1995) Aggrecan fragments terminating in the sequence NITEGE[323] are present within human OA and RA cartilage. *Trans. Orthop. Res. Soc.*, **20**, 328 (Abstr).

Basset, P., Bellocq, J.P., Wolf, C., Stoll, I., Hurtin, P., Limacher, J.M., Podhajcer, O.L., Chenard, M.P., Rio, M.C. and Chambon, P. (1990) A novel metalloproteinase gene specifically expressed in stromal cells of breast carcinomas. *Nature*, **348**, 699–704.

Breckon, J.J.W., Hembry, R.M., Reynolds, J.J. and Meikle, M.C. (1994) Regional and temporal changes in the synthesis of matrix metalloproteinases and TIMP-1 during development of the rabbit mandibular condyle. *J. Anat.*, **184**, 99–110.

Breckon, J.J.W., Hembry, R.M., Reynolds, J.J. and Meikle, M.C. (1995) Matrix metalloproteinases and TIMP-1 localization at sites of osteogenesis in the craniofacial region of the rabbit embryo. *Anat. Rec.*, **242**, 177–187.

Brown, C.C., Hembry, R.M. and Reynolds, J.J. (1989) Immunolocalization of metalloproteinases and their inhibitor in the rabbit growth plate. *J. Bone Joint Surg.*, **71-A**, 580–593.

Büttner, F.H., Chubinskaya, S., Margerie, D., Huch, K., Fletchtenmacher, J., Cole, A.A., Kuettner, K.E. and Bastrik, E. (1996) Expression of membrane type 1 matrix metalloproteinase in human articular cartilage. *Arthritis Rheum.*, **40**, 704–709.

Case, J.P., Sano, H., Lafyatis, R., Remmers, E.F., Kumkumian, G.K. and Wilder, R.L. (1989) Transin stromelysin expression in the synovium of rats with experimental erosive arthritis – *in situ* localization and kinetics of expression of the transformation-associated metalloproteinase in euthymic and athymic Lewis rats. *J. Clin. Invest.*, **84**, 1731–1740.

Cole, A.A., Chubinskaya, S., Schumacher, B., Huch, K., Cs-Szabo, G., Yao, J., Mikecz, K., Hasty, K.A. and Keuttner, K.E. (1996) Chondrocyte matrix metalloproteinase-8 – human articular chondrocytes express neutrophil collagenase. *J. Biol. Chem.*, **271**, 11023–11026.

Dayer, J.M., Krane, S.M., Russell, R.G.G. and Robinson, D.R. (1976) *Proc. Nat. Acad. Sci. USA*, **73**, 945–949.

Dean, D.D., Martel-Pelletier, J., Pelletier, J.-P., Howell, D.S. and Woessner, J.F. (1989) Evidence for metalloproteinase and metalloproteinase inhibitor imbalance in human osteoarthritic cartilage *J. Clin. Invest.*, **84**, 678–685.

Dean, D.D., Muniz, O.E., Woessner, J.F. and Howell, D.S. (1990) Production of collagenase and tissue inhibitor of metalloproteinases (TIMP) by rat growth plates in culture. *Matrix*, **10**, 320–330.

Edwards, J.C.W., Wilkinson, L.S., Soothill, P., Hembry, R.M., Murphy, G. and Reynolds, J.J. (1996) Matrix metalloproteinases in the formation of human synovial joint cavities. *J. Anat.*, **188**, 355–360.

Ehrlich, M.G., Tebor, G.B., Armstrong, A.L. and Mankin, H.J. (1985) Comparative study of neutral proteoglycanase activity by growth plate zone. *J. Orthop. Res.*, **3**, 269–276.

Firestein, G.S., Paine, M.M. and Littman, B.H. (1991) Gene-expression (collagenase, tissue inhibitor of metalloproteinases, complement, and HLA DR) in rheumatoid-arthritis and osteoarthritis synovium – quantitative-analysis and effect of intraarticular corticosteroids. *Arthritis Rheum.*, **34**, 1094–1105.

Flannery, C.R., Lark, M.W. and Sandy, J.D. (1992) Identification of a stromelysin cleavage site within the interglobular domain of human aggrecan – evidence for proteolysis at this site *in vivo* in human articular-cartilage. *J. Biol. Chem.*, **267**, 1008–1014.

Fosang, A.J., Neame, P.J., Hardingham, T.E., Murphy, G. and Hamilton, J.A. (1991) Cleavage of cartilage pro-teoglycan between G1 and G2 domains by stromelysins. *J. Biol. Chem.*, **266**, 15579–15582.

Fosang, A.J., Last, K., Knauper, V., Neame, P.J., Murphy, G., Hardingham, T.E., Tschesche, H. and Hamilton, J.A. (1993) Fibroblast and neutrophil collagenases cleave at 2 sites in the cartilage aggrecan interglobular domain. *Biochem. J.*, **295**, 273–276.

Fosang, A.J., Last, K., Neame, P.J., Murphy, G., Knauper, V., Tschesche, H., Hughes, C.E., Caterson, B. and Hardingham, T.E. (1994) Neutrophil collagenase (MMP-8) cleaves at the aggrecanase site E(373)–A(374) in the interglobular domain of cartilage aggrecan. *Biochem. J.*, **304**, 347–351.

Fosang, A.J., Last, K., Knäuper, V., Murphy, G. and Neame, P.J. (1996) Degradation of cartilage aggrecan by collagenase-3 (MMP-13). *FEBS Lett.*, **380**, 17–20.

Hasty, K.A., Jeffrey, J.J., Hibbs, M.S. and Welgus, H.G. (1987) The collagen substrate specificity of human neutrophil collagenase. *J. Biol. Chem.*, **262**, 10048–10052.

Hasty, K.A., Reife, R.A., Kang, A.H. and Stuart, J.M. (1990) The role of stromelysin in the cartilage destruction that accompanies inflammatory arthritis. *Arthritis Rheum.*, **33**, 388–397.

Hembry, R.M., Bagga, M.R., Murphy, G., Henderson, B. and Reynolds, J.J. (1993) Rabbit models of arthritis – immunolocalization of matrix metalloproteinases and tissue inhibitor of metalloproteinase in synovium and cartilage. *Am. J. Pathol.*, **143**, 628–642.

Hembry, R.M., Bagga, M.R., Reynolds, J.J. and Hamblen, D.L. (1995) Immunolocalization studies on 6 matrix metalloproteinases and their inhibitors, TIMP-1 and TIMP-2, in synovia from patients with osteoarthritis and rheumatoid-arthritis. *Ann. Rheum. Dis.*, **54**, 25–32.

Henriet, P., Rousseau, G.G. and Eeckhout, Y. (1992) Cloning and sequencing of mouse collagenase cDNA – divergence of mouse and rat collagenases from the other mammalian collagenases. *FEBS Lett.*, **310**, 175–178.

Hollander, A.P., Pidoux, I., Reiner, A., Rorabeck, C., Bourne, R. and Poole, A.R. (1995) Damage to type-ii col-lagen in aging and osteoarthritis starts at the articular surface, originates around chondrocytes, and extends into the cartilage with progressive degeneration. *J. Clin. Invest.*, **96**, 2859–2869.

Kinoh, H., Sato, H., Tsunezuka, Y., Takino, T., Kawashima, A., Okada, Y. and Seiki, M. (1996) MT-MMP, the cell-surface activator of proMMP-2 (pro-gelatinase-A), is expressed with its substrate in mouse tissue during embryogenesis. *J. Cell. Sci.*, **109**, 953–959.

Knäuper, V., López-Otin, C., Smith, B., Knight, G. and Murphy, G. (1996a) Biochemical characterization of human collagenase-3. *J. Biol. Chem.*, **271**, 1544–1550.

Knäuper, V., Will, H., Lopez-Otin, C., Smith, B., Atkinson, S.J., Stanton, H., Hembry, R.M. and Murphy, G. (1996b) Cellular mechanisms for human procollagenase-3 (MMP-13) activation – evidence that MT1-MMP (MMP-14) and gelatinase-A (MMP-2) are able to generate active enzyme. *J. Biol. Chem.*, **271**, 17124–17131.

Lark, M.W., Boyne, E.K. and Lohmander, L.S. (1995) Aggrecan degradation in osteoarthritis and rheumatoid-arthritis. *Acta Orthop. Scand.*, **66 (Suppl 266)**, 92–97.

Lefebvre, O., Regnier, C., Chenard, M.-P., Wendling, C., Chambon, P., Basset, P. and Rio, M.-C. (1995) Developmental expression of mouse stromelysin-3 messenger-RNA. *Development*, **121**, 947–955.

Lohmander, L.S., Hoerrner, L.A. and Lark, M.W. (1993) Metalloproteinases, tissue inhibitor, and proteoglycan fragments in knee synovial fluid in human osteoarthritis. *Arth. Rheum.*, **36**, 181–189.

Matrisian, L.M. and Hogan, B.L.M. (1990) Growth factor-regulated proteases and extracellular matrix remodel-ing during mammalian development. *Current Topics in Developmental Biology*, **24**, 219–259.

McCachren, S.S. (1991) Expression of metalloproteinases and metalloproteinase inhibitor in human arthritic synovium. *Arthritis Rheum.*, **34**, 1085–1092.

McDonnell, J., Hoerrner, L.A., Lark, M.W., Harper, C., Dey, T., Lobner, J., Eiermann, G., Kazazi, S.D., Singer, I.I. and Moore, V.L. (1992) Recombinant human interleukin-1-beta induced increase in levels of proteo-glycans, stromelysin, and leukocytes in rabbit synovial fluid. *Arthritis Rheum.*, **35**, 799–805.

Mehraban, F., Kuo, S.-Y., Riera, H., Chang, C. and Moskowitz, R.W. (1994) Prostromelysin and procollagenase genes are differentially up-regulated in chondrocytes from the knees of rabbits with experimental osteoarthritis. *Arthritis Rheum.*, **37**, 1189–1197.

Mitchell, P.G., Magna, H.A., Reeves, L.M., Lopresti-Morrow, L.L., Yocum, S.A., Rosner, P.J., Geoghegan, K.F. and Hambor, J.E. (1994) *J. Clin. Invest.*, **97**, 761–768.

Mohtai, M., Smith, R.L., Schurman, D.J., Tsuji, Y., Torti, F.M., Hutchinson, N.I., Stetler-Stevenson, W.G. and Goldberg, G.I. (1993) Expression of 92-KD type-IV collagenase gelatinase (gelatinase-B) in osteoarthritic cartilage and its induction in normal human articular cartilage by interleukin-1. *J. Clin. Invest.*, **92**, 179–185.

Murphy, G., Atkinson, S., Ward, R., Gavrilovic, J. and Reynolds, J.J. (1992) The role of plasminogen activators in the regulation of connective tissue metalloproteinases. *Ann. NY Acad. Sci.*, **667**, 1–12.

Murphy, G., Nguyen, Q., Cockett, M.I., Atkinson, S.J., Allan, J.A., Knight, C.G., Willenbrock, F. and Docherty, A.J.P. (1994) Assessment of the role of the fibronectin-like domain of gelatinase-A by analysis of a deletion mutant. *J. Biol. Chem.*, **269**, 6632–6636.

Murphy, G. and Willenbrock, F. (1995) Tissue inhibitors of matrix metalloendopeptidases. *Methods Enzymol.*, **248**, 496–510.

Okada, Y., Shinmei, M., Tanaka, O., Naka, K., Kimura, A., Nakanishi, I., Bayliss, M.Y., Iwata, K. and Nagase, H. (1992) Localization of matrix metalloproteinase-3 (stromelysin) in osteoarthritic cartilage and synovium. *Lab. Invest.*, **66**, 680–690.

Okada, Y., Gonoji, Y., Nakanishi, I., Nagase, H. and Hayakawa, T. (1990) Immunohistochemical demonstration of collagenase and tissue inhibitor of metalloproteinase (TIMP) in synovial lining cells of rheumatoid synovium. *Virchows. Archiv. B Cell Pathol.*, **59**, 305–312.

Poole, A.R., Alini, M. and Hollander, A. (1995) In: *Mechanisms and Models in Rheumatoid Arthritis* (eds. Henderson, B., Edwards, C.W. and Pettipher, E.R.) Academic Press, London, pp. 163–204.

Quinn, C.O., Scott, D.K., Brinckerhoff, C.E., Matrisian, L.M., Jeffrey, J.J. and Partridge, N.C. (1990) Rat collagenase – cloning, amino-acid-sequence comparison, and parathyroid-hormone regulation in osteoblastic cells. *J. Biol. Chem.*, **265**, 22342–22347.

Reboul, P., Pelletier, J.P., Tardif, G., Cloutier, J.M. and Martel-Pelletier, J. (1996) The new collagenase, collagenase-3, is expressed and synthesized by human chondrocytes but not by synoviocytes – a role in osteoarthritis. *J. Clin. Invest.*, **97**, 2011–2019.

Reponen, P., Sahlberg, C., Munaut, C., Thesleff, I. and Tryggvason, K. (1994) Expression of 92-KD type-IV collagenase (gelatinase-B) in the osteoclast lineage during mouse development. *J. Cell Biol.*, **124**, 1091–1102.

Sandy, J.D., Neame, P.J., Boynton, R.E. and Flannery, C.R. (1991) Catabolism of aggrecan in cartilage explants – identification of a major cleavage site within the interglobular domain. *J. Biol. Chem.*, **266**, 8683–8685.

Sato, H., Takino, T., Okada, Y., Cao, J., Shinagawa, A., Yamamoto, E. and Seiki, M. (1994) A matrix metalloproteinase expressed on the surface of invasive tumor cells. *Nature*, **370**, 61–65.

Sirum, K.L. and Brinckerhoff, C.E. (1989) Cloning of the genes for human stromelysin and stromelysin. 2. Differential expression in rheumatoid synovial fibroblasts. *Biochemistry*, **28**, 8691–8698.

Walakovits, L.A., Moore, V.L., Bhardwaj, N., Gallick, G.S. and Lark, M.W. (1992) Detection of stromelysin and collagenase in synovial-fluid from patients with rheumatoid arthritis and posttraumatic knee injury. *Arthritis Rheum.*, **35**, 35–42.

Welgus, H.G., Jeffrey, J.J. and Eisen, A.Z. (1981) Human-skin fibroblast collagenase – assessment of activation energy and deuterium-isotope effect with collagenous substrates. *J. Biol. Chem.*, **256**, 9511–9515.

Welgus, H.G., Grant, G.A., Sacchettini, J.C., Roswit, W.T. and Jeffrey, J.J. (1985) The gelatinolytic activity of rat uterus collagenase. *J. Biol. Chem.*, **260**, 13601–13606.

Wernicke, D., Seyfert, C., Hinzmann, B. and Gromnica-Ihle, E. (1996) Cloning of collagenase – from the synovial membrane and its expression in rheumatoid-arthritis and osteoarthritis. *J. Rheumatol.*, **23**, 590–595.

Will, H., Atkinson, S.J., Butler, G.S., Smith, B. and Murphy, G. (1996) The soluble catalytic domain of membrane type-1 matrix metalloproteinase cleaves the propeptide of progelatinase-A and initiates autoproteolytic activation – regulation by TIMP-2 and TIMP-3. *J. Biol. Chem.*, **271**, 17119–17123.

Wolfe, G.C., MacNaul, K.L., Buechel, F.F., McDonnell, J., Hoerrner, L.A., Lark, M.W., Moore, V.L. and Hutchinson, N.I. (1993) Differential in vivo expression of collagenase messenger-RNA in synovium and cartilage – quantitative comparisonwith stromelysin messenger RNA levels in human rheumatoid arthritis and osteoarthritis patients and in 2 animal models of acute inflammatory arthritis. *Arthritis Rheum.*, **36**, 1540–1547.

Woolley, D.E., Crossley, M.J. and Evanson, J.M. (1977) Collagenase at sites of cartilage erosion in the rheumatoid joint. *Arthritis Rheum.*, **20**, 1231–1239.

Yang, E.V. and Bryant, S.V. (1994) Developmental regulation of a matrix metalloproteinase during regeneration of axolotl appendages. *Dev. Biol.*, **166**, 696–703.

Yasui, N., Hori, H. and Nagai, Y. (1981) Production of collagenase inhibitor by the growth cartilage of embryonic chick bone – isolation and partial characterization. *Coll. Res.*, **1**, 59–72.

12 The Use of Monoclonal Antibody Technology for Studies of Cartilage Proteoglycan Metabolism with the Onset of Degenerative Joint Disease

B. Caterson, C.R. Flannery, D.R.R. Hiscock, C.E. Hughes and C.B. Little

Connective Tissue Biology Labs, Cardiff School of Biosciences, University of Wales, Cardiff, UK

INTRODUCTION

Adult articular cartilage is an avascular, aneural and hypocellular tissue with relatively slow turnover of its extracellular matrix components that are synthesised and maintained by chondrocytes. The chondrocytes of adult articular cartilage occur in four zones of the tissue where they exhibit distinct morphologies (see Chapter 1). The articular cartilage extracellular matrix consists primarily of proteoglycans, collagens, associated ions and water which collectively interact with one another to give the tissue its biophysical properties of resisting and dissipating mechanical loads applied to it during joint articulation (Ratcliffe and Mow, 1996). Chondrocyte's maintenance of this composite of organic molecules, ions and water is essential for the normal function of the tissue. Changes in the metabolism of the chondrocytes can significantly effect the normal maintenance and turnover of cartilage extracellular matrix components, ultimately leading to the onset of degenerative joint disease (see Hardingham and Fosang, 1992; Ratcliffe and Mow, 1996, for review).

Type II collagen is the major collagen present in articular cartilage with lesser amounts of types VI, IX and XI (see Chapter 9). Collagens II and XI form the major fibril structural architecture of the cartilage (Benninghoff Arcades – Benninghoff, 1925) with the type IX collagen molecules regulating fibril size through their interaction and alignment along the fibre periphery. Type VI collagen is found closely associated with the chondrocyte pericellular space (Poole *et al.*, 1992; Lee *et al.*, 1997) where it is involved in a fine microfibrillar meshwork within chondrons that form distinct morphological entities within the cartilage (Benninghoff, 1925; Poole *et al.*, 1987; Lee *et al.*, 1997). Aggrecan is the major proteoglycan present in hyaline articular cartilages. The aggrecan monomers $(2–2.5 \times 10^6$ dalton) form large macromolecular aggregates ($80–100 \times 10^6$ dalton) with hyaluronic acid through the specific association of their N-terminal G1 globular domains (Hardingham and Muir, 1972; Hascall and Heinegard, 1974). This association of aggrecan monomers with hyaluronic acid is stabilized by specific interactions with small glycoproteins called link proteins (Gregory, 1973; Heinegard and Hascall, 1974; Caterson and Baker, 1978; Baker and Caterson, 1979).

The entrapment of these large, highly hydrated, proteoglycan aggregates within the collagen fibril meshwork provides articular cartilage with its ability to resist compressive loads applied to the joint during articulation (see Ratcliffe and Mow, 1996 for review). Maintenance of these matrix interactions between cartilage macromolecules is essential for tissue homeostasis. Normal turnover of these molecules is controlled by the chondrocytes resident in the different morphological zones of the articular cartilage. The everyday turnover of the cartilage matrix macromolecules is currently believed to occur through the action of matrix metalloproteinases (MMPs) whose activities are closely regulated through the counteraction of naturally occurring tissue inhibitors of MMPs (TIMPs) that are also resident in the cartilage extracellular matrix (see Chapter 10).

Changes in the metabolism of the chondrocytes precede the onset of overt degenerative joint disease that is observed by the clinician. Early metabolic events in the pathogenesis of arthritis involve swelling of the cartilage and an increase in proteoglycan and collagen biosynthesis that is presumably an attempt at remodeling or repair of the tissue in response to its inadequate biomechanical environment (Muir, 1986). In addition, recent studies (Little *et al.*, 1996) have shown that anabolic and catabolic changes occur in the metabolism of the small interstitial proteoglycans, decorin and biglycan, with the onset of joint pathology. Histologically, the first events are seen as breakdown and removal of proteoglycans from the superficial zone of the articular cartilage surface – see Figure 12.1. This loss of proteoglycan from the joint surface compromises the cartilages' ability to resist compressive loads which eventually leads to the joint fibrillation at the surface that is depicted in Figure 12.1. In addition, this proteoglycan depletion at the articular cartilage surface also exposes the insoluble collagen fibrillar meshwork to degradation by matrix proteinases. Collectively, these events result in enzymatic and mechanical destruction of the cartilage and lead to the eventual joint space narrowing that is observed in radiological analysis of pathological joints (Ratcliffe and Mow, 1996). At the time of X-ray identification of joint pathology, the changes in the chondrocyte's metabolism are essentially irreversible in terms of induction of intrinsic cartilage repair. In order to combat this disease process, researchers need to better understand the early changes in cartilage metabolism that lead to joint pathology if they are to target therapeutic modes of intervention that can slow the progression of cartilage destruction. Whilst arthritis must be considered a degenerative *joint* disease (i.e. a disease involving all joint tissues), its earliest and overt metabolic changes are clearly seen as changes in cartilage proteoglycan metabolism.

Normal Cartilage

Osteoarthritic Cartilage
Early   Late

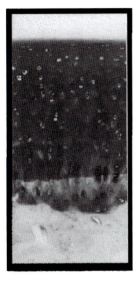
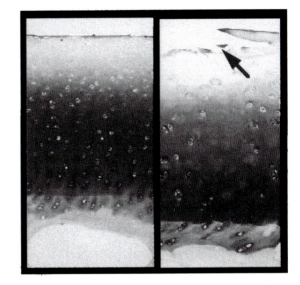

FIGURE 12.1   *Toluidine Blue staining of Normal and Osteoarthritic (Early and Later stage) canine articular cartilage.* Articular cartilage was harvested from the experimental (Osteoarthritic) and contralateral control (Normal) knees of Pond-Nuki dogs 6 (Early) and 12 months (Late) after severance of their anterior cruciate ligament in the experimental knee. Cartilage samples were fixed in paraformaldehyde and stained with Toluidine Blue for routine histology. Normal cartilage shows a strong Toluidine Blue staining pattern throughout the complete depth of the cartilage. The Osteoarthritic cartilage (Early and Late stage) shows a gradual loss and decrease of Toluidine Blue staining from the joint surface through to the mid and deep zones of the articular cartilage. This decrease in staining is due to gradual loss (catabolism) of proteoglycans from the tissue. This loss of proteoglycan compromises the cartilages' ability to resist and dissipate mechanical loads in joint articulation which leads to fibrillation (arrow) at the cartilage surface.

For the past 16 years, research in our laboratory has focused on the use of monoclonal antibody technology to study changes in cartilage proteoglycan metabolism in health and disease (Caterson *et al.*, 1981, 1985, 1986, 1987, 1995; Caterson and Hughes, 1995). Using monoclonal antibody technology we have been able to detect subtle biochemical changes that occur in both anabolic (attempted remodeling/repair) and catabolic (matrix destruction) aspects of cartilage metabolism in the pathogenesis of arthritis (Caterson *et al.*, 1990a, 1995; Carney *et al.*, 1992; Hughes *et al.*, 1992, 1995a; Visco *et al.*, 1993; Slater *et al.*, 1995; Carlson *et al.*, 1995; Caterson and Hughes, 1996). Recently, our laboratory has initiated new studies, using molecular biology techniques (RT-PCR), to monitor the expression of matrix proteinases in articular cartilage metabolism. This chapter summarises our past and recent work using these technologies to study changes in articular cartilage proteoglycan metabolism in the pathogenesis of degenerative joint disease.

ANABOLIC CHANGES IN CARTILAGE PROTEOGLYCAN METABOLISM

Several years ago, in collaborative studies with Drs. Tim Hardingham, Helen Muir and their co-workers at the Kennedy Institute of Rheumatology, London our laboratory performed studies describing subtle biochemical compositional differences in the chondroitin sulfate (CS) glycosaminoglycan chains of newly synthesised proteoglycan isolated from osteoarthritic cartilage (Caterson *et al.*, 1990a). These differences were detected by two monoclonal antibodies denoted **3-B-3**(−) and **7-D-4**. Antibody 3-B-3 recognises, as its epitope, a non-reducing terminal unsaturated uronic acid residue adjacent to N-acetylgalactosamine-6-sulfate that is produced after the CS chains have been digested with the bacterial enzyme chondroitinase (Couchman *et al.*, 1984; Caterson *et al.*, 1985, see Figure 2). This epitope is denoted as 3-B-3(+) since its use requires that CS-proteoglycans are pre-digested with chondroitinase to generate its specific epitope. However, this antibody also recognises a natural epitope, a *mimotope* (Geysen *et al.*, 1988), which is a structure that mimics the bacterial enzyme-generated epitope and contains a saturated glucuronic acid residue (rather than an unsaturated sugar residue) at the non-reducing terminal of the CS glycosaminoglycan chains of cartilage proteoglycans (Figure 12.2). When antibody 3-B-3 is used without chondroitinase pretreatment, immunoreactivity with the native mimotope structure is designated 3-B-3(−) – see Figure 12.2. Proteoglycans containing the 3-B-3(−) mimotope at the non-reducing terminal of CS glycosaminoglycans occur at low frequency in proteoglycans isolated from normal cartilage. However, its expression is much more prevalent in proteoglycans extracted from osteoarthritic tissue (Caterson *et al.*, 1990a; Carney *et al.*, 1992; Slater *et al.*, 1995; Caterson *et al.*, 1995). Proteoglycans containing CS glycosaminoglycans containing the 3-B-3(−) mimotope accumulate in CsCl density gradients at a lower buoyant density than the majority of the cartilage aggrecan subpopulation (Griffin, 1995; Hiscock, D.R.R., Griffin, J.P. and Caterson, B., unpublished work).

The epitope for antibody 7-D-4 is less well characterised (Caterson *et al.*, 1990b; Sorrell *et al.*, 1993). However, it appears to recognise subtle combinations of sulfated and non-sulfated disaccharide isomers within the native CS chain (Carney *et al.*, 1996) – see Figure 12.2. Expression of the 7-D-4 epitope in CS glycosaminoglycans is also more prevalent in proteoglycans extracted from osteoarthritic cartilage but differs in human compared to other animal species (Caterson *et al.*, 1990a; Visco *et al.*, 1993; Slater *et al.*, 1995; Carlson *et al.*, 1995). Since we first described antibodies recognising native CS epitopes, other researchers have now described another anti-CS monoclonal antibody, denoted 846, that recognises a similar native CS epitope which also has increased expression in OA cartilage (Rizkalla *et al.*, 1992). Antibody 846 was originally thought to recognise a protein epitope which is normally expressed in foetal proteoglycans that were believed to be re-expressed in cartilage pathology (Glant *et al.*, 1986); however, retrospectively (Poole, 1993) this antibody was characterised as recognising an epitope in native CS similar to our antibodies 3-B-3(−) and 7-D-4.

Expression of these anabolic neoepitopes in CS glycosaminoglycans of OA cartilage proteoglycans appears to result from the tissues attempt to repair or remodel the damaged

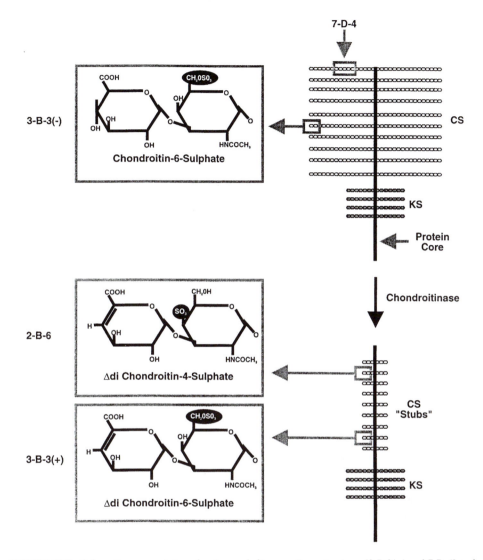

FIGURE 12.2   *Schematic representation of native anabolic neoepitope structures [3-B-3(−) and 7-D-4] and chondroitinase-generated epitopes [2-B-6 and 3-B-3(+)] found in chondroitin sulphate glycosaminoglycan chains.* Cartilage aggrecan monomer is simplistically represented as a central protein core with chondroitin sulphate (CS) and keratan sulphate (KS) glycosaminoglycan chains radiating from the core protein. Chondroitinase digestion of the CS produces CS "stubs" covalently attached to the aggrecan core protein which contain unsaturated disaccharide isomers of CS at their non-reducing termini (Caterson *et al.*, 1985). The native anabolic neoepitope [3-B-3(−)] occurs at the non-reducing termini of some of the CS glycosaminoglycan chains and consists of a disaccharide with a saturated glucuronic acid residue adjacent to N-acetylgalactosamine-6 sulphate. The 7-D-4 neoepitope is located within the native CS glycosaminoglycan chain; its exact structure has not been determined yet. Also shown are the disaccharide structures for the chondroitinase-generated epitopes of antibodies 2-B-6 and 3-B-3(+). Both of these epitopes have an unsaturated glucuronic acid residue at the non-reducing terminal adjacent to a 4-sulphated [2-B-6] or 6-sulphated [3-B-3(+)] N-acetylgalactosamine residue of the CS-unsaturated disaccharide. The 3-B-3(−) structure is a mimotope of the 3-B-3(+) epitope that is produced after chondroitinase digestion of 6-sulphated CS glycosaminoglycan chains.

cartilage extracellular matrix. In addition, their expression may also reflect a switch in the chondrocytes metabolism to a hypertrophic phenotype. Credence for this latter hypothesis is supported by; (i) expression of the 3-B-3(−) mimotope and the 7-D-4 epitope in the hypertrophic zone (but not other zones) of normal human and bovine growth plate (Byers *et al.*, 1992; Gibson *et al.*, 1996), and (ii) the observation that type X collagen is synthesised by hypertrophic cell clusters in osteoarthritic cartilage (von der Mark *et al.*, 1992).

Monitoring the expression of these anabolic markers of altered proteoglycan metabolism in arthritis has now been widely used in several animal models that mimic arthritic diseases in humans (Caterson *et al.*, 1990a; Carney *et al.*, 1992; Visco *et al.*, 1993; Ratcliffe *et al.*, 1993; Caterson and Hughes, 1995; Carlson *et al.*, 1995). Similarly, they have also been used in analysis of proteoglycans extracted from human arthritic tissue (Caterson *et al.*, 1990a; Rizkalla *et al.*, 1992; Slater *et al.*, 1995). Their potential use as diagnostic reagents for identifying proteoglycan metabolites in human body fluids has also been demonstrated (Hazell *et al.*, 1995). Collectively, these studies have established that subtle changes do occur in the biochemistry of the CS chains of cartilage proteoglycans during the pathogenesis of OA (i.e. their sulfation and chain termination). Furthermore, their detection can be used as "markers" of altered metabolism that is predictive of early changes that occur in the onset of degenerative joint disease.

CATABOLIC CHANGES IN ARTICULAR CARTILAGE PROTEOGLYCAN METABOLISM

In the past 6 years (Caterson, 1991; Hughes *et al.*, 1992, 1995a; Caterson *et al.*, 1992, 1995; Caterson and Hughes, 1995), our laboratory has developed and demonstrated the feasibility of using monoclonal antibody technology to study novel aspects of cartilage proteoglycan catabolism in health and disease. In 1992 (Hughes *et al.*, 1992), we described methods for producing monoclonal antibodies against catabolic neoepitopes on link protein metabolites generated by the action of different proteinases on cartilage proteoglycan aggregates. This publication validated our novel hypothesis that one could indeed produce monoclonal antibodies directed against catabolic neoepitopes on polypeptide degradation products that were specifically generated by different matrix proteases. More recently, we have used similar technologies to study the mechanisms involved in proteolytic degradation of aggrecan in normal turnover and arthritic diseases (Hughes *et al.*, 1992, 1994, 1995b, 1997; Fosang *et al.*, 1994; Lin *et al.*, 1995; Ilic *et al.*, 1995; Tortorella *et al.*, 1996).

The mechanisms underlying aggrecan catabolism in normal articular cartilage turnover and in diseases such as osteoarthritis and rheumatoid arthritis are thought to involve initial cleavage of aggrecan at two predominant sites within the interglobular domain (IGD) of the molecule located between the G1 and G2 globular domains of aggrecan – see Figure 12.3 (Maniglia *et al.*, 1991; Sandy *et al.*, 1991; Flannery *et al.*, 1992). These two catabolic cleavage sites occur between residues Asn341-Phe342 (Flannery *et al.*, 1992) and Glu373-Ala374 in the native human aggrecan sequence (Maniglia *et al.*, 1991; Sandy *et al.*, 1991; Sandy *et al.*, 1992). The former site is hydrolysed by many of the matrix metalloproteinases (MMPs 1, 2, 3, 7, 8, 9, 10 and 13), whilst the latter site results from an as yet unidentified proteolytic activity referred to as 'aggrecanase'. In recent publications (Hughes *et al.*, 1994,1995a; Caterson *et al.*, 1995), we have described two new mono-clonal antibodies (BC-3 and BC-4) which recognise the catabolic neoepitope N-terminal amino acid sequence (ARGSV...) in the IGD of aggrecan catabolites generated by the unknown enzyme 'aggrecanase', and also, the new C-terminal amino acid sequence (...DIPEN) in the aggrecan G1 domain with a small component of the IGD that is gener-ated by the action of MMP's, respectively (Figure 12.3). In addition (Caterson *et al.*, 1995), we have recently produced and characterised two new monoclonal antibodies (BC-13 and BC-14) that recognise the additional C- and N-terminal neoepitopes generated by 'aggrecanase' (...ITEGE) and the MMP's (FFGSV...), respectively – see Figure 12.3. Several other laboratories have now made analogous monoclonal and polyclonal antibodies that recognise most of these neoepitope sequences (Lark *et al.*, 1995, 1997; Singer *et al.*, 1995; Fosang *et al.*, 1995, 1996) but not the 'aggrecanase'-generated N-terminal neoepitope sequence (ARGSVI...) that is specifically recognised by monoclonal antibody BC-3 (Hughes *et al.*, 1995a).

In recent studies (Hughes *et al.*, 1995a, 1995b; Fosang *et al.*, 1994; Witt *et al.*, 1995; Lin *et al.*, 1995; Tortorella *et al.*, 1996; Arner *et al.*, 1997a, 1997c), we and others have used these catabolic neoepitope antibodies to identify specific catabolites of aggrecan produced by the unknown proteolytic activity 'aggrecanase'. An example of the use of

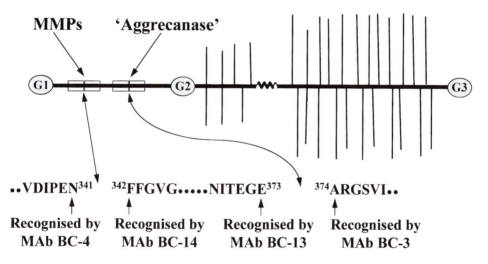

FIGURE 12.3 *Schematic representation of an aggrecan monomer molecule showing the matrix metallopro-teinase (MMP) and 'aggrecanase' cleavage sites within its interglobular domain and the amino acid sequences recognized by neoepitope monoclonal antibodies.* The interglobular domain (IGD) of aggrecan is located between the G1 and G2 globular domains at the N-terminal end of the aggrecan protein core. Within the IGD there are two major sites of proteolytic cleavage, Asn341-Phe342 and Glu373-Ala374 that are specifically cleaved by MMPs 1, 2, 3, 7, 8, 9, 10 and 13 and "aggrecanase", respectively, during aggrecan catabolism (Sandy *et al.*, 1991; Flannery *et al.*, 1992; Hardingham and Fosang, 1992). Cleavage by these proteolytic activities at these sites generates new C- and N-terminal neoepitope sequences that are specifically recognized by mono-clonal antibodies BC-3, BC-4, BC-13 and BC-14 as indicated in the cartoon.

this antibody technology to immunolocate specific 'aggrecanase'-generated catabolites in Western Blot analyses of cartilage explant media is shown in Figure 12.4. Bovine articular cartilage explants were cultured in the presence of the cytokine IL-1β for 48 h and aggrecan catabolites released into the medium were purified on associative CsCl density gradients, deglycosylated with chondroitinase, keratanase and keratanase II, and fractionated using SDS-PAGE prior to immunochemical analyses with monoclonal antibodies 2-B-6 (anti C-4-S 'stubs' – Caterson et al., 1985) and BC-3 (anti-'aggrecanase-generated neoepitope ARGSV ...). Immunolocation analyses with 2-B-6 shows multiple aggrecan degradation products that originally contained 4-sulphated CS glycosaminoglycans. In contrast, antibody BC-3 only recognises a few of these bands indicating that they contain the 'aggrecanase'-generated neoepitope with the N-terminal sequence ARGSV... The occurrence of several BC-3 positive bands in this Western Blot indicates that additional proteolytic cleavages have occurred at sites C-terminal to the major cleavage sites found in the interglobular domain of aggrecan (Maniglia et al., 1991; Sandy et al., 1991).

In our collaborative work with researchers at Dupont-Merck (Hughes et al., 1995b; Tortorella et al., 1996; Arner et al., 1997c) we have used similar bovine explant culture systems treated with a single dose of IL-1 or TNF-alpha as an in vitro model that mimics pathological degradation processes in arthritis. Immunochemical analyses of aggrecan metabolites with monoclonal antibody BC-3 has indicated that 'aggrecanase'-generated

Analysis of Proteoglycan Fragments
Released from Cartilage Explants

2-B-6   BC3

2-B-6 positive fragments indicate multiple proteolytic cleavage sites within the aggrecan core protein.

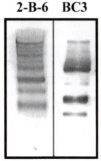

BC-3 positive bands detect those fragments with an ARGS.. N-terminal neoepitope resulting from 'aggrecanase'cleavage within the IGD of aggrecan.

FIGURE 12.4 *Immunolocation analyses of deglycosylated aggrecan metabolites from bovine articular cartilage explant culture medium, using antibodies 2-B-6 (anti- 4-sulphated CS "stubs") and BC-3 (anti- ARG...).* Culture medium from bovine articular cartilage explant cultures exposed to IL-1, to induce accelerated aggrecan catabolism was used as a source of aggrecan catabolites produced by 'aggrecanase' activity. The aggrecan catabolites in the medium were purified on associative CsCl gradients, deglycosylated with chondroitinase, keratanase and keratanase II, then subjected to SDS-PAGE prior to immunolocation analyses with antibodies 2-B-6 and BC-3. Immunolocation with antibody 2-B-6 identifies several aggrecan catabolites with 4-sulphated CS "stubs" attached (Caterson et al., 1985) whilst immunolocation with antibody BC-3 specifically identifies aggrecan metabolites derived from 'aggrecanase' proteolysis in the interglobular domain of aggrecan (Hughes et al., 1995a).

catabolites were first evident in the culture media after 8 hours of exposure to cytokines. This result suggested that 'aggrecanase' was a newly synthesised proteolytic activity or that it took time to activate the enzyme. In the untreated cultures the appearance of BC-3 positive catabolites occurred at very low levels, but only after 24 h of culture (Hughes *et al.*, 1995). Analysis, with monoclonal antibody BC-14 (anti FFG ..., see Figure 12.3) showed no evidence of MMP-generated degradation products in these bovine explant culture systems.

We have also used these catabolic neoepitope antibodies in studies aimed at identifying potential enzymes with 'aggrecanase' activity. In collaborative studies (Fosang *et al.*, 1994), we used monoclonal antibody BC-3 to demonstrate that neutrophil collagenase (MMP-8) could catalyze 'aggrecanase' proteolytic activity (cleavage) on aggrecan; this unexpected result suggesting that other MMPs may also exhibit this activity. This result also left open the question as to whether or not chondrocytes could synthesise MMP-8. Recently (Cole *et al.*, 1996), have used immunohistochemical analyses and *in situ* hybridisation techniques to demonstrate the presence and expression of MMP-8 in IL-1 stimulated and human osteoarthritic cartilage, these results supporting the consideration that MMP-8 might be 'aggrecanase'. However, recent publications challenge this conclusion (Arner *et al.*, 1997b).

Despite mounting evidence implicating the involvement of MMPs in the degradation of aggrecan, it has not been reported that a known MMP can exclusively cleave the Glu373-Ala374 bond (human sequence enumeration) of the aggrecan core protein, the specific peptide bond which is cleaved *in vivo* in human cartilage during the course of degenerative joint disease (Sandy *et al.*, 1992). In recent studies our laboratory has adopted the use of a "gene-family" PCR technique which was contrived to identify novel MMP gene-family members that were expressed in model systems that mimic cartilage degradation *in vivo*. For this study, minimally degenerate oligonucleotide primers were designed based on two protein sequences which are highly conserved amongst all known MMPs; i.e. the "cysteine switch" (amino acid sequence PRCGVPD) and the catalytic zinc-binding domain (amino acid sequence HE X GH X L). No new MMPs were discovered in our RT-PCR analyses using these primers. However, our results (Figure 12.5), demonstrated that mRNA for MMP-13 (or collagenase-3), a MMP not previously detected in cartilage, was preferentially upregulated in rat and bovine chondrocytes cultured under conditions of elevated matrix catabolism (Flannery and Sandy, 1995). These results were confirmed using primers designed to exclusively amplify MMP-3 (a MMP implicated in aggrecan degradation *in vivo* – Flannery *et al.*, 1992), MMP-13 and GAPDH (Figure 12.5). However, conventional N-terminal amino acid sequence analysis of the native aggrecan catabolites generated following digestion with purified MMP-13 had a predominant N-terminus corresponding to Phe342, consistent with hydrolysis of the Asn341-Phe342 bond which is preferentially cleaved by all MMPs examined to date. Collectively, these data suggest that there are at least two different mechanisms of aggrecan metabolism occurring in control versus cytokine or retinoic acid stimulated cultures i.e. normal turnover possibly utilising local and focal action of the MMPs versus the pathological, more general, cytokine-induced degradation elicited by 'aggrecanase'. These differences may possibly distinguish two distinct mechanisms of cartilage proteoglycan metabolism; normal turnover versus pathological degradation in degenerative joint diseases.

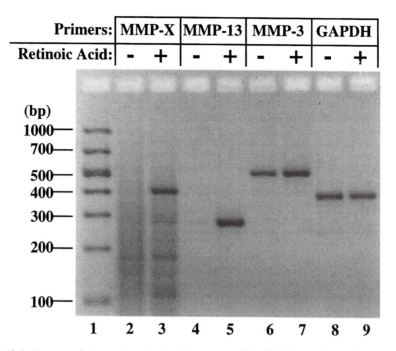

FIGURE 12.5 *Agarose gel electrophoresis of products generated by RT-PCR amplification of RNA isolated from rat chondrosarcoma chondrocytes.* Portions of RT-mRNA prepared from cells cultured in the absence (lanes 2, 4, 6, 8) or presence (lanes 3, 5, 7, 9) of 1 μM retinoic acid for 4 days were amplified using MMP "gene-family" degenerate primers (designated MMP-X) or primers which exclusively amplify MMP-3, MMP-13 or GAPDH. DNA size markers are shown in lane 1, with sizes in base pairs given on the left. The ~404 bp product shown in lane 3 was identified as rat MMP-13 by sequence analysis; all other PCR products were also sequenced to confirm identity. Results similar to those shown in this figure were obtained using RNA isolated from cultured bovine articular chondrocytes.

BIOCHEMICAL PROPERTIES OF 'AGGRECANASE'

As mentioned above, the identity of the proteolytic activity 'aggrecanase' has not yet been determined in spite of concerted efforts from numerous researchers located in academic and industry research laboratories in many countries. It is over six years since the proteolytic activity of 'aggrecanase' on aggrecan was first described (Maniglia *et al.*, 1991). In very recent work, our laboratory in collaboration with Drs. Bartnik, Büttner and Eidenmüller (Hoechst Marion Roussel, Weisbaden, Germany) have been able to synthesise, for the first time, a recombinant polypeptide substrate (rAgg1) that is catabolised by 'aggrecanase' in a novel cell culture system (Hughes *et al.*, 1997). In this system, identification of 'aggrecanase'-generated recombinant catabolites is specifically determined by using antibody BC-3 (Figure 12.3). Antibody BC-3 specifically detects 'aggrecanase'-generated rAgg1 degradation products in the media of agarose cultures containing rat chondrosarcoma or bovine chondrocytes that were exposed to retinoic acid or IL-1 to mimic pathological degradation pathways of aggrecan metabolism (untreated cultures

TABLE 12.1
Biochemical properties of 'Aggrecanase'.

---

1. Interleukin-1, tumor necrosis factor-alpha and retinoic acid all stimulate the expression of 'aggrecanase' in a dose dependent manner.
2. It takes time for chondrocytes in explant and agarose cultures to express cytokine-induced 'aggrecanase' activity i.e. 'aggrecanase' is unlikely to occur as an inactive proenzyme sequestered in the cartilage extra-cellular matrix.
3. Induction of 'aggrecanase' activity requires de novo protein synthesis.
4. 'Aggrecanase' activity can occur non-cell associated i.e. it is a stable activity found in conditioned media from cartilage explant and agarose cultures.
5. 'Aggrecanase' is a metalloproteinase (i.e. it is inhibited by EDTA and 1,10 phenanthroline) but it is not necessarily a known matrix metalloproteinase.
6. Drugs currently used for the treatment of arthritis symptoms (Indomethacin, Tenidap, Doxycycline, Naproxen and Dexamethasone) do not inhibit 'aggrecanase' activity in model culture systems.

Data summarized from Arner *et al.*, 1997a, b and c; Hughes *et al.*, 1995b, 1997; Ilic *et al.*, 1995; Tortorella *et al.*, 1996; Witt *et al.*, 1995.

serve as controls). Antibody BC-14 can also be used to detect rAgg1 catabolites with the neoepitope sequence FFG … which indicate the occurrence of MMP activity(ies) in these cell culture systems.

Although the identity of 'aggrecanase' is still not known, several interesting bio-chemical characteristics and properties of this unknown proteolytic activity have been determined using this novel system utilising a recombinant substrate for monitoring 'aggrecanase' activity. These conclusions, as well as those that resulted from our cartilage explant culture studies described above, are all summarised in Table 12.1. Important findings concerning the biochemical properties of 'aggrecanase' are: (i) it takes time to syn-thesis and/or activate 'aggrecanase' activity; (ii) induction of this activity or 'aggrecanase' activation requires de novo protein synthesis; and (iii) in spite of currently held beliefs, 'aggrecanase' is not necessarily a cell-associated activity since it can occur in extra-cellular compartments not associated with the chondrocyte (i.e. conditioned medium). Furthermore, this novel system utilising the recombinant rAgg1 substrate for detecting 'aggrecanase' activity, coupled with detection of specific aggrecan catabolites with neoepitope antibodies (Hughes *et al.*, 1997), offers considerable potential for facilitating the discovery and identification of 'aggrecanase' in the very near future. This discovery will undoubtedly influence our choice of therapeutic targets for slowing the progression of cartilage destruction in arthritis (i.e. 'aggrecanase' or MMPs, or both).

ACKNOWLEDGEMENTS

The research summarised in this chapter was supported by funding from the National Institutes of Health (USA), The Arthritis Foundation (USA), The Arthritis and Rheumatism Council (UK) and a grant from Hoechst Marion Roussel, Weisbaden (Germany).

REFERENCES

Arner, E.C., Decicco, C.P., Pratta, M.A., Copeland, R.A., Trzaskos, J.M., Magolda, R.L. and Tortorella, M.D. (1997a) Characterization of soluble bovine cartilage "aggrecanase". *Trans. Orthop. Res. Soc.*, **22**, 103.

Arner, E.C., Decicco, C.P., Pratta, M.A., Newton, R.C., Trzaskos, J.M., Magolda, R.L. and Tortorella, M.D. (1997b) "Aggrecanase", and not MMP-1, -2, -3, -8, -9, is critical for IL-1-induced cartilage aggrecan degradation. *Trans. Orthop. Res. Soc.*, **22**, 454.

Arner, E.C., Hughes, C.E., Decicco, C.P., Caterson, B. and Tortorella, M.D. (1997c) Cartilage proteoglycan degradation is mediated by "aggrecanase": an activity blocked by active-site and activation inhibitors of matrix metalloproteinases. *Osteoarthritis and Cartilage*, submitted.

Baker, J.R. and Caterson, B. (1979) The isolation and characterization of the link proteins from proteglycan aggregates of bovine nasal cartilage. *J. Biol. Chem.*, **254**, 1287–1292.

Benninghoff, A. (1925) Form und Bauder Gelenkknorpel in iheren Beziehungen zur Funktion. Der Aufbau des Gelenkknorpels in seinen Beziehungen zur Funktion. *Z. Zellforch Mikrosk Anat. Forsch.*, **2**, 783–862.

Byers, S., Caterson, B., Hopwood, J.J. and Foster, B.K. (1992) Immunolocation analysis of glycosaminoglycans in the human growth plate. *J. Histochem. Cytochem.*, **40**, 275–282.

Carlson, C.S., Loeser, R.F., Johnstone, B., Tulli, H.M., Dobson, D.B. and Caterson, B. (1995) Osteoarthritis in Cynomolgus Macaques II: Detection of modulated epitopes in cartilage and synovial fluid. *J. Orthop. Res.*, **13**, 399–409.

Carney, S.L., Billingham, M.E.J., Caterson, B., Ratcliffe, A., Bayliss, M.T., Hardingham, T.E. and Muir, H. (1992) Changes in proteoglycan turnover in experimental canine osteoarthritic cartilage. *Matrix*, **12**, 137–147.

Carney, S.L., Caterson, B. and Penticost, H.R. (1996) The investigation of glycosaminoglycan mimotope structure using capillary electrophoresis and other complimentary electrophoretic techniques. *Electrophoresis*, **17**, 384–390.

Caterson, B. and Baker, J.R. (1978) The interaction of link proteins with proteoglycan monomers in the absence of hyaluronic acid. *Biochem. Biophys. Res. Commun.*, **80**, 596–603.

Caterson, B., Baker, J.R., Christner, J.E., Kearney, J.F. and Stohrer, R.C. (1981) The characterization of clonal antibodies directed against bovine nasal cartilage proteoglycan and link protein. In: *Monoclonal Antibodies and T-cell Hybridomas: Perspectives and Technical Advances*. Hammerling, G.J., Hammerling, U. and Kearney, J.F., eds, A series of Research Monographs in Immunology. Vol. 3, pp. 259–267, Amsterdam, New York, Oxford: Elsevier/North Holland.

Caterson, B., Christner, J.E., Baker, J.R. and Couchman, J.R. (1985) The production and characterization of monoclonal antibodies directed against connective tissue proteoglycans. *Federation Proceedings*, **44**, 386–393.

Caterson, B., Calabro, T., Donohue, P.J. and Jahnke, M.R. (1986) Monoclonal antibodies against cartilage proteoglycan and link protein. In: *Articular Cartilage Biochemistry*. Kuettner, K.E., Schleyerbach, R. and Hascall. V.C., eds, pp. 59–73, New York: Raven Press.

Caterson, B., Calabro, T. and Hampton, A. (1987). Monoclonal antibodies as probes for elucidating proteoglycan structure and function. In: *Biology of the Extracellular Matrix: A series, "Biology of Proteoglycans"*, Wight, T. and Mecham, R., eds, pp. 1–26, New York: Academic Press.

Caterson, B., Mahmoodian, F., Sorrell, J.M., Hardingham, T.E., Bayliss, M.T., Carney, S.L., Ratcliffe, A. and Muir, H. (1990a) Modulation of native chondroitin sulfate structures in tissue development and in disease. *J. Cell. Science*, **97**, 411–417.

Caterson, B., Griffin, J.P., Mahmoodian, F. and Sorrell, J.M. (1990b) Monoclonal antibodies against chondroitin sulfate isomers: Their use as probes for investigating proteoglycan metabolism. *Biochem. Soc. Trans.*, **18**, 820–823.

Caterson, B. (1991) Immunological aspects of markers of joint disease. *J. Rheumatology*, **18**(Suppl. 27), 19–23.

Caterson, B., Hughes, C.E., Johnstone, B. and Mort, J.S. (1992) Immunological markers of cartilage proteoglycan metabolism in animal and human osteoarthritis. In: *Articular Cartilage and Osteoarthritis*, Kuettner, K.E., Schleyerbach, R., Peyron, J. and Hascall, V.C., eds, pp 415–427, New York: Raven Press.

Caterson, B. and Hughes, C.E. (1995) Anabolic and catabolic markers of proteoglycan metabolism in arthritis. In: *Osteoarthritic Disorders*, Kuettner, K.E. and Goldberg, V., eds, pp. 315–327, Rosemont, IL: AAOS Publications.

Caterson, B., Hughes, C.E., Roughly, P.R. and Mort, J.S. (1995) Anabolic and catabolic markers of proteoglycan metabolism in osteoarthritis. *Acta. Orthop. Scand.* (*Supp 266*), **266**, 121–124.

Cole, A.A., Chubinskaya, S., Schumacher, B., Huch, K., Cs-Szabo, G., Yao, J., Mikecz, K., Hasty, K.A. and Kuettner, K.E. (1996) Chondrocyte matrix metalloproteinase-8: Human articular chondrocytes express neutrophil collagenase. *J. Biol. Chem.*, **271**, 11023–11026.

Couchman, J.R., Caterson, B., Christner, J.E. and Baker, J.R. (1984) Mapping by monoclonal antibody detection of glycosaminoglycans in connective tissue. *Nature*, **307**, 650–652.

Flannery, C.R., Lark, M.W. and Sandy, J.D. (1992) Identification of a stromelysin cleavage site within the interglobular domain of human aggrecan. Evidence for proteolysis at this site *in vivo* in human articular cartilage. *J. Biol. Chem.*, **267**, 1008–1014.

Flannery, C.R. and Sandy, J.D. (1995) Identification of MMP-13 (collagenase-3) as the major matrix metalloproteinase expressed by chondrocytes during retinoic acid induced matrix catabolism. *Trans. Orthop. Res. Soc.*, **20**, 102.

Fosang, A.J., Last, K., Neame, P.J., Murphy, G., Knauper, V., Tschesche, H., Hughes, C.E., Caterson, B. and Hardingham, T.E. (1994) Neutrophil collagenase (MMP-8) cleaves at the aggrecanase site E373-A374 in the interglobular domain of cartilage aggrecan. *Biochem. J.*, **304**, 347–351.

Fosang, A.J., Last, K., Gardiner, P., Jackson, D.C. and Brown, L. (1995) Development of a cleavage-site-specific monoclonal antibody for detecting metalloproteinase-derived aggrecan fragments: detection of fragments in synovial fluids. *Biochem. J.*, **310**, 337–343.

Fosang, A.J., Last, K. and Maciewicz, R.A. (1996) Aggrecan is degraded by matrix metalloproteinases in human arthritis. *J. Clin. Invest.*, **98**, 2292–2299.

Geysen, H.M., Mason, T.J., Tribbick, G. and Edmundson, A.B. (1988) Mimotopes: Mimics of antibody epitopes. In: *Molecular Mimicry in Health and Disease*, Lernmark, A. Dyrberg, T. Terenius, T. and Hokfelt, B., eds, pp. 315–324, Amsterdam: Elsevier.

Gibson, G., Lin, D.L., Franckl, K., Caterson, B. and Foster, B. (1996) Type X collagen is colocalized with a proteoglycan epitope to form distinct morphological structures in bovine growth cartilage. *Bone*, **19**, 307–315.

Glant, T.T., Mikecz, K. and Poole, A.R. (1986) Monoclonal antibodies to different protein-related epitopes of human articular cartilage proteoglycans. *Biochem. J.*, **234**(1), 31–41.

Gregory, J.D. (1973) Multiple aggregation factors in cartilage proteoglycan. *Biochem. J.*, **133**, 383–386.

Griffin, J.P. (1995) The biochemical characterization of proteoglycans containing atypical chondroitin sulfate epitopes. PhD, Department of Biochemistry, University of North Carolina at Chapel Hill, Chapel Hill, North Carolina.

Hardingham, T.E. and Muir, H. (1972). The specific interaction of hyaluronic acid with cartilage proteoglycans. *Biochim. Biophys. Acta.*, **279**(2), 401–405.

Hardingham, T.E. and Fosang, A.J. (1992) Proteoglycans: many forms and many functions. *FASEB J.*, **6**, 861–870.

Hascall, V.C. and Heinegård, D. (1974) Aggregation of cartilage proteoglycans. I. The role of hyaluronic acid. *J. Biol. Chem.*, **249**, 4232–4241.

Hazell, P.K., Dent, C., Fairclough, J.A., Bayliss, M.T. and Hardingham, T.E. (1995) Changes in glycosaminoglycan epitope levels in knee joint fluid following injury. *Arthritis and Rheumatism*, **38**, 953–959.

Heinegård, D. and Hascall, V.C. (1974) Aggregation of cartilage proteoglycans: Characteristics of the proteins isolated from trypsin digests of aggregates. *J. Biol. Chem.*, **249**, 4250–4256.

Hughes, C.E., Caterson, B., White, R.J., Roughley, P.J. and Mort, J.S. (1992) Monoclonal antibodies recognizing protease-generated neoepitopes from cartilage proteoglycan dsegradation. Application to studies of human link protein cleavage by stromelysin. *J. Biol. Chem.*, **267**, 16011–16014.

Hughes, C.E., Caterson, B., Fosang, A.J., Roughley, P.R. and Mort, J.S. (1994) Production of monoclonal antibodies that specifically recognize neoepitope sequences generated by "aggrecanase" and matrix metalloproteinase catabolism of aggrecan. *Trans. Orthop. Res. Soc.*, **19**, 311.

Hughes, C.E., Caterson, B., Fosang, A.J., Roughley, P.J. and Mort, J.S. (1995a) Monoclonal antibodies that specifically recognize neoepitope sequences generated by aggrecanase and matrix metalloproteinase cleavage of aggrecan: Application to catabolism *in situ* and *in vitro*. *Biochem. J.*, **305**, 799–804.

Hughes, C.E., Wang, H., Caterson, B., Tortorella, M.D. and Arner, E.C. (1995b) Time course of IL-1 induced "aggrecanase" cartilage catabolism inficates the presence of both different rates of release and different pools of aggrecan metaboiites. *Trans. Orthop. Res. Soc.*, **20**, 329.

Hughes, C.E., Büttner, F., Eidenmuller, B., Caterson, B. and Bartnik, E. (1997) Utilization of a recombinant substrate (rAgg1) to study the biochemical properties of 'aggrecanase' in cell culture systems. *J. Biol. Chem.*, **272**, 20269–20274.

Ilic, M.Z., Mok, M.T., Williamson, O.D., Campbell, M.A., Hughes, C.E. and Handley, C.J. (1995) Catabolism of aggrecan by explant cultures of human articular cartilage in the presence of retinoic acid. *Arch. Biochem. Biophys.*, **322**, 22–30.

Lark, M.W., Gordy, J.T., Weidner, J.R., Ayala, J., Kimura, J.H., Williams, H.R., Mumford, R.A., Flannery, C.R., Carlson, S.S., Iwata, M. and Sandy, J.D. (1995) Cell-mediated catabolism of aggrecan. Evidence that cleavage at the "aggrecanase" site (Glu373-Ala374) is a primary event proteolysis of the interglobular domain. *J. Biol. Chem.*, **270**, 2550–2556.

Lark, M.W., Bayne, E.K., Flanagan, J., Harper, C.F., Hoerner, L.A., Hutchinson, N.I., Singer, I.I., Donatelli, S.A., Weidner, J.R., Williams, H.R., Mumford, R.A. and Lohmander, L.S. (1997) Aggrecan degradation in human cartilage: Evidence for both matrix metalloproteinase and aggrecanase activity in normal, osteoarthritic and rheumatoid joints. *J. Clin. Invest.*, **100**, 93–106.

Lee, G.M., Poole, C.A., Kelley, S.S., Chang, J. and Caterson, B. (1997) Isolated chondrons: a viable alternative for studies of chondrocyte metabolism *in vitro*. *Osteoarthritis and Cartilage*, **5**, 261–274.

Lin, P.P., Hughes, C.E., Clarke, J.B. and Caterson, B. (1995) Inhibitors of nitric oxide synthetase reverse the IL-1 induced inhibition of aggrecan synthesis but not degradation. *Trans. Orthop. Res. Soc.*, **20**, 217.

Little, C.B., Ghosh, P. and Bellenger, C.R. (1996) Topographic variation in biglycan and decorin synthesis by articular cartilage in the early stages of osteoarthritis: An experimental study in sheep. *J. Orthop. Res.*, **14**, 433–444.

Maniglia, C.A., Loulakis, P.P., Shrikhande, A.V. and Davis, G. (1991) IL-1 elevated proteoglycan degradation reveals amino-terminal sequence homology. *Trans. Orthop. Res. Soc.*, **16**, 193.

Muir, H. (1986) Current and future trends in articular cartilage research and osteoarthritis. In: *Articular Cartilage Biochemistry*. Kuettner, K.E., Schleyerbach, R. and Hascall, V.C., eds, pp. 423–440, New York: Raven Press.

Poole, A.R. (1993) Cartilage in Health and Disease. In: *Arthritis and Allied Conditions: A Textbook of Rheumatology*, McCarthy, D.J. and Koopman, W., eds, pp. 279–333, Philadelphia: Lea and Febiger.

Poole, C.A., Flint, M.H. and Beaumont, B.W. (1987) Chondrons in cartilage ultrastructural analysis of the pericellular microenviroment in adult human articular cartilage. *J. Orthopaed. Res.*, **5**, 509–522.

Poole, C.A., Ayad, S. and Gilbert, R.T. (1992) Chondrons from articular cartilage (V): Immunohistochemical and evaluation of type VI collagen organisation in isolated chondrons by light, confocal and electron microscopy. *J. Cell Sci.*, **103**, 1101–1110.

Ratcliffe, A. and Mow, V.C. (1996) Articular Cartilage. In: *Extracellular Matrix*. Comper, D.W., eds, Vol. 2, pp. 234–302, London: Harwood Academic Publishers.

Rizkalla, G., Reiner, A., Bogoch, E. and Poole, A.R. (1992) Studies of the articular cartilage proteoglycan aggrecan in health and osteoarthritis: Evidence for molecular heterogeneity and extensive molecular changes in disease. *J. Clin. Invest.*, **90**, 2268–2277.

Sandy, J.D., Neame, P.J., Boynton, R.E. and Flannery, C.R. (1991) Catabolism of aggrecan in cartilage explants. Identification of a major cleavage within the interglobular domain. *J. Biol. Chem.*, **266**, 8683–8685.

Sandy, J.D., Flannery, C.R., Neame, P.J. and Lohmander, L.S. (1992) The structure of aggrecan fragments in human synovial fluid: evidence for the involvement in osteoarthritis of a novel proteinase which cleaves the Glu373-Ala374 bond of the interglobular domain. *J. Clin. Invest.*, **89**, 1512–1516.

Singer, I.I., Kawka, D.W., Bayne, E.K., Donatelli, S.A., Weidner, J.R., Williams, H.R., Ayala, J.M., Mumford, R.A., Lark, M.W., Glant, T.T., Nabozny, G.H. and David, C.S. (1995). VDIPEN, a metalloproteinase-generated neoepitope, is induced and immunolocalized in articular cartilage during inflammatory arthritis. *J. Clin. Invest.*, **95**, 2178–2186.

Slater, R.R., Bayliss, M.T., Lachiewicz, P.F., Visco, D.M. and Caterson, B. (1995) Monoclonal antibodies that detect biochemical markers of arthritis in humans. *Arthritis and Rheumatism*, **38**(5), 655–659.

Sorrell, J.M., Carrino, D.A. and Caplan, A.I. (1993) Structural domains in chondroitin sulfate identified by anti-chondroitin sulfate monoclonal antibodies. Immunosequencing of chondroitin sulfates. *Matrix*, **13**, 351–361.

Tortorella, M.D., Hughes, C.E., Wang, H., Caterson, B., Decicco, C.P. and Arner, E.C. (1996) MMP inhibitors block IL-1 induced "aggrecanase" cleavage of cartilage proteoglycan. *Trans. Orthop. Res. Soc.*, **21**, 148.

Visco, D.M., Johnstone, B., Hill, M.A., Jolly, G.A. and Caterson, B. (1993) Immunohistochemical analysis of 3-B-3(−) and 7-D-4 epitope expression in canine and human osteoarthritis. *Arthritis and Rheumatism*, **36**, 1718–1725.

von der Mark, K., Kirsch, T., Nerlich, A., Kuss, A., Weseloh, G., Gluckert, K. and Stoss, H. (1992) Type X collagen synthesis in human osteoarthritic cartilage: Indication of chondrocyte hypertrophy. *Arthritis and Rheumatism*, **35**, 806–811.

Witt, M., Fosang, A.J., Hughes, C.E. and Hardingham, T.E. (1995) Changes in the patterns of aggrecan cleavage in cartilage explants following stimulation with IL-1 alpha or retinoate and inhibition of cleavage by a metalloproteinase inhibitor. *Trans. Orthop. Res. Soc.*, **20**, 122.

13 New Approaches to Articular Cartilage Repair and Regeneration

Joseph A. Buckwalter

01013 Pappajohn Pavilion, Department of Orthopaedics,
University of Iowa College of Medicine, Iowa City, IA 52242

For at least 250 years physicians and scientists have been seeking a way to restore synovial joint articular surfaces following articular cartilage loss or degeneration. They made little progress for the majority of these 250 years, but in the last three decades clinical and basic scientific investigations have shown that a variety of methods, including implantation of artificial matrices, growth factors, perichondrium, periosteum and transplanted chondrocytes and mesenchymal stem cells can stimulate formation of cartilaginous tissue in synovial joint osteochondral and chondral defects (Buckwalter, 1996a,b; Buckwalter and Lohmander, 1994; Buckwalter *et al.*, 1994). In addition, review of several operative procedures used to treat osteoarthritis, including osteotomies, penetration of subchondral bone and joint distraction and motion, has shown that these procedures can stimulate formation of new articular surfaces (Buckwalter, 1996c; Buckwalter and Lohmander, 1994; Johnson, 1986, 1990; Odenbring *et al.*, 1992; Valberg *et al.*, 1995). The apparent potential of these multiple methods for stimulating cartilage formation has created great interest on the part of patients, physicians and scientists, however the wide variety of methods and approaches to evaluating their results have made it difficult to evaluate their success in restoring joint function and to define their most appropriate current clinical applications.

Better understanding of articular cartilage lesions and degeneration and recognition of the limitations of current treatments have also contributed to the recent interest in cartilage repair and regeneration (Buckwalter, 1992; Buckwalter and Lohmander, 1994; Buckwalter and Martin, 1995; Buckwalter and Mow, 1992). Advances in synovial joint imaging and arthroscopic techniques have increased understanding of the frequency and types of chondral defects and made it possible for orthopaedic surgeons to diagnose and evaluate these lesions with great accuracy. It has become clear that isolated lesions of the articular surface must be distinguished from cartilage degeneration due to osteoarthritis

(Martin and Buckwalter, 1996). Isolated articular cartilage and osteochondral defects appear to result from trauma that often leaves the majority of the articular surface intact (Buckwalter, 1992). They commonly occur in adolescents and young adults who wish to maintain a high level of activity and in some of these individuals cause joint pain, effusions and mechanical dysfunction. Although the natural history of isolated chondral and osteochondral defects has not been well defined, clinical experience suggests that when left untreated these lesions fail to heal, and that they may progress to symptomatic joint degeneration. Conventional treatment by debridement and various methods of penetrating subchondral bone produces variable results (Buckwalter and Lohmander, 1994).

In contrast with isolated chondral or osteochondral defects, osteoarthritis or degenerative joint disease consists of progressive loss of articular cartilage that begins with fraying or fibrillation of the articular surface and progresses to exposure of subchondral bone: attempted repair of articular cartilage, remodelling of subchondral bone, and in many instances osteophyte formation accompany the articular cartilage degeneration (Buckwalter and Martin, 1995; Mankin and Buckwalter, 1996). Despite the attempted repair of the articular surface, once joint degeneration begins it usually progresses and eventually causes pain and loss of mobility. However, in some instances the degenerative process does not progress; and, rarely, spontaneous improvement occurs. Thus, even in osteoarthric joints the potential exists for slowing or possibly temporarily reversing the degeneration of articular cartilage.

Current treatments of osteoarthritis do not restore the articular surface (Buckwalter and Lohmander, 1994; Mankin and Buckwalter, 1996). Exercise programs, medications and physical therapy can decrease symptoms and improve mobility, but they do not detestably alter the course of the disease for most patients. Fusion of degenerated joints relieves pain; and, when necessary, restores stability and alignment; but this procedure necessarily sacrifices mobility and may increase the probability of degeneration of other joints that are subjected to increased loading and motion as a result of the loss of motion in the fused joint. Osteotomies of the hip and knee can decrease pain and in some patients lead to formation of a new articular surface; however, the results vary considerably among patients. Resection of osteoarthritic hips, knees, shoulders and elbows and replacement with implants fabricated from synthetic materials predictably relieves pain. Unfortunately, joint replacements have important limitations, especially for young active patients, primarily because they do not restore an articular surface with the mechanical properties and durability of articular cartilage and because synthetic materials must be fixed to the patient's bone. Thus, wear of implant surfaces limits their life-span and within this life-span the bond between the implant and the bone may fail.

Treatments that promote formation of new articular surfaces in isolated chondral and osteochondral defects and in joints with cartilage degeneration could potentially relieve symptoms and restore joint function. Evaluating these treatments depends to some extent on the methods of assessing articular cartilage repair and regeneration. Table 13.1 lists some of the reports of the results of treatments intended to restore articular surfaces, and shows that all of these reports describe clinical improvement for a majority of the patients and in most instances for more than 75% of the patients. Although these clinical studies

TABLE 13.1
Selected clinical reports of articular cartilage repair.

Authors	Number of patients/ joints/defects	Results	Comments
Excision of Damaged Cartilage and Underlying Bone (Spongialization)			
Ficat *et al.* [31]	85 patients (patellae)	• 67 (79%) good or excellent results	• used for treatment of patellar chondral lesions
Joint Debridement and Abrasion of Subchondral Bone			
Ewing [29]	223 joints (knees)	• 163 (73%) improved	• increased severity of joint disease decreased the probability of a good result
Friedman *et al.* [32]	73 joints (knees)	• 44 (60%) improved • 25 (34%) unchanged • 4 (5%) worse	• patients less than 40 years old had better results
Johnson [43, 44]	>400 Joints (knees)	• 75% satisfactory	• 12% of patients symptom free two years after surgery
Sprague [67]	69 joints (knees)	• 51 (74%) good • 7 (10%) fair • 11 (16%) poor	
Perichondrial Grafts			
Seradge *et al.* [64]	16 MCP joints	• 100% of patients age 20–29 and 75% of patients 30–39 good	• no patient over age 40 had a good result
	20 PIP joints	• 75% of patients 10–19, 66% of patients 20–29 good	
Homminga *et al.* [35]	25 patients/30 defects (knees)	• mean score on knee function scale improved • 28 (93%) of defects filled with cartilaginous tissue	• biopies showed hyaline tissue • results not related to patient age
Joint Distraction			
van Valburg *et al.* [69]	11 patients (11 ankles)	• at an average of 20 months all patients had less pain and five were pain free • three of six patients with radiographs had increased joint space	• none of the patients had a joint fusion
Osteotomy			
Weisl [74]	757 Hips	• joint space increased immediately in about one third and in another one third over 18 months • about two thirds of patients had pain relief for five years, after ten years only about one fourth had pain relief	• better results in patients with increased joint space • better results in patients under 70 years of age with unilateral hip disease
Reigstad *et al.* [62]	103 Hips	• 70% good results at one year, 51% good results at five years and 30% good results at ten years	

(Table Continued)

Authors	Number of patients/ joints/defects	Results	Comments
Bergenudd *et al.* [5]	19 Knees	• new fibrocartilaginous surface in nine patients, no change in eight patients and deterioration of the articular surface in two patients	• no correlation among histologic studies, radiographic appearance and clinical results
Insall *et al.* [39]	95 Knees	• 97% good or excellent results at two years, 85% good or excellent results at five years and 15% of knees pain free at nine years	
Carbon Fiber Matrix			
Muckle *et al.* [54]	47 patients (knees)	• 36 (77%) satisfactory at an average of three years after treatment	• no synovitis
Brittberg *et al.* [11]	36 patients (knees)	• 30 (83%) good or excellent results at an average of four years after treatment	• good pain relief • no adverse effects
Autologous Chondrocyte Transplantation			
Brittberg *et al.* [12]	23 patients (knees)	• 14/16 (88%) patients with femoral defects and 2/7 (29%) patients with patellar defects good or excellent results	• eliminated joint locking and reduced swelling and pain
Peterson [15]	66 patients (knees)	• 47 (71%) improved	

provide important information, they have significant limitations. The ages of patients treated and the types of articular surface defects treated vary considerably. Some series included patients with advanced degenerative disease while others only included patients with localised chondral defects in otherwise normal joints. None of them were controlled prospective studies and the lengths of follow-up and measures of outcome vary, thus it is difficult to compare the efficacy of these approaches to articular cartilage repair and regeneration. This paper first examines methods of evaluating cartilage repair and regeneration and then reviews current methods of restoring articular surfaces including penetration of subchondral bone, osteotomies, joint distraction, soft tissue grafts, growth factors, cell transplantation and artificial matrices.

EVALUATING ARTICULAR CARTILAGE REPAIR AND REGENERATION

The terms repair and regeneration are, at times, used interchangeably in discussions of approaches to restoring lost or damaged articular cartilage. To some extent this contributes to confusion in evaluating methods of stimulating cartilage formation. Repair refers to the replacement of lost or damage tissue with new tissue that may not duplicate the structure, composition and function of the original tissue; regeneration refers to the formation of new tissue that duplicates the structure, composition and function of the original tissue (Buckwalter *et al.*, 1996). Figure 13.1 shows the differences between normal articular cartilage (Figure 13.1A) and well formed repair cartilage (Figure 13.1B). Although the repair tissue has restored an articular surface, and when examined from the surface may appear nearly normal, the repair tissue does not duplicate structure, composition and material properties of normal articular cartilage (Athanasiou *et al.*, 1990; Buckwalter and Mow, 1992; Buckwalter *et al.*, 1990).

The capacity for regeneration of tissue varies among species and tissues, and with age (Buckwalter *et al.*, 1996). Humans have the capacity to regenerate bone tissue at any age following bone fracture or in some instances, even loss of bone tissue. Osteochondral fracture or degeneration of cartilage extending to bone can stimulate a formation of cartilaginous tissue in humans, but this tissue differs in matrix composition and mechanical properties from normal articular cartilage (Buckwalter and Mow, 1992; Buckwalter *et al.*, 1990) and thus is not the result of articular cartilage regeneration in the strictest sense. Infants and possibly even some older children may be an exception to the lack of articular cartilage regeneration in humans (Buckwalter *et al.*, 1996). In some instances

(A)

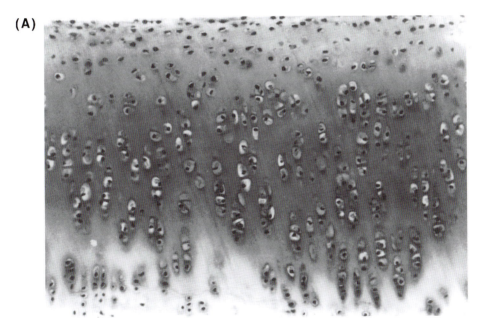

FIGURE 13.1 Light micrographs of rabbit patellar articular cartilage stained with Safranin O to demonstrate the presence of glycosaminoglycans. The joint surface is at the top, the calcified cartilage and subchondral bone at the bottom: (A) Normal rabbit articular cartilage. Notice the zonal organisation of the matrix: small ellipsoidal chondrocytes in the superficial zone next to the articular surface, isolated and clustered spheroidal chondrocytes in the transitional zone and spheroidal chondrocytes forming columns in the deep zone. The matrix has a homogeneous, hyaline, appearance. The matrix of the transitional and deep zones stains diffusely with Safranin O, i.e., the dark regions of the matrix, indicating a high concentration of glycosaminoglycans.

(B)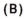

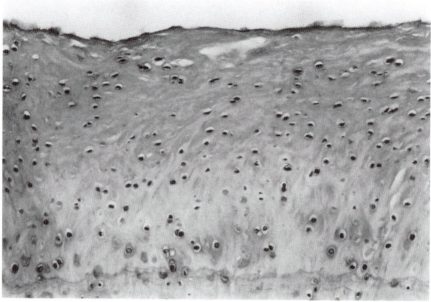

(B)   Well formed repair cartilage six months after creation of a osteochondral defect. Compared with normal articular cartilage the zonal organisation is less well defined, the matrix has a fibrous appearance and Safranin O staining concentrates near a few cells. The zone of calcified cartilage has reformed.

(C)

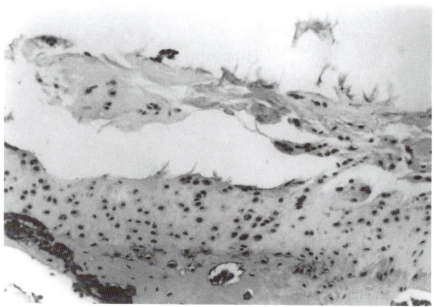

(C)   Fibillated repair cartilage one year after creation of an osteochondral defect. Only a thin layer of fragmented tissue covers the subchondral bone and the matrix lacks staining for Safranin O.

they heal osteochondral injuries with tissue that cannot be distinguished from normal articular cartilage by gross inspection and imaging studies. Although regeneration of normal articular cartilage would be an optimal result of treatment of cartilage loss or damage, and methods of regenerating human articular cartilage may be discovered, repair tissue can provide excellent function. For example, repair tissue can restore the function of lacerated or ruptured tendons and ligaments.

Determining which methods have the greatest promise of restoring and articular surface depends on comparing their results. Yet, one of the problems faced by physicians and scientists in comparing the multiple methods of stimulating articular cartilage repair is the variability in experimental models and clinical applications. For example, species differ in the thickness and mechanical properties of their articular cartilage (Athanasiou et al., 1991) and probably the type and quality of natural cartilage repair or effects of various methods of stimulating repair. Furthermore, methods which stimulate cartilage repair in a normal animal joint will not necessarily lead to similar success in an osteoarthritic human joint. In humans, patient age, condition of the joint including stability, alignment and extent of degenerative change, loading and motion of the joint following treatment, activity level and body weight may affect results (Buckwalter, 1995; Buckwalter et al., 1996; Buckwalter and Lohmander, 1994).

Considerable variability also exists in methods of measuring the results of attempts to stimulate articular cartilage repair. The ultimate measure of a method of articular cartilage repair or regeneration is the extent to which the method restores the long term function of a synovial joint, that is full painless low friction motion, distribution of loads across the joint and durability. Two years provides a reasonable minimum time necessary to assess restoration of joint function, and five years or more of improved joint function is a reasonable expectation for any procedure that would have significant value for large numbers of people. However, requiring that a method of restoring articular cartilage demonstrates long term restoration of joint function before proceeding with further studies, refinements and clinical trials would considerably delay development and clinical use of promising treatments. For this reason, short term evaluation is also necessary. The available experimental evidence suggests that chondral and osteochondral repair tissue formation is usually complete in six weeks or less following an attempt to stimulate restoration of an articular surface, but that remodelling of the repair tissue may continue for many months and probably years (Buckwalter et al., 1996; Buckwalter and Lohmander, 1994; Buckwalter and Mow, 1992). Degeneration of well formed articular cartilage repair tissue may occur within months, or years after apparent clinically successful improvement in joint function (Buckwalter et al., 1990) (Figure 13.1C). Thus the minimal time for short term evaluation of cartilage repair for most methods is in the range of four to six weeks, and for those methods that show promise at this earliest time period another evaluation after six months would be desirable. The best short term evaluation of a method of stimulating cartilage repair is the extent to which that method produces new tissue that restores joint function, structure and an articular surface that duplicates the volume, shape, structure, composition and mechanical properties of normal articular cartilage. Table 13.2 lists measures that can be used to evaluate the short term results of attempts to restore an articular cartilage surface. In addition to these measures, recent work suggests that expression of the proteoglycan epitope 7D4 distinguishes hyaline like repair cartilage from normal articular cartilage and from fibrous repair

TABLE 13.2
Evaluating cartilage repair.

Joint function	– Range of motion – Smoothness of motion (lack of catching, locking or creptus) – Pain – Stability
Joint structure	– Articular surface integrity, contour and congruity – Subchondral bone plate contour, shape, thickness and organisation – Synovial membrane thickness and cellularity (synovitis/effusion) – Osteophytes – Alignment
Chondral repair tissue structure	– Volume (thickness) – Integrity (presence or absence of fibrillation or tissues) – Binding to adjacent normal tissue – Matrix zonal organisation – Cellularity (cell density) – Cell morphology (chondrocytic *vs.* fibroblastic)
Chondral repair tissue matrix composition	– Type II collagen concentration – Type I collagen concentration – Water concentration – Aggrecan concentration, degree of aggregation, aggrecan size and composition – Dermatan sulfate proteoglycan concentration – Non-collagenous protein concentrations (fibronectin, tenascin)
Repair tissue mechanical properties	– Stiffness – Permeability – Strength

cartilage in the early stages of articular cartilage repair, and that with maturation and remodelling of hyaline like articular cartilage repair tissue the expression of 7D4 decreases (Lin *et al.*, 1993).

It has been generally assumed that cartilaginous repair tissue that more closely resembles normal articular cartilage will also have mechanical properties that more closely resemble normal articular cartilage, and that the volume, morphology and histochemical staining of repair tissue will correlate with the mechanical properties of the tissue. One recent study examined this latter assumption (Spirt, 1996). Spirt and colleagues using statistical evaluation of inter-rater reliability progressively refined a semi-quantitative scale for histologic evaluation of cartilage repair. This procedure produced a highly reliable scale for evaluation of cartilage repair consisting of four categories: thickness of the chondral repair tissue, degree of subchondal bone depression, intensity of Safranin-O staining in the chondral repair tissue and cell morphology in the chondral repair tissue. Comparison of scores on the refined articular cartilage repair scale with indentation stiffness of the repair tissue showed a strong correlation between better articular cartilage repair as measured by the scale and increased indentation stiffness: the scores on the scale accounted for more than 70% of the indentation stiffness of the repair tissue

($r^2 = 0.71$, $p < 0.002$). The results of this study suggest that the minimal evaluation of articular cartilage repair tissue should include the volume or thickness of the chondral repair tissue, when appropriate the restoration of the subchondral bone structure, the morphology of the chondral repair tissue and an estimate of the proteoglycan content of the chondral repair tissue.

PENETRATION OF SUBCHONDRAL BONE

Penetration of subchondral bone was the first method developed to stimulate formation of a new articular surface and is still the most commonly used (Buckwalter and Lohmander, 1994) (Table 13.1). In regions with full thickness loss or advanced degeneration of articular cartilage, penetration of the exposed subchondral bone disrupts subchondral blood vessels leading to formation of a fibrin clot over the bone surface (Buckwalter et al., 1996; Buckwalter and Lohmander, 1994). If the surface is protected from excessive loading, undifferentiated mesenchymal cells migrate into the clot, proliferate and differentiate into cells with the morphologic features of chondrocytes (Shapiro et al., 1993). In many instances they form a fibrocartilaginous repair tissue over the bone surface similar to that shown in Figure 13.1B (Johnson, 1986, 1990). Experimental studies have shown that the mesenchymal cells in the osseous portion of an osteochondral defect form bone and smaller amounts of cartilage while the cells in the chondral portion of the defect form a cartilaginous tissue that in some instances closely resembles articular cartilage (Buckwalter et al., 1996; Buckwalter et al., 1990; Metsaranta et al., 1996). However, the extent and quality of cartilage formed in the chondral portions of the defects varies considerably among defects and rarely fills more than 75% of the total volume of the chondral defect (Buckwalter et al., 1990).

Surgeons first debrided degenerated articular cartilage and drilled into the subchondral bone through arthrotomies and found that many patients reported a decrease in symptoms following recovery from the procedure (Bentley, 1978; Haggart, 1940; Insall, 1974; Magnuson, 1941). One group advocated treating patellar articular surface degeneration by excising damaged cartilage along with underlying subchondral bone, a procedure they referred to as "spongialisation." They found good or excellent results in a high percentage of their patients (Ficat et al., 1979) (Table 13.1). Surgeons have developed a variety of other methods of penetrating subchondral bone to stimulate formation of a new cartilaginous surface including arthroscopic abrasion of the articular surface and making multiple small diameter defects or fractures with an awl or similar instrument (Buckwalter and Lohmander, 1994). A number of surgeons have reported that arthroscopic abrasion of chondral and osteochondral lesions in osteoarthritic joints can decrease symptoms (Baumgertner et al., 1990; Ewing, 1990; Johnson, 1986, 1990). Examination of joint surfaces following arthroscopic abrasion has shown that in many individuals it results in formation of fibrocartilaginous articular surface that varies in composition from dense fibrous tissue with little or no type II collagen to hyaline cartilage like tissue with predominantly type II collagen (Johnson, 1986, 1990). In some patients this tissue persists for years.

Prospective randomised controlled trials of arthroscopic abrasion treatment of osteoarthritic joints have not been reported, but several authors have reviewed series of patients and found that these procedures can decrease the symptoms of osteoarthritis of the knee. One group of investigators treated 73 patients with arthroscopic debridement and abrasion of subchondral bone (Friedman *et al.*, 1984). At an average of 12 months following the procedure 60% of the patients were improved, 34% were unchanged and 6% were worse. Another investigator found that seventy-three percent of his patients had relief of pain and stiffness following arthroscopic debridement and abrasion (Ewing, 1990). He noted that the probability of a satisfactory clinical result decreased with increasing severity of the degenerative joint disease. Sprague found 84% good results following arthroscopic debridement of 78 knees (Sprague, 1981); and Johnson found that 75% of the patients with exposed subchondral bone treated by abrasion arthroplasty had satisfactory results, although only 12% of the patients in this series had no symptoms at two years following treatment (Johnson, 1986, 1990). Baumgaertner and associates reported less successful results: they found 39% early failures in a series of 49 knees, and 47% failures at final follow up examination (Baumgaertner, 1990). In this same series, excellent results decreased from 41% of the patients at the time of maximum improvement to 24% at the time of final follow up.

Johnson also found that in many patients with radiographic evidence of cartilage joint space narrowing, or no radiographically demonstrable joint space, the joint space increased following abrasion (Johnson, 1986, 1990). Although an increase in radiographic joint space following subchondral abrasion presumably indicates formation of a new articular surface, the development of this new surface does not necessarily result in symptomatic improvement. Bert and Maschka (Bert, 1993; Bert and Maschkta, 1989) found that 51% of 59 patients treated with abrasion arthroplasty had evidence of increased radiographic joint space two years after treatment, but 31% of these individuals either had no symptomatic improvement or more severe symptoms.

Some of the variability in the clinical results of attempts to restore an articular surface by penetrating subchondral bone may result from differences in the extent and quality of the repair tissue. However, no studies have documented a relationship between the extent and type of repair tissue and symptomatic or functional results suggesting that formation of a new articular surface following penetration of subchondral bone does not necessarily relieve pain. The lack of predictable clinical benefit from formation of cartilage repair tissue may result from variability among patients in the severity of the degenerative changes, joint alignment, patterns of joint use, age, perception of pain, pre-operative expectations or other factors. It may also result from the inability of the newly formed tissue to replicate the properties of articular cartilage. Examination of the tissue that forms over the articular-surface following penetration of subchondral bone shows that it lacks the structure, composition, mechanical properties and in most instances the durability of articular cartilage (Buckwalter *et al.*, 1996; Buckwalter and Lohmander, 1994; Buckwalter and Mow, 1992; Buckwalter *et al.*, 1990; Mitchell and Shepard, 1976). For these reasons, even though it covers the subchondral bone, it may fail to distribute loads across the articular surface in a way that avoids pain with joint loading and further degeneration of the joint.

Currently, it is not clear which method of penetrating subchondral bone produces the best new articular surface, and differences in patient selection and technique among surgeons using the same method may be responsible for variations in results making it difficult to compare techniques. However, comparison of bone abrasion with subchondral drilling for treatment of an experimental chondral defect in rabbits showed that while neither treatment predictably restored the articular surface, drilling appeared to produce better long term results than abrasion (Fenkel *et al.*, 1994). This observation fits well with previous experimental work showing that chondral repair tissue that grows up through multiple drill holes that pass from the articular surface into vascularised bone will spread over exposed subchondral bone between holes and form a fibrocartilaginous articular surface (Mitchell and Shepard, 1976). It also suggests that small diameter holes that leave the bone intact between defects lead to formation of more stable repair tissue than abraded bone surfaces (Fenkel *et al.*, 1994).

Despite the evidence that penetration of subchondral bone stimulates formation of fibrocartilaginous repair tissue, the clinical value of this approach remains uncertain. In contrast with reports of symptomatic improvement in patients with cartilage degeneration treated with penetration of subchondral bone (Ewing, 1990; Friedman *et al.*, 1984; Johnson, 1986, 1990; Sprague, 1981), one investigator has concluded that while joint debridement can improve symptoms in many patients, abrasion or drilling of subchondral bone does not benefit patients with osteoarthritis of the knee and may increase symptoms (Bert, 1993). In addition, the short periods of follow up, lack of well defined evaluations of outcomes, lack of randomised controlled trials and the possibility for a significant placebo effect (Moseley *et al.*, 1994) or an improvement in symptoms due to joint irrigation alone (Gibson *et al.*, 1992; Livesley *et al.*, 1991) make it difficult to define the indications for penetration of subchondral bone to stimulate formation of a new articular surface.

OSTEOTOMIES

Osteotomies of the hip and knee are a generally accepted method of treating joints with localised loss or degeneration of the articular surface. Osteotomies have not been commonly used for treatment of articular cartilage loss or degeneration in joints other than the hip and knee, but in one study tibial osteotomies produced good or excellent results in 15 of 18 patients with primary ankle osteoarthritis, a rare condition in which osteoarthritis develops in the absence of any history of trauma (Takakura *et al.*, 1995). In selected patients surgeons also perform osteotomies to correct skeletal deformities or joint incongruities that may lead to joint degeneration.

Treatment of an osteoarthritic joint or a joint with a large osteochondral defect with an osteotomy consists of cutting the bone adjacent to the involved joint and then stabilising the cut bone surfaces in a new position thereby changing the alignment of the joint. Some surgeons have combined joint debridement and penetration of subchondral bone with osteotomy, but this approach is not widely used. In general, surgeons plan osteotomies to decrease loads on the most severely damaged regions of the joint surface, bring regions of the joint surface that have remaining articular cartilage into opposition with regions that lack articular cartilage or correct joint malalignment that maybe contributing to symptoms and joint dysfunction. Most hip and knee osteotomies performed to treat osteoarthritis alter joint alignment in the coronal plane (varus and valgus osteotomies), however surgeons design some hip osteotomies to change joint alignment in the sagittal plane (flexion and extension osteotomies) or alter the relationship of the joint surfaces by rotation of the femoral head relative to the acetabulum (rotational osteotomies).

The optimal planes and degrees of joint realignment for specific osteoarthritic joints have not been defined, nonetheless, clinical experience shows that osteotomies of the hip and knee can decrease symptoms and stimulate formation of a new articular surface (Buckwalter and Lohmander, 1994). The decreased pain could result from decreasing stresses on regions of the articular surface with the most advanced cartilage degeneration, decreasing intraosseous pressure or formation of a new articular surface, but the mechanisms of symptomatic improvement and formation of new articular surfaces remain poorly understood (Buckwalter and Lohmander, 1994). Most clinical studies have shown that in at least some patients osteotomies lead to improvement in the radiographic signs of joint degeneration including resolution of subchondral cysts or lucencies, decreased subchondral bone density and increased radiographic joint space (Buckwalter and Lohmander, 1994) This latter change may result either from the altered relationship between the articular surfaces or the formation of a new articular surface. That is, osteotomies may alter joint alignment to separate previously opposed joint surfaces or they may rotate a cartilage covered articular surface into opposition with a surface consisting of exposed bone, thus creating a radiographically visible cartilage space where prior to the osteotomy bone opposed bone. In one series of 757 intertrochanteric osteotomies performed to treat osteoarthritis of the hip, the radiographic joint space increased immediately following the procedure in approximately one-third of the patients (Weisl, 1980). In these patients the increased joint space presumably resulted from alterations in the relationships between the joint surfaces. In another third of the patients the radiographic joint space increased during the next 18 months, and these individuals had better clinical results. This result suggests that over 18 months these patients developed a new articular surface in some areas of the joint as a result of the altered loading. Evidence that hip osteotomies stimulate formation of fibrocartilaginous tissue over articular surfaces that previously consisted of exposed bone supports this suggestion (Beyers, 1974; Itoman et al., 1992).

Reports of the treatment of degenerative disease of the knee with osteotomies also describe increased radiographic joint space accompanied by decreased subchondral sclerosis, and in some people formation of a new fibrocartilaginous articular surface (Buckwalter and Lohmander, 1994). One group of investigators biopsied the articular cartilage of the medial femoral condyle at the time of osteotomy and then again at an average of two years after osteotomy in 19 patients with degenerative disease of the medial side of the knee joint (Bergenudd et al., 1992). The biopsies showed formation of a new fibrocartilaginous articular surface in nine patients, no change in eight patients and deterioration of the articular surface in two patients. Radiographic examination showed that six knees had improved, 11 had remained unchanged and two had deteriorated. There was no correlation among the histologic studies, the radiographic appearance, the postoperative varus-valgus angle or the clinical results. A similar study of 14 patients found proliferation of a new fibrocartilaginous surface on the tibial condyle in eight patients and on the medial femoral condyle in nine patients two years following osteotomy (Odenbring, 1992). This study also did not find a correlation between regeneration of an articular surface and clinical outcome.

Long term follow up of patients treated with osteotomies for hip and knee osteoarthritis shows that the clinical results deteriorate with time (Insall *et al.*, 1984; Reistad and Gronmark, 1984; Weisl, 1980). Reigstad and Gronmark evaluated 103 hips treated by intertrochanteric osteotomy (Reigstad and Gronmark, 1984) One year following surgery 70% of the hips had a good result, at five years 51% had a good result and at ten years only 30% of the hips still showed a beneficial effect of the osteotomy. A study of 95 knees in 85 patients treated with a tibial osteotomies showed that the percent of patients with good or excellent results declined from 97% at two year follow up to 85% at five years, and that only 15% of the knees were pain free nine years or more following surgery (Insall *et al.*, 1984). A similar study of 39 knees in 35 patients showed that the percent of patients with good results declined from 87% at two years to 57% at fifteen years following surgery (Berman *et al.*, 1991). Matthews *et al.* (1988) followed 40 patients treated with knee osteotomies and found that 86% of the patients had useful function of the knee at one year, but this value progressively declined to 64% at three years, 50% at five years and 28% at nine years. Variables that appear to adversely affect the results of knee osteotomies include advanced patient age, obesity, severe joint degeneration, joint instability, limited joint motion, operative over correction or under correction and post operative loss of correction (Berman *et al.*, 1991; Coventry *et al.*, 1993; Insall *et al.*, 1984; Matthews *et al.*, 1988). However, even patients who appear to be optimal candidates for osteotomy and who have a good initial surgical outcome, tend to develop recurrent pain and evidence of advancing osteoarthritis with time.

Several studies indicate that the results of osteotomies could be improved through advances in technique and patient selection (Odenbring *et al.*, 1990, 1989a,b). Evaluation of pre-operative joint mechanics may also lead to improved results. Surgeons generally use radiographs that demonstrate joint alignment, subchondral bone density and cartilage space to plan osteotomies that will redistribute articular surface loading. They base this practice on the assumption that static joint alignment can be used to predict loading in different regions of a joint. One group of investigators showed that dynamic joint loading also should be considered (Prodromus *et al.*, 1985; Wang *et al.*, 1990). They studied patients with knee osteoarthritis and varus deformity using gait analysis and found that the patients could be separated into two groups: those with high adduction moments at the knee and those with low adduction moments. The two groups did not differ in preoperative knee score, initial knee alignment, post-operative knee alignment, age or weight; but those with high pre-operative adduction moments had only 50 percent good or excellent results at an average of 3.2 years following osteotomy compared with 100 percent good or excellent results for patients with low pre-operative adduction moments (Prodromos *et al.*, 1985). With increasing time the results for both groups deteriorated, but the patients with low pre-operative adduction moments maintained better clinical results (Wang *et al.*, 1990).

At present the overall clinical results of hip and knee osteotomies vary more than those of joint replacement, and the relationships among the degree of alteration of joint loading, type of osteotomy, quality and extent of articular surface repair, radiographic changes and clinical outcome remain unclear. Given the available information, identifying the patients most likely to benefit from osteotomy, planning the optimal osteotomy for a specific joint and predicting the outcome of the procedure for an individual patient are difficult. Better understanding of the effects of altering joint alignment on the articular surface and possibly combining procedures designed to alter joint alignment with new methods of stimulating cartilage formation could improve the results of these procedures.

JOINT DISTRACTION

Clinical experience with pseudarthroses following fractures and with some resection arthroplasties suggests that distraction and motion of bone or articular surfaces promotes cartilage formation over the opposing surfaces (Buckwalter et al., 1996, 1994; Buckwalter and Mow, 1992). A recent preliminary report describes encouraging results of joint distraction and motion as a treatment for patients with post-traumatic ankle osteoarthritis (Buckwalter, 1996b; Valburg et al., 1995). Van Valburg and colleagues treated advanced post-traumatic osteoarthritis of the ankle with joint distraction in 11 patients (Van Valburg et al., 1995). After application of an Ilizarov device, the authors distracted the joints 0.5 mm per day for five days and then maintained the distraction of the articular surfaces throughout the course of treatment. Patients were allowed to walk a few days after surgery, active joint motion was started between six and 12 weeks after surgery, and after 12 to 22 weeks the distraction device was removed. At an average of 20 months after treatment none of the patients had proceeded with an arthrodesis: all 11 patients had less pain, and five were pain free; six had more motion; and, three of six that had radiographic studies had increased joint space. The authors concluded that distraction of an osteoarthritic ankle joint delays arthrodesis, and that it may stimulate repair of osteoarthritic cartilage.

This preliminary study has important limitations. It included only 11 patients. The measures of pain, function and restoration of an articular surface were of uncertain reliability and validity. Although the mean follow up was nearly two years, nine of the 11 patients were followed for 20 months or less. Despite the limitations, the report of symptomatic improvement and delay, if not avoidance, of arthrodesis in all 11 patients show that joint distraction, including the concept of distraction arthroplasty, deserve further evaluation as a possible treatment of osteoarthritis. However, in addition to rigorous prospective clinical studies, before joint distraction should be accepted as an effective treatment for post-traumatic osteoarthritis, further work is needed to better define the patients most likely to benefit from this approach and the optimal method of joint distraction treatment including duration and extent of distraction and the role of joint motion.

SOFT TISSUE GRAFTS

Treatment of osteoarthritic joints by soft tissue grafts usually involves debriding the joint and interposing soft tissue grafts consisting of fascia, muscle, tendon, periosteum or perichondrium between debrided or resected articular surfaces (Buckwalter and Lohmander, 1994). The potential benefits of soft tissue grafts include introduction of a new cell popu- lation along with an organic matrix, a decrease in the probability of anklyosis before a new articular surface can form, and some protection of the graft or host cells from excessive loading. The success of soft tissue arthroplasty depends not only on the severity of the joint abnormalities and the type of graft, but on postoperative motion to facilitate generation of a new articular surface.

Animal experiments and clinical experience show that perichondrial and periosteal grafts placed in articular cartilage defects can produce new cartilage (Buckwalter and Lohmander, 1994). Recently O'Driscoll has described the use of periosteal grafts for the treatment of isolated chondral and osteochondral defects, and in preliminary evaluation of a small series of patients he has found good or excellent results in more than three quarters of the patients (Buckwalter, 1996a). He has stressed the need for further development of this procedure, careful selection of patients and exacting surgical technique. Homminga *et al.* treated 30 chondral lesions of the knee in 25 patients with rib perichondrial grafts (Homminga *et al.*, 1990). The mean score on a scale designed to evaluate knee function improved significantly and arthroscopic examination showed that 28 of the 30 chondral defects had filled almost completely with a tissue resembling articular cartilage. Engkvist and Johannson treated 26 patients with painful stiff small joints with rib perichondrial arthroplasty (Engkvist and Johansson, 1980). Some individuals had improved motion and decreased pain, but a roughly equal number were not improved. Seradge *et al.* studied the results of rib peri- chondrial arthroplasties in 16 metacarpophalangeal joints and 20 proximal interphalangeal joints at a minimum of three years following surgery (Seradge *et al.*, 1984). Patient age was directly related to the results. One hundred percent of the patients in their twenties and 75% of the patients in their thirties had good results following metacarpophalangeal joint arthroplasties. Seventy-five percent of the patients in their teens and 66% of the patients in their twenties had good results following proximal interphalangeal joint arthroplasties. None of the patients older than 40 years had a good result with either type of arthroplasty. The authors concluded that perichondrial arthroplasty could be used for treatment of post- traumatic osteoarthritis of the metacarpophalangeal joint and proximal interphalangeal joints of the hand in young patients.

The clinical observation that perichondrial grafts produced the best results in younger patients (Seradge *et al.*, 1984) agrees with the concept that age may adversely affect the ability of undifferentiated cells or chondrocytes to form an articular surface or that with age the population of cells that can form an articular surface declines (Buckwalter *et al.*, 1993). The age related differences in the ability of cells to form a new articular surface may also help explain some of the variability in the results of other procedures including osteotomies or procedures that penetrate subchondral bone, that is, younger people may have greater potential to produce a more effective articular surface when all other factors are equal.

GROWTH FACTORS

Growth factors influence a variety of cell activities including cell proliferation, migration, matrix synthesis and differentiation. Many of these factors, including the fibroblast growth factors, insulin like growth factors and transforming growth factor beta family, have been shown to affect chondrocyte metabolism and chondrogenesis (Buckwalter *et al.*, 1996; Buckwalter and Lohmander, 1994). Bone matrix contains a variety of these molecules including transforming growth factor beta, insulin like growth factors, bone morphogenic proteins, platelet derived growth factors and others (Buckwalter *et al.*, 1996, 1994). In addition, mesenchymal cells, endothelial cells and platelets produce many of these factors. Thus, osteochondral injuries and exposure of bone due to loss of articular cartilage may release these agents that affect the formation of cartilage repair tissue, and they probably have an important role in the formation of new articular surfaces after currently used surgical procedures including resection arthroplasty, penetration of subchondral bone, soft tissue grafts and possibly osteotomies.

Local treatment of chondral or osteochondral defects with growth factors has the potential to stimulate restoration of an articular surface superior to that formed after penetration of subchondral bone alone, especially in joints with normal alignment and range of motion and with limited regions of cartilage damage. A recent experimental study of the treatment of partial thickness cartilage defects with enzymatic digestion of proteoglycans that inhibit adhesion of cells to articular cartilage followed by implantation of a fibrin matrix and timed release of TGF-beta showed that this growth factor can stimulate cartilage repair (Hunziker and Rosenberg, 1994, 1996). The cells that filled the chondral defects migrated into the defects from the synovium and formed a fibrous matrix. Despite the promise of this approach, the wide variety of growth factors, their multiple effects, the interactions among them, the possibility that the responsiveness of cells to growth factors may decline with age (Buckwalter *et al.*, 1993; Martin and Buckwalter, 1996; Pfeilschifter, 1993) and the limited understanding of their effects in osteoarthritic joints make it difficult to develop a simple strategy for using these agents to treat patients with osteoarthritis. However, development of growth factor based treatments for isolated chondral and osteochondral defects and early cartilage degenerative changes in younger people appears promising.

CELL TRANSPLANTATION

The limited ability of host cells to restore articular surfaces (Buckwalter and Mow, 1992; Buckwalter *et al.*, 1990) has led investigators to seek methods of transplanting cells that can form cartilage into chondral and osteochondral defects. Experimental work has shown that both chondrocytes and undifferentiated mesenchymal cells placed in articular cartilage defects survive and produce a new cartilage matrix (Buckwalter and Lohmander, 1994). Wakitani and associates found that 80% of rabbit osteochondral defects treated with allograft articular chondrocytes embedded in collagen gels healed within twenty-four weeks (Waikitani *et al.*, 1989). Other investigators have reported similar results with chondrocyte transplantation (Itay *et al.*, 1987, 1988; Noguchi *et al.*, 1994; Robinson *et al.*, 1990). Recently, Brittberg and colleagues compared the results of treating chondral defects in rabbit patellar articular surfaces with periosteal grafts alone, carbon fiber scaffolds and periosteum, autologous chondrocytes and periosteum and autologous chondrocytes, carbon fiber scaffolds and periosteum (Brittberg, 1996; Brittberg *et al.*, 1996). They found that the addition of autologous chondrocytes improved the histologic quality and amount of repair tissue. Cultured mesenchymal stem cells also can repair large osteochondral defects (Wakitani *et al.*, 1994a,b). Within two weeks of transplantation they differentiate into chondrocytes and begin to produce a new articular surface.

In addition to these animal experiments with cell transplants, a group of investigators has reported using autologous chondrocyte transplants for treatment of localised cartilage defects of the femoral condyle or patella in 23 patients (Brittberg *et al.*, 1994b). The investigators harvested chondrocytes from the patients, cultured the cells for 14 to 21 days, and then injected them into the area of the defect and covered them with a flap of periosteum. At two or more years following chondrocyte transplantation 14 of 16 patients with condylar defects and two of seven patients with patellar defects had good or excellent clinical results. Biopsies of the defect sites showed hyaline like cartilage in 11 of 15 femoral and one of seven patellar defects. More recently this group of investigators has reported the results in a larger group of patients (Buckwalter, 1996a). They found that at more than two years after treatment for chondral defects of the knee 47 of 66 patients had improved knee function. These results indicate that chondrocyte transplantation combined with a periosteal graft can promote restoration of an articular surface in humans, but more work is needed to assess the function and durability of the new tissue and determine if it improves joint function and delays or prevents joint degeneration, and if this approach will be beneficial in osteoarthritic joints.

ARTIFICIAL MATRICES

Treatment of chondral defects with growth factors or cell transplants requires a method of delivering and in most instances at least temporarily stabilising the growth factors or cells in the defect. For these reasons, the success of these approaches often depends on an artificial matrix. In addition, artificial matrices may allow, and in some instances stimulate ingrowth of host cells, matrix formation and binding of new cells and matrix to host tissue. Investigators have found that implants formed from a variety of biologic and non-biologic materials including treated cartilage and bone matrices, collagens, collagens and hyaluronan, fibrin, carbon fiber, hydroxyapatite, porous polylactic acid, polytetrafluoro-ethylene, polyester and other synthetic polymers facilitate restoration of an articular surface (Buckwalter and Lohmander, 1994). Lack of studies that directly compare different types of artificial matrices makes it difficult to evaluate their relative merits, but the available reports show that this approach can contribute to restoration of an articular surface. For example, in animal experiments collagen gels have proven to be an effective way of implanting chondrocytes and mesenchymal stem cells and fibrin has been used to implant and allow timed release of a growth factor (Hunziker and Rosenberg, 1994). Treatment of osteochondral defects in rats and rabbits with carbon fiber pads resulted in restoration of a smooth articular surface consisting of firm fibrous tissue that filled the pads (Muckle and Minns, 1990). Use of the same approach to treat osteochondral defects of the knee in humans produced a satisfactory result in 77% of 47 patients evaluated clinically and arthroscopically three years after surgery (Muckle and Minns, 1990). Brittberg and colleagues also studied the use of carbon fiber pads for treatment of articular surface defects (Brittberg et al., 1994a). They found good or excellent results in 83% of 36 patients at an average of four years after treatment.

CONCLUSIONS

Over the next five years, physicians and patients will see a wide variety of exciting new methods and combinations of methods for stimulating repair and possibly even regeneration of articular cartilage. Chondrocyte and mesenchymal stem cell transplantation, periosteal and perichondrial grafting, synthetic matrices, growth factors and other methods of stimulating formation of articular cartilage represent only a part of the spectrum of new treatments of musculoskeletal diseases and injuries currently being developed. Other remarkable biotechnologies that have the potential to stimulate healing and tissue regeneration include combining growth factors with synthetic matrices and cell and tissue transplants, and use of electromagnetic fields, ultrasound and controlled loading and motion. It is unlikely any one of these methodologies will be uniformly successful in the restoration of articular surfaces. Instead, the available clinical and experimental evidence indicates that future optimal methods of restoring articular surfaces will begin with a detailed analysis of the structural and functional abnormalities of the involved joint, and the patient's expectations for future joint use. Based on this analysis the surgeon will develop a treatment plan that potentially combines correction of mechanical abnormalities (including malalignment, instability and intra-articular causes of mechanical dysfunction), debridement that may nor may not include limited penetration of subchondral bone and applications of growth factors or implants that may consist a synthetic matrix that incorporates cells or growth factors followed by a post-operative course of controlled loading and motion. At the same time these new technologies become available, increasing social concerns for the cost and quality of health care will hold all medical and surgical treatments to higher standards of safety, efficacy and cost efficiency. Physicians must carefully assess new technologies and expect the highest quality of scientific evidence before recommending new procedures to their patients. Not every treatment, and especially surgical treatments, can or should be evaluated by rigorous randomised double blind prospective controlled studies before acceptance by physicians. However, delaying widespread use of promising new treatments until their value has been unequivocally demonstrated by repeated long term large scale randomised prospective controlled studies would not serve patients well, and other types of well designed studies can provide evidence of clinical efficacy including demonstration that a treatment restores joint structure and function (Table 13.2). Nonetheless, physicians need to consider that few clinical study design features have the potential to improve the apparent results of a treatment as much as physicians evaluating their own results in the absence of reliable validated measures of outcome, lack of simultaneous control or comparison groups and short follow ups.

ACKNOWLEDGMENT

Some of the ideas and information presented in this article were also presented in a recent review published in the Journal of Bone and Joint Surgery (Buckwalter and Lohmander, 1994).

REFERENCES

Athanasiou, K.A., Rosenwasser, M.P., Buckwalter, J.A., Malinin, T.I. and Mow, V.C. (1991) Interspecies comparisons of *in situ* intrinsic mechanical properties of distal femoral cartilage. *J. Ortho. Res.*, **9**, 330–340.

Athanasiou, K.A., Rosenwasser, M.P., Spiker, R.L., Buckwalter, J.A. and Mow, V.C. (1990) Effects of passive motion on the material properties of healing articular cartilage. *Trans. Ortho. Res. Soc.*, **15**, 156.

Baumgaertner, M.R., Cannon, W.D., Vittori, J.M., Schmidt, E.S. and Maurer, R.C. (1990) Arthroscopic debridement of the arthritic knee. *Clin. Orth. Rel. Res.*, **253**, 197–202.

Bentley, G. (1978) The surgical treatment of chondromalacia patellae. *J. Bone Joint Surg.*, **60B**, 74–81.

Bergenudd, H., Johnell, O., Redlund-Johnell, I. and Lohmander, L.S. (1992) The articular cartilage after osteotomy for medial gonarthrosis: biopsies after 2 years in 19 cases. *Acta Orthop. Scand.*, **63**(4), 413–416.

Berman, A.T., Bosco, S.J., Kirshner, S. and Avolio, A. (1991) Factors influencing long-term results in high tibial osteotomy. *Clin. Orthop.*, **272**, 192–198.

Bert, J.M. (1993) Role of abrasion arthroplasty and debridement in the management of osteoarthritis of the knee. *Rheum. Dis. Clinics North America*, **19**(3), 725–739.

Bert, J.M. and Maschka, K. (1989) The arthroscopic treatment of unicompartmental gonarthoisis. *J. Arthroscopy*, **5**, 25.

Beyers, P.D. (1974) The effect of high femoral osteotomy on osteoarthritis of the hip. *J. Bone Joint Surg.*, **56B**, 279–290.

Brittberg, M. (1996) *Cartilage Repair*, Goteborg University, Sweden.

Brittberg, M., Faxen, E. and Peterson, L. (1994a) Carbon fiber scaffolds in the treatment of early knee osteoarthritis. *Clin. Ortho. Rel. Res.*, **307**, 155–164.

Brittberg, M., Lindahl, A., Nilsson, A., Ohlsson, C., Isaksson, O. and Peterson, L. (1994b) Treatment of deep cartilage defects in the knee with autologous chondrocyte transplantation. *New Eng. J. Med.*, **331**, 889–895.

Brittberg, M., Nilsson, A., Lindahl, A., Ohlsson, C. and Peterson, L. (1996) Rabbit articular cartilage defects treated with autologous cultured chondrocytes. *Clin. Ortho. Rel. Res.*, **326**, 270–283.

Buckwalter, J.A. (1995) Activity vs. rest in the treatment of bone, soft tissue and joint injuries. *Iowa Orthop. J.*, **15**, 29–42.

Buckwalter, J.A. (1996a) Cartilage researchers tell progress: Technologies hold promise, but caution urged. *Am. Acad. Ortho. Surg. Bulletin*, **44**(2), 24–26.

Buckwalter, J.A. (1996b) Joint distraction for osteoarthritis. *Lancet*, **347**, 279–280.

Buckwalter, J.A. (1992) Mechanical injuries of articular cartilage. In: *Biology and Biomechanics of the Traumatized Synovial Joint*, Finerman, G., Ed. pp. 83–96. Park Ridge IL: American Academy of Orthopaedic Surgeons.

Buckwalter, J.A. (1996c) Regenerating articular cartilage: why the sudden interest? *Orthopaedics Today*, **16**, 4–5.

Buckwalter, J.A., Einhorn, T.A., Bolander, M.E. and Cruess, R.L. (1996) Healing of musculoskeletal tissues. In: *Fractures* (Rockwood, C.A. and Green, D., Ed.) pp. 261–304. Lippincott.

Buckwalter, J.A. and Lohmander, S. (1994) Operative treatment of osteoarthrosis: Current practice and future development. *J. Bone Joint Surg.*, **76A**, 1405–1418.

Buckwalter, J.A. and Martin, J.A. (1995) Degenerative joint disease. In: *Clinical Symposia*, pp. 2–32. Summit NJ Ciba Geigy.

Buckwalter, J.A. and Mow, V.C. (1992) Cartilage repair in osteoarthritis. In: *Osteoarthritis: Diagnosis and Management 2nd edition*, (Moskowitz, R.W., Howell, D.S., Goldberg, V.M. and Mankin, H.J., Ed.) pp. 71–107. Philadelphia, Saunders.

Buckwalter, J.A., Mow, V.C. and Ratliff, A. (1994) Restoration of injured or degenerated articular surfaces. *J. Am. Acad. Ortho. Surg.*, **2**, 192–201.

Buckwalter, J.A., Rosenberg, L.A. and Hunziker, E.B. (1990) Articular cartilage: Composition, structure, response to injury, and methods of facilitation repair. In: *Articular Cartilage and Knee Joint Function: Basic Science and Arthroscopy* (Ewing, J.W., Ed.) pp. 19–56. New York: Raven Press.

Buckwalter, J.A., Woo, S.L.-Y., Goldberg, V.M., Hadley, E.C., Booth, F., Oegema, T.R. and Eyre, D.R. (1993) Soft tissue aging and musculoskeletal function. *J. Bone Joint Surg.*, **75A**, 1533–1548.

Coventry, M.B., Ilstrup, D.M. and Wallrichs, S.L. (1993) Proximal tibial osteotomy. A critical long-term study of eighty-seven cases. *J. Bone Joint Surg.*, **75A**, 196–201.

Engkvist, O. and Johansson, S.H. (1980) Perichondrial arthroplasty: a clinical study in twenty-six patients. *Scand. J. Plast. Reconstr. Surg.*, **14**, 71–87.

Ewing, J.W. (1990) Arthroscopic treatment of degenerative meniscal lesions and early degenerative arthritis of the knee. Chap 9 In: *Articular Cartilage and Knee Joint Function. Basic Science and Arthroscopy* (Ewing, J.W., Ed.) pp. 137–145. New York: Raven Press.

Fenkel, S.R., Menche, D.S., Blair, B., Watnik, N.F., Toolan, B.C. and Pitman, M.I. (1994) A comparison of abrasion burr arthroplasty and subchondral drilling in the treatment of full-thickness cartilage lesions in the rabbit. *Trans. Ortho. Res. Soc.*, **19**, 483.

Ficat, R.P., Ficat, C., Gedeon, P.K. and Toussaint, J.B. (1979) Spongialization: A new treatment for diseased patellae. *Clin. Orthop.*, **144**, 74–83.

Friedman, M.J., Berasi, D.O., Fox, J.M., Pizzo, W.D., Snyder, S.J. and Ferkel, R.D. (1984) Preliminary results with abrasion arthroplasty in the osteoarthritic knee. *Clin. Orthop.*, **182**, 200–205.

Gibson, J.N.A., White, M.D., Chapman, V.M. and Strachan, R.K. (1992) Arthroscopic lavage and debridement for osteoarthritis of the knee. *J. Bone Joint Surg.*, **74B**, 534–537.

Haggart, G.E. (1940) The surgical treatment of degenerative arthritis of the knee joint. *J. Bone Joint Surg.*, **22**, 717–729.

Homminga, G.N., Bulstra, S.K., Bouwmeester, P.M. and Linden, A.J.V.D. (1990) Perichondrial grafting for cartilage lesions of the knee. *J. Bone Joint Surg.*, **72B**, 1003–1007.

Hunziker, E.B. and Rosenberg, L.C. (1996) Repair of partial-thickness defects in articular cartilage: cell recruitment from the synovial membrane. *J. Bone Joint Surg.*, **78A**, 721–733.

Hunziker, E.B. and Rosenberg, R. (1994) Induction of repair partial thickness articular cartilage lesions by timed release of TGF-Beta. *Trans. Ortho. Res. Soc.*, **19**, 236.

Insall, J. (1974) The Pridie debridement operation for osteoarthritis of the knee. *Clin. Orthop.*, **101**, 61–67.

Insall, J.N., Joseph, D.M. and Msika, C. (1984) High tibial osteotomy for varus gonarthrosis. A long-term follow-up study. *J. Bone Joint Surg.*, **66A**, 1040–1048.

Itay, S., Abramovici, A. and Nevo, Z. (1987) Use of cultured embryonal chick epiphyseal chondrocytes as grafts for defects in chick articular cartilage. *Clin. Orthop.*, **220**, 284–303.

Itay, S., Abramovici, A., Ysipovitch, Z. and Nevo, Z. (1988) Correction of defects in articular cartilage by implants of cultures of embryonic chondrocytes. *Trans. Orthop. Res. Soc.*, **13**, 112.

Itoman, M., Yamamoto, M., Yonemoto, K., Sekiguchi, M. and Kai, H. (1992) Histological examination of surface repair tissue after successful osteotomy for osteoarthritis of the hip. *Int. Orthop.* (Germany), **16**, 118–121.

Johnson, L.L. (1986) Arthroscopic abrasion arthroplasty. Historical and pathologic perspective: Present status. *Arthroscopy*, **2**, 54–59.

Johnson, L.L. (1990) The sclerotic lesion: Pathology and the clinical response to arthroscopic abrasion arthroplasty. Chap 22. In: *Articular Cartilage and Knee Joint Function. Basic Science and Arthroscopy* (Ewing, J.W., Ed.) pp. 319–333. New York: Raven Press.

Lin, P., Buckwalter, J.A., Olmstead, M. and Caterson, B. (1993) Monoclonal antibody 7D4 is a marker for articular cartilage repair in rabbits and monkeys. *Ortho. Trans.*, **18**, 262.

Livesley, P.J., Doherty, M., Needoff, M. and Moulton, A. (1991) Arthroscopic lavage of osteoarthritic knees. *J. Bone Joint Surg.*, **73B**, 922–926.

Magnuson, P.B. (1941) Joint debridement: surgical treatment of degenerative arthritis. *Surg. Gynecol. Obstet.*, **73**, 1–9.

Mankin, H.J. and Buckwalter, J.A. (1996) Restoring the osteoarthritic joint. *J. Bone and Joint Surg.*, **78A**, 1–2.

Martin, J.A. and Buckwalter, J.A. (1996) Fibronectin and cell shape affect age related decline in chondrocyte synthetic response to IGF-I. *Trans. Ortho. Res. Soc.*, **21**, 306.

Matthews, L.S., Goldstein, S.A., Malvitz, T.A., Katz, B.P. and Kaufer, H. (1988) Proximal tibial osteotomy. Factors that influence the duration of satisfactory function. *Clin. Orthop.*, **229**, 193–200.

Metsaranta, M., Kujala, U.M., Pelliniemi, L., Osterman, H., Aho, H. and Vuorio, E. (1996) Evidence for insufficient chondrocytic differentiation during repair of full-thickness defects of articular cartilage. *Matrix Biology*, **15**, 39–47.

Mitchell, N. and Shepard, N. (1976) The resurfacing of adult rabbit articular cartilage by multiple perforations through the subchondral bone. *J. Bone Joint Surg.*, **58A**, 230–233.

Moseley, J.B., Wray, N.P., Kuykendall, D., Willis, K. and Landon, G.C. (1994) Arthroscopic treatment of osteoarthritis of the knee: a prospective, randomized, placebo-controlled trail: results of a pilot study. In: *American Academy of Orthopaedic Surgeons 61st Annual Meeting*. New Orleans LA: American Academy of Orthopaedic Surgeons.

Muckle, D.S. and Minns, R.J. (1990) Biological response to woven carbon fiber pads in the knee: A clinical and experimental study. *J. Bone and Joint Surg.*, **72B**, 60–62.

Noguchi, T., Oka, M., Fujino, M., Neo, M. and Yamamuro, T. (1994) Repair of osteochondral defects with grafts of cultured chondrocytes. Comparison of allografts and isografts. *Clin. Ortho. Rel. Res.*, **302**, 251–258.

Odenbring, S., Egund, N., Knutson, K., Linstrand, A. and Larsen, S.T. (1990) Revision after osteotomy for gonarthrosis. A 10–19 year follow-up of 314 cases. *Acta Ortho. Scand.*, **61**, 128–130.

Odenbring, S., Egund, N., Lindstand, A., Lohmander, L.S. and Wilen, H. (1992) Cartilage regeneration after proximal tibial osteotomy for medial gonarthrosis. *Clin. Ortho. Rel. Res.*, **277**, 210–216.

Odenbring, S., Egund, N., Linstrand, A. and Tjornstrand, B. (1989a) A guide instrument for high tibial osteotomy. *Acta Ortho. Scand.*, **60**, 449–451.

Odenbring, S., Tjornstrand, B., Egund, N., Hagstedt, B., Hovelius, L., Linstrand, A., Luxhoj, T. and Svanstrom, A. (1989b) Function after tibial osteotomy for medial gonarthrosis below aged 50 years. *Acta Ortho. Scand.*, **60**, 527–531.

Pfeilschifter, J., Diel, I., Brunotte, K., Naumann, A. and Ziegler, R. (1993) Mitogenic responsiveness of human bone cells *in vitro* to hormones and growth factors decreases with age. *J. Bone Miner. Res.*, **8**, 707–717.

Prodromos, C.C., Andriacchi, T.P. and Galante, J.O. (1985) A relationship between gait and clinical changes following high tibial osteotomy. *J. Bone Joint Surg.*, **67**A, 1188–1194.

Reigstad, A. and Gronmark, T. (1984) Osteoarthritis of the hip treated by intertrochanteric osteotomy. A long-term follow up. *J. Bone Joint Surg.*, **66A**, 1–6.

Robinson, D., Halperin, N. and Nevo, Z. (1990) Regenerating hyaline cartilage in articular defects of old chickens using implants of embryonal chick chondrocytes embedded in a new natural delivery substance. *Calcif. Tissue Int.*, **46**, 246–253.

Seradge, H., Kutz, J.A., Kleinert, H.E., Lister, G.D., Wolff, T.W. and Atasoy, E. (1984) Perichondrial resurfacing arthroplasty in the hand. *J. Hand Surg.*, **9A**, 880–886.

Shapiro, F., Koide, S. and Glimcher, M.J. (1993) Cell origin and differentiation in the repair of full-thickness defects of articular cartilage. *J. Bone Joint Surg.*, **75A**, 532–553.

Spirt, A.A., Brand, R.A., Buckwalter, J.A. and Mohler, C.G. (1996) Enhancing the reliability of a valid histologic grading scale for articular cartilage repair. *Trans. Ortho. Res. Soc.*, **21**, 542.

Sprague, N.F. (1981) Arthroscopic debridement for degenerative knee joint disease. *Clin. Orthop.*, **160**, 118–123.

Takakura, Y., Tanaka, Y., Kumai, T. and Tamai, S. (1995) Low tibial osteotomy for osteoarthritis of the ankle. Results of a new operation in 18 patients. *J. Bone Joint Surg.*, **77B**, 50–54.

Valburg, A.Av., Roermund, P.Mv., Lammens, J., Melkebeek, Jv., Verbout, A.J., Lafeber, F.P.J.G. and Bijlsma, J.W.J. (1995) Can Ilizarov joint distraction delay the need for an arthrodesis of the ankle? A preliminary report. *J. Bone Joint Surg.*, **77A**, 720–725.

Wakitani, S., Goto, T., Mansour, J.M., Goldberg, V.M. and Caplan, A.I. (1994a) Mesenchymal stem cell-based repair of a large articular cartilage and bone defect. *Trans. Ortho. Res. Soc.*, **19**, 481.

Wakitani, S., Goto, T., Pineda, S.J., Young, R.G., Mansour, J.M., Caplan, A.I. and Goldberg, V.M. (1994b) Mesenchymal cell-based repair of large, full-thickness defects of articular cartilage. *J. Bone Joint Surg.*, **76A**, 579–592.

Wakitani, S., Kimura, T., Hirooka, A., Ochi, T., Yoneda, M., Natsuo, N., Owaki, H. and Ono, K. (1989) Repair of rabbit articular surfaces with allograft chondrocytes embedded in collagen gel. *J. Bone Joint Surg.*, **71B**, 74–80.

Wang, J.-W., Kuo, K.N., Andriacchi, T.P. and Galante, J.O. (1990) The influence of walking mechanics and time on the results of proximal tibial osteotomy. *J. Bone Joint Surg.*, **72A**, 905–909.

Weisl, H. (1980) Intertrochanteric osteotomy for osteoarthritis. A long-term follow-up. *J. Bone Joint Surg.*, **62B**, 37–42.

Section 3
Synovium

14   The Biology of Synovial Cells

Jo C.W. Edwards*

University College London

THE BIOLOGY OF SYNOVIAL CELLS

Although synovium is traditionally thought of as a connective tissue, it could more accurately be described as disconnective tissue. Even to call it a tissue may be inappropriate, since synovium is a functional unit, the outer anatomical boundaries of which are hard to define. Perhaps synovium could be defined as that part of mesenchyme involved in the development and maintenance of disconnection between locomotor elements at sites of maximal internal shear.

The development of disconnection between locomotor elements is addressed by Dr Pitsillides in this volume. The following discussion will deal with the maintenance of that disconnection. Recent studies have indicated that the process is highly sophisticated, making use of multiple interactions between resident fibroblasts and immigrant macrophages. Moreover, these interactions are mediated by cell surface ligands also involved in regulation of the humoral immune response. Thus, it is beginning to become clear why the commonest disease of synovium, rheumatoid arthritis, should also be characterised by disordered regulation of antibody production.

Maintenance of disconnection may be considered at two levels. Firstly, fibroblasts at the tissue surface maintain the plane of disconnection by secreting, on one side, soluble hyaluronan, and on the other, solid matrix, to which they adhere through integrin ligands. Secondly, the response to injury at the synovial surface appears to be modulated in such a way that disconnection is not abrogated by accumulation of debris in the synovial space and consequent adhesion during tissue repair. This modulation is characterised by the permission of granulocyte egress into the synovial cavity, but retention of macrophages with specialised receptor and effector function at the tissue surface.

* Corresponding author. Rheumatology Unit, Arthur Stanley House, Tottenham Street, London W1P 9PG, UK.

SYNOVIAL STRUCTURE

The detailed microanatomy of synovium is reviewed elsewhere (Key, 1932; Edwards, 1987). Cell populations can be divided into those of the surface or intimal layer and those of the deeper subintima. The intima consists almost entirely of fibroblasts and macrophages. It covers most synovial surfaces, but in some areas of fibrous synovium is absent. The subintima can comprise a variety of tissue types and may contain fibroblasts, macrophages, mast cells, adipocytes and vascular wall cells, including endothelial cells, smooth muscle cells and pericytes. Again, the subintima may be absent, with intimal cells lying directly on another tissue such as periosteum, muscle or tendon. The vascular net within synovial subintima is rich and specialised in terms of capillary fenestrations and microarchitecture (Davies and Edwards, 1948; Suter and Majno, 1964). Its significance is discussed by Levick in this volume. The present discussion will focus on two cell types; the fibroblast and the macrophage.

SYNOVIAL INTIMAL CELLS

In the past, the extent of the intimal layer was hard to define, since conventional histological stains did not discrimate between intimal and adjacent subintimal cells. A number of techniques are now available for identifying intimal cells by specialised cytochemical features (see Table 14.1), allowing a more precise definition of intimal boundaries. The normal intima appears as being one or two cells thick, although electronmicroscopy may reveal a greater degree of overlapping of cell bodies and processes. In disease, intimal cell numbers are increased, but grosser estimates of intimal cellularity usually relate to oblique sectioning. Capillaries may lie adjacent to intimal cells, but are probably never completely surrounded by intimal cells or matrix and are, therefore, considered subintimal, at least by convention.

Intimal cells are a mixture of macrophages and fibroblasts (Barland, 1962; Edwards, 1987). The two are best distinguished using a cytochemical assay for non-specific esterase activity, for which intimal macrophages, but not fibroblasts, are strongly positive. Other markers are often unsatisfactory, either because they label cell membranes, which are too closely apposed to those of adjacent cells to resolve with the light microscope, or because of convergence of function of the two cell types. Thus, CD68, which is a lysosomal marker, distinguishes poorly between the intimal cells, at least in inflamed tissue, since intimal fibroblasts can develop relatively large numbers of lysosomes. Cells other than macrophages and fibroblasts are very scarce in normal tissue, but include a few cells with features of interdigitating dendritic cells (Wilkinson *et al.*, 1990). In disease, a few polymorphs and lymphocytes may occur within the intimal boundaries.

INTIMAL FIBROBLASTS

Intimal fibroblasts have, for several decades, been attributed with the ability to synthesise large quantities of soluble hyaluronan. Direct evidence for specialised metabolic machinery

Table 14.1
Properties of synovial macrophage and fibroblast populations.

Normal	CD68	NSE	CD14	FcγRI	FcγRIIIa	CR1	CR2	CR3	UDPGD	VCAM-1	DAF
Macrophage											
intimal	++	++	+	+	++	−/+	−	++	−	−/?+	+
subintimal	++	+	++	++	−	++	−	−/+	−	−	+
Fibroblast											
intimal (SIF)	−/+	−	−	−	−	−	−/++*	−	++	++	++
subintimal	−	−	−	−	−	−	−	−	−	−/++*	−/++*

* = may be induced in inflammatory disease.

for hyaluronan synthesis in cells of the intimal layer was obtained by Pitsillides and coworkers, in 1992, using a cytochemical assay for uridine diphosphoglucose dehydrogenase activity. Double labelling studies confirmed that high uridine diphosphoglucose dehydrogenase activity was present in the fibroblast population (Wilkinson *et al.*, 1992). There is also some evidence to indicate that synovial intimal fibroblasts carry large amounts of hyaluronan synthase, but better probes for this molecule are still needed.

The functions of hyaluronan are probably multiple, but two properties have emerged as of particular relevance to the maintenance of disconnection. Hyaluronan confers thixotropic and elastic properties to synovial fluid which encourage the maintenance of a fluid film between moving surfaces, even at high loads and low speeds (Unsworth, 1993). Hyaluronan molecules also have the capacity to impact in filter meshes with a porosity at the submicron level, resulting in dramatic reduction in the hydraulic conductance of the filter. This is almost certainly crucial to the maintenance of a minimum volume of fluid within synovial spaces, and is reviewed by Levick (1995).

Intimal fibroblasts are surrounded by a matrix which contains several elements found in basal laminae. These include collagen type IV, laminin, and chondroitin-6-sulphate containing proteoglycans (Revell *et al.*, 1995). Collagens V and VI are also present (Ashhurst *et al.*, 1991). No true basement lamina structure is detectable by electron microscopy, although something approaching this may be seen as a halo around individual cells. The absence of a basal lamina has been attributed to the absence of entactin from the matrix (Zvaifler, verbal communication). Intimal cells carry relatively large amounts of $\beta 1$ integrins, chiefly the $\alpha 3$, $\alpha 5$ and $\alpha 6$ forms, which are capable of mediating adhesion through binding to a range of matrix components (El-Gabalawy and Wilkins, 1992).

Thus, intimal fibroblasts appear to be adapted to the production both of the soluble matrix of synovial fluid and the specialised solid matrix of the tissue surface. How the cells maintain the polarity between these matrices remains a mystery, and is perhaps the key unsolved problem in synovial biology.

Synovial intimal fibroblasts also express two molecules which appear to be specifically involved in interactions with macrophages. These are vascular cell adhesion molecule-1 (VCAM-1) and complement decay-accelerating factor (DAF) (Medof *et al.*, 1987; Stevens *et al.*, 1990; Morales-Ducret *et al.*, 1992; Wilkinson *et al.*, 1993; Edwards and Wilkinson, 1994; Edwards and Cambridge, 1995). VCAM-1 is a molecule expressed chiefly on resident cells and mediates intercellular adhesion through binding to $\alpha 4$ $\beta 1$ integrin on mononuclear leucocytes. It is also present on myoblasts and mediates myoblast fusion through homotypic adhesion. VCAM-1 is inducible at low levels on vascular wall cells, including some endothelial cells, but is expressed at much higher levels on four cell populations; synovial intimal fibroblasts, haemopoietic bone marrow stromal fibroblasts, the follicular dendritic cells (FDC) of lymphoid germinal centres and the epithelial cells of the parietal component of Bowman's capsule (Edwards and Wilkinson, 1994).

DAF is expressed at low level on endothelium and all blood cells, but, again, at much higher levels on a restricted number of resident cell populations (Medof *et al.*, 1987). These include amniotic epithelial cells, synovial intimal fibroblasts, bone marrow stromal cells, FDC, some pulmonary epithelial cells and the epithelial cells of the parietal component of Bowman's capsule. DAF inhibits C3 convertases, thereby diverting the complement cascade away from the generation of C5a and membrane attack complex.

This diversion may protect cells from damage by membrane attack complex, especially in the amniotic cavity. However, it is thought that this may not be the most significant effect of DAF, since complement-mediated damage is not a major problem in DAF deficient individuals. More important may be the ability of DAF to allow generation of C3 fragments such as C3dg and C3bi in the absence of chemotactic signals from C5a. C3dg and C3bi play key roles in the handling of immune complexes in the regulation of the humoral immune response.

Sites of co-expression of VCAM-1 and DAF appear to fall into two categories. The first includes bone marrow and lymph node where both molecules are involved in B lymphocyte survival and differentiation. The second includes synovial intima and Bowman's capsule, where the molecules appear to be involved in the control of macrophage function at sites where a space needs to be preserved, free of debris or adhesion. The function of VCAM-1 appears to be to limit macrophage egress into the space, while allowing the passage of granulocytes. The advantage of this would seem to be that granulocytes can be used as scavengers within the space, but can then be reabsorbed, with their ingested contents, into the tissue by macrophages held at the tissue surface. This is likely to avoid the accumulation of sequestered cell debris within the synovial space. The contribution of DAF to macrophage function is probably more subtle and will be returned to after a discussion of the functional specialisation of intimal macropahges.

The control of synovial fibroblast behaviour is still not understood, but a working hypothesis is emerging. DAF is expressed by fibroblasts along the presumptive joint or tendon sheath line even before cavity formation in human synovial spaces (Edwards and Wilkinson, 1996). The expression of DAF may depend on predetermined morphogenetic information carried by these cells alone; what Wolpert described as "positional information". There is evidence of precommitment of all interzone (presynovial) and perichondrial fibroblasts to a particular phenotype at a very early stage, in terms of expression of high levels of CD44 (Edwards et al., 1994). However, information from immobilised chick embryos suggests that the specialised features of synovial intimal cells may also be dependent on shear stresses generated by muscle activity prior to cavity formation (Dowthwaite and Pitsillides, work in progress). It seems likely that synovial fibroblasts have a specific potential to express DAF, and this potential is realised under the influence of shear stresses along the presumptive joint line and maintained by shear stresses at the tissue surface once the space has formed. The same would appear to apply for VCAM-1, but VCAM-1 expression is delayed in respect to DAF (Edwards et al., 1994) and may require a signal from macrophages. It is conceivable that shear stresses act on cells through an intercellular CD44-hyaluronan-CD44 link.

Two pieces of evidence support this model. Firstly, fibroblasts from synovium lose VCAM-1 and DAF in culture, but can be induced to re-express these molecules with stimuli which fail to induce expression on fibroblasts from other sources (Leigh et al., 1996). Secondly, bone marrow stromal cells derive from the same CD44-rich "envelope" (Edwards et al., 1994) which surrounds early cartilage elements, suggesting that these cells also carry the propensity to express VCAM-1 and DAF, which is activated by other signals present within developing marrow.

Preliminary studies in vitro (Leigh, unpublished) indicate that in synovial explants cultured under conditions of continued medium flow fibroblasts lining artefactual cut surfaces will also express DAF. This is consistent with the idea that the intimal phenotype is maintained by the local microenvironment and that subintimal cells can take on the intimal phenotype under appropriate conditions. This suggests that the increase in intimal fibroblast numbers seen in inflammatory disease may represent acquisition of an intimal phenotype by adjacent subintimal fibroblasts as much as cell division within the intima.

INTIMAL MACROPHAGES

Intimal macrophages, like other macrophages, are almost certainly bone marrow derived. There is no evidence that they are derived from a pre-committed "synoviotropic" subset of monocytes, but once they have arrived in the intima they show functional specialisation. None of the individual features of synovial intimal macrophages is unique, but the combination of features may be. These features are summarised in Table 14.1. Bröker et al. (1990) noted that in diseased tissue intimal macrophages tended to express more of the immunoglobulin G Fc receptor FcγRIIIa than other synovial macrophages. Recently, Blades (in preparation) has shown that normal intimal macrophages express high levels of FcγRIIIa. Palmer and coworkers demonstrated that these cells also express high levels of and the complement receptor CR3 (Palmer, 1995). They express relatively low levels of two other receptors, FcγRI (Broker et al., 1990) and CR1 (Palmer, 1995). They express low levels of CD14 and have high non-specific esterase activity, and in a number of other respects have the hall marks of "mature" macrophages. CD14 bright cells with features more suggestive of immature macrophages are found immediately beneath the intima in inflamed tissue, suggesting that monocytes enter the tissue in the subintimal region and mature as they migrate to the intima (Broker et al., 1990; Palmer, 1995).

As will be discussed later, the FcγRIIIa bright/CR3 bright/FcγRI dull/CR1 dull phenotype may be significant both to normal function and susceptiblity to disease. What is not clear is just how unusual this phenotype is. FcγRIIIa is expressed by macrophages from many tissues in tissue culture, and in sections of tissue affected by certain diseases, including tumours (van-Ravenswaay-Claasen et al., 1992). However, it may be relatively unusual for macrophages to express FcγRIIIa in normal tissues other than primary and secondary lymphoid organs. FcγRIIIa is certainly present on macrophages in lymph node, spleen and bone marrow (Tuijnman, 1993). Recent studies at UCL indicate that FcγRIIIa is totally restricted to synovial intimal macrophages within fetal limbs at 10–12 weeks gestation. In normal adult synovium FcγRIIIa is restricted to the intimal layer, and is absent from all types of associated subintimal connective tissue. Reports of FcγRIIIa expression by macropahges in other tissues vary. Peritoneal macrophages appear to express significant amounts. However, peritoneal macropahges appear to differ in that they express low levels of CR3 (Hart et al., 1992).

FcγRIIIa has little affinity for monomeric IgG but binds the Fc portion of IgG molecules bound as small immune complexes. Binding through FcγRIIIa leads to intracellular signalling with the production of reactive oxygen species and cytokines such as tumour necrosis factor alpha (TNFα). Binding may also involve an interaction with CR3 and C3bi. A third molecule, mannose binding protein, may also be implicated. Both FcγRIIIa and CR3 are inducible by transforming growth factor beta (TGFβ) whereas FcγRI and CR1 are not (van de Winkel and Capel, 1993).

The role of FcγRIIIa and CR3 in normal synovium probably relates to the advantage of having a row of macrophages on the tissue surface capable of rapid interaction with foreign or degraded material. The precise reasons for the expression of these, rather than other, receptors are not entirely clear but may relate to an ability to retrieve granulocytes and associated bacteria or tissue debris from the joint space. DAF may well play a role in this process by modulating the involvement of complement components.

CO-REGULATION OF CELL PHENOTYPES IN SYNOVIAL INTIMA

The sequence of signals which maintain both fibroblast and macrophage phenotypes in the intima is not yet known. As indicated above, DAF may be induced on fibroblasts initially by shear stress acting through hyaluronan and CD44. Macrophages do not appear in the intimal layer until the joint space has formed. As soon as they do they express FcγRIIIa. This may be in response to TGFβ. TGFβ may be secreted by a number of cells, but mast cells may be specifically implicated. Mechanical stimulation of neuropeptidergic fibres leads to secretion of mediators such as histamine and TGFβ by mast cells in the skin in the generation of the triple response. A similar axon reflex-based mechanism may operate in synovium. Neuropeptidergic fibres are present with endings in proximity to the intimal layer (Mapp, 1995). Interestingly, DAF expression is also induced by histamine in some cell types. Mast cells occur in a regular array just beneath the intimal cells of both joint and tendon sheath synovium. Thus FcγRIIIa expression may be induced by mechanical forces acting through TGFβ. In both fetal and adult synovium there is a very striking co-localisation of FcγRIIIa and DAF, the latter probably on matrix fibres as well as fibroblast cell membranes. This suggests some further interaction between FcγRIIIa and DAF, yet to be established.

The expression of VCAM-1 by intimal fibroblasts has not been seen in fetal synovium and may occur significantly after the arrival of FcγRIIIa-expressing macrophages. This raises the possibility that ligation of FcγRIIIa leads to the production of TNFα and that TNFα is necessary for induction of VCAM-1 expression by intimal fibroblasts. *In vitro* TNFα will induce expression of VCAM-1 by synovial fibroblasts. It will contribute to the expression of DAF if other cytokines such as gamma interferon (γ-IFN) are also present. However, since γ-IFN is unlikely to be present in normal synovium, and DAF expression antedates the presence of FcγRIIIa expressing macrophages in fetal synovium, the role of TNFα in the maintenance of DAF expression in the intima is uncertain.

SUBINTIMAL CELLS

As indicated above, the subintima is populated by a variety of cell types, including fibroblasts and macrophages. As far as has been established, within normal subintima, these cells are indistinguishable cytochemically from their counterparts in other types of connective tissue. The fibroblasts lack VCAM-1 and DAF expression and the macrophages carry surface ligands typical of macrophages elsewhere. In diseased tissue the picture is more complex. VCAM-1 and, in particular, DAF expression in subintima is more extensive than that seen in inflammatory states in tissues such as skin. This is consistent with the concept of a common commitment to expression of these molecules by all synovial fibroblasts, as described above. Patterns of surface ligand expression on macrophages vary considerably from place to place within inflamed tissue, but the general pattern is as noted in the discussion of intimal macrophages.

THE DANGERS OF IMMUNE DEVIATION IN SYNOVIUM

The co-expression of FcγRIIIa, VCAM-1 and DAF by synovial intimal cells may be considered a form of what has become known as immune deviation. Immune deviation describes a modulation in the behaviour of cellular or humoral components of the immune response within a specific tissue. The anterior chamber of the eye is perhaps the best described site of immune deviation (Streilein, 1995). Delayed hypersensitivity responses to intraocular antigens are suppressed by a mechanism which probably also involves neuropeptides and TGFβ. The blood brain barrier may be considered another mechanism for immune deviation, as may the expression of specific adhesion molecules on the endothelium of different organs. Immune deviation commonly appears to involve regulating the types of leucocyte which are permitted to cross tissue interfaces and function in specific microenvironments, as described above for synovium.

The co-expression of FcγRIIIa, VCAM-1 and DAF by synovial intimal cells appears to expose the synovium to a peculiar problem in the context of certain types of circulating immune complexes. Small complexes which are not cleared from the circulation, but can gain access to the extravascular fluid space may interact with synovial FcγRIIIa and generate inflammatory signals including reactive oxygen species and TNFα. In the presence of TNFα and immigrant lymphocytes synovial fibroblasts appear to be able to support both T and B lymphocyte survival, through expression of VCAM-1, DAF and also complement receptor 2 (Edwards and Cambridge, 1995). Thus, in the persistent presence of small circulating complexes synovium may become ectopic lymphoid tissue. If this ectopic lymphoid tissue generates immunoglobulins capable of forming immune complexes the problem may become self-perpetuating. It is likely that rheumatoid factors, which are immunoglobulins capable of forming complexes by self-association, are particularly likely both to interact with FcγRIIIa in this way and to be synthesised within ectopic lymphoid tissue. Thus, rheumatoid arthritis may be the inevitable Achilles heel of the strategy by which the synovial intimal microenvironment protects the synovial space from pathogens, debris and adhesion and, thereby, maintains tissue disconnection.

REFERENCES

Ashhurst, D.E., Bland, Y.S. and Levick, J.R. (1991) An immunohistochemical study of the collagens of rabbit synovial interstitium. *J. Rheumatol.*, **18**, 1669–1672.

Barland, P., Novikoff, A.B. and Hamerman, D. (1962) Electron microscopy of the human synovial membrane. *J. Cell Biol.*, **14**, 207–216.

Bröker, B., Edwards, J.C.W., Fanger, M. and Lydyard, P. (1990) The prevalence and distribution of macrophages bearing FcRI, FcRII and FcRIII in synovium. *Scand. J. Rheumatol.*, **19**, 123–135.

Davies, D.V. and Edwards, D.A.W. (1948) The blood supply of the synovial membrane and intra-articular structures. *Ann. R. Coll. Surg.*, 142–156.

Edwards, J.C.W. (1987) Structure of synovial lining. In: *The Synovial Lining in Health and Disease* (Henderson, B. and Edwards, J.C.W. authors), London: Chapman and Hall, 17–40.

Edwards, J.C.W. and Cambridge, G. (1995) Is rheumatoid arthritis a failure of B cell death in synovium? *Ann. Rheum. Dis.*, **54**, 696–700.

Edwards, J.C.W. and Wilkinson, L.S. (1994) Cell adhesion in autoimmune rheumatic disease. In: *Autoimmune Disease* (D.A. Isenberg and A. Horsefall Eds.), Bios, Oxford.

Edwards, J.C.W. and Wilkinson, L.S. (1996) Distribution in human tissues of the synovial lining associated epitope recognised by monoclonal antibody 67. *J. Anatomy*, **188**, 119–127.

Edwards, J.C.W., Wilkinson, L.S., Jones, H.M., Soothill, P., Henderson, K.J., Worrall, J.G. and Pitsillides, A.A. (1994) The formation of human synovial joint cavities: a possible role for hyaluronan and CD44 in altered interzone cohesion. *J. Anat.*, **185**, 355–367.

El-Gabalawy, H. and Wilkins, J. (1992) β1(CD29) integrin expression in rheumatoid synovial membranes: an immunohistologic study of distribution patterns. *J. Rheumatol.*, **20**, 231–237.

Hart, P.H., Jones, C.A. and Finlay Jones, J.J. (1992) Peritoneal macrophages during peritonitis. Phenotypic studies. *Clin. Exp. Immunol.*, **88**, 484–491.

Key, J.A. (1932) The synovial membrane of joints and bursae. In: *Special Cytology*, Vol. 2, pp. 1055–76, New York: PB Hoeber Inc.

Leigh, R.D., Cambridge, G. and Edwards, J.C.W. (1996) Epression of B cell survival cofactors on synovial fibroblasts. *B. J. Rheumatol. Abst. Suppl.*, **1**, 110.

Levick, J.R. (1995) Fluid movement across synovium in healthy joints: role of synovial fluid macromolecules. *Ann. Rheum. Dis.*, **54**, 417–423.

Mapp, P.I. (1995) Innervation of synovium. *Ann. Rheum. Dis.*, **54**, 398–403.

Medof, M.E., Walter, E.I., Rutgers, J.L., Knowles, D.M. and Nussenzweig, V. (1987) Identification of the complement decay accelerating factor on epithelium and glandular cells and in body fluids. *J. Exp. Med.*, **165**, 848–64.

Morales Ducret, J., Wayner, E., Elices, M.J., Firestein, G. and Zvaifler, N. (1992) a4/b1 integrin (VLA-4) ligands in arthritis: Vascular cell adhersion molecule expression in synovium and on fibroblast-like synoviocytes. *Arthr. Rheum.*, 1424–1431.

Palmer, D.G. (1995) The anatomy of the rheumatoid lesion. *Br. Med. Bull.*, **51**, 286–295.

Revell, P.A., Al-Saffar, N., Fish, S. and Osei, D. (1995) Extracellular matrix of the synovial intimal cell layer. *Ann. Rheum. Dis.*, **54**, 404–407.

Stevens, C.R., Mapp, P.I. and Revell, P.A. (1990) A monoclonal antibody (Mab 67) marks type B synoviocytes. *Rheumatology Int.*, **10**, 103–106.

Streilein, J.W. (1995) Immunological non-responsiveness and acquisition of tolerance in relation to immune privilege in the eye. *Eye*, **9**, 236–240.

Suter, E.R. and Majno, G. (1964) Ulstrastructure of the joint capsule in the rat: presence of two kinds of capillaries. *Nature*, **202**, 920–921.

Tuijnman, W.B., Van-Wichen, D.F. and Schuurman, H.J. (1993) Tissue distribution of human IgG Fc receptors CD16, CD32 and CD64: an immunohistochemical study. *APMIS*, **101**, 319–29.

Unsworth, A. (1993) Lubrication of human joints. In: *Mechanics of human joints* (Wright, V. and Radin, E.L. Eds.), pp. 137–162. Marcel Dekker, New York.

van de Winkel, J.G.J. and Capel, P.J.A. (1993) Human IgG Fc receptor heterogeneity. *Immunology Today*, **14**, 215–221.

van-Ravenswaay-Claasen, H.H., Kluin, P.M. and Fleuren, G.J. (1992) Tumor infiltrating cells in human cancer. On the possible role of CD16$^+$ macrophages in antitumor cytotoxicity. *Lab. Invest*, **67**, 166–74.

Wilkinson, L.S., Edwards, J.C.W., Poston, R. and Haskard, D.O. (1993) Cell populations expressing VCAM-1 in normal and diseased synovium. *Lab. Invest*, **68**, 82–88.

Wilkinson, L.S., Pitsillides, A.A., Worrall, J.G. and Edwards, J.C.W. (1992) Light microscopic characterisation of the fibroblastic synovial lining cell (synoviocyte). *Arthr. Rheum.*, **35**, 1179–1184.

Wilkinson, L.S., Worrall, J.G., Sinclair, H.S. and Edwards, J.C.W. (1990) Immunohistochemical reassessment of accessory cell populations in normal and diseased human synovium. *B. J. Rheumatol.*, **29**, 259–263.

15 Physiology of Synovial Fluid and Trans-synovial Flow

J.R. Levick[1,*], R.M. Mason[2], P.J. Coleman[1] and D. Scott[1]

[1]*Department of Physiology, St. George's Hospital Medical School, London;*
[2]*Department of Biochemistry, Charing Cross and Westminster Medical School, London*

INTRODUCTION

OVERVIEW

The biochemistry of the synovial fluid–synovial interstitium system is reviewed in the preceding paper by Mason *et al.* Here a number of related physiological issues are described, namely:

- organization of the lining and its microcirculation,
- effect of microvascular Starling 'forces' on fluid transfer across joint lining,
- effect of intra-articular pressure and joint movement on trans-synovial flow,
- effect of intra-articular colloids and bidirectional trans-synovial flow in stationary joints,
- effect of intra-articular hyaluronan; do macromolecules necessarily escape freely across the synovial lining?

Before considering these issues in more depth, however, it is useful to consider briefly the value of understanding trans-synovial fluid and macromolecular transport.

NEED TO KNOW: CONCENTRATION OF 'MARKERS' IN SYNOVIAL FLUID

There is a self-evident fundamental scientific value to understanding the regulation of a fluid that is central to joint function as a lubricant, as a medium transmitting nutrients to

* Corresponding author.

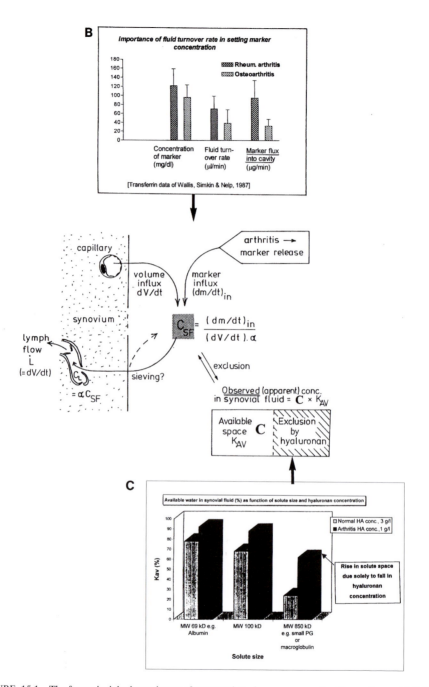

FIGURE 15.1   The four principle determinants of measured marker mass per unit volume of synovial fluid in the steady state are marker input rate, fluid turnover rate, fractional available water and possibley partial reflection by lining (for very large macromolecules). *Inset B* shows how analysis of marker concentration alone (difference not significant between rheumatoid arthritis and osteoarthritis) can mislead with regard to marker flux (difference three-fold; Wallis *et al.*, 1987) unless differences in fluid turnover rate are also taken into account. *Inset C* shows how marker concentration as analysed can mislead for large macromolecules (less so for albumin-size molecules) when hyaluronan concentration and therefore available water fraction varies between conditions (e.g., rheumatoid arthritis versus osteoarthritis). Calculated from Ogston's steric exclusion expression.

cartilage, and as a medium that flushes degraded solutes from the joint into the lymphatic system (review, Levick, 1995). Synovial fluid regulation is also central to joint swelling in clinical effusions. Interest in this area has sharpened recently, however, for a practical reason. This is the use of concentration of biochemical markers of arthritis in synovial fluid as a quantitative index of the activity of the disease process. The factors that govern marker concentration in synovial fluid in the steady state are illustrated in Figure 15.1a. They include not only the *rate of marker input* by the diseased tissue but also the *rate of synovial fluid volume turnover*. In any dynamic system (one that is turning over) solute concentration in the continually replaced intra-articular water is determind by the *ratio* of solute input rate (mass per unit time) to volume input rate, i.e. by microvascular filtration rate into the cavity (Levick, 1992). The latter equals volume drainage from the cavity and into the lymphatic system (lymphatic clearance rate) if there is a steady state over a period of time. Since fluid turnover rate is increased in most arthritides, and by a variable degree (see inset B of Figure 15.1), steady state marker concentration alone is not an ideal measure of disease activity. A better index is provided, in principle, by marker flux (mass/time), as shown by the results in inset B. In order to calculate the marker flux from the apparent concentration of marker as analyzed biochemically, the apparent concentration must be multiplied by the fluid clearance rate (turnover rate), e.g. Jensen *et al.* (1993). Fluid turnover rate can be estimated by radiolabelled albumin clearance as described by Wallis *et al.* (1987) and Myers *et al.* (1995).

The relations between the various factors that potentially influence marker concentration (depending on marker properties) are summarized in Figure 15.1a. It should be noted that the exclusion of a very large marker from part of the synovial fluid water by hyaluronan can be substantial. Consequently, the rise in available space that accompanies hyaluronan dilution (as in an effusion) can itself cause a fall in effective concentration, especially for very large macromolecules (inset C, Figure 15.1), and not a rise in measured concentration as stated in error by Levick (1992). An additional factor that could possibly influence the intra-articular concentration of very large markers might be partial reflection by the lining i.e. very large macromolecular markers may possibly not escape through the lining as freely as water or albumin, as reviewed previously (Levick, 1992). This potential effect is represented as a sieving fraction, α, in Figure 15.1a. New information relating to sieving will be considered further under 'Do all macromolecules escape freely through synovial interstitium?' later.

ORGANISATION OF THE LINING AND ITS MICROCIRCULATION

The synovial lining has a distinct organizational pattern normal to its free surface. Wide interstitium-filled spaces between the lining cells facilitate exchange with the joint cavity, but the pathway is nevertheless narrowest at this interface; the fraction of the tissue occupied by interstitium increases progressively with depth, from about 40% at the free surface to >90% on the subsynovial aspect in rabbit synovium (Price *et al.*, 1995, rabbit; no human data known). The permeability of the matrix greatly influences transport into and out of the joint cavity (see below). The matrix is a dense fibrous one and its glycosaminoglycan (GAG) composition is reviewed in the preceding article. It has a very distinctive fibrillar organization; a network of fine type VI collagen microfibrils predominates near the free surface, while coarser type I–III–V fibrils in bundles become increasingly abundant with distance from the surface. Heterogeneity in a lateral plane may also exist, since a higher concentration of hyaluronan (judged by immunohistological stain density) appears to exist around the synovial capillary than in the inter-capillary zones (Worrall *et al.*, 1991). Moderately fenestrated capillaries are abundant and are located only 5–10 μm (rabbit) to 35 μm (man) beneath the free surface, and their fenestrations (thin, membrane-spanned windows through the wall) are preferentially orientated towards the joint cavity (Levick, 1995). This facilitates fluid and solute exchange with the cavity because it minimizes the transport distance to the surface. Lymphatics capillaries lie deeper, in the subsynovium (Yamashita and Ohkubo, 1993), much of which is loose areolar connective tissue. A rich venular plexus is also found at this level. The subsynovium connects with connective tissue planes up and down the limb. This enables subsynovium to act as a sink of very large compliance for fluid driven across the lining from the joint cavity, as in many of the animal experiments described below.

EFFECT OF MICROVASCULAR STARLING 'FORCES' ON FLUID TRANSFER ACROSS JOINT LINING

The experimental method used to study trans-synovial flow in our laboratory has been to infuse the solution of interest into the knee cavity in an anaesthetised laboratory animal (rabbit) and to control the intra-articular pressure by adjusting the height of an infusion reservoir. A drop counter records flow into the cavity, and in the steady state after >15 min at constant pressure the sustained rate of absorption into the cavity equals net rate of fluid transfer out of the cavity across the synovial lining, after a small correction for viscous creep of the cavity wall.

Using the above approach four pressure terms – the 4 'Starling pressures' – have been shown experimentally to govern the direction and magnitude of net fluid flow across synovium. The term 'net' flow is used advisedly here, because the observed trans-synovial flow represents the sum of two flows – flow between joint cavity and plasma (which can be in either direction depending on the balance of pressures) and flow from joint cavity to subsynovium, bypassing the capillaries (which is outwards when IAP is raised above subsynovial pressure as in infusion experiments). The 4 classical pressures referred to above are:

- capillary blood pressure (P_c),
- plasma colloid osmotic pressure (π_p),
- intra-articular fluid pressure (P_j), and
- intra-articular colloid osmotic pressure (π_j).

The last of these is created chiefly by plasma proteins that have escaped into the synovial fluid. The osmotic pressure of hyaluronan itself is less than $1 \, \text{cmH}_2\text{O}$ at normal concentrations ($\sim 3 \, \text{mg ml}^{-1}$). The fifth relevent pressure, subsynovial fluid pressure, is difficult to access or investigate.

The actions of the intravascular pressures P_c and π_p have been demonstrated by perfusing the synovial microcirculation at various blood pressures with solutions of varying albumin concentration. Raising synovial capillary colloid osmotic pressure (COP) in this way linearly increases the rate of absorption of fluid from the joint cavity, while raising synovial capillary blood pressure has the opposite effect, linearly reducing net absorption rate, or even reversing it to net filtration into the cavity if intra-articular pressure is not too high. Trans-synovial flow is thus a 'passive' transport process that is governed, at least partially, by the classical Starling principle of fluid exchange. The effect of changing π_p on trans-synovial flow ($d\dot{Q}_s/d\pi_p$) is about 80% of that of changing P_c (i.e. $d\dot{Q}_s/dP_c$), indicating that the fenestral membrane is about 80% reflective to plasma albumin. Thus although the fenestra confers high permeability to water and nutrients like glucose, it is not simply a 'hole' in the capillary wall but functions as a semipermeable membrane across which proteins can generate osmotic pressure.

INTRA-ARTICULAR FLUID PRESSURE AND TRANS-SYNOVIAL FLOW

The effect of intra-articular fluid pressure (IAP) is pivotal in joint fluid exchange. IAP is the only term affected directly by joint angle, and consequently it couples fluid exchange to joint movement. Also, because IAP influences flow that passes *in between* capillaries into the subsynovium and lymphatic system (Darcy flow through interstitium) *as well as* affecting flow across the capillary wall (Starling flow), it has a much bigger effect on net trans-synovial flow than have the other 3 pressure terms, cmH$_2$O for cmH$_2$O – in fact around four times bigger.

THE EDLUND CURVE (ABSORPTION RATE VERSUS IAP)

Figure 15.2 shows how positive (supra-atmospheric) intra-articular pressures increase the trans-synovial efflux of plain Krebs solution from the joint cavity (no hyaluronan or extravascular protein present). Flow passes from the joint cavity partly into the microcirculation and to a greater degree into the subsynovial region where the lymphatic plexus is located. The shape of the relation varies considerably but there is commonly a marked, 3–6 fold steepening as pressure is raised, as described by Edlund in 1949. Classically this increase in conductance takes off at IAPs around 7–11 cmH$_2$O. This is a pathological pressure level, because in extended rabbit knees (and in human ones too) the pressure is normally several cmH$_2$O subatmospheric, while in flexed knees without effusions IAP normally rises only to between atmospheric pressure and $+5$ cmH$_2$O (see Figure 15.4 later). Similar pressure – flow curves are found post mortem, albeit with lower absolute flows (because transcapillary exchange is eliminated), so the steepening is clearly due to increases in the hydraulic conductance of the interstitial pathway rather than the microvascular wall. The substantial hydraulic resistance of the lining (resistance is 1/conductance) is readily demonstrated experimentally by perforating it from within by an intra-articular needle; trans-synovial flow at a given IAP immediately increases

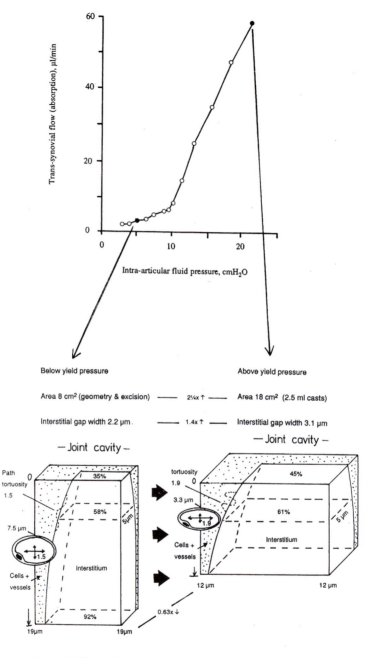

FIGURE 15.2 Nonlinear effect of intra-articular pressure on rate of absorption of saline (here) or plasma protein solution (similar) from cavity of rabbit knee (the 'Edlund curve'). Lower pair of sketches summarize morphometric measurements on rabbit knee synovium fixed at indicated pressures; dotted zone represents
intracelluar space, clear zone extracellular space. Stretch as pressure and volume rise leads to increased surface
area and interstitial gap size and reduce transport distances i.e. thinning (data summarized in Levick, 1991).
These geometrical deformations, however, account only partially for the increased hydraulic conductance seen
in the pressure-flow relation; see text.

by several 100% (unpublished results, Figure 15.3a). The relatively high resistance of the lining enables it to act as an internal 'skin' (albeit a leaky one) that holds the vital synovial fluid within the joint cavity. The resistance of the lining arises chiefly from the biopolymers that interlace the intercellular spaces, as indicated by theoretical considerations (Levick, 1987a; Price *et al.*, 1996a) and as confirmed by a dramatic rise in permeability after intra-articular injection of hyaluronidases or chondroitin ABC'ase (unpublished results, Figure 15.3b). The permeability of the lining does not appear to depend very much on synovial cell activity in the short term (minutes-hours), because intra-articularly administered metabolic inhibitors such as iodoacetate and azide have relatively minor effects on net trans-synovial absorption rate (Figure 15.3c). A small reduction following metabolic inhibition may be the result of increased capillary filtration due to endothelial damage (unpublished data).

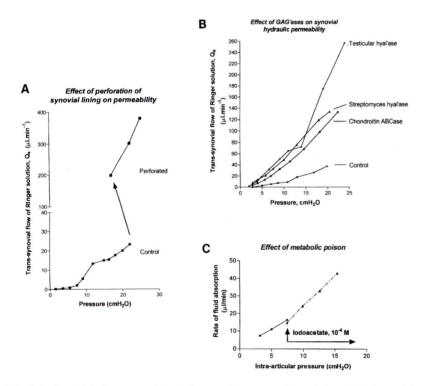

FIGURE 15.3 Unpublished recent studies of the synovial pressure-flow relation (Edlund curve) in rabbit knees. (A) Perforation of the synovial lining from within by an intra-articular needle causes an order-of-magnitude increase in hydraulic conductance; note scale change on ordinate. This simple experiment demonstrates the high-resistance, skin-like property of the normal joint lining. (B) Large increases in hydraulic conductance also follow selective digestion of GAG components of the interstitial matrix; note the scale difference compared with figure 2. Each curve represents a separate knee. The hydraulic resistance of the lining thus arises in part from its GAG content. (C) Metabolic poisons such as iodoacetate and azide cause relatively minor reductions in net trans-synovial absorption rate upon application; this may be due to capillary damage, leading to increased filtration. There is no marked overall effect on the Edlund relation, indicating that the lining's biophysical properties are dominated by the extracellular matrix chiefly and are not, in the short term, dependent on active cell function/metabolism.

STRETCH

Two factors are known to contribute to the conductance increases. The first (stretch) is illustrated in the lower part of Figure 15.2, which summarizes morphometric measurements on light and electron micrographs of rabbit knee synovium fixed *in situ* at low and high IAPs (Levick, 1991). With an increase in IAP there is an increase in synovial surface area, increased interstitial gap size, reduced distance between cavity and subsynovium, and reduced distance between cavity and capillary wall. As a result the geometric factor governing hydraulic conductance, namely the ratio of path area to thickness, more than doubles between 5 and 25 cm H_2O.

MATRIX HYDRATION

The second change is a decrease in the concentration of biopolymers in the interstitial matrix upon raising IAP. Collagen fibrils and GAG chains are important contributors to interstitial hydraulic resistance as shown by enzyme experiments (Figure 15.3b). At approximately 4 mg per ml of extrafibrillar space the GAGs however may not be the only significant resistive elements (Levick, 1987a; Price *et al.*, 1996a). The net GAG concentration (inclusive of chondroitin and heparan sulphates plus hyaluronan) falls to 54% of control level in synovium perfused to 25 cm H_2O, which is sufficient to generate a 3–4 fold rise in hydraulic permeability (Price *et al.*, 1996b). Since the concentration of collagen, a fixed component, decreases by a similar amount, it is inferred that matrix hydration increases. Mean hyaluronan concentration, however, does *not* decrease, which seems to indicate a relatively fast hyaluronan synthetic response. The rate of secretion of hyaluronan into the matrix (cf. into the cavity) calculated from the above observations was 2–3 μg/h per joint. This could be an underestimate if concomittant washout was occurring.

JOINT ANGLE, INTRA-ARTICULAR PRESSURE AND FLUID TURNOVER

IAP is the only pressure term directly affected by joint angle and may therefore couple trans-synovial fluid exchange to movement. IAP depends on both joint angle and fluid volume, as illustrated in Figure 15.4; this composite figure is based partly on rabbit and canine studies (Knight and Levick, 1982; Nade and Newbold, 1984) and partly on studies by Eyring and Murray (1964), Jayson and Dixon (1970), Baxendal *et al.* (1985), Todd *et al.* (1991) and others on human joints. At endogenous synovial fluid volume, pressure is subatmopheric in extension, and a very slow rise with time indicates that slight net trans-synovial flow is directed into the joint cavity under these conditions (lower left inset, Figure 15.4). The rate is approximately 2–4 μl/h/cm^2 synovium or 20–40 μl/h for the rabbit knee, as reviewed elsewhere (Levick, 1987b). The IAP is not very sensitive to angle at low endogenous volumes, but flexion can nevertheless raise it to slightly supra-atmospheric values. It is known from the Edlund curve and other evidence (lower right inset, Figure 15.4) that at supra-atmospheric pressure the net trans-synovial flow is directed out of the cavity. Thus joint movement probably provides one mechanism for generating a turnover of synovial fluid. In support of this, trans-synovial flow patterns

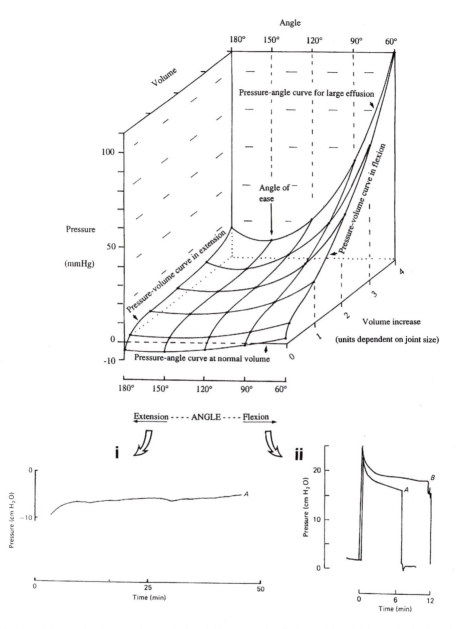

FIGURE 15.4   Relation between intra-articular fluid pressure (vertical, *y* axis) and joint angle (horizontal, *x* axis) at various intra-articular volumes that range from normal to marked effusions (third dimension, *z* axis). The *y–z* relation is the sigmoidal compliance curve of a joint (pressure–volume relation), which varies in steepness according to the joint's angle. The plot is a generalized one; see text for references. Insets show time course of pressure in rabbit knee (i) when subatmospheric in extension (ii) when flexed on a small effusion. The slow rise in pressure with time in (i) is attributed to net filtration into the joint; the slow decline in (ii), line A, is attributed to net outflow from the cavity; line B is a control using nonabsorbable oil. Changes in joint angle may therefore produce 'ebb-and-flow' fluid turnover.

computed by a mathematical model (see below) predict that switching between sub- and supra-atmospheric pressures will indeed generate an ebb-and-flow pattern of fluid turnover. This still leaves open the question, however, as to whether stationary joints can achieve fluid turnover too. Recent evidence that bears on this issue is considered in the next section.

Figure 15.4 also shows that IAP increases as a sigmoidal function of effusion volume; and that the presence of an effusion renders IAP far more sensitive to angle than is the case at normal fluid volume. Indeed acute flexion can transiently generate pressures sufficient to compress the synovial vessels, and several groups have shown an impairment of synovial blood flow and oxygenation under these circumstances. This tends to exaccerbate the intra-articular acidosis in such joints, and may possibly lead to free oxygen radical damage on reperfusion (Blake *et al.*, 1989; Geborek *et al.*, 1989; James *et al.*, 1990). There is a minimum, however, on the pressure-angle relation for an effusion and the swollen joint is predominantly held in this characteristic 'angle of ease' when at rest.

INTRA-ARTICULAR COLLOIDAL OSMOTIC PRESSURE (COP)

EFFECT ON NET ABSORPTION RATE FROM CAVITY

Intra-articular COP can be varied by infusing albumin solutions intra-articularly at controlled IAPs. Raising the intra-articular COP is found to reduce net trans-synovial absorption from the joint cavity, and can even reverse it against an outward directed IAP provided the latter is not too high. The reduction in outflow is partly the effect of increased fluid viscosity, which accompanies any rise in plasma protein concentration. A more important factor, however, is that the intra-articular albumin permeates the interstitial pathway to reach the pericapillary space, where it acts osmotically at the fenestral outer surface to raise capillary filtration rate. Capillary filtration towards the cavity then reduces the net outflow of fluid from the joint cavity (see below) or even reverses it. In support of this interpretation, the reversal of net trans-synovial flow can be abolished by arresting the circulation (Levick and McDonald, 1994).

DILUTION OF INTRA-ARTICULAR INFUSATE AND 'BIDIRECTIONAL FLOW' CONCEPT

We raised the question earlier as to whether a *stationary* joint is capable of fluid turnover – a question relevant to prolonged limb immobilisation by casts or paralysis. An observation during the above study indicated that bulk turnover can still occur, at least under certain conditions. It was noted that when intra-articular fluid was sampled after 20 min or so of continuous albumin infusion (preceded by multiple washes with the infusate), the intra-articular concentration was lower than that of the infusate, despite the fact that the absorbed fluid was continuously being replaced by fresh infusate. The higher the infused COP, the greater was the degree of dilution. Also, the lower the intra-articular pressure, the greater was the degree of dilution (Levick and McDonald, 1994). These features suggested the following explanation. Intra-articular albumin diffuses to the pericapillary space, where it raises the ultrafiltration rate by the Starling mechanism. Some of this plasma ultrafiltrate passes into the joint cavity and thereby dilutes the infusate. The measured trans-synovial flow is thus a net flow representing the difference between (i) input from the microcirculation via immediately overlying interstitium and (ii) a simultaneous outflow through the interstitium further from the capillary's sphere of hydraulic influence (see Figure 15.5a). In other words, the observations implied that flow can occur simultaneously in opposite directions at different points in space over the synovial surface. The dilution observation thus raised the possibility that fluid might turn over even in a stationary joint at fixed angle, given appropriate boundary (i.e. pressure) conditions.

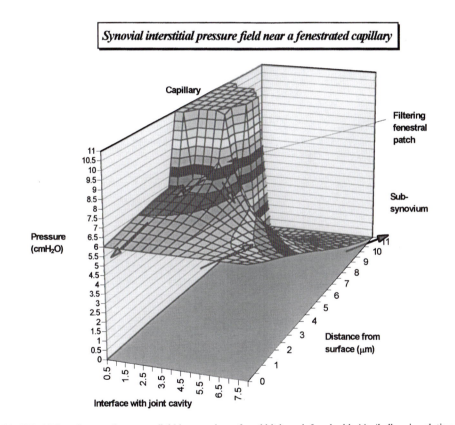

FIGURE 15.5a   Computed pressure field in synovium of a rabbit knee infused with 44 g/l albumin solution at 6 cmH$_2$O intra-articular pressure in the steady state. The half-cylinder of high pressure is a half capillary, with part of its associated block of synovium at lower pressure (basic repeating unit of the model; some of field to right is omitted here). The x axis runs along the interface with the joint cavity at right angles to the capillary axis. The z axis shows distance into the synovium (0 = interface with cavity), with the subsynovium at its far border. Pressure isobars are shown as horizontal contours. Flow occurs at right angles to the pressure isobars as indicated by the arrows.

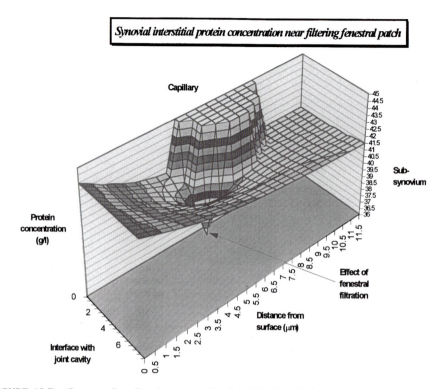

FIGURE 15.5b Corresponding albumin concentration field. The sharp dip in concentration near the fenestral patch on the capillary wall is the diluting effect of plasma ultrafiltrate. The steep gradient here serves to drive interstitial albumin towards the wall by diffusion, counteracting the 'wash-away' effect of the outward filtration stream.

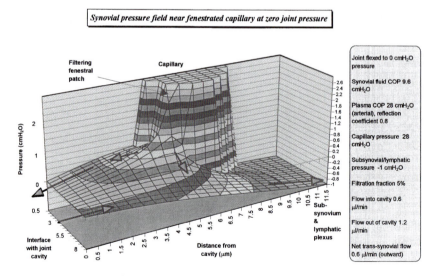

FIGURE 15.5c The above solutions correspond to the experimental situation or to a moderate effusion. The pressure field and flow arrows in frame C represent a stationary nonswollen joint flexed at such an angle that intra-articular pressure is zero. The model predicts almost zero net trans-synovial flow (slight net outflow), but this is seen to be the result of simultaneous inflows and outflows of comparable magnitude.

MATHEMATICAL MODEL TO ASSESS 'BIDIRECTIONAL FLOW' CONCEPT

For the above explanation to work, however, the diffusion rate of intra-articular albumin towards the capillary fenestrations has to be fast enough to maintain an effective concentration there despite the countergoing filtration stream, which is washing albumin away from the wall. To assess the physical feasibility of substantial upstream diffusion, a mathematical model of passive fluid and protein transport across rabbit knee synovium was constructed, based on morphometric data and incorporating restricted interstitial albumin diffusion against the local filtration stream. Steady state solutions were obtained by an iterative, finite difference method (Levick, 1994). An example is shown in Figure 15.5a; the boundary conditions here (IAP $6\,cmH_2O$, intra-articular protein $44\,g/l$) correspond to a modest clinical effusion. The vertical axis is pressure, and pressure isobars are shown as shaded bands. The half-cylinder of high pressure is a half capillary, with its associated block of synovium at lower pressure (the basic repeating unit of the model). The interface with the joint faces the reader, and the z axis represents distance into the synovium from the free surface towards subsynovium. Flow occurs at right angles to the isobars. Because there is rapid filtration through the patch of fenestrations in the capillary wall, which characteristically face the joint cavity, a ridge of high interstitial fluid pressure is generated outside the fenestrations, extending locally towards the joint cavity. This drives a fraction of the capillary ultrafiltrate into the cavity via interstitium directly overlying the capillary. However, away from the effective sphere of influence of the capillary, the pressure gradient is directed from cavity to subsynovium (because the experimenter infused fluid into the cavity; or because *in vivo* the joint is at a flexed angle); and flow here is outwards from the cavity. Flow is thus bidirectional under these conditions and the net observed flow represents the difference between inflow and outflow components. The corresponding protein concentration gradients are shown in Figure 15.5b, where the vertical axis is now protein concentration. Fenestral ultrafiltration creates a dip in protein concentration near the wall, and the steep local concentration gradient drives intra-articular albumin towards the wall against the filtration stream – rather like a dye in a slowly moving river that keeps station with the bank by continuously diffusing upstream. The model thus confirms the physical feasibility of bidirectional fluid turnover given appropriate boundary conditions.

The model, developed to help interpret experimental results, can also be used to predict flow patterns occurring naturally *in vivo*. Figure 15.5c shows the computed flow pattern for a joint containing a normal intra-articular protein concentration and flexed sufficiently for IAP to be 'zero' (i.e. atmospheric pressure), while the subsynovial lymphatic pump is assumed to maintain a slightly lower pressure in subsynovium. Under these boundary conditions the pressure field again reveals bidirectional flow, indicating that it is indeed biophysically possible that synovial fluid may turn over even without joint motion. As indicated earlier, volume turnover is one of several factors influencing 'marker' concentration in the joint cavity.

EFFECT OF INTRA-ARTICULAR HYALURONAN ON FLUID ABSORPTION

In the above experiments the hydraulic situation was deliberately simplified by washing or diluting out the endogenous hyaluronan normally present in synovial fluid. The effect

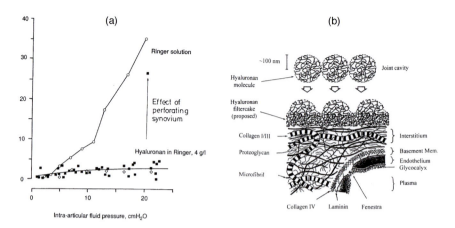

FIGURE 15.6   (a) Effect of hyaluronan (rooster comb, $4\,g/l$, MW 2×10^6, filled squares) or native bovine synovial fluid (open diamonds) on the 'Edlund curve' (open circles). Hyaluronan greatly buffers the outflow. Arrow shows the sharp rise in lining permeability when the hyaluronan-caked lining is deliberately perforated by a hypodermic needle. Unpublished results. (b) Schematic illustration of 'filtercake' working hypothesis, showing partial sieving of hyaluronan by synovial interstitial matrix. If local fenestral filtration is occurring, it is possible that the filtercake may be uneven, unlike that sketched here.

of hyaluronan itself on trans-synovial fluid absorption is a dramatic and complex one, as shown in Figure 15.6. Hyaluronan greatly reduces outflow from the joint cavity and raising the IAP causes little rise in outflow, especially above $\sim 10\,cmH_2O$; there is virtually a flow 'plateau'. One might speculate that the biological value of this massive hydraulic buffering lies in preventing the joint from wringing itself dry during periods of flexion and high pressure, thereby retaining (i) a major lubricating macromolecule and (ii) the volume needed for hydrodynamic lubrication and the convective transport functions of synovial fluid. The mechanism underlying the flattening of the Edlund curve appears not to be viscous (McDonald and Levick, 1994, 1995) but involves a rise in outflow resistance with each rise in IAP. The rise in outflow resistance counteracts the effect of the pressure rise, so outflow rate changes little. If outflow resistance is reduced by deliberately perforating the synovial lining with a cannula tip, there is an immediate rise in outflow by an order of magnitude (Figure 15.6a).

DO ALL MACROMOLECULES ESCAPE FREELY THROUGH SYNOVIAL INTERSTITIUM?

THE FILTERCAKE HYPOTHESIS

Flow plateaux are very characteristic of sieving membranes that 'silt up' owing to the formation of a filtercake of retained particles, and this has often been described for artificial macromolecular sieves (e.g. Parker and Winlove, 1984). Our working hypothesis, illustrated in Figure 15.6b, is that the porosities of the interstitial matrix *partially* reflect and sieve out the gigantic hyaluronan molecules relative to water, so that a 'filtercake' of hyaluronan chains forms near the surface. Resistance to flow through hyaluronan chains is known to be high, so the effect of a hyaluronan filtercake would be to raise outflow resistance, and this could produces the observed flow plateau. If this working hypothesis turns out to be correct (and it is unproven), it could have important implications for large 'markers' of arthritis in synovial fluid, such as proteoglycans. As pointed out in the introduction (Figure 15.1), if large macromolecules do *not* escape across the lining interstitium with the same freedom (i.e. velocity) as water and small proteins, then partial reflection will be an additional factor affecting their concentration in synovial fluid. Two lines of evidence reinforce the feasibility of macromolecular sieving by synovial interstitium, at least for hyaluronan, as follows.

HOW BIG ARE THE SYNOVIAL INTERSTITIAL 'PORES'?
MEAN HYDRAULIC RADIUS

One way to characterize the average effective size of the irregular porosities within an interstitial matrix is by the mean hydraulic radius of the matrix. This is, by definition, the ratio of void volume (water space) to surface area of the 'solid' molecular chains in the matrix, the biopolymer chains being represented as cylindrical structures for the purpose of surface area calculation. Figure 15.7 shows mean hydraulic radii calculated from biochemical data for a wide variety of interstitia ranging from aqueous humor to articular cartilage (Levick, 1987a). Not surprisingly the smaller the mean hydraulic radius, the less the hydraulic permeability of the matrix. The radius covers a wide range; in articular cartilage it is small enough to exclude albumin-size proteins almost totally (as Maroudas, 1970, has shown experimentally) whereas in less dense interstitia there is lesser exclusion and freer transport. The estimate of mean hydraulic radius for synovial matrix has a wide range of uncertainty but from the quantitative biochemical results of Mason *et al.* (preceding review) and from physiological estimates of synovial lining resistance, synovial mean hydraulic radius is calculated to lie between 15 nm and 45 nm. By comparison the radius of gyration of individual rooster comb hyaluronan molecule used in the experiment of Figure 15.6 is of the order 100 nm. Moreover at physiological concentration (>1 g/l) the adjacent molecular domains of hyaluronan overlap to produce a quasi-continuous network of chains. Thus, even allowing for the ability of GAG chains to permeate small spaces slowly by reptation (snake-like wriggling), dimensional considerations appear to support the view that hyaluronan molecules should escape through synovium less easily than do water molecules. Indeed, Parker and Winlove (1984) showed this to be the case for Millipore membranes with a pore width as big as 450 nm.

EFFECT OF MACROMOLECULAR SIZE ON HALF-LIFE OR
TURNOVER TIME IN JOINT SPACE

The other class of evidence pointing to partial macromolecular sieving by rabbit synovial interstitial matrix arises from studies of intra-articular half-life or turnover time for very large versus smaller macromolecular solutes. The intra-articular half-life of a proteoglycan fragment of molecular mass 2.5×10^6 is 12.4 h in the rabbit knee, in contrast to 3.9 h for albumin (Page-Thomas *et al.*, 1987). The intra-articular half-life of hyaluronan of

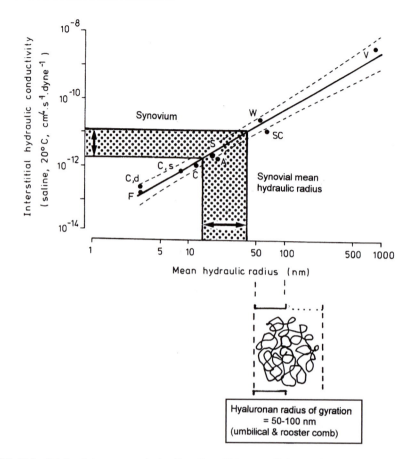

FIGURE 15.7   Relation between mean hydraulic radius within extracellular matrix and the hydraulic conductivity of a unit cube of the matrix to saline, for a wide range of tissues. The two parameters both depend on the density of biopolymers in the matrix. Dotted band shows estimated range for synovial matrix of rabbit knee. Radius of gyration of commercial hyaluronan preparations shown for comparison. V, vitreous humor; W, Wharton's jelly; SC, subcutis; S, scleral stroma; A, aortic interstitium; C, corneal stroma; Cs, Cd, F, articular cartilage from various sites (see Levick, 1987a for references).

molecular mass 6×10^6, namely 13 h, is significantly longer than that of hyaluronan of molecular mass 0.9×10^6, namely 10 h, in volume-expanded rabbit knees (Brown *et al.*, 1991). Denlinger (1982) found the half-life of hyaluronan to be longer still, 27–32 h, in the rabbit knee at normal volume.

In recent unpublished studies of endogenous hyaluronan by Scott, Ray and Coleman in our laboratory a washout technique was used to measure endogenous hyaluronan mass in the rabbit knee fluid. By means of further washes after 4 h, hyaluronan secretion rate *in vivo* was measured. Endogenous hyaluronan mass ($\sim$180 µg) divided by the measured secretion rate ($\sim$5–6 µg/h) gave an estimated turnover time of $\geqslant$31 h (equivalent to a half-life of $\geqslant$22 h). Similarly Knox *et al.* (1988) estimated the turnover time for endogenous hyaluronan in rabbit shoulder joints to be 20–28 h. An analogous approach was used to measure plasma protein permeation rate into the cavity and hence plasma protein turnover time in the same joints. This, however, was only 1–2 h. The latter result is very close to estimates of plasma protein turnover time in the normal human knee cavity, and also to estimates of volume turnover time based on filtration rate into the rabbit knee (review; Levick, 1987b).

In view of the above results it seems likely that the residence time for very large macromolecules in the joint cavity is an order of magnitude longer than that of plasma proteins and water (bulk volume). The implication of the various lines of evidence reviewed above is, therefore, that very large macromolecules (relative molecular mass $> 10^6$) do not escape freely through the lining. If this is correct, the value of the sieving ratio 'α' in Figure 15.1 may not necessarily be unity (it will vary with fluid velocity), and this may influence the intra-articular concentration of the larger markers of joint disease activity, such a proteoglycan fragments, compared with smaller ones. A caveat must be added however; the biophysical properties of the interstitial matrix in inflammed, oedematous human joints are unknown and may differ substantially from those of the healthy rabbit knee. There remains a dearth of quantitative biochemical and hydraulic information for human synovial matrix which precludes further inferences in this direction at present.

REFERENCES

Baxendale, R.H., Ferrell, W.R. and Wood, L. (1985) Intra-articular pressure during active and passive movement of normal and distended knee joints. *J. Physiol.*, **369**, 179P.

Blake, D.R., Merry, P., Unsworth, J. *et al.* (1989) Hypoxic reperfusion injury in the inflammed human joint. *Lancet* (i), **8633**, 289–293.

Brown, T.J., Laurent, U.B.G. and Fraser, J.R.E. (1991) Turnover of hyaluronan in synovial joints: elimination of labelled hyaluronan from the knee joint of the rabbit. *Exp. Physiol.*, **76**, 125–134.

Denlinger, J.L. (1982) Metabolism of sodium hyaluronate in articular and ocular tissues. Doctoral dissertation, Université de Sciences et Techniques de Lille.

Edlund, T. (1949) Studies on the absorption of colloids and fluid from rabbit knee joints. *Acta Physiol. Scand.*, **18**, Supplement 62, 1–108.

Eyring, J.E. and Murray, W.R. (1964) The effect of joint position on the pressure of intra-articular effusions. *J. Bone Joint Surg.*, **46A**, 1235–1241.

Geborek, P., Forslind, K. and Wollheim, F. (1989) Direct assessment of synovial blood flow and its relation to induced hydrostatic pressure changes. *Ann. Rheum. Dis.*, **48**, 281–286.

James, M.J., Cleland, L.G., Roffe, A.M. and Leslie, A.L. (1990) Intra-articular pressure and the relationship between synovial perfusion and metabolic demand. *J. Rheumatol.*, **17**, 521–527.

Jayson, M.I.V. and Dixon, A.St.J. (1970) Intra-articular pressure in rheumatoid arthritis of the knee. 1. Pressure changes during passive joint distension. *Ann. Rheum. Dis.*, **29**, 261–265.

Jensen, L.T., Henriksen, J.H., Olesen, H.P., Risteli, J. and Lorenzen, I.B. (1993) Lymphatic clearance of synovial fluid in conscious pigs; the aminoterminal propeptide of type III procollagen. *Eur. J. Clin. Invest.*, **23**, 778–784.

Knight, A.D. and Levick, J.R. (1982) Pressure–volume relationships above and below atmospheric pressure in the synovial cavity of the rabbit knee. *J. Physiol.*, **328**, 403–420.

Knox, P., Levick, J.R. and McDonald, J.N. (1988) Synovial fluid – its mass, macromolecular content and pressure in major limb joints of the rabbit. *Quart. J. Exp. Physiol.*, **73**, 33–46.

Levick, J.R. (1987a) Flow through interstitium and other fibrous matrices. *Quart. J. Exp. Physiol.*, **72**, 409–438.

Levick, J.R. (1987b) Synovial fluid and trans-synovial flow in stationary and moving joints. In: *Joint Loading: Biology and Health of Articular Structures*, Helminen, H., Kiviranta, I., Tammi, M., Saamaren, A.M., Paukonnen, K. and Jurvelin, J., Ed. pp. 149–186. Bristol, Wright and Sons.

Levick, J.R. (1991) A two-dimensional morphometry-based model of interstitial and transcapillary flow in rabbit synovium. *Exp. Physiol.*, **76**, 905–201.

Levick, J.R. (1992) Synovial fluid; determinants of volume and material concentration. In: *Articular Cartilage and Osteoarthritis*, pp. 529–541. Kuettner, K.E., Hascall, V.C. and Schleyerbach, R., Ed. NY, Raven Press.

Levick, J.R. (1994) An analysis of the interaction between extravascular plasma protein, interstitial flow and capillary filtration; application to synovium. *Microvasc. Res.*, **47**, 90–125.

Levick, J.R. (1995) Microvascular architecture and exchange in synovial joints. *Microcirculation*, **2**, 217–233.

Levick, J.R. and McDonald, J.N. (1994) Viscous and osmotically mediated changes of interstitial flow induced by extravascular albumin in synovium. *Microvasc. Res.*, **47**, 68–89.

Maroudas, A. (1970) Distribution and diffusion of solutes in articular cartilage. *Biophys. J.*, **10**, 365–379.

McDonald, J.N. and Levick, J.R. (1994) Hyaluronan reduces fluid escape rate from joints disparately from its effect on fluidity. *Exp. Physiol.*, **79**, 103–106.

McDonald, J.N. and Levick, J.R. (1995) Effect of intra-articular hyaluronan on pressure – flow relation across synovium in anaesthetized rabbits. *J. Physiol.*, **485**, 179–193.

Myers, S.L., Brandt, K.D. and Eilam, O. (1995) Even low grade synovitis significantly accelerates the clearance of protein from the canine knee. Implications for measurement of synovial fluid "markers" of osteoarthritis. *Arth. Rheum.*, **38**, 1085–1091.

Nade, S. and Newbould, P.J. (1984) Pressure–volume relationships and elastance in the knee joint of the dog. *J. Physiol.*, **357**, 417–439.

Ogston, A.G. (1970) On the interaction of solute molecules with porous networks. *J. Phys. Chem.*, **74**, 668–669.

Page-Thomas, D.P., Bard, D., King, B. and Dingle, J.T. (1987) Clearance of proteoglycan from joint cavities. *Ann. Rheum. Dis.*, **46**, 934–937.

Parker, K.H. and Winlove, C.P. (1984) The macromolecular basis of the hydraulic conductivity of the arterial wall. *Biorheology*, **21**, 181–196.

Price, F.M., Levick, J.R. and Mason, R.M. (1996a) Glycosaminoglycan concentration in synovium and other tissues of rabbit knee in relation to hydraulic resistance. *J. Physiol.*, **495**, 803–820.

Price, F.M., Levick, J.R. and Mason, R.M. (1996b) Changes in glycosaminoglycan concentration and synovial permeability at raised intra-articular pressures in rabbit knees. *J. Physiol.*, **495**, 821–833.

Price, F.M., Mason, R.M. and Levick, J.R. (1995) Radial organization of interstitial exchange pathway and influence of collagen in synovium. *Biophys. J.*, **69**, 1429–1439.

Todd, B.D., Venner, R.M. and Hutchinson, T.F. (1991) Pressure–volume relationships above and below atmospheric pressure in the human knee. The filling curve is sigmoidal. *J. Orthop. Rheumatol.*, **4**, 129–134.

Wallis, W.J., Simkin, P.A. and Nelp, W.B. (1987) Protein traffic in human synovial effusions. *Arth. Rheum.*, **30**, 57–63.

Worrall, J.G., Bayliss, M.T. and Edwards, J.C.W. (1991) Morphological localization of hyaluronan in normal and diseased synovium. *J. Rheumatol.*, **18**, 1466–1472.

Yamashita, S. and Ohkubo, M. (1993) Distribution and three-dimensional reconstruction of lymphatic vessels of the elbow joint capsule of rabbits. *Acta Anat. Nippon*, **68**, 513–521.

16   Biochemistry of the Synovium and Synovial Fluid

Roger M. Mason[1], J. Rodney Levick[2],
Peter J. Coleman[2] and David Scott[2]

[1]*Division of Biomedical Sciences, Imperial College School of Medicine,
Charing Cross Hospital, Fulham Palace Road, London, W6 8RF, UK;*
[2]*Department of Physiology, St. George's Hospital
Medical School, Cranmer Terrace, London, SW17 0RE, UK*

INTRODUCTION

The synovium is a thin sheet of tissue which lines all parts of the joint cavity except the articular cartilage and some ligaments. It is populated by two types of cell and has an extensive extracellular matrix (ECM) permeated by capillaries. The synovium is about 50–60 µm thick in the normal human knee joint (Stevens *et al.*, 1991) and between 10–20 µm thick in the rabbit knee joint (Levick and McDonald, 1989), the subject of our investigations. It rests on an underlying layer of loose connective tissue, the subsynovium, which is backed by skeletal muscle, fibrous capsule, tendon or fat. The synovium is also called the "synovial intima" or "synovial lining" and in older texts it was referred to as the "synovial membrane".

The synovium has a number of functions. An ultrafiltrate of plasma passes across its capillary walls, through the ECM, and into the joint cavity. Hyaluronan, a very long glycosaminoglycan (GAG), is synthesized by type B cells of the synovium and passes into the joint cavity. The ultrafiltrate and hyaluronan form the synovial fluid which is contained within the joint cavity and which has a major function in lubricating the joint surfaces. The synovial fluid also acts as a vehicle for transfer of small solute molecules such as glucose and dissolved oxygen from the capillary ultrafiltrate to the chondrocytes of the articular cartilage. The cartilage has no blood supply of its own, so this function of the synovial fluid is very important. Similarly, solutes passing from the cartilage into the joint cavity, find their way out via the synovial fluid, and then through the synovial

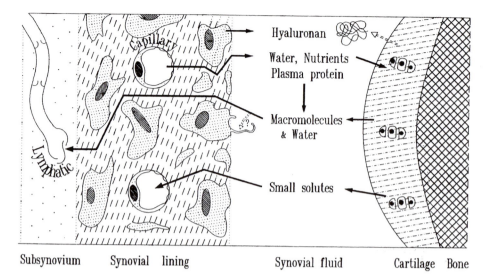

FIGURE 16.1 Overview of the relationship between the synovial lining, synovial fluid and articular cartilage in a synovial joint (reproduced from Levick *et al.*, 1997).

interstitium to the lymphatics in the subsynovium. Synovial fluid is also removed from the joint cavity by the phagocytic action of type A cells located in the superficial layer of the synovium. Some synovial fluid hyaluronan (Worrall *et al.*, 1991), as well as any foreign material or debris, leaves the joint cavity by this route.

The synovium and its fluid may be thought of as a functionally continuous system connecting the cartilage, vascular and lymphatic systems. However, as well as allowing for solute transfer, the synovium must also contain synovial fluid within the joint cavity. Hence a major requirement of synovial ECM is that it must provide hydraulic resistance. These features are summarised in Figure 16.1. The aim of this chapter will be to review the structure of this matrix and to relate it to the biophysical properties of the synovium.

MACROMOLECULAR COMPOSITION OF THE SYNOVIUM

Electron microscopy of the synovium shows that it contains large numbers of collagen fibre bundles (Figure 16.2). These are found predominantly in the lower two thirds of the synovium, whilst cells and microvessels predominate in the superficial layer adjacent to the joint cavity. Even so, there are substantial amounts of interstitial matrix in the superficial layer, and numerous microfibrils. On the basis of microfibril ultrastructure, Levick and McDonald (1990) predicted that the microfibrils were type VI collagen and immunoelectron microscopy confirms this (Okada *et al.*, 1990). Type VI collagen binds to several other types of matrix macromolecules including hyaluronan (Kielty *et al.*, 1992), fibronectin (Kielty *et al.*, 1992) and decorin (Bidanset *et al.*, 1992). It also promotes adhesion of cultured synoviocytes (Wolf and Carsons, 1991). Type VI collagen

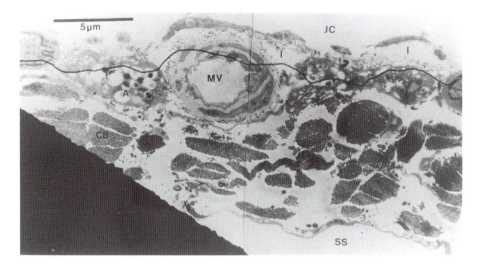

FIGURE 16.2   Composite electron micrograph of microdissected synovium. JC, joint cavity; I, interstitium; A, macrophage or A cell; MV, microvessel; CB, collagen bundle; SS, subsynovium. The line shows how the tissue was demarcated for morphometric analysis (reproduced from Price *et al.*, 1995).

is therefore likely to have a key role in ordering matrix architecture in the first 2–3 μm of the synovium and in anchoring the synoviocytes in this region to the matrix.

Type III collagen appears to be the major striated fibrillar collagen in the synovium and its distribution extends into the subsynovial connective tissue. Type I collagen is less prominent (Ashhurst *et al.*, 1991). Type V collagen is also present. The large collagen bundles in the synovium occupy interstitial space and other macromolecules such as hyaluronan, proteoglycans and fibronectin which are present in the synovial intima (Worrall *et al.*, 1991; Price *et al.*, 1996a; Linck *et al.*, 1983) are effectively excluded from this space (Price *et al.*, 1995). Thus the extrafibrillar concentration of these proteins and proteoglycans is much higher than their apparent concentration in synovium (see below).

Although the synovium lacks a formal basement membrane, its cells nevertheless synthesize some typical basement membrane type components such as the network-forming type IV collagen, and laminin. These surround the B-type synovial cells (Pollock *et al.*, 1990). The significance of this is not appreciated at the present time. Type IV collagen is also associated with the basement membrane of synovial blood vessels (Linck *et al.*, 1983; Scott *et al.*, 1984).

Several different types of proteoglycan have been identified in the synovium. These include decorin and biglycan (Worrall *et al.*, 1992), two members of the "leucine-rich" proteoglycan family. Decorin and biglycan carry chondroitin sulphate or dermatan sulphate chains as their GAG components. Using the monoclonal antibody 5D4 (Caterson *et al.*, 1983), we have detected keratan sulphate reactivity in the synovial intima and sub-synovium (Price *et al.*, 1994). This may indicate the presence in synovial interstitium of fibromodulin, a keratan sulphate-bearing member of the small leucine-rich proteoglycan family. No information is currently available about whether large chondroitin sulphate proteoglycans such as versican are present in the synovial interstitial matrix. Heparan sulphate proteoglycans are present in greater concentration than chondroitin sulphate proteoglycans (Price et al., 1996a), but again we do not know which types of proteoglycan, carrying heparan sulphate chains (e.g. perlecan, syndecans, glypican), are synthesized by synovial cells.

The non-sulphated GAG, hyaluronan, is present in the synovium as well as in the synovial fluid (Worrall et al., 1991; Balazs and Denlinger, 1985). The cells responsible for its synthesis are the type B synoviocytes since they show evidence of abundant UDP-glucose dehydrogenase activity (Pitsillides et al., 1993). This enzyme is required for synthesizing UDP-glucuronate, an essential precursor for making hyaluronan and other GAGs. Collagen VI probably provides an anchoring point for some of the hyaluronan molecules made by the synoviocytes, as discussed above. Moreover, type B synoviocytes also express CD44, a hyaluronan binding protein, on their cell surfaces (Henderson et al., 1993). Thus it seems likely that some of the hyaluronan synthesized by the cells is tethered in the synovium whilst other newly polymerised hyaluronan molecules pass directly into the synovial fluid, perhaps from cells which are polarised for this purpose. It is unlikely that significant numbers of hyaluronan molecules which are located initially in the synovial matrix move later into the synovial fluid. Experiments with joints obtained at post mortem support the view that passage of hyaluronan into the synovial fluid is an active process and that leaching from the synovial intimal interstitium does not occur to any significant extent (see below). Several other ECM macromolecules are present in the synovium. These include fibrillin, tenascin, and entactin. We have reviewed the evidence for this and their properties, elsewhere (Levick et al., 1996).

The hydraulic conductance or resistance of a tissue, i.e. its properties in permitting, or resisting, the flow of water and solute molecules through it, is thought to be governed primarily by the concentration and arrangement of proteoglycans, hyaluronan, collagen fibrils, and other proteins in its interstitial matrix (Levick, 1987a). Interstitial hydraulic resistance, which in the synovium is required to maintain the synovial fluid in the joint space, arises from hydraulic drag of the various biopolymers. Thus to understand the properties of the synovium more fully, we have investigated the concentration of these macromolecules in the synovial interstitium.

SYNOVIAL INTERSTITIAL VOLUME AND EXTRAFIBRILLAR SPACE

The structure of the rabbit synovium changes with its depth. Cells and their processes predominate at the surface, whilst the interstitium increases in volume with increasing depth. Moreover, the number of collagen bundles in the synovium increase with depth (Figure 16.2). Morphometric analysis enabled us to quantify these parameters (Price et al., 1995). At the synovium-joint cavity interface, $21.6 \pm 4.9\%$ of the synovial surface consisted of interstitial matrix in direct contact with the synovial fluid. Interstitial area as a fraction of the tissue, en face, rose steeply to 0.440 ± 0.095 at a depth of $2\,\mu m$ and to 0.938 ± 0.022 at $10\,\mu m$ from the surface. The harmonic mean thickness of the rabbit synovium in this series of experiments was $10.4 \pm 0.7\,\mu m$. The volume of the interstitium occupied by collagen bundles increased from $13.6 \pm 2.4\%$ in the most superficial $2\,\mu m$ slice to $\sim 49\%$ in the slice $4-6\,\mu m$ below the surface. This value was maintained at deeper levels.

We have estimated the minimal internal hydraulic resistivity of collagen bundles (range, 3.6×10^{10} to $21 \times 10^{10}\,dyn.s.cm^{-4}$) and compared it with the minimal value for the interstitial matrix not occupied by bundles (range, 0.12×10^{10} to $3.6 \times 10^{10}\,dyn.s.cm^{-4}$) (Price *et al.*, 1995). Given the difference, we conclude that each collagen bundle in the synovial interstitium will act as an obstruction to trans-synovial flow. Thus flow through the synovial interstitium will divert around the collagen bundles, in a manner analogous to water flowing around a rock in a stream, rather than through the obstruction. The effect of the collagen bundles in the synovium then is to reduce the cross-sectional area available for flow, to increase the flow pathway length and tortuosity, and to create hydraulic drag.

Since other matrix macromolecules such as GAGs are excluded from the space occupied by collagen fibrils, their effective hydrodynamic concentration in the extrafibrillar space where they are confined will be higher than their apparent concentration in the whole tissue, enhancing the synovium's resistance to flow and its ability to retain synovial fluid. In practice, the increasing interstitial volume in the synovium with depth is offset by decreasing bundle-free matrix. We calculate that from just below the surface ($2-4\,\mu m$ slice), about 50% of the tissue volume is available for trans-synovial flow and that this fraction is constant throughout the remaining depth of the tissue. At the surface ($0-2\,\mu m$ slice) the available space is reduced to $\sim 38\%$ of the tissue, due to the large volume (35%) occupied by synoviocytes in this zone (Price *et al.*, 1995).

GLYCOSAMINOGLYCAN CONCENTRATION IN THE EXTRAFIBRILLAR SPACE OF THE SYNOVIAL INTERSTITIUM

We used several ultrasensitive assays to measure the concentration of various GAGs in rabbit synovium. Chondroitin-4-sulphate and chondroitin-6-sulphate assays utilised capillary electrophoresis to separate their respective disaccharides after digesting with chondroitinase ABC (Price *et al.*, 1996a). Heparan sulphate was measured using a [103]Ruthenium red method (Gaffen *et al.*, 1994) and hyaluronan was assayed by an ELISA using a biotinylated hyaluronan-binding protein, G1 domain of aggrecan (Fosang *et al.*, 1990). These methods enabled reliable measurements to be made on the very small amounts of microdissected synovium obtained from a rabbit knee joint. Since the fraction of the tissue occupied by interstitium, and the fraction of the interstitium occupied by collagen fibre bundles was known (see above), it was possible to calculate the extrafibrillar concentration of individual GAGs (Table 16.1). The total GAG concentration in the

TABLE 16.1
Biopolymer concentrations in rabbit synovium.

Biopolymer	Measured in tissue $mg.g^{-1}$	Interstitial concentration $mg.ml^{-1}$	Extrafibrillar concentration $mg.ml^{-1}$
Ch-4-SO$_4$	0.345 ± 0.031	0.89	1.16
Ch-6-SO$_4$	0.053 ± 0.011		
Hep SO$_4$	0.664 ± 0.071	1.49	1.94
HA	0.265 ± 0.039	0.60	0.78
Collagen	72.53 ± 10.15	162.6	–

Measurements were made as described in Price *et al.*, 1996a.
Ch-4-SO$_4$, Chondroitin-4-sulphate; Ch-6-SO$_4$, chondroitin-6-sulphate; HepSO$_4$, heparan sulphate; HA, hyaluronan.

extrafibrillar space is about 4.1 mg.ml^{-1}, with heparan sulphate being the most abundant polymer (Price *et al.*, 1996a). Keratan sulphate, which on the basis of immunocyto-chemistry appears to be a component of the synovial ECM, was not measured by our assays. Thus the total GAG concentration may be an underestimate but this is unlikely to be of significant magnitude.

Interstitial conductivity can be predicted from biochemical data. Similarly, knowing the observed conductance of rabbit synovium (1.8×10^{-3} cm^3.min^{-1}.cm H$_2$O^{-1}), it is possible to calculate the GAG concentration which would be required to give this conductance. Levick (1994) predicted a uniform extrafibrillar GAG concentration of 13.9 mg.ml^{-1} in rabbit synovium to account for its conductance. Clearly the measured concentration of 4.1 mg.ml^{-1} indicates that GAGs are important contributors to the conductance of the synovium, but even if their concentration was marginally underestimated, they cannot solely account for the flow properties of the tissues.

One possibility that must be considered is whether the GAGs are highly concentrated in one layer of the synovium. If so their effective concentration could be higher than that estimated. However, we have no immunohistochemical evidence suggesting concentration of any of the GAGs into a narrow zone of the synovium.

The hydraulic conductivity of many tissues is lower than that predicted by their GAG concentration (Levick, 1987a) so the synovium is not exceptional in this. However, this poses the question as to what is responsible for the additional hydraulic drag. We measured the total protein content of rabbit synovium and, knowing the collagen content, were able to extrapolate the non-collagen protein content. This is ~44 mg.ml^{-1} of tissue. On the other hand, the estimated deficit of polymeric material required to account for synovial conductance is only ~5.0 mg.ml^{-1} tissue (~10 mg.ml^{-1} extrafibrillar space) (Price *et al.*, 1996a). Thus, whilst a significant proportion of the non-collagenous protein is probably cellular, only a small percentage (~11%) would need to be in the extrafibrillar space to give the observed conductivity of the tissue. We conclude that extrafibrillar space proteins, for example glycoproteins such as fibronectin and proteoglycan core protein, are important contributors to the conductance properties of the synovium. The fine microfibrils of type VI collagen in the superficial layer may also contribute to the hydraulic drag of the tissue (Price *et al.*, 1996a).

EFFECTS OF RAISED INTRA-ARTICULAR PRESSURE ON TRANS-SYNOVIAL FLOW AND THE INTERSTITIUM

Joint pathology is frequently accompanied by an effusion in the joint space which raises the intra-articular pressure. It has been known for many years that the conductance of the synovium increases at such pressures, at least in the short term (Edlund, 1949). Infusion of rabbit knee joints with saline under constant pressure indicates that above 7–10 cm H_2O there is a very marked increase in trans-synovial flow and hydraulic conductance (Price et al., 1996b). Stretching of the synovium under raised intra-articular pressure reduces its thickness and therefore the length of the flow pathway from the joint cavity to the subsynovium. However, this mechanical factor has been shown, quantitatively, to be insufficient to account for the increased conductance above pressures of 10 cm H_2O. Thus we must look for additional changes in the synovial intima to explain this. We postulated that the increased conductance could be due to a decreased concentration of extrafibrillar space macromolecules. This could result from either increased hydration of the synovium at higher pressures or to washout of some macromolecular components as fluid velocity increases.

We measured the concentration of synovium interstitial components in rabbit knee joints at an intra-articular pressure of 25 cm H_2O and compared them with concentrations in the opposite non-perfused joints which served as controls (Price et al., 1996b). There was a marked reduction in the concentration of collagen, heparan sulphate and chondroitin sulphate, but the concentration of hyaluronan remained unchanged at high intra-articular pressure. When the whole tissue concentrations were extrapolated to give the concentrations in the interstitium, that for collagen was 53% of the control synovium, chondroitin-4- and 6-sulphate were 60% and 52%, respectively, and heparan sulphate was 53%. Collagen is fixed in tissues and essentially insoluble. Thus the marked reduction in its concentration in the synovial interstitium at high intra-articular pressure indicates that an increase in hydration of the interstitium occurs under these conditions. This proposal is supported by the observation that the reduction in GAG concentrations are very similar to that of collagen. The fall in collagen concentration equates to an interstitial volume increase of 1.9 times at an intra-articular pressure of 25 cm H_2O. The 0.54-fold decrease in sulphated GAG concentration would result in a 2.8–4.2-fold rise in hydraulic conductivity and is able to account for the observed increase in conductivity (Price et al., 1996b).

In contrast to sulphated GAGs and collagen, the concentration of hyaluronan in the synovium remains virtually unchanged after increasing the intra-articular pressure (Price et al., 1996b). If there is an increase in interstitial volume under these conditions, as proposed above, the hyaluronan concentration must be maintained by a concurrent increase in its synthesis by the B-type synoviocytes. Since we know the volume expansion of the interstitium (i.e. 1.0 ml to 1.9 ml) and the hyaluronan concentration in the expanded interstitium (0.53 mg.ml^{-1}), we can calculate the rate of hyaluronan synthesis in vivo required to achieve this. This is ~91 µg hyaluronan per hour per ml of synovial interstitium. This calculation does not take account of any hyaluronan leaching out of the synovium during the experiment, so it may be an underestimate. Moreover, hyaluronan synthesis may occur at a much higher level at raised intra-articular pressure than it does at normal pressure Nevertheless, it is noteworthy that a synthetic rate of 91 µg.h^{-1}.ml^{-1} would replace the total mass of hyaluronan in the synovium within 3.6 hours! The significance of this and the signalling mechanism by which the B-type synoviocytes respond to raised pressure are unknown, and are interesting questions.

BIOCHEMISTRY OF THE SYNOVIAL FLUID

The biochemistry of the synovial fluid has received much attention from researchers (see Levick *et al.*, 1996; Balazs, 1982; Levick, 1987b, 1989 for a selection of reviews on this topic). Thus its composition and function will be summarised only briefly here. There is only a small volume of the fluid in normal joint cavities, for example about 1.0 ml in the human knee joint and 0.05 ml in the rabbit knee joint. The composition of the fluid reflects the fact that it is an ultrafiltrate of plasma which passes across the walls of the capillaries in the synovial intima, through the interstitium of the synovium and into the joint cavity. Thus the concentration of electrolytes and small solutes such as urea is the same in plasma and synovial fluid. The concentration of glucose is lower than that of plasma since it is utilised by the articular cartilage chondrocytes. Plasma proteins are present, but at a much lower concentration in the synovial fluid due to the sieving action of the synovial capillary walls. Albumin is the most prominent plasma protein in the synovial fluid and is the main contributor of colloid osmotic pressure (Table 16.2).

Synovial fluid also contains molecules secreted from B-type synoviocytes, notably hyaluronan and lubricin. These are of key importance for one of the main functions of the fluid, which is to act as a lubricant of the joint surfaces. Hyaluronan may also contribute to the hydraulic resistance of the synovial intima by forming a thin film over it. The other main function of the synovial fluid is to act as a medium for the transport of nutrient molecules, and oxygen from the blood to the cartilage and of metabolites from the cartilage out of the joint (Figure 16.1).

Hyaluronan is an unusual macromolecule. It is a linear non-sulphated GAG chain of great length. Using a TSK G6000 PW_{XL} HPLC column which had been calibrated with well-characterised hyaluronan standards, we found the molecular weight of rabbit synovial fluid hyaluronan to be 2.95×10^6 Daltons, with a range of $2.35–3.69 \times 10^6$ Daltons

TABLE 16.2
Synovial fluid composition.

Component	Synovial fluid	Plasma	Species
Na$^+$ (mM)	145	156	Cow
Cl$^-$ (mM)	111	110	Cow
Urea (mg/100 ml)	8.2	8.5	Cow
Glucose (mg/100 ml)	66	91	Cow
Protein (g/100 ml)	1.90	6.77	Human
Albumin (g/100 ml)	1.20	3.27	Human
Hyaluronan (g/100 ml)	0.2–0.4	4.2×10^{-6}	Human
Lubricin (g/100 ml)	0.005	?	Cow
Volume (ml)	1.0		Human
	0.05		Rabbit

(95% confidence interval). Hyaluronan is the main GAG synthesized by normal synovio-cytes in culture (Clarris et al., 1984). Cytochemical evidence indicates that it is a product of B-type synoviocytes (Wilkinson et al., 1992). Any hyaluronan detected in A-type synoviocytes is likely to be the result of phagocytosis of synovial fluid by those cells. Unlike other GAGs, hyaluronan is not synthesized on a protein core (Mason et al., 1982). Rather it is polymerised by addition of UDP-sugars to the non-reducing end of the chain. The enzyme responsible for this, hyaluronan synthase, is located at the plasma membrane and the growing chain is directly extruded into the extracellular compartment (Prehm, 1989).

Hyaluronan is extremely viscous (Balazs and Denlinger, 1985). Synovial fluid forms a thin viscous film over the surface of the synovium and articular cartilage in the joint space, and at low shear rates this provides an effective hydrodynamic lubricant (Radin et al., 1971; McCutcheon, 1978). However, hyaluronan is not an effective lubricant at high loads. Here, the 225 kDa glycoprotein, lubricin, has an important role (Swann, 1982). It is noteworthy that there is still no comprehensive theory to explain the lubrication of joints under all operating conditions (Mow et al., 1993).

Synovial fluid undergoes continual turnover by trans-synovial flow into synovial lymph vessels, estimated at about $2-4\,\mu l.h^{-1}.cm^2$ synovium in normal human and rabbit knees (Levick, 1987b). As a result, water and protein in the synovial fluid are replaced within a period of 2 h or less. The turnover time for hyaluronan appears to be consider-ably longer (Knox et al., 1988). In recent experiments we have washed out the rabbit knee joint exhaustively with repeated injections of Ringer solution. This allowed measurements of the total hyaluronan present in the joint ($182\pm9.9\,\mu g$) and, knowing the hyaluronan concentration in the synovial fluid ($3.6\,mg.ml^{-1}$), calculation of the total fluid volume ($50\,\mu l$). The replacement rate of hyaluronan into the joint over the subsequent 4 hours depended on whether it was left "dry", or was expanded by injection of a 2 ml bolus of Ringer solution. Hyaluronan secretion into "dry" joints was $4.80\pm0.77\,\mu g.h^{-1}$, but was significantly higher ($p=0.011$) into expanded joints, $5.80\pm0.84\,\mu g.h^{-1}$ ($n=5$). These secretion rates are equivalent to a complete replacement of synovial fluid hyaluro-nan in 38 h in the dry joint and 31 h in the expanded joint. No significant differences were found in the molecular weight of the hyaluronan synthesized in the two joint conditions. However, if circulatory arrest was induced and the joint treated with the metabolic poisons, sodium iodoacetate and sodium azide, no hyaluronan secretion occurred into the joint. These experiments demonstrate clearly that synovial fluid hyaluronan is synthesized and secreted by an active process and is not due to passive leaching of synovial intima hyaluronan into the joint space.

SYNOVIAL FLUID MARKERS OF JOINT DISEASE ACTIVITY

Products released from articular cartilage appear in the synovial fluid and leave the joint space by diffusing through the synovial intimal interstitium, as show in Figure 16.1. Synovial fluid can be sampled readily by the rheumatologist in the clinic. Thus a consid-erable effort has been made to determine whether the concentration or composition of synovial fluid molecules originating from the cartilage can serve as markers for disease activity (Lohmander *et al.*, 1995). Rigorous interpretation of such measurements requires an understanding of the rate of synovial fluid volume turnover in the joint as well as of the rate of marker input into it. These points are addressed in the following chapter by Levick *et al.* (1998).

CONCLUDING REMARKS

Ultrastructural and morphometric analysis enabled the synovial interstitial matrix and extrafibrillar volumes to be measured. Thus it was possible to calculate the effective hydrodynamic concentrations of GAGs in the extrafibrillar space of the synovium. The total GAG concentration is insufficient to account for the observed synovial hydraulic conductance, inferring that other macromolecules present must make an important contribution to the conductance. Measurements indicate that non-collagenous proteins are present in sufficient amount in the synovium to fulfil this role.

Perfusion at raised intra-articular pressure leads to increased hydration of synovial interstitial matrix. The effective concentration of sulphated GAGs in the extrafibrillar space falls, easily accounting for the observed increase in synovial conductance. However the concentration of hyaluronan in the interstitium is maintained, indicating increased synthesis of this GAG by the synoviocytes in the perfused joint. Finally, secretion of hyaluronan into the synovial fluid is an active process and its rate depends on the joint state.

ACKNOWLEDGEMENT

We are grateful to the Wellcome Trust for financial support.

REFERENCES

Ashhurst, D.E., Bland, Y.S. and Levick, J.R. (1991) Immunohistochemical study of the collagens of the rabbit synovial interstitium. *J. Rheumatol.*, **18**, 1669–1672.
Balazs, E.A. (1982) The physical properties of synovial fluid and the special role of hyaluronic acid. In: *Disorders of the Knee* (Helfet, A.J. Ed.,) pp. 61–75. Philadelphia: Lippincott.
Balazs, E.A. and Denlinger, J.L. (1985) Sodium hyaluronate and joint function. *J. Equine. Vet. Sci.*, **5**, 217–228.
Bidanset, D.J., Guidry, C., Rosenberg , L.C., Choi, H.U., Timpl, R. and Hook, M. (1992) Binding of the proteoglycan decorin to collagen type VI. *J. Biol. Chem.*, **267**, 5250–5256.
Caterson, B, Christner, J.E. and Baker, J.R. (1983) Identification of a monoclonal antibody that specifically recognizes corneal and skeletal keratan sulphate. *J. Biol. Chem.*, **258**, 8848–8854.
Clarris, B.J., Fraser, J.R.E., Muirden, K.D., Malcolm, L.P., Holmes, M.W.A. and Rogers, K. (1984) Stimulation of glycosaminoglycan production and lysosomal activity of human synovial cells in culture by low environmental pH. *Ann. Rheum. Dis.*, **43**, 313–319.
Edlund, T. (1949) Studies on the absorption of colloids and fluid from rabbit knee joints. *Acta Physiol. Scand.*, **18**, suppl. 62, 1–108.
Fosang, A.J., Hey, N.J., Carney, S.L. and Hardingham, T.E. (1990) An ELISA plate based assay for hyaluronan using biotinylated proteoglycan G1 domain (HA binding region). *Matrix*, **10**, 306–313.

Gaffen, J.D., Price, F.M., Bayliss, M.T. and Mason, R.M. (1994) A ruthenium103 red dot blot assay specific for nanogram quantities of sulfated glycosaminoglycans. *Anal. Biochem.*, **217**, 1–7.

Henderson, K.J., Pitsillides, A.A., Edwards, J.C.W. and Worrall, J.G. (1993) Reduced expression of CD44 in rheumatoid synovial cells. *Br. J. Rheumatol.*, **32**, suppl. 1, 25.

Kielty, C.M., Whittaker, S.P., Grant, M.E. and Shuttleworth, C.A. (1992) Type VI collagen microfibrils: evidence for a structural association with hyaluronan. *J. Cell Biol.*, **118**, 979–990.

Knox, P., Levick, J.R. and McDonald, J.N. (1988) Synovial fluid – its mass, macromolecular content and pressure in major limb joints of the rabbit. *Q. J. Exp. Physiol.*, **73**, 33–46.

Levick, J.R. (1987a) Flow through interstitium and other fibrous matrices. *Q. J. Exp. Physiol.*, **72**, 409–438.

Levick, J.R. (1987b) Synovial fluid and trans-synovial flow in stationary and moving joints. In: *Joint Loading: Biology and Health of Articular Structures*, (Helminen, H., Kiviranta, I., Tammi, M., Saamaren, A.K., Paukonnen, K. and Jurvelin, J., Ed) pp. 149–186. Bristol: Wright & Sons.

Levick, J.R. (1989) Synovial fluid exchange – a case of flow through fibrous mats. *News in Physiol. Sci.*, **4**, 198–202.

Levick, J.R. (1994) An analysis of the interaction between extravascular plasma protein, interstitial flow and capillary filtration; application to synovium. *Microvasc. Res.*, **47**, 90–125.

Levick, J.R. and McDonald, J.N. (1989) Ultrastructure of transport pathways in stressed synovium of the knee in anaesthetized rabbits. *J. Physiol.*, **419**, 493–508.

Levick, J.R. and McDonald, J.N. (1990) The microfibrillar meshwork of the synovial lining and associated broad-banded collagen – a clue to identity. *Ann. Rheum. Dis.*, **49**, 31–36.

Levick, J.R., Mason, R.M., Coleman, P.J. and Scott, D. (1998) Physiology of synovial fluid and trans-synovial flow. Chapter 15, this volume.

Levick, J.R., Price, F.M. and Mason, R.M. (1996) Synovial matrix-synovial fluid systems of joints. In: *Extracellular matrix, Volume 1: Tissue Function*, (Comper W. Ed) pp. 328–377. Harwood Academic Publishers.

Linck, G., Stocker, S., Grimaud, J.A. and Porte, A. (1983) Distribution of immunoreactive fibronectin and collagen (type I, III, IV) in mouse joints. *Histochemistry*, **77**, 323–328.

Lohmander, S., Saxne, T. and Heinegård, D. (1995) (eds) Molecular Markers for Joint and Skeletal Diseases. *Acta Orthopaed. Scand.*, **66**, suppl. 266.

Mason, R.M., d'Arville, C., Kimura, J.H. and Hascall, V.C. (1982) Absence of covalently linked core protein from newly synthesized hyaluronate. *Biochem. J.*, **207**, 445–457.

McCutcheon, C.W. (1978) Lubrication of Joints. In: *The Joints and Synovial Flow*, (Sokoloff L., Ed) pp. 4348–477. New York: Academic Press.

Mow, V.C., Ateshian, G.A. and Spilker, R.L. (1993) Biomechanics of diarthrodial joints: A review of twenty years of progress. *J. Biomech. Eng.*, **115**, 460–467.

Okada, Y., Naka, K., Minamoto, T., Ueda, Y., Oda, Y., Nakanishi, I. and Timpl, R. (1990) Localization of type VI collagen in the lining cell layer of normal and rheumatoid synovium. *Lab. Invest.*, **63**, 647–656.

Pitsillides, A.A., Wilkinson, L.S., Mehdizadeh, S., Bayliss, M.T. and Edwards, J.C.W. (1993) Demonstration of uridine diphosphoglucose dehydrogenase activity in normal and rheumatoid synovial lining cells. *Int. J. Exp. Pathol.*, **74**, 27–34.

Pollock, L.E., Lalor, P. and Revell, P.A. (1990) Type IV collagen and laminin in the synovial intimal layer: an immunohistochemical study. *Rheumatol. Int.*, **9**, 227–280.

Prehm, P. (1989) Identification and regulation of the eukaryotic hyaluronate synthase. In: *The Biology of Hyaluronan. Ciba Foundation Symposium*, **143**, Wiley: Chichester, pp. 21–40.

Price, F.M., Levick, J.R. and Mason, R.M. (1994) Quantification and localisation of the glycosaminoglycans of rabbit synovium. *Int. J. Exp. Pathol.*, **75**, A27.

Price, F.M., Levick, J.R. and Mason, R.M. (1996a) Changes in glycosaminoglycan concentration and synovial permeability at raised intra-articular pressure in rabbit knees. *J. Physiol.*, **495**, 821–833.

Price, F.M., Levick, J.R. and Mason, R.M. (1996b) Glycosaminoglycan concentration in synovium and other tissues of rabbit knee in relation to synovial hydraulic resistance. *J. Physiol.*, **495**, 803–820.

Price, F.M., Mason, R.M. and Levick, J.R. (1995) Radial organization of interstitial exchange pathway and influence of collagen in synovium. *Biophys. J.*, **69**, 1429–1439.

Radin, E.L., Paul, I.L., Swann, D.A. and Schottstaedt, E.S. (1971) Lubrication of synovial membrane. *Ann Rheum. Dis.*, **30**, 322–325.

Scott, D.L., Salmon, M., Morris, C.J., Wainwright, A.C. and Walton, K.W. (1984) Laminin and vascular proliferation in rheumatoid arthritis. *Ann. Rheum. Dis.*, **43**, 551–555.

Stevens, C.R., Blake, D.R., Merry, P., Revell, P.A. and Levick, J.R. (1991) A comparative study by morphometry of the microvasculature in normal and rheumatoid synovium. *Arthritis. Rheum.*, **34**, 1508–1513.

Swann, D.A. (1982) Structure and function of lubricin, the glycoprotein responsible for the boundary lubrication of articular cartilage. In: *Articular Synovium*, (Franchimont P., Ed) pp. 45–58. Karger: Basel.

Wilkinson, L.S., Pitsillides, A.A., Worrall, J.G. and Edwards, J.C.W. (1992) Light microscopic characteristics of the fibroblast-like synovial intimal cell (synoviocyte). *Arthritis. Rheum.*, **35**, 1179–1184.

Wolf, J. and Carsons, S. (1991) Distribution of type VI collagen expression in synovial tissue and cultured synoviocytes: relation to fibronectin expression. *Ann. Rheum. Dis.*, **50**, 493–496.

Worrall, J.G., Bayliss, M.T. and Edwards, J.C.W. (1991) Morphological localization of hyaluronan in normal and diseased synovium. *J. Rheumatol.*, **18**, 1466–1472.

Worrall, J.G., Wilkinson, L.S., Bayliss, M.T. and Edwards, J.C.W. (1992) Synovial expression of the chondroitin sulphate proteoglycans decorin and biglycan. *Br. J. Rheumatol.*, **31**, suppl. 2, 68.

Section 4
The Joint Capsule –
Tendons and Ligaments

17 Cell and Matrix Organisation in Tendons and Ligaments

J.R. Ralphs and M. Benjamin

Connective Tissue Biology Laboratory, School of Molecular and Medical Biosciences, University of Wales Cardiff, PO Box 911, Cardiff CF1 3US, United Kingdom

Tendons and ligaments are classified histologically as regular dense fibrous connective tissues – they contain many more-or-less parallel bundles of collagen fibres giving them great tensile strength. They are critical to, and often intrinsic parts of, synovial joints (Ralphs and Benjamin, 1994). Generally, tendons transfer the pull of mucles to bone, producing movement at a synovial joint. Conversely, ligaments restrict and control movements of synovial joints. Tendons sometimes form integral parts of the joint capsule – in the digits, they form the dorsal parts of the capsule of the interphalangeal joints; the patellar tendon forms the anterior part of the knee joint capsule; the rotator cuff tendons form and support the shoulder joint. Ligaments may be also intrinsic parts of the joint capsule (e.g. collateral ligaments of the finger joints) or may be positioned outside the capsule (lateral collateral ligament of the knee) or within the boundaries of the capsule (cruciate ligaments of the knee). The capsule and its associated ligaments or tendons is just as important as the articular surfaces in joint function and, in many cases, in joint pathology – e.g. damage to cruciate ligaments leading to osteoarthritis in the knee, capsule weakening leading to finger deformity in rheumatoid arthritis (Louis, 1987), bone deposition in ankylosing spondylitis (Resnick and Niwayama, 1981) and many others. In this review we concentrate mostly on tendons, as this is where most of our research has been performed.

ANATOMICAL ORGANISATION

Tendons are usually rounded or oval in cross section, but can be in the form of flattened sheets, in which case they are known as aponeuroses. Whilst the basic organisation of tendons linking a muscle to bone is well known, there are a number of variations in the relationship between muscle, tendon and bone. Not all muscles have tendons; those that do contract and make bones change their relative angles at a joint (Jones, 1941). Where there is no change in angle and the muscle pull is perfectly straight, the muscle attaches directly to the periosteum with no tendon. Tendons may link two muscle bellies, for example in the digastric muscles of the lower jaw, or may occur within a muscle, splitting the muscle belly up into small sections; a single muscle may have several tendons, allowing it to act on several bones, for example in the actions of tibialis posterior in the foot; alternatively a single tendon may focus the actions of two or more muscles onto a single bone, for example the Achilles tendon acting on the calcaneus. Tendons also allow muscles to be remote from the sites at which they act. This is necessary where there is insufficient space for the necessary muscle bulk and where the muscle pull has to pass through a confined space – a good example being the major muscles that move the fingers – the bulky muscle bellies are in the forearm, long tendons extend from them, pass through confined spaces at the wrist, and fan out to enter the individual fingers. Tendons also give the opportunity of changing the direction of pull of a muscle, wrapping around bony or ligamentous pulleys – muscle bellies cannot tolerate being pressed against such pulleys – for example the tendons wrapping around the malleoli of the ankle. It is important to realise that the tendon is part of the integrated muscle–tendon unit. The relative amount of non-contractile tendon and contractile muscle within a muscle–tendon unit will determine the extent of contraction of the unit – the greater the length of muscle relative to tendon, the greater proportionate contraction is possible. Also, the tendon itself is important to the mechanical properties of the muscle–tendon unit. Tendons have a limited, but important ability to stretch which allows them to act as energy stores in locomotion – their stretch and recoil results in less energy being required for movement. The importance of this can be seen in the Achilles tendon, where 17–34% of the total work done by the calf muscles is stored in the Achilles tendon during jumping exercises (Fukashiro et al., 1995). The extent of stretching of tendons varies – in the wrist, the tendon of flexor carpi ulnaris lengthens by 3.7% at maximum load, whereas that of extensor carpi radialis longus stretches by just 1.7% (Loren and Lieber, 1995). The Achilles tendon is highly compliant, with elongation to failure being approximately 16% (Nakagawa et al., 1996). These results show that there is subtle matching of physical characteristics of tendons to function in different muscle–tendon units, and clearly demonstrate that one tendon is not necessarily like another. The basis for such differences must lie in the precise anatomical, histological and biochemical organisation of the tendon and its extracellular matrix (ECM).

HISTOLOGICAL ORGANISATION

Tendons and ligaments are made up of fibroblasts arranged in rows lying between longitudinally oriented bundles of collagen fibrils. In conventional histology of tendons, the fibroblasts appear elongate in longitudinal section and stellate in transverse section. As we will show later, the cells have a very complex interconnected morphology which relates to the way in which the extracellular matrix was deposited (see Birk and Zycband,

1994) and to a probable cell to cell communicating network in certain adult tendons (McNeilly *et al.*, 1996).

At a higher level of structure, bundles of cells and collagen fibres are grouped into small, usually microscopic, fascicles (Figures 17.1, 17.2). Depending on the tendon, the microscopic fascicles may be assembled into larger, macroscopic fascicles which are bundled together to form the tendon or ligament, or, particularly in smaller tendons, the microscopic fascicles may make up the whole structure. There may be just a single fasicle, or up to several hundred fascicles making up the whole tendon. Macroscopic fascicles often

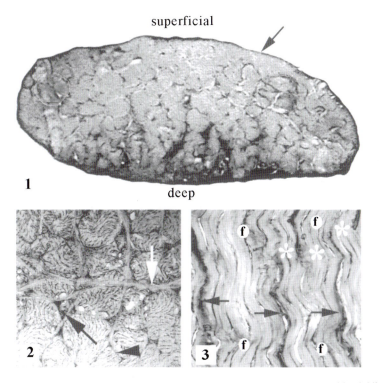

FIGURES 17.1–17.3   Histology of adult chicken digital flexor tendon; sections stained with toluidine blue.

1   Low power view of transverse section. The tendon is bounded by the epitenon (arrow) and the main body of the tendon is divided into approximately 120 rounded microscopic fascicles separated by endotenon. At its deep surface, this part of the tendon is pressed against the bone of the digit and is fibrocartilaginous – hence the section appears darker, with toluidine blue metachromasia indicating the presence of large quantities of glycosaminoglycans, towards the deep surface. ×30.

2   Medium power view of transverse section. Fasicles (f) can be seen as rounded structures containing transversely sectioned tendon cells and bounded by epitenon (arrows). This takes various forms – in some positions it is a very thin film (arrowhead); in others it contains prominent collagen fibres running across, rather than along, the tendon (white arrow), giving lateral reinforcement; finally it may appear as strongly metachromatic fibrocartilaginous material acting as a space filler between fascicles (black arrow). The latter is particularly prominent where the tendon has fibrocartilage on its deep surface. ×120.

3   Medium power view of longitudinal section. Fasicles (f) can be seen running longitudinally between dark streaks of endotenon (arrows). The fascicles are open ended, so that fibres from one fascicle enter 2 or more fascicles longitudinally (asterisks). ×120.

spiral along the length of the tendon, for example in human Achilles, patellar and finger flexor tendons (Barfred, 1973; Semple, 1980; Amiel et al., 1995). In flexor tendons from chicken toes, there are no macroscopic fascicles but in excess of 100 microscopic fascicles may be seen in transverse sections (Figure 17.1; McNeilly, 1996). In the rat tendons we have examined, there is no obvious fasicular organisation at all (McNeilly et al., 1996).

There is some confusion as to the precise histological terminology used to describe the fasicular structure, and here we outline the terminology we favour and will use in this review (see also Figure 17.1). The whole tendon is bounded by the *epitenon*, which is of variable thickness. Cells of the epitenon tend to be rather flatter than those of the tendon proper, and produce an extracellular matrix containing interwoven, rather than parallel, collagen fibres. We regard the connective tissue enclosing fascicles as the *endotenon*. It is loose connective tissue organised radially around fascicles and brings blood vessels and nerves in to the tendon; it can occur in single fasicle tendons simply as a wrapping of blood vessels amongst the tendon fibres.

In longitudinal sections of chicken digital flexor tendons, microscopic fascicles do not extend the length of the tendon, but are relatively short and open ended, with collagen fibres from the open ends entering other fascicles along the tendon; the fascicles are laterally staggered so that fibrils from one fasicle enter two or more others (Figure 17.3). Functionally, the macroscopic fascicles may allow some sliding relative to one another and give flexibility to the tendon. They may also allow distribution of force across a tendon. The organisation of smaller fascicles means that there is a continuity and interconnection of collagen fibre bundles throughout the tendon (or the macroscopic fasicle bundle) that probably spreads muscle pull across the whole structure and reduces the tendency for microtearing due to uneven loading.

At some sites there are further structures associated with the tendon. The tendon sheath is a synovial sheath enclosing tendons where they undergo considerable changes in direction or run through a confined space, allowing free movement (e.g. tendons at the wrist and the ankle). The *paratenon* is a specialisation of the loose connective tissues that tendons often pass through (e.g. the tendons in the forearm, or the Achilles tendon).

SPECIALISED STRUCTURES WITHIN TENDONS

Where tendons change direction around bony or fibrous pulleys, they experience compressive as well as tensile loads and often change their characteristics and become fibrocartilaginous. These have been the subject of considerable biochemical study, and have been shown to contain molecules typical of cartilage as well as of tendon – thus in addition to their usual components they contain elevated levels of the large proteoglycan aggrecan, which confers the ability to resist compression, and in some cases the collagen typical of cartilage, type II collagen (Vogel and Koob, 1989; Benjamin and Ralphs, 1995; see also Vogel, this volume). Tendons compressed *in vitro*, or surgically translocated around a bony pulley, develop fibrocartilage; conversely, if tendons that wrap around bony pulleys are surgically translocated away from them, they tend to lose their fibrocartilaginous nature (Ploetz, 1938; Gillard, 1979; Malaviya et al., 1996). In a study of human wrap-around tendons, we demonstrated that there were considerable differences in the extent of fibrocartilaginous differentiation in different tendons or in the same tendon associated with different pulleys (Benjamin *et al.*, 1995). The greatest extent of fibrocartilaginous differentiation has highly metachromatic ECM (indicative of high glycosaminoglycan content) with a basketweave arrangement of collagen fibres and large rounded fibrocartilage cells, in the tendon proper, the epitenon and the endotenon. The least extent of differentiation shows weakly metachromatic extracellular matrix, parallel collagen fibres and elongate cells that are only marginally plumper that pure tendon cells. There is a graded range of appearance between these two extremes. In some cases, fibro-cartilage differentiation is restricted to particular tendon components – thus the fibro-cartilage may only be in the epitenon, or the endotenon (see Figure 17.2). The extent of differentiation must reflect the magnitude of the compressive load experienced by the tendon, and has a number of components. These relate to the power of the muscle, the change in angle of the tendon around the pulley, the precise biomechanical characteristics of the tendon itself (see above) and the nature of the pulley – tendons wrapping around bony pulleys are more fibrocartilaginous than those wrapping around fibrous pulleys (Benjamin *et al.*, 1995).

Tendons and ligaments generally also contain fibrocartilage at their attachments to bone – the enthesis. Structurally, cells in the enthesis fibrocartilage become rounded, and the fibre orientation remains more or less parallel, with some splaying out towards the bony attachment (Benjamin and Ralphs, 1995). The functions of fibrocartilage in wrap around tendons is clear, in resisting compression against the pulley. Fibrocartilage at the enthesis also probably has a compression resisting component, as secondary compressive stresses build up in the tendon as it approaches the non-compliant bony interface. Angular motion of the tendon or ligament relative to the bone is also important, as where there is a large relative change in angle there is a large quantity of fibrocartilage, and where there is a small change a small quantity. These and other functions of the enthesis are discussed in Benjamin and Ralphs elsewhere in this volume.

There have been few developmental studies of tendon fibrocartilage, but there are at least two possible developmental origins which relate to the structural types outlined above. Fibrocartilage can develop from a cell population at the periphery of the tendon, which is probably the developing epitenon, or by metaplasia of the tendon cells them-selves (Evanko and Vogel, 1990; Ralphs *et al.*, 1992; Rufai *et al.*, 1992). In either case, development appears to be triggered by onset of movement of the animal, increasing load on the tendon (Ralphs *et al.*, 1992). Enthesial fibrocartilage initially develops from rem-nants of the embryonic cartilage of the bone rudiment, but with continued growth forms by metaplasia of tendon or ligament cells (Ralphs *et al.*, 1992; Rufai *et al.*, 1992; Gao *et al.*, 1996), again probably driven by forces exerted on the tendon during locomotion.

The extent to which fibrocartilage formation is pre-programmed developmentally, is unclear. One feature of highly developed fibrocartilage is the high degree of organisation of the collagen fibres of the ECM. As already indicated above, in tendon fibrocartilage this is the formation of a complex basketweave of collagen fibres in the fibrocartilages. It is relatively easy to envisage how simpler forms of fibrocartilage, i.e those with more-or less parallel fibre bundles, can form simply in response to compressive load – the cells start to make a new set of ECM molecules. It is harder to envisage how cells might dismantle a parallel arangement of fibres and reform a basketweave arrangement whilst still under load. The extent to which tendons can structurally remodel is unclear at present. It could be that the interwoven structure is preformed in early development at the same time as the parallel arrangement of the pure tendon is formed, giving a pre-formed fibrous organisation which subsequently differentiates into fibrocartilage under load.

BIOCHEMICAL COMPOSITION OF THE ECM

The major component of tendon and ligament ECM is collagen, predominently type I collagen. Smaller quantities of types III, V and VI are present (Benjamin and Ralphs, 1995; Waggett et al., 1996). In specialised regions of tendons and ligaments other collagens may be present, notably type II collagen where they wrap around bony pulleys and are fibrocartilaginous or types II and X collagen in the fibrocartilage at the attachment to bone; the amount of type II collagen, in particular, appears to increase with age and probably load at both sites (Benjamin et al., 1991a; Rufai et al., 1992; Koch and Tillmann, 1995). The presence of type X collagen probably relates to the formation of the sequence of tissue at an enthesis – the tendon runs into fibrocartilage, which then calcifies before it reaches the bone surface. The fibrocartilage and calcified fibrocartilage are dynamic in nature, may vary according to load and are of considerable importance in early growth of bones, at least in epiphyseal attachments (Evans et al., 1990; Benjamin et al., 1991b; Ralphs et al., 1992; Gao et al., 1996). For a more detailed discussion, see Benjamin and Ralphs, this volume.

Tendons have a considerable water content, which is mostly associated with glycosaminoglycans (GAGs) on proteoglycans. Tensional regions of tendons or ligaments contain the large proteoglycan versican and small quantities of aggrecan which lacks the G1 domain of the core protein in comparison with cartilage aggrecan (Campbell et al., 1996; Vogel et al., 1994). They also contain the small leucine rich proteoglycans lumican, fibromodulin and decorin (Roughley and Lee, 1994; Waggett et al., 1997), which are thought to be important in controlling collagen fibrillogenesis. In comparison, compressive regions and enthesial fibrocartilage are rich in aggrecan, which by analogy with articular cartilage confers compression resistance. The predominant small proteoglycan is biglycan, although the significance of this is not known (Vogel, 1995).

CELL ORGANISATION IN TENDONS AND LIGAMENTS

Tendon and ligament cells have attracted relatively little interest; most work has concentrated on the extracellular matrix, as this accounts for the mechanical properties of the tendon. However, it is important to recognise that, as in any other connective tissue, the cells make and maintain the extracellular matrix, which then performs the functions of the tissue. It is well known that tendon cells modify the ECM according to the load they experience. Immobilisation of tendons, experimentally or as part of treatment for other injuries, leads to depletion of the ECM and substantial weakening; remobilisation eventually results in regaining of strength (reviewed by Amiel *et al.*, 1995). Also, tendons respond to the type of load they experience – under compressive loads, such as where they change direction around bones, tendon cells synthesise ECM components more typical of cartilage, to form fibrocartilage (see above). Thus tendon cells sense the type and magnitude of loads they experience and coordinate an appropriate response to those stimuli.

Recently, we have made studies on the 3D shape of tendon cells that enable us to take new approaches to understanding tendon cell behaviour, and indeed fibrous connective tissue cell behavior, in general (Ralphs *et al.*, 1996; McNeilly *et al.*, 1996). Using fluorescent membrane dyes (Dil and $DiOC_7$), immunolabelling and confocal microscopy we have discovered the following. Firstly, tendon cells have complex, interconnected morphology. An individual tendon cell has elaborate cell processes not readily appreciated using conventional methodology (Figure 17.4). Laterally, cells send out broad flat cell processes which wrap around collagen fibre bundles and meet similar processes from laterally adjacent cells. Each cell has associations with around 5–9 collagen fibre bundles. Longitudinally, cells have long, thin processes which interact with cells anteriorly and posteriorly. There is, therefore, a 3D interconnected network of cell processes throughout a tendon, intimately associated with the extracellular matrix. There have been suggestions that tendon cells may be interconnected, based on ultrastructural studies (Senga *et al.*, 1995; Squier and Magnes, 1995; Tangi *et al.*, 1995), but the extent of cell/cell interactions described here has not been reported previously. Secondly, gap junctions occur on all cell processes where they meet and between cell bodies where they are next to one another in their longitudinal rows, as shown by immunolabelling for two of the gap junction proteins, connexin (cxn) 43 and cxn32. The 3D network of cell processes is therefore a communicating network (Figure 17.5). Thirdly, cxn43 and cxn32 occur at different contact points between tendon cells – cxn43 occurs between all cell processes and between cell bodies, whereas cxn32 only occurs between cell bodies – suggesting that there are 2 distinct junctional networks. This is supported by very recent studies where we have shown cxn43 junctions are largely absent in regions of tendons experiencing compressive loads, but cxn32 is to some extent retained (Gao *et al.*, 1997). In experimental *in vitro* systems, cxn43 and 32 can have very different communication characteristics, as shown by differing abilities to transfer molecular markers from cell to cell and in electrical connectivity and gating (e.g. Veenstra *et al.*, 1992; Elfgang *et al.*, 1995). We have also recently shown that knee ligament cells have similar structure and gap junctional connections to tendon cells (Benjamin and Ralphs, unpublished observations).

The discovery of a gap junctional network throughout tendons, which provides a mechanism that allows cells to couple electrically and biochemically, gives a new way of approaching the problem of how tendon cells sense and coordinate responses to load. For example, the effects of mobilisation on tendon maintenance, matrix modification and healing could be mediated by junctional communication. *In vitro* studies strongly suggest that junctional communication is important to tendon cells. Firstly, a single tendon cell in a confluent sheet propagates calcium transients to adjacent cells via an IP_3 dependant mechanism thought to involve gap junctions, in response to a mechanical stimulus (membrane deformation with a microelectrode; Banes *et al.*, 1995). Secondly, synthesis and phosphorylation of cxn43 is upregulated in tendon cells subjected to cyclical tensile

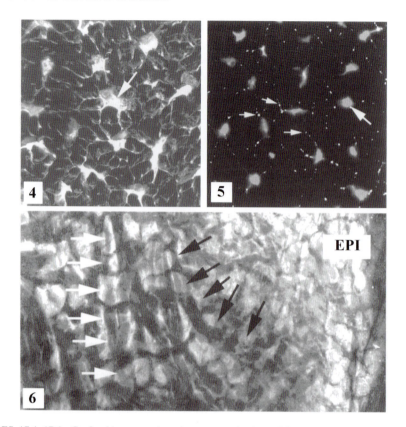

FIGURES 17.4–17.6   Confocal laser scanning microscope projections of fluorescently labelled tendon cells in rat digital flexor tendons. Images based on McNeilly *et al.* (1996).
4   Transverse cryosection stained with the fluorescent membrane dye DiI. Bright staining cell bodies send off flattened lateral cell processes that interact with similar processes from adjacent cells. The cell processes wrap up collagen fibre bundles, which appear in the image as dark spaces. The cell at centre (arrow) is associated with ca. 8 collagen fibre bundles. ×750.
5   Transverse cryosection immunolabelled for connexin 43 and counterstained with propidium iodide to show nuclei (large arrow). Gap junctions appear as bright foci of immunolabel (examples shown with small arrows) distributed on the interconnecting transverse cell processes. ×750.
6   Confocal optical section of whole mount preparation stained with DiI. Because of the curved shape of the specimen, the left part of the image is fairly deep within the tendon (40–50 μm from the surface) whereas as the image moves towards the right the tendon is sampled progressively closer to the surface. The extreme right hand part of the image is sampling the epitenon cells (epi), which form a covering for the tendon proper. In the deeper part of the tendon, dark spaces, representing collagen fibre bundles, pass from cell to cell longitudinally (left side row of white arrows indicates the cells), and are the major tensile load bearing structures. In the right hand side of the image, fibre bundles run obliquely just underneath the epitenon, forming a braided layer of collagen fibres at the periphery of the tendon; These fibre bundles are also passed from cell to cell (centre/right row of black arrows). ×600.

load *in vitro* (Banes *et al.*, 1995; see also Banes *et al.*, this volume). This result matches our observations on regional differences in connexin distribution in intact tendons – connexin 43 occurs in tensional regions but tends to disappear in compressive regions.

Taken together, the *in vivo* and *in vitro* results suggest that the transfer of information concerning mechanical deformation is likely to occur via gap junctions in tendons.

Indeed, the network of cytoplasmic processes could be a sensor for mechanical load, as one would expect deformation of cell processes with tendon movement. This is also thought to be the case in bone, where osteocyte cell processes interact through canaliculi, are linked by gap junctions and form a 3D network throughout the tissue (e.g. Jones *et al.*, 1993; Lanyon, 1993).

The organisation of cells in the tendon has important implications in development and organisation of the extracellular matrix. In whole mount preparations of rat digital flexor tendons, it has proved possible to use whole cell labelling techniques, allied to optical sectioning and 3D modelling using the confocal microscope, to examine cellular organisation at the tissue level (McNeilly *et al.*, 1996). Using this methodology, we showed that tendon cells, visible as brightly fluorescent structures, have non-fluorescent tracks corresponding to collagen fibre bundles running longitudinally through them (Figure 17.6). The tracks are passed from cell to cell along the tendon. At the periphery of the tendon, the tracks run oblique to the long axis of the tendon, representing the weave of fibres in the outermost part. Deeper in the tendon, the tracks run longitudinally, as the major load bearing components of the tendon. Thus many tendon cells are responsible for a given collagen fibre bundle along its length. In the deposition of their oriented matrices during development, cells use a series of three compartments to deposit oriented fibres Birk and Zycband, 1994). Firstly, 1–3 fibres form in narrow channels linked to the cell surface that originate deep in the cytoplasm. Secondly, these channels fuse together to form bundles of collagen fibres in close association with the cell surface. Thirdly, bundles become laterally associated to form macroaggregates, in a compartment defined by the apposition of 2–3 fibroblasts. In addition, we can define a fourth compartment. Our studies clearly demonstrate that fibre bundles, contained in the third compartment delineated by laterally adjacent cells, pass from cell to cell longitudinally in the tendon so that each fibre bundle is completely enclosed in wrappings of the fine sheet-like lateral cell processes. The fourth compartment, therefore, is that defined by longitudinal rows of cells associated with the same fibre bundle (McNeilly *et al.*, 1996). It is clearly important that cells must communicate to coordinate deposition and maintenance of the long collagen fibre bundles.

It seems likely that the initial organisation and interaction of cells is important in establishing the orientation of fibre bundles laid down cooperatively within the early tendon. Such cooperation would be necessary in laying down the parallel tensile fibres deep in the tendon, the "braided" arrangement of epitenon fibres peripherally, and the complex basketweave of fibres seen in the highly developed tendon fibrocartilages. It seems likely to us that this could mean that the most complex fibrocartilages are either developmentally pre-programmed, or certainly become established before there is any major onset of deposition of the organised tendon matrix. Certainly, early cell organisation is of key importance in development of fibrocartilage at other sites with high degrees of fibre organisation, for example in the formation of the annulus fibrosus of the intervertebral disc (Rufai *et al.*, 1995). In early development, tendon blastemas form independently of muscle (Milare, 1963; Shellswell and Wolpert, 1977; Kieny and Chevalier, 1979) but then require muscle activity to proceed to full development – in the absence of muscle the blastemas regress. Recently, cell–cell interactions have been implicated in early stages of tendon development, as Patel *et al.* (1996) have shown the expression of *Cek-8*, a cell to cell signalling receptor (a receptor tyrosine kinase) in early developing chick digital tendons. The receptor is present in tendon condensations and disappears in subsequent development. It may be that signalling via this receptor is important in initial organisation of cells to form the organised tendon blastemas, and that other signalling mechanisms, possibly involving mechanical signals from the muscle and gap junctional communication between presumptive tendon cells, take over with subsequent matrix deposition.

REFERENCES

Amiel, D., Chu, C.R. and Lee, J. (1995) Effect of loading on metabolism and repair of tendons and ligaments. In: *Repetitive motion disorders of the upper extremity* (Ed. S.L. Gordon, S.J. Blair and L.J. Fine), pp. 217–230. Rosemont, Illinois: American Academy of Orthopaedic Surgeons.

Banes, A.J., Hu, P., Xiao, H., Sanderson, M.J., Boitano, S., Brigman, B., Fischer, T., Tsuzaki, M., Brown, T.D., Almekinders, L.C. and Lawrence, W.T. (1995) Tendon cells of the epitenon and internal tendon compartment communicate mechanical signals through gap junctions and respond differentially to mechanical load and growth factors. In: *Repetitive motion disorders of the upper extremity* (Ed. S.L. Gordon, S.J. Blair and L.J. Fine), pp. 231–245. Rosemont, Illinois: American Academy of Orthopaedic Surgeons.

Barfred, T. (1973) Achilles tendon rupture. *Acta. Orthop. Scand. Suppl.*, **152**, 1–126.

Benjamin, M., Evans, E.J., Rao, R.D., Findlay, J.A. and Pemberton, D.J. (1991a) Quantitative differences in the histology of the attachment zones of the meniscal horns in the knee joint of man. *J. Anat.*, **177**, 127–134.

Benjamin, M., Tyers, R.N.S. and Ralphs, J.R. (1991b) Age-related changes in fibrocartilage of the rat quadriceps tendon. *J. Anat.*, **179**, 127–136.

Benjamin, M., Qin, S. and Ralphs, J.R. (1995) Fibrocartilage associated with human tendons and their pulleys. *J. Anat.*, **187**, 625–633.

Benjamin, M. and Ralphs, J.R. (1995) Functional and developmental anatomy of tendons and ligaments. In: *Repetitive Motion Disorders of the Upper Extremity* (Ed. S.L. Gordon, S.J. Blair and L.J. Fine), American Association of Orthopaedic Surgeons, Rosemont, Illinois, pp. 185–203.

Birk, D.E. and Zycband, E. (1994) Assembly of the tendon extracellular-matrix during development. *J. Anat.*, **184**, 457–463.

Campbell, M.A., Tester, A.M., Handley, C.J., Checkley, G.J., Chow, G.L., Cant, A.E., Winter, A.D. and Cain, W.E. (1996). Characterization of a large chondroitin sulfate proteoglycan present in bovine collateral ligament. *Arch. Biochem. Biophys.*, **329**, 181–190.

Elfgang, C., Eckert, R., Lichtenbergfrate, H., Butterweck, A., Traub, O., Klein, R.A., Hulser, D.F. and Willecke, K. (1995) Specific permeability and selective formation of gap junction channels in connexin-transfected HeLa cells. *J. Cell Biol.*, **129**, 805–817.

Evanko, S.P. and Vogel, K.G. (1990) Ultrastructure and proteoglycan composition in the developing fibrocartilaginous region of bovine tendon. *Matrix*, **10**, 420–436.

Evans, E.J., Benjamin, M. and Pemberton, D.J. (1990) Fibrocartilage in the attachment zones of the quadriceps tendon and patellar ligament of man. *J. Anat.*, **171**, 155–162.

Fukashiro, S., Komi, P.V., Järvinen, M. and Miyashita, M. (1995) *In vivo* Achilles tendon loading during jumping in humans. *Eur. J. Appl. Physiol. Occupat. Physiol.*, **71**, 453–458.

Gillard, G.C., Reilly, H.C., Bell-Booth, P.G. *et al.* (1979) The influence of mechanical forces on the glycosaminoglycan content of the rabbit flexor digitorum profundus tendon. *Conn. Tiss. Res.*, **7**, 37–46.

Gao, J., Messner, K., Ralphs, J.R. and Benjamin, M. (1996) An immunohistochemical study of enthesis development in the medial collateral ligament of the rat knee joint. *Anat. Embryol.*, **194**, 399–406.

Gao, J., Benjamin, M., Banes, A.J., Hill, B., Messner, K. and Ralphs, J.R. (1997) Regional differences in cell shape and gap junction expression in the Achilles tendon relate to fibrocartilage differentiation. *Trans. Orthop. Res. Soc.*, **22**, 449.

Jones, F.W. (1941) The principles of anatomy as seen in the hand. Bailliere, Tindall & Cox, London, pp. 283–297.

Jones, S.J., Gray, C., Sakamaki, H., Arora, M., Boyde, A. and Gourdie, R. (1993) The incidence and size of gap junctions between the bone cells in rat cavaria. *Anat. Embryol.*, **187**, 343–352.

Kieny, M. and Chevalier, A. (1979) Autonomy of tendon development in the embryonic chick wing. *J. Embryol. Exp. Morph.*, **49**, 153–165.

Koch, S. and Tillmann, B. (1995) The distal tendon of the biceps brachii. Structure and clinical correlations. *Ann. Anat.*, **177**, 467–474.

Lanyon, L.E. (1993) Osteocytes, strain detection, bone modeling and remodeling. *Calc. Tiss. Int.*, **53**, 102–107.

Loren, G.J. and Lieber, R.L. (1995) Tendon biomechanical properties enhance human wrist muscle specialization. *J. Biomech.*, **28**, 791–799.

Louis, D.S. (1987) Degenerative arthritis and allied conditions involving the interphalangeal joints. In: *The Interphalangeal Joints* (Ed. W.H. Bowers) pp. 142–155. Edinburgh: Churchill Livingstone.

Malaviya, P., Butler, D.L., Smith, F.N.L., Boivin, G.P., Vogel, K.G. and Quigley, S.D. (1996) Adaptive *in vivo* remodeling of the flexor tendon fibrocartilage-rich region in response to altered loading. *Trans. Orthop. Res. Soc.*, **21**, 4.

Milaire, J. (1963) Etude morpholoique et cytochimique du developpment des membres ches la souris et chez la taupe. *Arch. Biol.* (Liege) **74**, 129–317.

McNeilly, C.M. (1996) Structural studies on the interphalangeal joints of the toe and their associated tendons. PhD Thesis, University of Wales Cardiff, UK.

McNeilly, C.M., Banes, A.J., Benjamin, M. and Ralphs, J.R. (1996) Tendon cells *in vivo* form a three dimensional network of cell processes linked by gap junctions. *J. Anat.*, **189**, 593–600.

Nakagawa, Y., Hayashi, K., Yamamoto, N. and Nagashima, K. (1996) Age-related changes in biomechanical properties of the Achilles tendon in rabbits. *Europ. J. Appl. Physiol. Occupat. Physiol.*, **73**, 7–10.

Patel, K., Nittenberg, R., D'Souza, D., Irving, C., Burt, D., Wilkinson, D.G. and Tickle, C. (1996) Expression and regulation of *Cek-8*, a cell to cell signalling receptor in developing chick limb buds. *Development* **122**, 1147–1155.

Ploetz, E. (1938) Funktioneller bau und funktionelle anpassung der gleitsehnen. *Z. Orthop Ihre Grenzeb*, **67**, 212–234.

Ralphs, J.R., McNeilly, C.M., Hayes, A.J., Banes, A.J. and Benjamin, M. (1996) 3D modelling of tendon cell shape *in vivo* by confocal microscopy – cell–cell communication and the role of gap junctions. *Trans. Orth. Res. Soc.*, **21**, 5.

Ralphs, J.R. and Benjamin, M. (1994) The joint capsule: structure, composition, ageing and disease. *J. Anat.*, **184**, 503–509.

Ralphs, J.R., Tyers, R.N.S. and Benjamin, M (1992) Development of functionally distinct tendon fibrocartilages in the quadriceps tendon of the rat: the suprapatella and the attachment to the patella. *Anat. Embryol.*, **185**, 181–187.

Resnick, D. and Niwayama, G. (1981). Calcium pyrophosphate dihydrate (CPPD) crystal deposition disease. In: *Diagnosis of Bone and Joint Disorders*, Vol. 2 (Ed. D. Resnick and G. Niwayama), pp. 1521–1574. Philadelphia: WB Saunders.

Roughley, P.J. and Lee, E.R. (1994) Cartilage proteoglycans: structure and potential functions. *Microsc. Res. Tech.*, **28**, 385–397.

Rufai, A., Benjamin, M. and Ralphs, J.R. (1992) Development and ageing of phenotypically distinct fibrocartilages associated with the rat Achilles tendon. *Anat. Embryol.*, **186**, 611–618.

Rufai, A., Benjamin, M. and Ralphs, J.R. (1995) The development of fibrocartilage in the rat intervertebral disc. *Anat. Embryol.*, **192**, 53–62.

Semple, C. (1980) The design of tendons and their sheaths. In: *Scientific Foundations of Orthopaedics and Traumatology* (Owen, R., Goodfellow, J. and Bullough, P. Eds). Heinemann. London. pp. 74–78.

Senga, K., Kobayashi, M., Hattori, H., Yasue, K., Mizutani, H., Ueda, M. and Hoshino, T. (1995) Type VI collagen in mouse masseter tendon, from osseous attachment to myotendinous junction. *Anatomical Record*, **243**, 294–302.

Shellswell, G.B. and Wolpert, L. (1977) The pattern of muscle and tendon development in the chick wing. In: *Vertebrate Limb and Somite Morphogenesis* (Ede. D.A. Hinchliffe, J.R., Balls, M. Eds) Cambridge, MA: Cambridge University Press, pp. 71–86.

Squier, C.A. and Magnes, C. (1995) Spatial relationships between fibroblasts during the growth of rat tail tendon. *Cell and Tissue Research*, **234**, 17–29.

Tangi, K., Shimizu, T., Satou, T., Hashimoto, S. and Bonilla, E. (1995) Gap junctions between fibroblasts in rat myotendon. *Archives of Histology and Cytology*, **58**, 97–102.

Veenstra, R.D., Wang, H.Z., Westphale, E.M. and Beyer, E.C. (1992) Multiple connexins confer distinct regulatory and conductance properties of gap junctions in developing heart. *Circulation Research*, **71**, 1277–1283.

Vogel, K.G., Sandy, J.D., Pogany, G. and Robbins, J.R. (1994) Aggrecan in bovine tendon. *Matrix Biology*, **14**, 171–179.

Vogel, K.G. (1995) Fibrocartilage in tendon: a response to compressive load. In: *Repetitive Motion Disorders of the Upper Extremity* (Ed. S.L. Gordon, S.J. Blair and L.J. Fine), pp. 205–230. Rosemont, Illinois: American Academy of Orthopaedic Surgeons.

Vogel, K.G. and Koob, T.J. (1989) Structural specialisation in tendons under compression. *International Review of Cytology*, **115**, 267–293.

Waggett, A.D., Kwan, A.P.L., Woodnut, D.J., Rufai, A., Ralphs, J.R. and Benjamin, M. (1996) Collagens in fibrocartilages at the Achilles tendon insertion – a biochemical, molecular biological and immunohisto-chemical study. *Trans. Orthop. Res. Soc.*, **21**, 25.

Waggett, A.D., Kwan, A.P.L., Flannery, C.R., Woodnut, D.J., Rufai, A., Ralphs, J.R. and Benjamin, M. (1997) A biochemical molecular biological and immunohistochemical study of proteoglycans in fibrocartilages at the Achilles tendon insertion. *Trans. Orthop. Res. Soc.*, **22**, 451.

18 The Connexin 43 Gap Junction is a Mechanosensitive Gene in Avian Flexor Tendon Cells

A.J. Banes[1,*], G. Horesovsky[2], M. Tsuzaki[1], S. Boitano[3], W.T. Lawrence[4], T. Brown[5], P. Weinhold[1], C. Kenamond[1], M. Benjamin[6], J.R. Ralphs[6], C. McNeilly[6], J. Burt[7] and L. Miller[2]

[1]*Department of Orthopaedics, University of North Carolina, Chapel Hill, NC 27599-7055, USA;*
[2]*Molecular Pharmacology, GlaxoWellcome, Research Triangle Park, NC 27709, USA;*
[3]*Cell Biology and Anatomy, UCLA, Los Angeles, CA 90095-1361, USA;*
[4]*Department of Surgery, U. Massachusetts Medical Center, Worcester, MA 01655, USA;*
[5]*Orthopaedics Department, U. Iowa, Iowa City, IA 52242,USA;*
[6]*CTBL, Cardiff School of Biosciences, University of Wales Cardiff, Wales, UK;*
[7]*Physiology Department, University of Arizona, Tuscon, AZ 85721, USA;*

INTRODUCTION

Tendons are fibrous connective tissues designed to transmit the force of muscle contraction to bone to effect movement. They have a complex architecture: tendon is comprised of highly aligned matrix containing 70–80% type I collagen to provide tensile strength, 10–40% elastin yielding compliance and elasticity, proteoglycans as pulse dampeners, and lipids, especially in the tendon epitenon where they may reduce shear stress-induced friction (Oakes and Bialkower, 1977; Vogel and Evanko, 1988; Banes *et al.*, 1988a; Tsuzaki *et al.*, 1993; Brigman *et al.*, 1994). Two cell populations are represented in the

---

* Corresponding author. Acting Director of Research, Orthopaedics Department, 253 Burnett-Womack Bldg. 7055, University of North Carolina, Chapel Hill, NC 27599-7055, USA.

major compartments of tendon (Banes *et al.*, 1988b). The surface epitenon contains large, polygonal cells (tendon surface cells – TSC) embedded in a matrix containing 25% collagen, proteoglycan and 43% lipid, while the internal portion is comprised of a matrix containing 95% type I collagen and fibroblasts (tendon internal fibroblasts – TIF) in syncytial sheets amidst linear and branching collagen fascicles and bundles (Greenlee and Ross, 1967; Chaplin and Greenlee, 1975; Kastelic *et al.*, 1978; Riederer-Henderson *et al.*, 1983; Rowe, 1985a,b; Banes *et al.*, 1988a). As well as types I and III collagens, TSC store in their matrix fibronectin, TGF-β, and positive (IGF-I) and negative (possibly IGF-I binding proteins), modulators of cell division (Banes *et al.*, 1988a,b; Clemmons, 1991; Tsuzaki *et al.*, 1993, 1994; Brigman *et al.*, 1994). TSC are most active in migrating into and populating a wound bed in tendon following injury (Gelberman *et al.*, 1980, 1983, 1985; Hughes *et al.*, 1992; Banes *et al.*, 1993, 1994). TIF are less prepared to migrate and divide in response to injury (Banes *et al.*, 1993, 1994). TIF in mature tendon are positioned in syncytial arrays, intimately connected to each other; this arrangement appears optimal to promote junctional communication through connexin 43 gap junctions (McNeilly *et al.*, 1996). Their stores of TGF-β and IGF-I in the tendon internal compartment may be for possible recruitment of TSC and utilization by both cell types after injury (Tsuzaki *et al.*, 1994).

Traumatic injury to tendon constitutes an emergency. Injury results in: (1) bleeding, clotting and release of PDGF and TGF-β from platelets, accumulation of IGF-I from plasma, and release of IGF-I and TGF-β1 from TIF matrix at the wound site; (2) inflammation; (3) epitenon cell migration into the wound site; followed by (4) cell division and matrix synthesis (see Figure 17.8; Banes *et al.*, 1981, 1993, 1994; Gelberman *et al.*, 1985; Tsuzaki *et al.*, 1994). Passive progressive motion speeds recovery and promotes increased range of motion, but the mechanism by which this phenomenon occurs remains conjectural (Gelberman *et al.*, 1985). It may relate to response to load by TIF and TSCs in the healing process.

Tissues connected to tendon are known to respond to mechanical signals. Bone cells in the avian ulna can maintain bone mass in response to 300 repetitions of 300 microstrain per day (Rubin and Lanyon, 1985). In culture, osteoblasts respond to applied strain by elaborating cAMP, PGE_2, Ca^{2+} and increasing DNA synthesis (Harell *et al.*, 1977; Binderman *et al.*, 1988; Hasegawa *et al.*, 1985; Buckley *et al.*, 1988, 1990). Recently, Brighton and coworkers have shown that osteoblasts can respond to as little as 100 microstrain, elaborating inositol phosphates and increasing DNA synthesis (Brighton *et al.*, 1991). Muscle cells also respond to load, by rapid hypertrophy, contraction and actin polymerization (Vandenburgh, 1987). Cell response to load is particularly well characterised in vascular cell models, including endothelial and smooth muscle cells. Endothelial cells demonstrate a dose response to increasing shear stress by increasing secretion of plasminogen activator (Diamond *et al.*, 1989). These cells have a shear stress response element found in the promoter for several growth factors (Resnick *et al.*, 1993). Earlier, Komuro had shown that smooth muscle cells subjected to load increased cFOS expression within 15 min and activated a response element that mapped near the serum response element (Komuro *et al.*, 1990, 1991). Tendon cells also respond instantly to load by releasing intracellular calcium stores, altering their cytoplasmic filament content, polymerizing actin and altering their protein expression (Banes *et al.*, 1985, 1990; Banes, 1993). However, TSC and

TIF do not always respond in the same way to load. It is likely that all cells in mechanically active tissues detect, process and relay the signal to surrounding cells in a feedback loop designed to regulate tissue maintenance functions in accord with mechanical demand on the tissue (proper matrix type and cell/matrix ratio). This signal transduction scenario is an adaptive response to the load environment. The diversity of the tendon cell responses may be related to their functions and the way they receive and process chemical and mechanical signals.

What is the evidence that tendon cells intercommunicate with each other, respond to mechanical loads and that such responses are important *in vivo*? Firstly, results of light and transmission electron microscopy studies have shown that cells in both the epitenon and internal compartment of whole tendon, are physically connected to each other (Greenlee and Ross, 1967; Chaplin and Greenlee, 1975; Gillard *et al.*, 1979; McNeilly *et al.*, 1996). Gap junctions, as shown by the presence of connexin 43 (see below) occur at points of contact of cells in rat tendons (McNeilly *et al.*, 1996). In fact, internal fibroblasts are aligned in syncytial arrays that seem optimal for rapid, repeated electrical coupling. Secondly, *in vitro*, both TSC and TIF are biochemically and electrically coupled – they respond to a mechanical perturbation with a micropipet indentation of a target cell plasma membrane by increasing intracellular calcium stores and propagating the calcium wave to adjacent cells for up to 4–7 cell diameters (Banes *et al.*, 1995a). Sanderson and coworkers have developed a single cell stimulation model in ciliated tracheal epithelial cells (Sanderson *et al.*, 1988). They have shown that indenting a target cell membrane with a 1 μm wide pipet tip causes an increase in intracellular calcium concentration whose wave is propagated to adjoining cells by IP_3 through gap junctions (Sanderson *et al.*, 1990; Boitano *et al.*, 1992). Heparin blocks IP_3 receptors and blocks the wave propagation from cell to cell (Boitano *et al.*, 1992). Likewise, the gap junction blocker halothane also ablates the signal propagation. Loss of connexin 43 expression results in poor junctional competence and loss of the ability to transmit a calcium signal to a neighboring cell (Charles *et al.*, 1991). Transfection of junctionally incompetent c6 glioma cells with connexin 43 cDNA restored intercellular communication (Charles *et al.*, 1991, 1992). Thirdly, *in vivo*, tendon under tension, that is fixed with glutaraldehyde, contains cells that are dramatically indented, like marshmallows squeezed between reinforcing rods (Merrilees and Flint, 1980). Fourthly, as with every other cell type tested thus far, avian tendon cells contain gap junctions (Beyer *et al.*, 1990; Bennett *et al.*, 1991; Haefliger *et al.*, 1992; Willecke *et al.*, 1991).

Gap junctions are assemblies of individual 1.2 nm channels in the plasma membranes of contacting cells (Robertson, 1963; Revel and Karnovsky, 1967). Gap junctions pass ions and molecules with a molecular weight of below 1000 kDa (Bennett *et al.*, 1991; Goodenough *et al.*, 1996 reviews). Larger molecules such as proteins and nucleic acids are excluded from passage through the channels but smaller molecules like inositol phosphates and molecules of intermediate metabolism or ions such as Ca^{2+} can pass through (Saez *et al.*, 1989). Coupled cells constitute a functional syncytium so that electrical and chemical signals may be transmitted between and among partners to buffer metabolites and transmit regulatory molecules. The biochemistry of the hexameric subunits has only been understood over the last 10 years (Beyer *et al.*, 1990 review). Gap junction channels are composed of 26 kDa to 70 kDa protein subunits, the connexins (Beyer *et al.*, 1987), assembled into a hexamer at the plasma membrane surface; this forms a cylindrical hemichannel spanning the membrane and meeting up with a similar hemichannel in the adjacent cell. The hemichannel is termed a connexon (Robertson, 1963). A connexon of one connexin type may form a junction with a connexon comprised of 6 connexins of another molecular weight species. Approximately 13 types of connexins, divided into groups I and II, have been identified (Beyer et al., 1990; Bennett et al., 1991). Of special relevance here is Group II, which contains Xenopus, chicken, rat and human connexin 43, a 43 kDa monomer (Beyer et al., 1987, 1990). The connexins have a common structure, with a cytoplasmic n-terminus, an extracellular loop, a central cytoplasmic loop, a further extracellular loop, and an intracellular carboxy terminus. The cDNA structure for connexin 43 is most conserved between species in the membrane spanning domains and extracellular loops (Beyer et al., 1990). The cytoplasmic C-terminal domain also varies but the central cytoplasmic loop is altered less. The cytoplasmic N-terminus and extracellular loops vary in at most one residue. Connexin 43s from chicken and Xenopus are shorter by 3 and 1 residues respectively, but otherwise all domains are the same length (Bennett et al., 1991). It is known that ser-233 of rat connexin 32 is phosphorylated by a cAMP-dependent protein kinase but this characteristic is not shared by other connexins and little is known about their genetic regulation (Bennett et al., 1991). Gap junctions are not static structures, but turn over at the cell surface, with a half-life of about 2 h. They are protease resistant, but may require up to 72 h for re-expression after cells are passaged (Laird et al., 1991).

Gap junctions show gating characteristics – they can be switched on and off. Gating of the gap junction is hypothesized to be regulated by pH at the cytoplasmic tail region (Liu et al., 1993); acidification initially caused an increase in channel conductance followed by uniform channel closure upon further acidification. Low calcium ion concentration [0.05 mM], also closes the gate but higher concentrations, [1.2 mM], open the gate. Previously, it had been postulated that closure was due to tilting of the channel proteins (Unwin, 1989). If the connexin subunits are tilted towards each other, then the "gate" is closed, whereas if the subunits are not tilted, the "gate" is open. However, recent X-ray diffraction evidence renders the tilting subunit hypothesis unlikely (Caspar et al., 1988). Blockers of junctional communication such as acetylcholine (ACh) or the anesthetics, halothane, heptanol, isoflurane or octanol close the junction without affecting subunit tilt, probably by altering calcium homeostasis in the case of the anesthetics and by a protein kinase C (PKC)-mediated mechanism with ACh (Peracchia, 1991; Mody et al., 1991; Sill et al., 1991; Randriamampita et al., 1988).

The phosphorylation state of the channel protein subunits also affects gap junction behaviour. Phosphorylation may regulate connexin subunit trafficking (Musil et al., 1990; Mege et al., 1988). Musil has shown that connexin 43 proteins are not phosphorylated completely in L929 and S180 mouse cell lines, which lack functional gap junctions (Musil et al., 1990). However, S180 cells transfected with an avian cadherin gene (L-CAM) demonstrate normal connexin 43 phosphorylation and have functional gap junctions. Other results suggest that phosphorylation may regulate localization of connexin subunits to junctional complexes. Phosphorylated connexin 43 is Triton-X100 insoluble and is found in junctional complexes at the cell surface; nonphosphorylated connexin 43 is soluble and in the intracellular compartment (Musil and Goodenough, 1991); phosphorylation probably occurs after connexin 43 assembly into junctions. Alternatively, phosphorylation may affect channel conductance: blocking kinase activity or preventing dephosphorylation altered the frequency of single channel conductances from 65 and 100 to 100 or 65 pSiemens respectively (Moreno *et al.*, 1994). Avian cells have at least three forms of connexin 43: a 42–43 kDa nonphosphorylated form and two intermediate forms from 44–45 to 47 kDa that are phosphorylated at serine (Musil *et al.*, 1990; Laird *et al.*, 1991). Also, the relative amounts of connexin 43 in a cell are important since vole NIH 3T3 cells have 8 times more connexin protein than do mouse NIH 3T3 cells and have an increased capacity for intercellular communication as well, as judged by dye passage to neighboring cells. In addition, Rous sarcoma virus-transformed cells have impaired intercellular communication and a concomitant reduction in connexin 43 (Crow *et al.*, 1990). Paralleling the virus-induced impaired signalling result, it has been shown that a transformation-induced increase in v-src results in a reduction in cell–cell communication by increasing kinase activity and inactivation of connexin 43.

MATERIALS AND METHODS

CELL CULTURE

Tendon epitenon synovial cells (TSC) and internal fibroblasts (TIF) were isolated from avian flexor tendons by the method of Banes and coworkers (Banes *et al.*, 1988b). Briefly, the method involved sequential trypsin and collagenase treatment of the dissected flexor tendons of the legs to first isolate TSC, followed by mechanical scraping with a rubber policeman to remove residual epitenon. The remaining tendon samples were minced and treated with 0.5% collagenase to free TIF. Cells were washed in complete medium (10% fetal calf serum in DMEM-H with 0.5 mM ascorbate and antibiotics then plated at 25 kcells/cm^2 in 83 mm diameter collagen bonded growth surface culture plates for cell expansion. Cells were passaged in 0.01% trypsin in PBS, pH 7.2, after washing in 0.1 M phosphate buffered saline (PBS) pH 7.2. Cells were used from passes 2–3. For experiments involving cyclic mechanical loading, cells were plated in complete medium at 25 kcells/cm^2 onto type I collagen bonded Flex I^{TM}, flexible bottom culture plates (Flexcell Intl. Corp. McKeesport, PA). For experiments involving mechanical challenge with a glass micropipet (membrane indentation model), cells were plated either on collagen-coated glass cover slips or BioFlex^{TM} collagen bonded rubber membranes (0.020 inch thick, with 85% homogeneous radial strain, circumferential strain gradient, biaxial load when subjected to cyclic strain) at 25 kcells/cm^2 in complete medium (Pederson *et al.*, 1992, 1993; Gilbert *et al.*, 1989, 1990, 1994).

MEMBRANE INDENTATION MODEL

The effect of mechanical stimulation on calcium signalling was investigated using the membrane indentation model of Sanderson and coworker. This was used to challenge single cells in a cell sheet with a mechanical stimulus (Sanderson and Dirkson, 1986; Sanderson *et al.*, 1988; Sanderson and Dirkson, 1989; Sanderson *et al.*, 1990;

Boitano et al., 1992). Briefly, TSC and TIF were plated on collagen-coated glass coverslips or BioFlex, 0.020 inch thick, collagen bonded rubber membranes in complete medium at 25 kcells/cm^2 and grown to confluence and quiescence for 5 days without a medium change (Pledger et al., 1978). Medium was aspirated, the cells washed free in DMEM with HEPES pH 7.2, then loaded with 5 µM FURA-2AM in DMEM with 0.01% pleuronic detergent for 45 min at room temperature. Cells were washed in DMEM without FURA-2AM for 5–10 min, then placed in a holding jig on the stage of an Olympus OM-2 upright, fluorescence microscope equipped with a long working distance, water immersion, 40×, high transmission 340 nm UV objective (Olympus Corp. Tokyo, Japan), filter wheel system with 340 and 380 nm filters, 510 nm and above emission cutoff filter, CCD camera, intensifier screen, and Image-1 image analysis hardware with fura-2 signal collection software (Universal Imaging, West Chester, PA). A target cell in a monolayer was selected at random for mechanical challenge with a 0.5–1 micrometer diameter tip glass micropipet controlled by a Narishige micromanipulator. The pipet was positioned to a point just touching the plasma membrane and then advanced rapidly a distance of 2 micrometer with the micromanipulator (Sanderson and Dirkson, 1986; Sanderson et al., 1988). Intracellular calcium ion increase, $[Ca^{2+}]_{ic}$, was quantitated by ratio imaging the 340 and 380 nm excitation fields with 510 nm emission. Absolute calcium quantitation was performed by comparison to intensities of standard calcium solutions. Electroporation of heparin (an IP$_3$ receptor blocker) and Texas Red dextran (a positive control label to assure entry of heparin into the cell) was accomplished by pulsed field electroporation (Sill et al., 1991; Boitano et al., 1992). Halothane at 4.3 mM in DMEM, was incubated with cultures for 15 min prior to testing a response to a mechanical challenge. Data were expressed as the rise in $[Ca^{2+}]_i$ from a basal level of 35–50 nM to 350–1000 nM in 5 different cell arrays per culture. Cultures from three different isolations were used in the experiments.

CYCLIC MECHANICAL LOADING OF CELLS GROWN ON FLEXIBLE MEMBRANES

TSC or TIF were plated at 25 kcells/cm^2 in complete medium on Flex I, collagen bonded, flexible bottom culture plates as described above. Cells were subjected to 1, 3, 5 or 7 days of cyclic load at 1 Hz and 0.05 or 0.1 maximum strain using a FX2000 Flexercell Strain Unit (Banes et al., 1990). After loading, cultures were aspirated of fluid and placed on ice. For total RNA collection, were scraped from wells in guanidine thiocyanate buffer, two wells pooled per sample and samples frozen at −80°C. For protein collection, cells received, were scraped from the wells in SDS buffer and frozen at −20°C.

REVERSE TRANSCRIPTION AND POLYMERASE CHAIN REACTION FOR DETECTION OF CONNEXIN 26, 32, 37, 42, 43, 45, 45.6 AND 50 mRNAs

Total RNA was prepared from pectoralis major muscle, flexor profundus tendon and diaphyseal metatarsal bone from 52-day old White Leghorn chickens by the method of Chirgwin et al., 1979. Briefly, tissues were dissected, removed and frozen on dry ice at the abbatoire then ground to a fine powder in liquid nitrogen and RNA isolated using

RNA Stat60 followed by isopropanol precipitation. An aliquot of the RNA was treated with DNAase I, phenol-chloroform extracted then precipitated with ethanol and sodium acetate, washed and reconsituted in dH_2O at 1 mg/ml. Oligonucleotide primers to mouse connexin 26, 32 and 37 were synthesized after analysis of the sequences in the oligonucleotide program in MacVector. Likewise, sequences for avian connexin 42, 43, 45, 45.6 and 50 were also synthesized after computer analysis.

Reverse transcription of avian mRNAs to cDNAs was carried out using a Perkin Elmer kit with MULV enzyme (Mullis and Faloona, 1987). cDNAs were used under stringent PCR conditions (hot start, 95°C denaturing temperature, 72°C extension and 65°C annealing conditions for 40 cycles with a 4°C stop temperature. A portion of each sample was subjected to electrophoresis at 100 V for 20 min in a 1.5% agarose gel containing ethidium bromide in TAE buffer (Lehrach et al., 1977). cDNA sizes were estimated by comparing their migration position to that of a PCR standard cDNA ladder (AvaII and EcoRI digested pBR322). Product sizes for the connexins were 539 bp for connexin 26; 402 bp for connexin 32; 471 bp for connexin 37; 339 bp for connexin 42; 438 or 469 bp for connexin 43; 382 bp for connexin 45; 482 bp for connexin 45.6; 476 bp for connexin 50. Primers for connexin 26, 32 and 37 were based on mouse sequences. The remainder of the connexin sequences were based on chick sequences.

IDENTIFICATION OF CONNEXIN 43 PROTEINS BY WESTERN BLOT

Avian tendon cells were subjected to cyclic mechanical load in flexible bottom culture plates for 1, 3, 5 or 7 days at 1 Hz 0.05 or 0.1 maximum strain for 8 h/day and rested for 16 h/day. Cells were collected in lysis buffer then subjected to electrophoresis in a 10% SDS denaturing gel, transferred to nitrocellulose then blotted with anti-connexin 43 antibody and reacted with an enzyme-linked reporter antibody. Bands were visualized using a chemiluminescence technique and semi-quantitated using an Image-I image analyzer.

STATISTICS

Levels of significance were determined using SigmaStat software and analysis of variance with a Neuman–Kuehls t test for gauging confidence intervals.

CONFOCAL LASER SCANNING MICROSCOPY OF IMMUNOHISTOCHEMICALLY LABELED TENDON SECTIONS

Avian flexor profundus tendons were frozen on dry ice and cryosectioned at 20 μm, transferred to glass slides and stained by indirect immunofluorescence using monoclonal antibody to connexin 43 (McNeilly et al., 1996; Zymed or Chemicon) and fluorescein conjugated second antibody (Sigma). Nuclei were counterstained with propidium iodide (Molecular Probes). Samples were examined by confocal laser scanning microscopy with a Molecular Dynamics Sarastro 2000 confocal microscope set for dual channel excitation and emission. Section series were taken through the cryosections, the datasets gaussian filtered to remove noise and then 3D projections were produced, all using Molecular Dynamics ImageSpace™ software running on Silicon Graphics workstations.

RESULTS

Data in Table 18.1 indicate the levels of force that have been measured from tendon during normal activity and for peak loads. Kear and Smith (1975) reported minima and maxima for digital extensor tendons for slow walks to fast trots yielding ratios of maxima to minima of 3.4 to 6.0. Others reported ratios for flexor tendons from horses to be 1.4 to 9. Flexor tendons *in vivo*, can withstand up to 4–5% elongation as tension in the elastic range. Strains beyond 5% may result in loss of the crimp pattern but do not result otherwise in plastic deformation and failure. Tendon is designed to withstand approximately three times, on average, the maximum load delivered in the normal work range. The principle strain on flexor or extensor tendons is tensile, but the tendon surface experiences shear stress as well. In addition, the secondary strain is compressive in the normal direction to tension.

The cartoon in Figure 18.1a depicts the model of a 1 μm wide pipet tip pressed into the plasma membrane the target cell (cell 1). Extracellular calcium, shown as open triangles, enters the cell through calcium channels and reacts with FURA-2 in the cell to yield a fluorescence emission signal. Ca^{2+} from intracellular stores is released from bound stores (closed triangles) by an inositol trisphosphate (IP_3)-dependent mechanism (Boitano *et al.*, 1992). IP_3 diffuses through gap junction ion channels joining adjacent

TABLE 18.1

Authors	Tendon type	Measurement method	Activity/load level	% Strain (min–max)
Kear and Smith, 1975	ovine lateral. digital extensor	clip strain gauge (*in vivo*)	slow walk medium walk fast walk trot	1.0 (0.5–1.7) 1.1 (0.3–1.8) 1.3 (0.6–2.1) 1.5 (0.6–2.6)
Lochner *et al.*, 1980	equine superficial digital flexor	liquid metal strain gauge (*in vivo*)	standing with hoof angle (40–70°) walking with hoof angle (40–70°)	(7.1–9.8) (3.5–8.0) greater than standing
Stephens *et al.*, 1989	equine superficial digital flexor	Hall-effect strain sensor (*in vivo*)	walk with rider trot with rider canter with rider gallop with rider	4.3 7.9 9.6 16.1
Goldstein *et al.*, 1987	human fresh frozen flexor digital profundus	clip strain gauge (*in situ*)	23–65 N (simulating tendon forces in hand during poultry processing)	(0.2–1.8) *strains can increase 40% with creep
Best *et al.*, 1995	rabbit tibialis ant. muscle-tendon unit	noncontact optical method (*ex vivo*)	failure strain	<6.0
Abrahams, 1967	Human flex. and achilles; equine flex. and ext.	strain gauge extensometer (*in vitro*)	elastic limit	2.0–4.0%

cells and is responsible for the spread of a calcium wave from the target cell to neighboring cells. Data in Figure 18.1 panel b indicate that TIF respond to a single cell mechanical challenge with a pipet indentation of the plasma membrane by increasing intracellular calcium concentration in the target cell from a resting level of 50 nM to over 1000 nM. Moreover, the calcium wave was propagated to adjacent cells within seconds in a range of 4–5 cell diameters from the target cell. Both TIF and TSC (data not shown) responded in a similar fashion. Moreover, the rate of calcium wave propagation was approximately the same in both cell types. Data in Figure 18.1 panel c indicate that tendon cells infiltrated with heparin to block IP_3 receptors, yield an increase in intracellular calcium only in the target cell and were unable to communicate a mechanical load signal to neighboring cells via a calcium wave. Treatment of cells with halothane, an anesthetic that blocks gap junction channels, produced the same effect as heparin (data not shown).

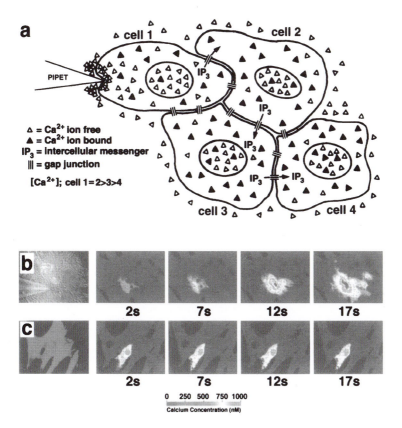

FIGURE 18.1   Panel (a) depicts a micropipet indenting the plasma membrane of a target cell loaded with the calcium ion sensitive compound, FURA-2AM. As the pipet mechanically stimulates the target cell (cell 1) with a "poke", extracellular calcium enters the cell, raising the fluorescence signal. Inositol trisphosphate is released, passing through gap junctions, and eliciting a calcium ion wave in neighboring cells. The calcium wave spreads at least 4–5 cell diameters from the target cell. Panel (b) shows a FURA-2AM-loaded tendon cell (TSC or TIF) stimulated with a micropipet, increasing in fluorescence signal and transducing the mechanical signal to neighbouring cells. Panel (c) shows that if cells are electroporated with heparin to block IP_3 receptors, the mechanical signal is not transduced from cell to cell, indicating the importance of IP_3 in the signal transduction process.

The picture in Figure 18.2 shows a longitudinal section of avian flexor profundus tendon stained immunochemically for connexin 43. The image shows that cells in the epitenon (TSC) are linked through gap junction connections with each other as are the cells in the tendon interior (TIF). Moreover, TSC are also linked with TIF with connexin 43 gap junctions. Connexin 43 (cn 43) is a major connexin protein expressed in avian tendon surface and internal cells.

Data in Figure 18.3 indicate that connexin mRNA expression increased by days 2–3 then decreased by day 5 in passage 2, log phase avian TSC and TIF after disaggregation and replating the cells at 25 kcells/cm^2, feeding and measuring daily connexin expression. Connexin 43 protein expression as measured by Western blot steadily increased after plating following the rise in mRNA. By day 5 cells were in stationary phase (quiescence), were not dividing, had a high degree of connexin protein expression and had functional gap junctions as gauged by an increase in $[Ca^{2+}]_{ic}$ in response to a membrane indentation with a micropipet (latter data not shown).

Figure 18.4 presents the connexin mRNA expression profile of avian pectoralis muscle, flexor profundus tendon and metatarsal bone from the diaphysis of 52-day old

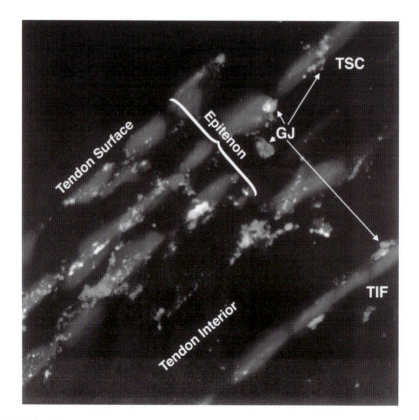

FIGURE 18.2   This longitudinal section of flexor tendon shows the association of cells in the epitenon (TSC) and internal compartments (TIF) with connexin 43 gap junctions (0.5 to 1 micron diameter punctate areas indicated as GJ, between cell processes). Epitenon cells connect with each other and with internal fibroblasts. The same is true for TIF. ×750.

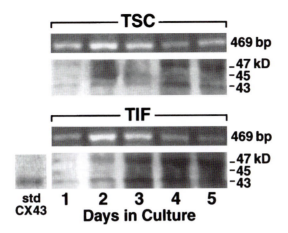

FIGURE 18.3   The top lane shows the pixel intensity for a 469 bp cDNA for connexin 43 amplified by
RT-PCR. The lower bands are for connexin 43 protein as identified by Western blot and represent the nonphosphorylated (connexin 43) and phosphorylated connexin bands (connexin 45 and 47) from TSC and TIF cultured from
avian flexor tendon for 1 to 5 days. The connexin 43 standard is from human umbilical vein smooth muscle cells.

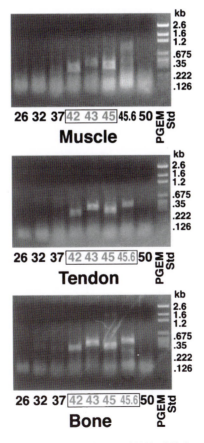

FIGURE 18.4   The cDNA patterns in this figure are from total RNA of 52-day old avian White Leghorn chicken
pectoralis major muscle, Flexor digitorum profundus tendon and metatarsal bone from the midshaft. Tendon and
bone express messages for connexins 42, 43, 45 and 45.6, whereas muscle expressed connexins 42, 43 and 45.

White Leghorn chickens. Muscle expressed connexin 42, 43 and 45 while both tendon and bone expressed connexin 42, 43, 45 and 45.6.

Western blots in Figure 18.5 indicate that connexin 26, 32 and 43 are present in avian tendon cells. However, TIF appear to express connexin 26 and 32 to a higher degree than do TSC. Moreover, in each experiment conducted, TIF consistantly expressed more detectable connexin 43 as well. In addition, analyses of Western blots of parts of tendons confirmed that these connexins were identified in epitenon and the internal compartment of whole tendons (data not shown).

Data in Figure 18.6a show that tendon cells plated at 25 kcells/cm^2 on collagen type I bonded rubber bottom culture plates and subjected to continuous cyclic deformation (1 Hz 0.1 strain) in a Flexercell Strain UnitR have decreased connexin expression after 1 day of loading but are not significantly different in protein expression levels at days 3 or 5 compared to those of non-loaded control counterparts. Data in Figure 18.6b indicate the results for tendon cells subjected to discontinuous cyclic loading at 1 Hz and 0.05 strain. Cells were loaded for 8 h per day and rested for the balance of the day (16 h). Cells subjected to this loading regime also demonstrated decreased connexin 43 expression after one day of load in either TSC (9% reduced NS) or TIF (40% reduced, $p < 0.05$). However TSC showed a 3 fold increase in connexin expression at day 7 after discontinuous cyclic load ($p < 0.01$). TIF showed increased connexin expression at days 3, 5 and 7 (1.6 fold, $p < 0.05$, 1.4 fold, $p < 0.05$; 1.9 fold, $p < 0.01$ respectively). The general trend of connexin

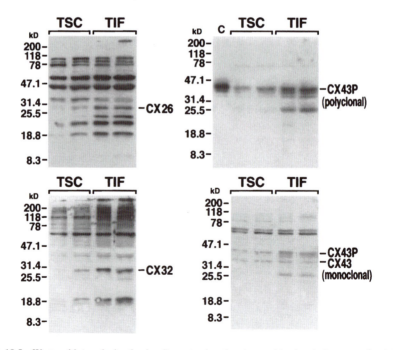

FIGURE 18.5 Western blot analysis of avian flexor tendon showing positive bands for connexins 26, 32 and 43 in both TSC and TIF.

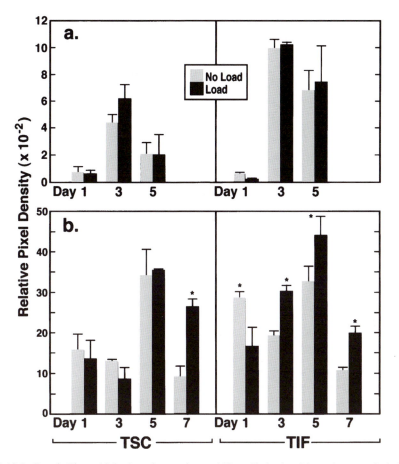

FIGURE 18.6   Data in Figure 18.6a show that continuous 1 Hz cyclic load at 0.1 maximum strain (cell elongation) decreases initial connexin 43 protein expression and does not stimulate connexin expression through 5 days in culture. Data in Figure 18.6b show that discontinuous cyclic tension at 1 Hz but 0.05 strain (maximum elongation) also decreases initial connexin expression but thereafter stimulates connexin expression.

expression levels followed the same pattern as observed in the experiment outlined in Figure 18.3.

DISCUSSION

Cells from both the surface (TSC) and interior (TIF) of flexor tendon respond to a physiologic level of mechanical load *in vitro* in a number of ways. Each cell type responds within milliseconds to a plasma membrane perturbation of a single cell in a cell sheet by increasing their intracellular calcium content. This increase is due to the influx of calcium ions from the bathing medium because if the experiment is conducted in the absence of extracellular calcium ions, the target cell most often does not sustain an increase in intracellular calcium concentration (Boitano et al., 1992). Next, the target cell signals the primary load event to its nearest neighbors by passing a chemical mediator through gap junctions. This mediator is most likely inositol trisphosphate (IP_3) since the load signal can be ablated by electroporating heparin, an IP_3 receptor blocker, into the cell (Boitano et al., 1992). Pretreating the cell with gap junction inhibitors such as halothane, octanol or microinjection with specific antibodies to connexins blocks the calcium wave propagation, showing the role of gap junctions in the transmission of the mechanical load signal from cell to cell (Boitano et al., 1992 and Boitano, personal comunication).

Connexin 43 is expressed by many fibroblasts and is a key connexin expressed by tendon cells (McNielly et al., 1996; Banes et al., 1995a,b). A hemichannel from each of two cells dock with each other at an intermembrane gap distance of about 1.2 nm to form a functional channel (Goodenough et al., 1996). Several hundred channels associate in one region of the plasma membrane to form a structure recognizable after phospho-tungstic acid staining and electron microscopy visualization as a gap junction. It is thought that phosphorylation of connexin monomers may mark the monomer for shuttling from the cytoplasm to a membrane site for junction assembly (Goodenough et al., 1996). Connexins from tendon TSC or TIF cells have several bands that are recognized by anti-connexin 43 antibody: a primary band is that at approximately 43 kDa representing the nonphosphorylated connexin form, with one or usually two higher molecular weight forms that may represent the mono- and di-phosphorylated forms of the protein. Unpublished work from our laboratory indicates that avian tendon cells express mRNAs for multiple connexins, including connexin 45 and 45.6. These data and the fact that alkaline phosphatase treatment of tendon cell extracts does not cause a major band shift from the higher, potentially phosphorylated forms of connexin 43 (molecular weight of 45 to 47 kDa), to a position of the nonphosphorylated form (43 kDa) suggests that other connexin proteins are expressed by tendon cells (Tsuzaki and Banes, unpublished). Nevertheless, connexin 43 protein expression, as semiquantitated by Western blot, increased in tendon cells subjected to discontinuous cyclic mechanical load (Figure 18.6b). The increase was greater in internal fibroblasts than in epitenon cells perhaps reflecting a greater need to intercommunicate mechanical signals within and between cells in the matrix of tendon – the internal compartment of tendon is where the majority of the tensile load is borne. Increased connexin protein expression required several days to be manifest, indicating that this phenomenon is an adaptive change. In fact, in both TSC and TIF subjected to continuous or discontinuous cyclic stretching in vitro, the initial effect of cyclic tension was to reduce connexin 43 protein expression. In experiments in which tension was cycled continuously, load did not stimulate increased connexin expression. Results of preliminary experiments designed to test for effects of excessive strain, i.e. greater than 5% cell elongation at 1 Hz for 3 to 7 days, on connexin protein expression indicated that connexin 43 gap junctions were smaller (approximately 0.1 micron diameter rather than 0.5 to 1 micron and less numerous than in control, nonstretched cells; unpublished observation; Figure 18.7). Moreover, excessive cyclic load decreased the number of dye coupled cells, that is cells that could transfer the dye, Lucifer Yellow, from an injected target cell to an attached potential recipient cell (Dr Jan Burt, personal communication). Taken together, these results indicate that: (1) acute load breaks gap junctions, (2) enough connections

NO LOAD

LOAD

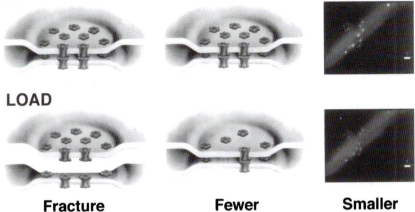

Fracture   **Fewer**   **Smaller**

FIGURE 18.7   Model of how excessive strain may act to fracture gap junctions between neighboring cells.

remain intact so that cells can still intercommunicate and that, (3) stretching cells discontinuously, allowing at least 18 h of nonload, stimulates connexin protein expression.

The model presented in Figure 18.8 is a compendium of how tendon cells may respond to a wound which alters the intrinsic strain in a tendon. In this model, we propose that tendon cells in normal tendon are in a nondividing, maintenance state in which they model and remodel tendon matrix and process routine mechanical load signals. Trauma causes a break in the tendon and subsequent loss of cell–cell and gap junction contacts. Bleeding from capillaries introduces growth factors such as platelet-derived growth factor (PDGF) and transforming growth factor b1 (TGF-β_1). PDGF, TGF-β_1 from platelets and insulin-like growth factor 1 (IGF-1) from plasma stimulate tendon cell division and act synergistically with load during convalescence to stimulate healing (Banes et al., 1995c,d). When the concentration of growth factors diminishes, then mechanical load applied to the tendon through normal ambulation or physical therapy may stimulate interconnection of cells with gap junctions to reestablish the maintenance program. Without the proper amount of applied motion during convalescence, the repair program runs out of control leading to fibrosis and other pathologies.

The general model shown in Figure 18.9 depicts several strategies cells may use to transduce mechanical deformation events and respond via known biochemical pathways (Banes et al., 1995c,d). Load signals that are detected by one or more cells may be transduced down a kinase pathway and on to the nucleus to induce or repress transcription or DNA synthesis. The deformation event most likely elicits an increase in intracellular calcium concentration both from extracellular sources and from IP3-dependent intracellular stores (Boitano et al., 1992). The signal then travels from the initial cell to neighbouring cells via gap junctions. We know that tendon cells can respond within milliseconds to one second to a mechanical deformation by increasing intracellular calcium ion or phosphorylating proteins. Tyrosine phosphorylation increases after a single deformation of a flexible membrane.

Events in Homeostasis and Wound Repair in Flexor Tendon: Growth Factor and Mechanical Load Effects

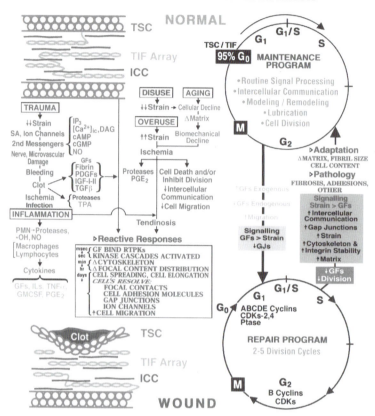

FIGURE 18.8   Model of how cells in tendon react to changes in strain after a wound and how intercellular signalling may be reestablished to return cells to a maintenance program.

Are gap junctions essential for intercellular communication given that other cell–cell connections exist such as cytoskeletally-connected integrins? Ingber has postulated in his tensegrity model that cells are connected and signal through direct mechanical linkage from the matrix via integrins through the cytoskeletal system to the nucleus (Ingber *et al.*, 1991, 1993; Wang *et al.*, 1993). Gap junction proteins may not have cytoskeletal connections but are known to pass signalling molecules intercellularly (Bennett *et al.*, 1991; Sanderson *et al.*, 1990). No one has yet shown a direct response in a cell by perturbing matrix and signalling through an integrin. However, direct evidence that connexins are involved in signalling derives from experiments with the c6 glioma cell line that is poorly electrically coupled (Charles *et al.*, 1992). If the cells are transfected with connexin 43 cDNA and express the protein, they gain the ability to communicate with neighbors both electrically and with a propagated calcium wave in response to a mechanical stimulation (Zhu *et al.*, 1991; Charles *et al.*, 1991). Loss of connexin 43 and gap junctions leads to

General Model of Mechanical Load Signal Transduction and Cell Response

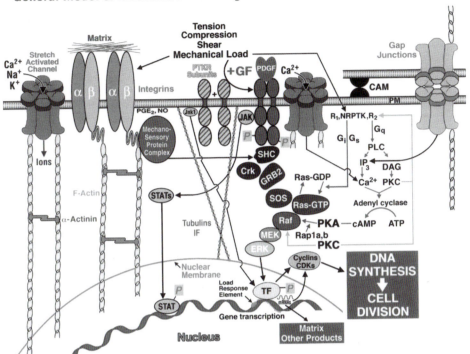

FIGURE 18.9   General model of mechanical load signal transduction and cell response. The systems are multifold and can be separated into detection, response and modulation pathways. The detection systems involve an example of a mechanically sensitive ion channel (stretch-activated channel) that is linked to the cytoskeleton. A principle detection system is the matrix-integrin-mechanosensory protein complex-cytoskeleton machinery (Clark and Brugge, 1995) that is linked to a kinase cascade (tyrosine or nontyrosine kinase cascade or the JAK/STAT kinase cascade) system that provides amplification, diversity, selectivity and modulation capabilities (mechanosensory protein complex contains talin, vinculin, tensin, paxillin, Src and focal adhesion kinase (FAK); SHC is a Src homology protein complex; Crk is a Src homology adaptor protein that binds paxillin and C3G; GRB2 is a growth factor receptor binding adaptor protein linking receptors to the Ras pathway through FAK and SOS, a guanine nucleotide exchange factor; Ras is a GTPase that regulates activation of Raf; MEK is a mitogen activated kinase; ERK is an extracellularly regulated kinase. Activated ERKs enter the nucleus and upregulate transcription factor expression (jun, fos, myc, erg-1) and activate nuclear binding proteins such as NF-kB. Specific regulation may occur at load response elements in promoters of certain genes such as PDGF. Alternatively, a load signal may activate a growth factor receptor (p for phosphorylation) with or without ligand and activate the same or a similar sequence of kinases (PTKR is protein tyrosine kinase receptor, GF is growth factor, PDGF is platelet derived growth factor). Load may act in synergy with a ligand to stimulate the kinase pathway. Mechanical load may also induce a conformational change in a nonreceptor protein tyrosine kinase receptor (R_1, NRPTK, R_2), regulated by g proteins (G_i or G_q) leading to activation of phospholipase C (PLC) stimulating production of second messengers inositol tris phosphate (IP_3) and diacylglycerol (DAG) stimulating an increase in intracellular calcium ion (Ca^{2+}) and protein kinase C activity (PKC). PKC and Ca^{2+} activate adenyl cyclase activity yielding cAMP that stimulates cAMP-dependent protein kinase A. PKA may act at Raf in the kinase cascade. Rap 1 a,b, Ras-like proteins, regulate the PKA stimulation of Raf. Specific genes are expressed that drive the cell toward DNA synthesis (cyclins and cyclin-dependent kinases, CDKs) and cell division or toward matrix expression or some other downstream response. The ion channel could also be a gap junction channel (GJ) with another hemichannel on top. GJs pass IP_3 which propagates a Ca^{2+} wave from cell to cell after a mechanical signal is detected. CAM is a cell adhesion molecule. IF is an intermediate filament. PGE_2 is prostaglandin E_2, NO is nitric oxide.

loss of regulation of DNA synthesis and cell division (Zhu *et al.*, 1991). Bennett and others believe that the connexins are intimately involved in regulating embryogenesis and development (Bennett *et al.*, 1991). Therefore, it is likely that gap junction regeneration is also essential for an organized wound healing response.

We hypothesize that during the initial phase of tendon healing, cells are driven by exogenous growth factors to migrate and divide, but regain autonomous control of cell division and maintenance functions as migration halts and gap junction communication is reestablished. It is appreciated that physical manipulation of limbs containing operated tendons results in a greater range of motion, better vascularization, more organized matrix and less time in convalescence (Gelberman *et al.*, 1983). We hypothesize that mechanical loading applied to tendon cells increases gap junction protein expression and intercellular communication that results in positive attributes after injury.

ACKNOWLEDGEMENTS

Supported by NIH AR38121, AR24845, Hunt Foundation. Special thanks to Ms. Jean McKinney for preparation of the manuscript.

REFERENCES

Abrahams, M. (1967) Mechanical properties of tendon *in vitro*, a preliminary report. *Med. Biol. Eng.*, **5**, 433–443.

Banes, A., Link, G.W., Bevin, A.G., Peterson, H.D., Gillespie, G.Y., Bynum, D., Watts, S. and Dahners, L. (1988a) Tendon synovial cells secrete fibronectin *in vivo* and *in vitro*. *J. Orthop. Res.*, **6**, 73–82.

Banes, A.J., Donlon, K., Link, G.W., Gillespie, G.Y., Bevin, A.G., Peterson, H.D., Bynum, D., Watts, S. and Dahners, L. (1988b) A simplified method for isolation of tendon synovial cells and internal fibroblasts: conformation of origin and biological properties. *J. Orthoped. Res.*, **6**, 83–94.

Banes, A.J., Enterline, D., Bevin, A.G. and Salisbury, R.E. (1981) Repair of flexor tendon: Effects of trauma and devascularization on collagen synthesis. *J. Trauma.*, **21**, 505–512.

Banes, A.J. (1993) Mechanical strain and the mammalian cell. In: *Physical Forces and the Mammalian Cell* (Frangos, J., Ed.), Orlando: Academic Press.

Banes, A.J., Link, G.W., Gilbert, J.W. and Monbureau, O. (1990) Culturing cells in a mechanically active environment: I. The Flexercell Strain Unit can apply cyclic or static tension or compression to cells in culture. *Am. Biotech. Lab.*, **8**, 12–22.

Banes, A.J., Sanderson, M., Boitano, S., Hu, P., Brigman, B., Tsuzaki, M., Fischer, T. and Lawrence, W.T. (1994) Mechanical load $+\backslash-$ growth factors induces $[Ca^{2+}]_{ic}$ release, cyclin D_1 expression and DNA synthesis in avian tendon cells. In: *Cell Mechanics and Cellular Engineering* (Ed. Mow, V.C., Guilak, F., Tran-Son-Tay, R., Hochmuth, R.M.) pp. 210–232. Springer-Verlag, New York.

Banes, A.J., Brigman, B., Yin, H., Tsuzaki, M., Almekinders, L. and Lawrence, W.T. (1993) Stimulation of DNA synthesis in tendon synovial and internal fibroblasts released from quiescence by serum, growth factors or mechanical loading. *Trans. Orth. Res. Soc.*, **18**, 161.

Banes, A.J., Gilbert, J., Taylor, D. and Monbureau, O. (1985) A new vacuum-operated stress-providing instrument that applies static or variable duration cyclic tension or compression to cells *in vitro*. *J. Cell Sci.*, **75**, 35–42.

Banes, A.J., Hu, P., Xiao, H., Sanderson, M., Boitano, S., Brigman, B., Fischer, T., Tsuzaki, M., Brown, T., Almekinders, L. and Lawrence, W.T. (1995a) Tendon cells of the epitenon and internal tendon compartment communicate mechanical signals through gap junctions and respond differentially to mechanical load and growth factors. In: *Repetitive Motion Disorders of the Upper Extremity* (Ed. S. Gordon, L. Fine, S. Blair) Amer. Acad. Orth. Surg., Chapter 16, pp. 1231–1246.

Banes, A.J., Tsuzaki, M., Yamamoto, J., Fischer, T., Brown, T. and Miller, L. (1995b) Mechanoreception at the cellular level: The detection, interpretation and diversity of responses to mechanical signals. *Biochem. Cell Biol.*, **73**, 349–365.

Banes, A.J., Xiao, H., Hu, P., Brigman, B., Tsuzaki, M., Van Wyk, J., Fischer, T. and Lawrence, W.T. (1995c) Cyclic mechanical load and growth factors act synergistically to stimulate DNA synthesis in tendon cells. *Trans. Orth. Res. Soc.*, **20**, 504.

Banes, A.J., Tsuzaki, M., Hu, P., Brigman, B., Brown, T., Almekinders, L., Lawrence, W.T. and Fischer, T. (1995d) Cyclic mechanical load and growth factors stimulate NA synthesis in avian tendon cells. *J. Biomechanics*, **28** (Special Issue on Cytomechanics), 1505–1513.

Bennett, M.V.L., Barrio, L.C., Bargiello, T.A., Spray, D.C., Hertzberg, E. and Saez, J.C. (1991). Gap junctions: New tools, new answers, new questions. *Neuron*, **6**, 305–320.

Best, T.M., McElhaney, J.H., Garret, W.E. and Myers, B.S. (1995) Axial strain measurements in skeletal muscle at various strain rates. *J. Biomech. Engr.*, **117**, 262–265.

Beyer, E.C., Paul, D.L. and Goodenough, D.A. (1990) Connexin family of gap junction proteins. *J. Membrane Biol.*, **116**, 187–194.

Beyer, E.C., Paul, D.L. and Goodenough, D.A. (1987) Connexin 43: A protein from rat heart homologous to a gap junction protein from liver. *J. Cell Biol.*, **105**, 2621–2629.

Binderman, I., Zor, U., Kaye, A.M., Shimshoni, Z., Harell, A. and Somjen, D. (1988). The transduction of mechanical force into biochemical events in bone cells may involve activation of phospholipase A2. *Calcif. Tissue Int.*, **42**, 261–266.

Boitano, S., Dirkson, E.R. and Sanderson, M.J. (1992) Intercellular propagation of calcium waves mediated by inositol triphosphate. *Science*, **258**, 292–295.

Brighton, C.T., Strafford, B., Gross, S.B., Leatherwood, D.F., Williams, U.L. and Pollack, S.R. (1991) The proliferative and synthetic response of isolated calvarial bone cells of rats to cyclic biaxial mechanical strain. *J. Bone Joint Surg.*, **73**(A), 320–331.

Brigman, B.E., Yin, H., Tsuzaki, M., Lawrence, W.T. and Banes, A.J. (1994) Fibronectin levels are elevated in avian flexor tendon synovium and isolated cells compared with tissue and cells from the internal tendon compartment. *J. Orth. Res.*, **12**, 253–261.

Buckley, M.J., Banes, A.J., Levin, L.G., Sumpio, B.E., Sato, M., Jordan, B., Gilbert, J., Link, G.W. and Tay, R.T.S. (1988) Osteoblasts increase their rate of division and align in response to cyclic, mechanical tension *in vitro. Bone and Mineral*, **4**, 225–236.

Buckley, M.J., Banes, A.J. and Jordan, R. (1990) Effects of mechanical strain on osteoblasts *in vitro. J. Oral. Maxofac. Surg.*, **48**, 276–282.

Caspar, D., Sosinsky, G., Tibbits, T., Philips, W. and Goodenough, D. (1988) In: *Gap Junctions*, (Ed. E.L. Hertzberg, R.G. Johnson) pp. 117–133, New York, Liss.

Chaplin, D.M. and Greenlee, T.K. (1975) Development of human digital tendons. *J. Anat.*, **120**, 253–274.

Charles, A.C., Merrill, J.E., Dirksen, E.R. and Sanderson, M.J. (1991) Intercellular signalling in glial cells: Calcium waves and oscillations in response to mechanical stimulation and glutamate. *Neuron*, **6**, 983–992.

Charles, A.C., Merrill, J.E., Dirksen, E.R. and Sanderson, M.J. (1992) Intercellular calcium signaling via gap junctions in glioma cells. *J. Cell Biol.*, **118**, 195–201.

Chirgwin, J.M., Pryzbyla, A.E., MacDonald, R.J. and Rutter, W.J. (1979) Isolation of biologically active ribonucleic acid from sources enriched in ribonuclease. *Biochemistry*, **18**, 5294–5299.

Clark, E.A. and Brugge, J.S. (1995) Integrins and signal transduction pathways: the road taken. *Science*, **268**, 233–239.

Clemmons, D.R. (1991) Insulin-like growth factor binding protein control secretion and mechanisms of action. *Adv. Exp. Med. Biol.*, **293**, 113–123.

Crow, D.S., Beyer, E.C., Paul, D.L., Kobe, S.S. and Lau, A.F. (1990) Phosphorylation of connexin 43 gap junction protein in uninfected and Rous sarcoma virus-transformed mammalian fibroblasts. *Mol. Cell Biol.*, **10**, 1754–1763.

Diamond, S.L., Eskin, S.G. and McIntire, L. (1989) Fluid flow stimulates tissue plasminogen activator secretion by cultured human endothelial cells. *Science*, **243**, 1483–1485.

Gelberman, R.H., Menon, J., Gonsalves, M. and Akeson, W.H. (1980) The effects of mobilization on the vascularization of healing flexor tendons in dogs. *Clin. Orthop. Rel. Res.*, **153**, 283–289.

Gelberman, R.H., Vandeberg, J.S., Lundborg, G.M. and Akeson, W.H. (1983) Flexor tendon healing and restoration of the gliding surface. An ultrastructural study in dogs. *J. Bone Joint Surg.*, **65A**, 70–80.

Gelberman, R.H., Vandeberg, J.S., Manske, P.R. and Akeson, W.H. (1985) The early stages of flexor tendon healing: A morphologic study of the first fourteen days. *J. Hand Surg.*, **10A**, 776–784.

Gilbert, J.A., Banes, A.J., Link, G.W. and Jones, G.J. (1989) Surface strain on living cells in a mechanically active *in vitro* environment. *ANSYS Conf. Proc.* (Ed. D.E. Dietrich), Swanson Analysis Systems: Houston, PA. pp. 13.2–13.7.

Gilbert, J.A., Banes, A.J., Link, G.W. and Jones, G.J. (1990) Video analysis of membrane strain: an application in cell stretching. *Exp. Tech. Sept./Oct.*, 33–45.

Gilbert, J.A., Banes, A.J., Weinhold, P.S., Link, G.W. and Jones, G.L. (1994). Strain profiles for circular plates and membranes employed to mechanically deform cells *in vitro*. *J. Biomech.*, **27**, 1169–1177.

Gillard, G.C., Reilly, H.C., Bell-Booth, P.G. and Flint, M.H. (1979) The influence of mechanical forces on the glycosaminoglycan content of the rabbit flexor digitorum profundus tendon. *Conn. Tiss. Res.*, **7**, 37–46.

Goldstein, S.A., Armstrong, T.J., Chaffin, D.B. and Matthews, L.S. (1987) Analysis of cumulative strain in tendons and tendon sheaths. *J. Biomech.*, **20**, 1–6.

Goodenough, A., Goliger, J.A. and Paul, D.L. (1996) Connexins, connexons and intercellular communication. *Ann. Rev. Biochem.*, **65**, 475–502.

Greenlee, T.K. and Ross, R. (1967) The development of the rat flexor digital tendon, a fine structure study. *J. Ultrastruc. Res.*, **18**, 354–376.

Haefliger, J.A., Bruzzone, R., Jenkins, N.A., Gilbert, D.J., Copeland, N.G. and Paul, D.L. (1992). Four novel members of the connexin family of gap junction proteins. *J. Biol. Chem.*, **267**, 2057–2064.

Harrell, A., Dekel, S. and Binderman, I. (1977) Biochemical effect of mechanical stress on cultured bone cells. *Calcif. Tiss. Int.*, **22**, 202–209.

Hasegawa, S., Sata, S., Saito, S., Suzuki, Y. and Brunette, D.M. (1985) Mechanical stretching increases the number of cultured bone cells synthesizing DNA and alters their pattern of protein synthesis. *Calc. Tiss. Int.*, **37**, 431–436.

Hughes, F.J., Aubin, J.E. and Hersche, J.N.M. (1992) Differential chemotactic responses of different population of fetal rat calvaria cells to platelet-derived growth factor and transforming growth factor. *Bone and Mineral*, **19**, 63–74.

Ingber, D.E. (1991) Control of capillary growth and differentiation by extracellular matrix. Use of a tensegrity (tensional integrity) mechanism for signal processing. *Chest*, **99**, 34s–40s.

Ingber, D.E. (1993) Cellular tensegrity: defining new rules of biological design that govern the cytoskeleton. *J. Cell Sci.*, **104**, 613–627.

Kastelic, J., Galeski, A. and Baer, E. (1978) The multicomposite structure of tendon. *Conn. Tiss. Res.*, **6**, 11–23.

Kear, J. and Smith, R.N. (1975) A method for recording tendon strain in sheep during locomotion. *Acta Orthop. Scand.*, **46**, 896–905.

Komuro, I., Katoh, Y., Shibazaki, Y., Kurabayashi, M., Hoh, E., Takaku, F. and Yakaki, Y. (1991). Mechanical loading stimulates cell hypertrophy and specific gene expression in cultured rat cardiac myocytes. *J. Biol. Chem.*, **266**, 1265–1268.

Komuro, Y., Kaida, T., Shibazaki, Y., Kurabayashi, M., Katoh, Y., Hoh, E., Takaku, F. and Yazaki, Y. (1990). Stretching cardiac myocytes stimulates prooncogene expression. *J. Biol. Chem.*, **265**, 3595–3598.

Laird, D.W., Puranam, K.L. and Revel, J.P. (1991) Turnover and phosphorylation dynamics of connexin 43 gap junction protein in cultured cardiac myocytes. *Biochem. J.*, **273**, 67–72.

Lehrach, H., Diamond, D., Wozney, J.M. and Boedtker, H. (1977) RNA molecular weight determinations by gel electrophoresis under denaturing conditions: a critical reexamination. *Biochemistry*, **16**, 4743.

Liu, S., Taffet, S., Stoner, L., Delmar, M., Vallano, M.L. and Jalife, J. (1993) A structural basis for the unequal sensitivity of the major cardiac and liver gap junctions to intracellular acidification: The carboxyl tail length. *Biophys. J.*, **64**, 1422–1433.

Lochner, F.K., Milne, D.W., Mills, E.J. and Groom, J.J. (1980) *In vivo* and *in vitro* measurements of tendon strain in the horse. *Am. J. Vet. Res.*, **41**, 1929–1937.

McNeilly, C., Banes, A.J., Benjamin, M. and Ralphs, J.R. (1996) Tendon cells *in vivo* form a three dimensional network of cell processes linked by gap junctions. *J. Anat.*, **189**, 593–600.

Mege, R.M., Matsuzaki, F., Gallin, W.J., Goldberg, J.I., Cunningham, B.A. and Edelman, G.A. (1988) Construction of epithelioid sheets by transfection of mouse sarcoma cells with cDNAs for chicken cell adhesion molecules. *Proc. Natl. Acad. Sci.*, **85**, 7274–7278.

Merrilees, M.J. and Flint, M.H. (1980) Ultrastructural study of tension and pressure zones in a rabbit flexor tendon. *Am. J. Anat.*, **157**, 87–106.

Mody, I., Tanelian, D.L. and MacIver, M.B. (1991). Halothane enhances tonic neuronal inhibition by elevating intracellular calcium. *Brain Res.*, **538**, 319–323.

Moreno, A.P., Saez, J.C., Fishman, G.I. and Spray, D.C. (1994) Human connexin 43 gap junction channels: regulation of unitary conductances by phosphorylation. *Circ. Res.*, **74**, 1050–1057.

Mullis, K.B. and Faloona, F.A. (1987) Specific synthesis of DNA *in vitro* via a polymerase-catalyzed chain reaction. In: *Methods in Enzymology* (Ed.,Wu, R.) **155**, 335–350.

Musil, L.S. and Goodenough, D.A. (1991) Biochemical analysis of connexin 43 intracellular transport, phosphorylation and assembly into gap junctional plaques. *J. Cell Biol.*, **115**, 1357–1374.

Musil, L.S., Cunningham, B.A., Edelman, G.M. and Goodenough, D.A. (1990) Differential phosphorylation of the gap junction protein connexin 43 in junctional communication-competant and deficient cell lines. *J. Cell Biol.*, **111**, 2077–2088.

Oakes, B. and Bialkower, B. (1977) Biomechanical and ultrastructural studies on the elastic wing tendon from the domestic fowl. *J. Anat.*, **123**, 369–387.

Pedersen, D.R., Brown, T.D. and Banes, A.J. (1992). Mechanical behavior of a new substratum for strain-mediated cell culture experiments. NACOB II:355–356. *The Second North American Congress on Biomechanics*. Chicago, IL, Aug. 24–28.

Pederson, D.R., Bottlang, M., Brown, T.D. and Banes, A.J. (1993) Hyperelastic constitutive properties of poly-dimethylsiloxane cell culture membranes. *BED Ad. Bioengin. ASME*, **26**, 607–609.

Peracchia, C. (1991) Effects of the anesthetics heptanol, halothane and isoflurane on gap junction conductance in crayfish septate axons: A calcium- and hydrogen-independent phenomenon potentiated by caffeine and theophylline, and inhibited by 4-aminopyridine. *J. Membrane Biol.*, **121**, 67–78.

Pledger, W.J., Stiles, C.D., Antoniades, H.N. and Scher, C.D. (1978) An ordered sequence of events is required before BALB/c-3T3 cells become committed to DNA synthesis. *Proc. Natl. Acad. Sci.*, **75**, 2839–2843.

Randriamampita, C., Giaume, C., Neyton, J. and Trautmann, A. (1988) Acetylcholine-induced closure of gap junction channels in rat lacrimal glands is probably mediated by protein kinase C. *Pflugers Arch.*, **412**, 462–468.

Resnick, N., Collins, T., Atkinson, W., Bonthron, D.T., Dewey, C.F. Jr. and Gimbrone, M.A. Jr. (1993) Platelet-derived growth factor B chain promoter contains a cis-acting fluid shear-stress-responsive element *Proc. Natl. Acad. Sci.*, **90**, 4591–4595.

Revel, J.P. and Karnovsky, J.J. (1967) Hexagonal array of subunits in intercellular junctions of the mouse heart and liver. *J. Cell Biol.*, **33**, C7–C12.

Riederer-Henderson, M.A., Gauger, A., Olson, L., Robertson, C. and Greenlee, T.K. Jr. (1983) Attachment and extracellular matrix differences between tendon and synovial fibroblastic cells. *In Vitro*, **19**, 127–133.

Robertson, J.D. (1963) The occurrence of a subunit pattern in the unit membrane of club ending in Mauthner cell synapses in goldfish brains. *J. Cell Biol.*, **19**, 201–221.

Rowe, R.W.D. (1985a) The structure of rat tail tendon. *Conn. Tiss. Res.*, **14**, 9–20.

Rowe, R.W.D. (1985b) The structure of rat tail tendon fascicles. *Conn. Tiss. Res.*, **14**, 21–30.

Rubin, C. and Lanyon, L. (1985) Regulation of bone mass by mechanical strain magnitude. *Calcif. Tiss. Int.*, **37**, 411–417.

Saez, J.C., Connor, J.A., Spray, D.C. and Bennett, M.V. (1989) Hepatocyte gap junctions are permeable to the second messenger, inositol 1,4,5-trisphosphate, and to calcium ions. *Proc. Natl. Acad. Sci.*, **86**, 2708–2712.

Sanderson, M.J., Charles, A.C. and Dirksen, E.R. (1990) Mechanical stimulation and intracellular communication increases intracellular Ca^{2+} in epithelial cells. *Cell Reg.*, **1**, 585–596.

Sanderson, M.J., Chow, I. and Dirksen, E.R. (1988) Intercellular communictaion between ciliated cells in culture. *Am. J. Physiol.*, **254**, C63–C74.

Sanderson, M.J. and Dirksen, E.R. (1986) Mechanosensitivity of cultured ciliated cells from the mammalian respiratory tract: implications for the regulation of mucociliary transport. *Proc. Natl. Acad. Sci.*, **83**, 7302–7306.

Sanderson, M.J. and Dirksen, E.R. (1989) Inositol trisphosphate mediates intercellular communication between ciliated epithelial cells. *J. Cell Biol.*, **109**, 304a.

Sill, J.C., Uhl, C., Eskuri, S., VanDyke, R. and Tarara, J. (1991) Halothane inhibits agonist-induced inositol phosphate and Ca^{2+} signaling in A7r5 cultured vascular smooth muscle cells. *Mol. Pharm.*, **40**, 1006–1013.

Stephens, P.R., Nunamaker, D.M. and Butterweck, D.M. (1989) Application of a hall-effect transducer for measurement of tendon strain in horses. *Am. J. Vet. Res.*, **50**, 1089–1095.

Tsuzaki, M., Brigman, B., Xiao, H., Lawrence, W.T. and Banes, A.J. (1994) IGF-I and TGF-β drive tendon cell DNA synthesis. *Trans. Orth. Res. Soc.*, **19**, 18.

Tsuzaki, M., Yamauchi, M. and Banes, A.J. (1993) Tendon Collagens: Extracellular matrix composition in shear stress and tensile components of flexor tendon. *Conn. Tiss. Res.*, **29**, 141–152.

Unwin, N. (1989) The structure of ion channels in membranes of excitable cells. *Neuron*, **3**, 665–676.

Vandenburgh, H.H. (1987) Motion into mass: how does tension stimulate muscle growth? *Med. Sci. Sports Ex.*, **19**, S142–S149.

Vogel, K. and Evanko, S.P. (1988) Proteoglycans of fetal bovine tendon. *Trans. Orthop. Res. Soc.*, **13**, 182.

Wang, N., Butler, J.P. and Ingber, D.E. (1993) Mechanotransduction across the cell surface and through the cytoskeleton. *Science*, **260**, 1124–1127.

Willecke, K., Hennemann, H., Dahl, E., Jungbluth, S. and Heynkes, R. (1991) The diversity of connexin genes encoding gap junctional proteins. *Eur. J. Cell Biol.*, **56**, 1–7.

Zhu, D., Caveney, S., Kidder, G.M. and Naus, C.C.G. (1991). Transfection of C6 glioma cells with connexin 43 cDNA: Analysis of expression, intercellular coupling, and cell proliferation. *Proc. Natl. Acad. Sci.*, **88**, 1883–1887.

19 What Proteoglycan Content Says about the Mechanical History of Tendon

Kathryn G. Vogel*, Stephen P. Evanko[1] and James R. Robbins[2]

*Department of Biology, The University of New Mexico,
Albuquerque, NM/USA 87131*

INTRODUCTION

Tendon is a soft connective tissue that usually experiences purely longitudinal/tensional forces as it transmits muscle action to bone. Tendon is composed primarily of type I collagen and it is the ordered arrangement of collagen fibrils that provides for the extraordinary strength that the tissue has in tension. Because tendon injuries are notoriously slow to heal, the tissue is often considered more as a substance with relevant material properties than as a living tissue with important biological properties. However, this static view of tendon is inaccurate. This paper deals with the ability of cells in tendon to modify the composition and organisation of tendon matrix and form fibrocartilage when the tissue is subjected to altered mechanical loads.

The ability of mechanical forces to affect tendon composition was pointed out in morphological studies nearly 60 years ago (Ploetz, 1938). Current study of the phenomenon began with a series of seminal papers published by Michael Flint and co-workers between 1975 and 1980. Flint described a 'sesamoid-like pad' at the point where the rabbit flexor digitorum profundus tendon wraps under the calcaneus and talus. Cells in the pressure-bearing region were round and their cytoplasm was characterised by a dense array of intermediate filaments (Merrilees and Flint, 1980). Glycosaminoglycan (GAG) content was ~15 fold higher in the sesamoid region than in the tensional region and most of this was chondroitin sulphate (Gillard *et al.*, 1977).

* Corresponding author.
Current address: [1] Univ. of Washington SOM, Dept. of Pathology, Seattle WA 98195.
[2] Department of Cell Biology and Physiology, University of New Mexico, Albuquerque, NM 87131.

The forces involved in maintaining these distinct regions of tendon were investigated by surgical translocation of the flexor digitorum profundus tendon in 6–8 week old New Zealand white rabbits followed by analysis of the amount and type of GAG. When the tendon was translocated onto the extensor aspect of the leg, removing both tensional and compressive load, $>60\%$ of the GAG (mainly chondroitin sulphate) was lost from the pressure-bearing region in the first 8 days. Significant loss of GAG from the pressure-bearing region of tendon was measured 8 days after severing the Achilles tendon and removing a 1 cm segment of the sciatic nerve, after sciatic neurectomy alone, and 30 days after immobilisation of one leg in a plaster cast (Gillard et al., 1979). Each of these procedures was expected to diminish compressive loading on the tendon and thus these findings support the conclusion that biochemical change in the tendon was due to diminished compressive load.

The structural and functional properties of fibrocartilage lie between dense fibrous connective tissues that are strong in tension, and hyaline cartilage with its remarkable ability to withstand compressive loading. This tissue is found at two distinct locations in tendons (Benjamin and Evans, 1990). It is found at tendinous insertions, where it is embryonically derived from the cartilaginous primordia of bone (Rufai et al., 1992, 1995) and in the midsubstance of tendon at points where tendon wraps around bone and is subjected to compressive loading (Vogel and Koob, 1989). At midsubstance sites the fibrocartilage appears to develop by metaplasia of tendon cells. Fibrocartilage in midsubstance regions of vertebrate tendon has been described in the flexor digitorum profundus tendon of rabbit (as discussed above, Merrilees and Flint, 1980), cow (Koob and Vogel, 1987a) and dog (Okuda et al., 1987), the suprapatella of the quadriceps tendon in rat (Ralphs et al., 1991, 1992), and human tibialis posterior tendon (Vogel et al., 1993). It is common in vertebrate tendon.

PROTEOGLYCANS OF BOVINE TENDON

TISSUE MORPHOLOGY

It is useful to compare the morphology and composition of the proximal region of bovine deep flexor tendon, which is subjected only to tensional forces, with the more distal region of this tendon that passes under sesamoid bones of the metacarpo-phalangeal joint and is subjected to compressive, shear and frictional forces in addition to tension (Figure 19.1). Collagen fibres in the proximal/tensional region are arranged in longitudinal bundles and elongated cells are found among the fibres (Figure 19.1d). In contrast, collagen fibres in the region of compressive fibrocartilage are arranged in a basket-weave configuration with a great deal of interfibrillar space (Figure 19.1e,f) and the collagen fibrils are of thinner mean diameter (Evanko and Vogel, 1990). Cells of the distal/compressed tendon are round and often appear to be enclosed in lacunae. In addition to type I collagen, a lesser amount of type II collagen (the collagen type found in cartilage) was demonstrated by immunohistochemistry to be present in the extracellular matrix of this region of tendon (Vogel and Koob, 1989).

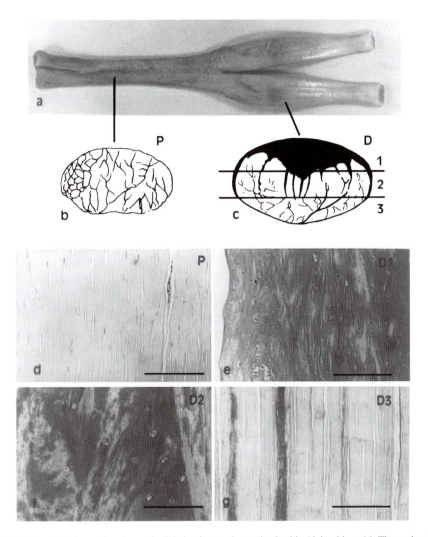

FIGURE 19.1   Histology of regions of adult bovine tendon stained with Alcian blue. (a) The entire deep flexor tendon is shown in a posterior view after removal from the joint. Cross-sections were cut from (b) the proximal/tensional and (c) the distal/compressed region, and longitudinal divisions of the distal slices made as indicated in (c). D1 is the compressed/anterior surface of the tendon and D3 is the opposite/posterior surface. The appearance of longitudinal sections from proximal/tensional (d), and distal/compressed regions D1 (e), D2 (f) and D3 (g) are shown after staining with Alcian blue. The darker staining in D1 and D2 sections corresponds to higher content of proteoglycan. Bars – 100 µm. (From Vogel *et al.*, *Eur. J. Cell Biol.*, **41**, 102–112 (1986))

PROTEOGLYCANS – TENSIONAL TENDON

Proteoglycans (PGs) are a minor constituent of proximal/tensional tendon, making up <1% of the tissue dry weight. The predominant PG is a small molecule (MW $= 10^5$) with a core protein having MW ~45,000 Da and one dermatan sulphate chain attached near the N-terminal end (Day *et al.*, 1986; Vogel and Heinegard, 1985). This molecule is now known as decorin. The core protein of this PG binds to fibrillar collagen (Brown and Vogel, 1989) and the molecule was named because collagen fibrils are 'decorated' by the PG. A small amount of large PG ($MW > 10^6$) was also found in tensional tendon. These molecules showed minimal aggregation with hyaluronan and did not have keratan sulphate chains (Vogel and Heinegard, 1985).

PROTEOGLYCANS – COMPRESSED TENDON

The GAG content of distal/compressed regions of bovine deep flexor tendon is 5 to 10 fold higher than tensional tendon and consists primarily of large proteoglycans. These large PGs were like aggrecan of articular cartilage because they were of similar large size by Sepharose chromatography, they demonstrated the ability to aggregate with hyaluronan (Vogel and Heinegard, 1985) and both chondroitin sulphate and keratan sulphate chains were present (Vogel and Thonar, 1988). It was presumed for some time, however, that they could not be aggrecan because they were in tendon. Based on tryptic peptide maps we have now demonstrated that large PGs in the compressed region of bovine tendon are, in fact, identical to aggrecan from bovine articular cartilage (Vogel et al., 1994). Throughout the rest of this chapter we will use the name 'aggrecan' to refer to large PG when we have identified it based on core protein analysis or mRNA expression. Otherwise we will refer only to 'large PG', although we believe it is likely that this will also be demonstrated to be aggrecan.

A second small PG carrying two dermatan sulphate chains was identified in fetal tendon and in the compressed region of adult bovine tendon (Fisher et al., 1989; Vogel and Evanko, 1987). This molecule is now known as biglycan. Although the core protein of biglycan is highly homologous to decorin, it did not show binding to type I collagen (Brown and Vogel, 1989; Hedbom and Heinegard, 1993). Biglycan is particularly abundant in regions of fetal tendon that are destined to receive compressive force after birth (Vogel and Evanko, 1987). Modulation of biglycan synthesis appears to be a sensitive indicator of changes in the differentiation of cells in tendon but the function of this molecule is not yet known. A third small PG carrying keratan sulphate chains, fibromodulin, was identified in fetal tendon; the fibromodulin core protein lacking GAG chains was present in both tensional and compressed regions of adult tendon (K. Vogel and P. Chevalier, unpublished result).

PG synthesis in cultured fresh tissue explants closely mimicked the type of PG found in that tissue. That is, cultured pieces of tissue from the tensional region synthesised small PG molecules and cultured pieces of tissue from the compressed region synthesised primarily large PG (Koob and Vogel, 1987b; Vogel et al., 1986). After two weeks in culture, however, cells in pieces of compressed tendon had switched their synthetic phenotype so that synthesis of small PGs was predominant (Koob and Vogel, 1987b). Cells from the compressed region of tendon expressed mRNA for aggrecan at a level similar to expression in articular chondrocytes (Robbins and Vogel, 1994). Aggrecan has often been called the 'cartilage-specific PG'. However, demonstration of aggrecan and type II collagen in tendon means that cells in a particular region of tendon have become, by most definitions, chondrocytes. It makes mechanical sense for tendon to accumulate a high level of aggrecan, the molecule that is primarily responsible for giving cartilage its compressive stiffness, right where the tissue needs to resist compression. It makes sense also that this chondrocytic synthesis would be lost when cells are no longer compressed, just as the molecules were lost from tissue when the tissue was no longer compressed (Gillard *et al.*, 1979).

GENE EXPRESSION

Gene expression for various PGs and collagen was measured in cells of each region of fresh bovine tendon from both fetal and adult animals (Robbins and Vogel, 1994). Messenger RNA for aggrecan and type II collagen was highly expressed in cells from the compressed region of adult tendon, indicating that this tissue contains cells with a chondrocytic phenotype. In contrast, only mRNA for decorin was highly expressed in cells from the tensional region of adult tendon. As might be expected, expression of mRNA for type I collagen was very high in the growing fetal tissue. The major developmental changes in mRNA expression in the compressed region of tendon included a ~25 fold increase in aggrecan expression between fetal and adult tissue and an increase in type II collagen mRNA from undetectable in fetal tendon to expression in adult tendon that was nearly as high as the level expressed in cells from adult articular cartilage. Developmental change in the tensional region, in addition to reduced expression of type I collagen, consisted of a 4 fold increase in decorin expression.

SUMMARY

This descriptive work on PG composition, synthesis, and mRNA expression in bovine tendon has provided a dynamic picture of tendon as a tissue. Correlation of the biochemical description with tissue anatomy allows us to conclude that decorin is the primary type of PG in tendon subjected to tensional load. In contrast, regions of tendon that wrap around a bony prominence contain aggrecan and biglycan as prominent components. Synthesis and accumulation of aggrecan, mRNA expression of aggrecan and type II collagen, and a rounded cellular morphology, are the criteria used to call this tissue a fibrocartilage and the cells chondrocytes. The implications of cellular transition as a result of mechanical load from fibroblast to chondrocyte, and tissue transition from tendon to fibrocartilage, are profound. The message is that differentiation of a connective tissue cell is not determined solely by its genetics but is also influenced by its environment. Environment includes the mechanical forces seen by the cell as well as the composition of the extracellular matrix that surrounds the cell. This matrix is the product of earlier cells. In tissue development, as in raising children, both nature and nurture are important.

REGULATION OF PROTEOGLYCAN SYNTHESIS BY CYCLIC COMPRESSION *IN VITRO*

Because culture of adult fibrocartilage without load led to diminished synthesis of large PG, we wondered whether imposition of a compressive load under controlled *in vitro* conditions could maintain aggrecan synthesis during culture. An additional question was whether load could induce aggrecan expression in tissue where it was not a prominent component.

ADULT TENDON FIBROCARTILAGE

A device was constructed to apply cyclic uniaxial compressive loads to unconfined discs (5 mm in diameter × 3 mm thick) of fibrocartilage from adult bovine tendon (Koob et al., 1992). The tendon bifurcates prior to passing under the bones of the foot, thereby providing two essentially identical fibrocartilaginous regions. Three discs were excised from each branch of the tendon; one disc received daily unconfined cyclic, uniaxial compressive load (544 kPa, 5 s/min, 20 min/day) while the equivalent disc from the other branch was cultured in parallel without applied load.

All discs synthesised predominantly large PG when first placed in culture. After two weeks in culture the nonloaded discs synthesised predominantly small PGs whereas loaded discs continued to produce predominantly large PG. The ratio of large/small ^{35}S-labeled PG synthesised on day 14 was nearly twofold higher in compressed tissue compared to noncompressed tissue (1.06 ± 0.09 vs. 0.57 ± 0.07). In addition, discs were maintained in culture for 21 days without applied loads and then one of each pair of discs was subjected to daily 20 min cyclic compression for 4 days. Large PG synthesis was elevated by 52% in the compressed discs compared to controls and the ratio of large to small PG synthesis in loaded discs was twice as high as that in matched discs that received no compressive stimulus in culture (Koob et al., 1992). Autoradiography demonstrated that cell proliferation during culture was minimal and confined to the disc edges, whereas ^{35}S-labeled PG synthesis occurred throughout the discs.

These experiments demonstrated that mechanical compression can regulate synthesis of distinct PG types in tendon fibrocartilage. The result is a significant demonstration, under controlled culture conditions, that cells in a differentiated adult connective tissue will alter their PG synthesis as a result of changed mechanical loading. It is notable also that a minimal loading regimen (as little as ten loading cycles in a 10 min period each day) was sufficient to maintain aggrecan synthesis.

FETAL TENDON

Experiments with fetal tendon were undertaken for both developmental and practical reasons. Because the fetal tendon has not yet fully developed a fibrocartilage at the point of future compression it was possible to ask whether application of load in vitro to the pre-fibrocartilaginous region would stimulate aggrecan synthesis. In addition, the fetal tendon is more cellular and more uniform than adult tissue (Evanko and Vogel, 1990), making it possible to measure synthesis and isolate RNA from small pieces of tissue. The device constructed for these experiments allowed us to apply continuous cyclic unconfined compression to six 8 mm segments of living tendon; matched segments were cultured in the same vessel without load (Evanko and Vogel, 1993). Segments were compressed to 70% of original thickness at a frequency of 1 cycle every 6 s (0.17 Hz) for three days. Compression was perpendicular to the long axis of the tendon. Duration of piston–tissue contact was ~0.2 s.

The primary effect of compression was to stimulate selectively synthesis of large PG and biglycan (Evanko and Vogel, 1993; Figure 19.2). Incorporation of [^{35}S]sulphate into large PG was increased 100–300% and incorporation into biglycan was increased 50–150% in compressed tissue compared to matched uncompressed tissue segments. Incorporation into decorin was unchanged. PGs synthesised by compressed tissue were larger, due to slightly longer GAG chains. Disaccharide analysis showed that the C6S/C4S ratio was higher in both the large and small PG populations from compressed tissue. In addition, Northern blot analysis showed that aggrecan mRNA levels were increased more than fivefold in loaded tissue. We feel that these results are highly significant, not just

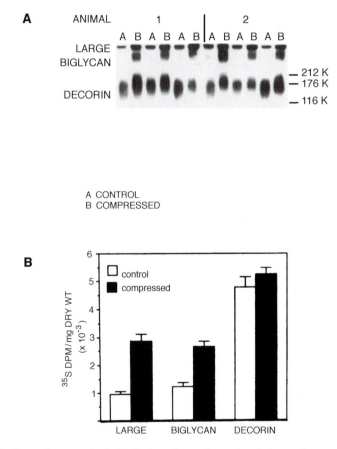

FIGURE 19.2 Proteoglycan synthesis by fetal tendon explants after 3-day cyclic compression loading. (A) Segments of the distal pre-fibrocartilaginous region of fetal tendon from two animals were subjected to 72 h of cyclic compression and allowed to incorporate [^{35}S]sulphate for 12 h. Radiolabeled proteoglycans extracted from the tissue were separated by 5.5–20% SDS/PAGE and visualised by fluorography. The migration positions of large proteoglycan, biglycan, and decorin are indicated. Molecular weight standards were myosin (212K), a2 macroglobulin (176K), and b galactosidase (116K). (B) Replicate gels were cut, solubilised and counted to quantitate the radioactivity of each type of proteoglycan. Open bars, control. Filled bars, compressed. Error bars indicate SEM ($n = 6$). (Modified from Evanko and Vogel, *Archiv. Biochem. Biophys.*, **307**,153–164, 1993)

because PG synthesis was stimulated but because the compressive regimen induced a number of alterations that are similar to the differences we had previously documented between tensional and compressed regions of tendon. Increased synthesis of large PG and biglycan, a higher chondroitin sulphate C6S/C4S sulfation ratio, and longer GAG chains are all characteristics of PGs in the compressed, as compared to the tensional, region of bovine tendon.

Similar *in vitro* loading was carried out with segments of fetal tendon from the tensional region – a tissue that does not normally experience transverse loading nor develop into fibrocartilage. The compression regimen stimulated increased synthesis of large PG and biglycan (Evanko and Vogel, 1993). This result is significant because it suggests that fetal cells from a region of tissue that would not normally become fibrocartilage are nonetheless capable of selectively responding to a compression regimen with altered PG synthesis that would lead toward fibrocartilage formation. This may be a capacity shared among cells in a wide variety of connective tissues.

EFFECTS OF TGF-β

A remarkably similar series of changes in PG synthesis was induced in fetal tendon segments subjected to cyclic compression *in vitro* and in fetal tendon segments incubated in the presence of added TGF-β1. In both cases synthesis of large PG and biglycan was enhanced whereas synthesis of decorin was not affected (Robbins *et al.*, 1997). In addition, both treatments resulted in synthesis of longer GAG chains and increased C6S/C4S ratio. These synthetic changes were also reflected in mRNA levels quantitated by slot-blot analysis of RNA isolated from cells of fetal tendon segments subjected to cyclic mechanical load. Following loading the level of aggrecan mRNA was increased 200–450%, the level of biglycan mRNA increased 100%, and the level of versican mRNA increased 130%. The level of decorin mRNA remained virtually unchanged, while expression of α1(I) collagen increased 40%. Segments cultured in the presence of 1 ng/ml TGF-β also demonstrated increased levels of mRNA for aggrecan (140%) and biglycan (120%) without change in decorin level.

The similarity of effects induced by compression and TGF-β suggested a possible causal relationship. The level of mRNA for TGF-β1 was assessed on Northern blots (for probe specificity) and on slot blots (for quantitation). In these experiments the relative level of TGF-β1 mRNA was normalised to the level of a housekeeping gene, glyceraldehyde3 phosphodehydrogenase (G3PDH). The level of TGF-β1 mRNA showed an increase of 40% after 3-day compression, compared to nonloaded control segments (Robbins *et al.*, 1997). Experiments to directly measure the amount of newly-synthesised TGF-β were then undertaken. To accomplish this, segments of fetal tendon were subjected to load, labeled with ^{35}S-cysteine, extracted, and the radioactive TGF-β collected by immunoprecipitation and quantitated after SDS/PAGE and autoradiography. The amount of newly-synthesised TGF-β immunoprecipitated from extracts of loaded tissue was several-fold greater than from nonloaded tissue. The experiments of this study support an hypothesis suggesting that one aspect of the response of cells in fetal tendon to compressive load is increased TGF-β synthesis which, in turn, stimulates synthesis of extracellular matrix PG and leads toward fibrocartilage formation.

SUMMARY

The *in vitro* loading experiments have provided evidence that fetal tendon cells respond to compressive load with rapid and appropriate changes in PG synthesis – changes which if continued over a period of time will give the tissue increased compressive stiffness. In addition, we have shown that synthesis of the large PG of fibrocartilage in adult tendon is maintained by minimal loading, but is lost when loading ceases. These observations greatly strengthen the hypothesis that tendon cells are capable of a rapid and appropriate response to mechanical stimuli.

PROTEOGLYCANS IN HUMAN TENDONS

TIBIALIS POSTERIOR

In the proximal/tensional region of human tibialis posterior tendon collagen bundles were organised in a strictly linear manner with elongate cells between the fibre bundles (Vogel *et al.*, 1993). In contrast, the collagen arrangement in the more distal region that passes under the medial malleolus was less linear and often swirled, and the cells had a more rounded appearance. The proximal/tensional region was not stained at all with Alcian blue whereas the distal/compressed region showed definite staining that was particularly prominent surrounding the cells. GAG content was 3.3 fold higher in the region of tibialis posterior tendon that passes under the medial malleolus than in adjacent proximal/tensional regions (Vogel *et al.*, 1993). By SDS/PAGE and Western blot analysis the compressed region of this tendon contained large PG and biglycan in addition to decorin whereas the tensional region contained only decorin. In addition, decorin from the compressed region of the tendon migrated more slowly in the gel, indicating that it was larger than decorin from the tensional region. Because the decorin core proteins migrated to the same position we conclude that the GAG chains on decorin from the compressed region were longer.

ROTATOR CUFF

Longitudinal midsubstance sections of human rotator cuff tendons revealed a tissue that was quite different from the tibialis posterior tendon. The rotator cuff tendons were characterised by dense bundles of linear collagen fibres with a few highly elongated cells. Between these bundles of collagen was an irregular loose matrix that stained darkly with Alcian blue, indicating that this is the location of most of the glycosaminoglcyans. Blood vessels were embedded in this material. The GAG content of supraspinatus, infra-spinatus and subscapularis tendons was determined in left and right shoulders of seven individuals ranging in age from 22 to 72 years (Berenson *et al.*, 1996). For comparison, GAG content was measured in the distal/tensional region of the biceps tendons of the same shoulders and the proximal portion that runs over the head of the humerus receiving transverse pressure in addition to tension. All tendons were free of gross pathology. The GAG content for all three tendons of the rotator cuff was generally similar and in every case the level was higher (mean = 2.5 fold higher) than in the tensional region of biceps tendon (Berenson *et al.*, 1996). Approximately half of the GAG in each tendon was determined to be hyaluronan. PG extracted from the tensional region of biceps tendon was exclusively decorin. In contrast, PGs extracted from tendons of the rotator cuff included large PG and biglycan, as well as decorin. The large PG was probably aggrecan, based on size and the presence of both chondroitin sulphate and keratan sulphate GAG chains. The core proteins of two other small PGs, fibromodulin and lumican, were also found in the cuff tendons; these proteins did not have associated GAG chains.

These studies demonstrate that the PG content of rotator cuff tendons and the region of human tibialis posterior that passes under the medial malleolus includes biglycan and large PG in addition to decorin, and therefore, in terms of PG type, these tendons are similar to the fibrocartilaginous region of bovine deep flexor tendon. However, Alcian blue staining of histological sections revealed intriguing distinctions among PG-rich regions of the three tendons that are the subject of this paper. (1) In the region of bovine deep flexor tendon that wraps under bone, the matrix stains uniformly dark with Alcian blue; lacunae containing round cells are embedded in this matrix. In short, it looks like articular cartilage. (2) Alcian blue staining of the region of human tibialis posterior that contacts the medial malleolus was not found throughout the matrix. Instead, staining was localised around individual cells in the tissue which appeared to have synthesised a surrounding layer of PGs. (3) In tendons of the rotator cuff, seams of an irregular matrix material that stained with Alcian blue were located between the longitudinal collagen bundles. The material in these seams was often separated from the collagen bundles beside it, suggesting that these layers were not tightly attached to each other.

CONCLUSIONS AND SPECULATION

This work has led us to conclude that it is possible to say something about the mechanical environment in tissue by examining the amount and type of PGs that are present. Cells in a collagen-rich connective tissue that contain elevated GAG levels, and both large PGs and biglycan in addition to decorin, have responded to a mechanical environment that is distinct from pure tension and includes hydrostatic stress/compression.

We suggest that the function of the large PG (aggrecan) in tendon, by analogy to its role in cartilage, is to resist compressive load by providing the fixed negative charge density that holds counterions and water in the tissue. To accomplish this in tendons under high load, the PG is dispersed throughout the collagenous matrix, as in bovine tendon. Where load is less, as in the human tibialis posterior, PG surrounds some cells but does not permeate all of the collagenous matrix. PG accumulation in the rotator cuff tendons had a different localisation. The rotator cuff tendons, as described by Clark and Harryman (1992), consist of several layers in which tendon fasicles run longitudinally and also at an angle of 45° to each other. PGs were concentrated in material between the collagenous bundles. In this location, the large PGs could function to separate and lubricate the collagen bundles as they slide relative to each other during the normal and complex motions of the shoulder. This function is not the same as providing direct resistance to compressive load, but it may also be based on the hydrophilic nature of the GAG chains of aggrecan.

The appearance of PG in layers of loose tissue that separate the collagen bundles of rotator cuff tendons could be a response designed to minimise shear stress by allowing collagen fibres to move easily relative to each other. In support of the latter suggestion we note that the uniform proteoglyan-rich, fibrocartilaginous matrix of bovine deep flexor tendon is found only on the inner curvature of this tendon (i.e. near the point of contact with bone and extending several mm into the tissue) where hydrostatic forces are highest. However, deeper into this tissue and at the outer curvature (where collagen fibres must be displaced a greater distance relative to each other as the tendon bends) longitudinal sections reveal linear collagen bundles separated by layers of loosely organised PG-rich material (Vogel *et al.*, 1986; compare Figures 19.1e–g). Cross-sectional images of this tissue show that the endotenon is expanded (Figure 19.3B). The region of this tendon subjected only to tension does not have a PG-rich layer of material around collagen bundles (Figure 19.3A).

As we continue to investigate the transitions of which tendon is capable, the thesis so eloquently stated by Nathan and Sporn (1991) takes on increasing significance. They said 'the extracellular matrix of a cell reflects its metabolic history'. That is, the biochemical composition and organisation of tissue matrix contains both a record of the past history of that tissue, and information that regulates its cellular response to stimuli in the present. We believe that the PG content of tendon is a relevant part of its metabolic history, written in biochemical language and thus available to become a useful marker of the tissue's current functional status.

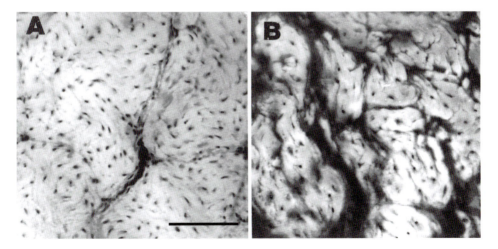

FIGURE 19.3 Histology of adult bovine deep flexor tendon – cross section. Collagen bundles and cells of the (A) proximal/tensional region and (B) distal/compressed region at the D2 level (see Figure 19.1). Note that the endotenon is indistinct in the tensional region, but contains a great deal of stained extracellular matrix in the compressed region. Bar = 100 μm.

ACKNOWLEDGEMENTS

This manuscript is based on a paper that was awarded the 1996 Elizabeth Winston Lanier Kappa Delta Award for Basic Science by the American Academy of Orthopaedic Surgeons. Many colleagues have contributed to developing the ideas and performing the experiments of this project. We wish to specifically acknowledge Dr. Dick Heinegard, Dr. Thomas Koob, Dr. John Trotter, Dan Hernandez, Dr. Alice Maroudas, Dr. Field Blevins, Matthew Berenson, Dr. David Thompson, and Kevin Hollander.

Grant support was provided by the National Institutes of Health (AR36110).

REFERENCES

Benjamin, M. and Evans, E.J. (1990) Fibrocartilage. *J. Anat.*, **171**, 1–15.

Berenson, M.C., Blevins, F.T., Plaas, A.H.K. and Vogel, K.G. (1996) Proteoglycans of human rotator cuff tendons. *J. Orthop. Res.*, **14**, 518–525.

Brown, D.C. and Vogel, K.G. (1989) Characteristics of the *in vitro* interaction of a small proteoglycan (PGII) of bovine tendon with type I collagen. *Matrix*, **9**, 468–478.

Clark, J.M. and Harryman, D.T. (1992) Tendons, ligaments, and capsule of the rotator cuff. *J. Bone Joint Surg.*, **74-A**, 713–725.

Day, A.A., Ramis, C.I., Fisher, L.W., Geheron-Robey, P., Termine, J.D. and Young, M.F. (1986) Characterization of bone PG II cDNA and its relationship to PG II mRNA from other connective tissues. *Nuc. Acid Res.*, **14**, 9861–9876.

Evanko, S.P. and Vogel, K.G. (1990) Ultrastructure and proteoglycan composition in the developing fibrocartilaginous region of bovine tendon. *Matrix*, **10**, 420–436.

Evanko, S.P. and Vogel, K.G. (1993) Proteoglycan synthesis in fetal tendon is differentially regulated by cyclic compression *in vitro*. *Archiv. Biochem. Biophys.*, **307**, 153–164.

Fisher, L.W., Termine, J.D. and Young, M.F. (1989) Deduced protein sequence of a bone small proteoglycan I (biglycan) shows homology with proteoglycan II (decorin) and several nonconnective tissue proteins in a variety of species. *J. Biol. Chem.*, **264**, 4571–4576.

Gillard, G.C., Merrilees, M.J., Bell-Booth, P.G., Reilly, H.C. and Flint, M.H. (1977) The proteoglycan content and the axial periodicity of collagen in tendon. *Biochem. J.*, **163**, 145–151.

Gillard, G.C., Reilly, H.C., Bell-Booth, P.G. and Flint, M. (1979) The influence of mechanical forces on the glycosaminoglycan content of the rabbit flexor digitorum profundus tendon. *Connect. Tiss. Res.*, **7**, 37–46.

Hedbom, E. and Heinegard, D. (1993) Binding of fibromodulin and decorin to separate sites on fibrillar collagens. *J. Biol. Chem.*, **268**, 27307–27312.

Koob, T.J. and Vogel, K.G. (1987a) Site related variations in glycosaminoglycan content and swelling properties of bovine flexor tendon. *J. Orthop. Res.*, **5**, 414–424.

Koob, T.J. and Vogel, K.G. (1987b) Proteoglycans synthesis in organ cultures from regions of bovine tendon subjected to different mechanical forces. *Biochem. J.*, **246**, 589–598.

Koob, T.J., Clark, P.E., Hernandez, D.J., Thurmond, F.A. and Vogel, K.G. (1992) Compression loading *in vitro* regulates proteoglycan synthesis by tendon fibrocartilage. *Arch. Biochem. Biophys.*, **298**, 303–312.

Merrilees, M.J. and Flint, M.H. (1980) Ultrastructural study of tension and pressure zones in a rabbit flexor tendon. *Amer. J. Anat.*, **157**, 87–106.

Nathan, C. and Sporn, M. (1991) Cytokines in context. *J. Cell Biol.*, 113, 981–986.

Okuda, Y., Gorski, J.P. and Amadio, P.C. (1987) Effect of postnatal age on the ultrastructure of six anatomical areas of canine flexor digitorum profundus tendon. *J. Orthop. Res.*, **5**, 231–241.

Ploetz, E. (1938) Functioneller Bau und functionelle Anpassung der Gleitsehnen. *Z. Orthop.*, **67**, 212–234.

Ralphs, J.R., Benjamin, M. and Thornett, A. (1991) Cell and matrix biology of the suprapatella in the rat: A structural and immunocytochemical study of fibrocartilage in a tendon subject to compression. *Anat. Rec.*, **231**, 167–177.

Ralphs, J.R., Tyers, R.N.S. and Benjamin, M. (1992) Development of functionally distinct fibrocartilages at two sites in the quadriceps tendon of the rat: the suprapatella and the attachment to the patella. *Anat. Embryol.*, **185**, 181–187.

Robbins, J.R. and Vogel, K.G. (1994) Regional expression of mRNA for proteoglycans and collagen in tendon. *Eur. J. Cell Biol.*, **64**, 264–270.

Robbins, J.R., Evanko, S.P. and Vogel, K.G. (1997) Mechanical loading and TGF-β regulate proteoglycan synthesis in tendon. *Arch. Biochem. Biophys.*, **342**, 201–211.

Rufai, A., Benjamin, M. and Ralphs, J.R. (1992) Development an ageing of phenotyically distinct fibrocartilages associated with the rat Achilles tendon. *Anat. Embryol.*, **186**, 611–618.

Rufai, A., Ralphs, J.R. and Benjamin, M. (1995) The structure and histopathology of the insertional region of the human Achilles tendon. *J. Orthop. Res.*, **13**, 585–593.

Vogel, K.G. and Evanko, S.P. (1987) Proteoglycans of fetal bovine tendon. *J. Biol. Chem.*, **262**, 13607–13613.

Vogel, K.G. and Heinegard, D. (1985) Characterization of proteoglycans from adult bovine tendon. *J. Biol. Chem.*, **260**, 9298–9306.

Vogel, K.G., Keller, E.J., Lenhoff, R.J., Campbell, K. and Koob, T.J. (1986) Proteoglycan synthesis by fibroblast cultures initiated from regions of adult bovine tendon subjected to different mechanical forces. *Eur. J. Cell Biol.*, **41**, 102–112.

Vogel, K.G. and Koob, T.J. (1989) Structural specialization in tendons under compression. *Int. Rev. Cytol.*, **115**, 267–293.

Vogel, K.G., Ordog, A., Pogany, G. and Olah, J. (1993) Proteoglycans in the compressed region of human tibialis posterior tendon and in ligaments. *J. Orthop. Res.*, **11**, 68–77.

Vogel, K.G., Sandy, J.D., Pogany, G.L. and Robbins, J.R. (1994) Aggrecan in bovine tendon. *Matrix Biol.*, **14**, 171–179.

Vogel, K.G. and Thonar, E.J.-M.A. (1988) Keratan sulfate is a component of proteoglycan in the compressed region of adult bovine flexor tendon. *J. Orthop. Res.*, **6**, 434–442.

20 Ageing and Pathology of the Rotator Cuff

Graham Riley

Rheumatology Research Unit, Box 194, Addenbrooke's Hospital, Cambridge CB2 2QQ

INTRODUCTION

Synovial joints consist of a variety of tissues, including bone, cartilage, synovium, capsule, ligament and tendon. Each tissue has a specific and important role; bone provides the main structural component, cartilage cushions the bony interface and the synovium lubricates the tissue surfaces. Ligaments and capsule hold the joint together, and tendons transmit force from muscle to bone. Although heterogeneous in structure and composition, these tissues do not function in isolation. In a normal joint, they act together to support and maintain pain-free motion, and the structure and function of each tissue is finely tuned to meet the mechanical requirements of the joint. Thus the synovial joint is best thought of as a complex 'organ', comprising both hard and soft tissues. In the arthritides, although the pathology might have its origins in any one of these tissues, all of the joint tissues will be involved to some degree. Studies of arthritic disease however, have concentrated largely on bone, cartilage and synovium. The soft tissues of the joint – the tendons, ligaments and capsule – have been largely ignored, even though it is increasingly recognised that many arthritides are caused primarily by lesions affecting them. This chapter focuses on the rotator cuff tendon complex in the shoulder; a collection of soft tissues which is frequently involved in synovial joint pathology.

OVERVIEW OF ROTATOR CUFF 'TENDINITIS' AND SOFT TISSUE RHEUMATISM

Lesions of tendons, tendon sheaths, and their insertions ('entheses') are a common cause of soft tissue rheumatism and associated with much pain and chronic disability. These and other soft tissue problems are responsible for an estimated four million general practitioner consultations a year, and comprise up to twenty-five percent of all referrals to rheumatology clinics (Wood *et al.*, 1979; Bamji *et al.*, 1990).

'Tendinitis' is the clinical term often used to describe any condition causing pain when a tendon is placed under tension. A number of different tendons are commonly affected by tendinitis, including the calcaneal (Achilles) tendon and the common extensor tendon at its origin from the lateral epicondyle ('tennis elbow'). However the most frequent site of tendinitis, often leading to tendon rupture, is the rotator cuff complex in the shoulder (Codman, 1934).

Tendinitis is not often treated surgically and frequently does not have an obvious cause such as trauma to explain the pathology. It affects the main body of the tendon and is not necessarily associated with inflammation of the tendon sheath (tenosynovitis) – often affecting tendons that lack a tendon sheath (Leadbetter, 1992). The name presupposes an inflammatory component, although evidence of inflammation from histopathological studies is often lacking.

Rotator cuff tendinitis is the most common of the regional musculoskeletal disorders, and a major problem in the community (Chard and Hazleman, 1987; Bjelle, 1989). Pain, dysfunction and ultimately tendon rupture most frequently affect the supraspinatus tendon in the superior portion of the rotator cuff, and this tendon is the main focus of this paper.

CLINICAL PERSPECTIVE

Rotator cuff tendinitis often presents with the onset of pain localised to the insertion of deltoid. Pain is often worse at night and exacerbated when the arm is raised, typically between 60 and 120 degrees of elevation (Kessel and Watson, 1977). Active voluntary motion is often restricted, but passive elevation of the arm is generally possible. There may be a distinct catch during elevation as a result of an impingement between the soft tissues of the joint and the under surface of the acromion or coraco-acromial ligament (Dalton, 1989).

Although considered a self limiting condition, which slowly resolves with time, the prognosis is poor in a significant number of patients (Binder *et al.*, 1984; Bulgen *et al.*, 1984). The factors that influence recovery are poorly understood and the response to treatment is extremely variable. Conventional conservative therapies of rest, physiotherapy and non-steroidal anti-inflammatory therapy are often of limited benefit and many patients do not respond to corticosteroid injection (Berry *et al.*, 1980; Fearnley and Vadasz, 1969).

As affected tendons are not biopsied, our understanding of the disease process is relatively poor. Most patients present in middle-age and often without any remembered incident of shoulder injury or trauma (Hazleman, 1989). It is generally believed that age-related 'degenerative' changes of the tendon are important. However it is not known whether such changes are uniform throughout the population, or whether some individuals are predisposed to tendinitis. Certain occupations, sports and activities are all associated with shoulder pain, although no single specific offending activity has yet been described. Some individuals appear to be predisposed to soft tissue lesions, as syndromes as diverse as rotator cuff tendinitis, tennis elbow, de Quervain's tenosynovitis and Dupuytren's contracture tend to occur more frequently in the same individuals (Nirschl and Pettrone, 1973; Day *et al.*, 1978; Binder and Hazleman, 1983). The anatomical shape and disposition of the structures comprising the shoulder joint has been cited as a primary cause of much shoulder pain and tendon degeneration (Neer, 1983). Thus an understanding of the physiology and anatomy of the shoulder is important in any consideration of rotator cuff tendinitis.

PHYSIOLOGY AND ANATOMY OF THE ROTATOR CUFF

The human shoulder is adapted to allow a wide range of movement of the upper limb and the overhead activity of the hand. The shoulder is a complex of joints, the most important of which are the glenohumeral joint, the acromioclavicular joint and the scapulothoracic joint. Normal shoulder activity requires the synchronous functioning of each of these joints and their related muscle groups to accomplish pain free movement (Constant, 1989).

The glenohumeral joint between the head of the humerus and the flat glenoid fossa of the scapula is functionally a ball and socket type joint, but lacks the bony stability that characterises the hip joint. The great mobility of the shoulder has thus been obtained at the expense of joint stability. Functional stability is maintained by the soft tissues which surround the joint – the joint capsule, the glenohumeral ligaments and the rotator cuff, a group of muscles with tendons that insert onto the head of the humerus (Kessel and Bayley, 1986).

Movement of the arm is initiated and stabilised by the co-ordinated contraction of the muscles of the rotator cuff. Supraspinatus lies superiorly, the long head of biceps inferiorly, subscapularis anteriorly and infraspinatus and teres minor posteriorly. The rotator cuff tendons are fused together in the adult, occupying the superior portion of the glenohumeral joint and separating it from the subacromial bursa. The tendons and their corresponding muscle form a precisely controlled complex which acts co-operatively in the healthy shoulder to assure pain-free movement (de Palma, 1983).

The shoulder joint capsule, reinforced by the rotator cuff tendons is lax and allows considerable movement of the glenohumeral joint. It is strengthened at certain points by the glenohumeral ligaments below and the coracohumeral and transverse humeral ligaments above. These ligaments assist the rotator cuff tendons in supporting the joint. The external superior surface of the cuff tendons forms the floor of the subacromial bursa, a fluid filled cavity that acts to lubricate and facilitate joint movement – a function that may often be compromised in pathologic lesions and trauma affecting these tissues (Bywaters, 1979). In the normal healthy shoulder, the joint cavity and subacromial bursa do not communicate, but may do so as a result of degenerative changes or injury to the tendons. The acromion forms an arch over the superior part of the glenohumeral joint and the supraspinatus tendon, articulating with the clavicle at the acromioclavicular joint. The coracohumeral ligament stretches between the coracoid process of the scapula and the medial border of the acromion. Both these structures have been implicated in the pathology of rotator cuff tendinitis, because of the association of 'impingement' [on the tendon] with many rotator cuff tears (Neer, 1983).

PATHOLOGY OF TENDINITIS

Normal tendon is immensely strong under tension and does not normally rupture in mid-substance under normal physiological load unless prior degeneration has occurred (Cronkite, 1936). Consequently it is generally believed that 'degenerative' changes of the tendon matrix are important in the pathology of tendinitis.

The supraspinatus tendon on the superior aspect of the cuff is most often affected by tendinitis and tendon rupture. Most lesions are typically found in a region approximately 1.0 cm from the bony insertion – an area which has been described as the 'critical zone' (Codman, 1934). Vascular injection studies have correlated the critical zone with a region of anastomosis between bone-derived and muscle-derived blood vessels (Moseley and Goldie, 1963). The tendon was otherwise relatively well vascularised, although Moseley and Goldie (1963) reported no change in the anastomotic network with age.

A hypovascular region was identified in the majority (63%) of supraspinatus tendons, but only found in a small proportion of infraspinatus and subscapularis tendons (37% and 7% respectively; Rothman and Parke, 1965). There was also a reduction in the size of the vascular bed with age. Thus avascularity of the supraspinatus was correlated directly with degenerative changes in the tendon, and it has been suggested there is a 'wringing out' of the blood vessels when the arm is in a resting position of adduction and neutral rotation (Rathbun and MacNab, 1970). In an animal model, similar degenerative changes – including the breakdown of the collagen fibril structure, a reduction in cell density, lipid accumulation and calcification – could be induced in rabbit Achilles tendon, using a plastic insert that impinges on the tendon and reduces tendon blood flow (MacNab, 1973).

More recent studies have questioned the clinical significance of these observations. Brooks et al. (1992), used quantitative histological analysis to show that there was no significant difference in the size of the vascular bed in infraspinatus and supraspinatus tendons and that both had zones of relative hypovascularity. Laser doppler flow studies have demonstrated that the 'critical zone' remains well perfused (Chansky and Ianotti, 1991). Tendon cells are also substantially more resistant to hypoxia than other cell types, and tendon explants can be maintained by diffusion of nutrients alone, without the need for blood perfusion (Webster and Burry, 1982; Lundborg et al., 1980). Therefore it is thought unlikely that vascular changes alone can precipitate supraspinatus tendon degeneration.

One theory, which has gained general acceptance more recently, suggests that 95% of rotator cuff tears can be attributed to an 'impingement' of the supraspinatus tendon against the overlying acromion or acromioclavicular joint (Neer, 1983). In some individuals, the shape and slope of the overlying acromion causes a narrowing of the free space through which the tendon must pass, predisposing to impingement. In many cases, rotator cuff tears are associated with an osteophytic outgrowth from the acromion or acromioclavicular joint (Neer, 1983). Impingement is thus considered a unifying concept, in which the various pathological entities – of tendon strain, inflammation, fibrosis and rupture – are viewed as different stages of a common pathological process (Cofield, 1985). However, radiological studies of normal and painful shoulders have shown no association of rotator cuff tears with osteoarthritic changes in the joint and little evidence of osteophytic bone formation on the acromial margin (Cotton and Rideout, 1964). Ozaki (1988) examined 200 shoulders and found no direct association of partial tears of the tendons with any acromial abnormalities. In addition, many of the earliest degenerative changes are found in the central part of the tendon (Olson, 1953). Other studies have found that small tears are found within the main body of the tendon and at the articular surface more frequently than the bursal surface (Fukuda et al., 1990). Impingement may be secondary to tendon pathology, which reduces the functional ability of the rotator cuff to maintain the position of the humeral head during rotation, allowing the humerus to rise up, and pinch the tendon against the acromial arch. Alternatively, swelling of the tendon may occur after injury, causing impingement which would then further exacerbate the tendon injury.

In summary, an accumulation of tissue damage occurring in an area which is hypovascular, and therefore relatively hypoxic, has been proposed to account for tendon degeneration and rupture. It is not known to what extent the aged tendon fibroblast (tenocyte) is able to mount an effective repair response and whether the chronicity of supraspinatus tendon lesions is essentially a problem of poor tissue repair. In the absence of any convincing animal models, very little is known about the cellular processes involved in tendinitis and tendon degeneration. There is little understanding of the relative contribution of 'intrinsic factors', such as tenocyte viability and synthetic activity, and 'extrinsic factors' such as trauma and mechanical forces (tension, compression and shear). Changes in the structure and composition of the tendon matrix are presumed to predispose to tendinitis and tendon rupture, although exactly what matrix changes are involved has only recently been the subject of investigation.

HISTOPATHOLOGY

A number of studies have described an increased incidence of 'degenerative change' in cadaver supraspinatus tendons with advancing age (Keyes, 1935; Lindblom, 1939; Wilson and Duff, 1943; Simmonds, 1943; Olson, 1953). These early studies typically reported degenerative features such as abnormality in the tendon collagen structure, with a granularity and loss of the normal clearly defined, wavy outline of the collagen fibre bundles (Wilson and Duff, 1943). Cellular changes were evident, with a loss of the normal parallel alignment, and many cells had a rounded, shrunken nucleus. The tendon fascicles were separated by a more homogenous, sclerotic tissue and the distinct inter-fascicular (endotenon) structure seen in younger individuals was lost (Lindblom, 1939).

In a recent study of ageing cadaver tendons we confirmed these observations, but reported a number of other degenerative changes including the presence of calcification, lipid deposits and blood vessel changes (intimal thickening; Chard et al., 1994). The most frequent observation, found in 18% of specimens, was glycosaminoglycan (GAG) infiltration between the collagen fibrils, frequently associated with cell rounding and fibrocartilaginous metaplasia. Similar increases in GAG were observed in degenerative tendinitis, though much more frequently, affecting 75% of tendons. These studies showed how rare it was to find a normal supraspinatus tendon in individuals over the age of thirty.

We have developed a scoring system to grade the severity of degenerative change, based on the structure and organisation of the collagen fibrils and the appearance of the tenocytes (Goddard *et al.*, 1992). On a four point scale of increasing degeneration, we classified normal tendon as grade 1 and the most severely degenerate tendon grade 4. An analysis of over 100 supraspinatus tendons showed that only 23% [of tendons] under 40 years of age were normal (grade 1). This proportion declined steadily with age, with less than 10% normal tendons over 80 years of age. The proportion of tendons most severely affected (grade 4) increased from 18% in tendons under 40 years, to peak at 45% in tendons between 60 and 80 years of age. In contrast, a sample of age-matched tendons from the insertion of biceps brachii – a flexor tendon that is rarely affected by any pathology – were predominantly normal (grade 1; 79%), with the remainder showing only mild degeneration (grade 2). Out of 40 supraspinatus tendons coming to surgery for degenerative tendinitis, all showed either moderate or severe degeneration of the collagen fibre network (grades 3 and 4). These observations are consistent with the hypothesis that accumulated changes in the tendon matrix, which are common in the supraspinatus tendon, are more severe in patients with tendinitis and predispose to tendon rupture. Although it involves extensive remodelling of the collagen fibre network, the mechanism of change is not yet known, but presumably involves an altered pattern of collagen synthesis, or collagen breakdown, (or both) mediated by the tenocytes within the tendon substance. The biochemical changes of the tendon matrix with age and degeneration have only recently been investigated, and some of this data is summarised below.

CHANGES IN COLLAGEN COMPOSITION

Connective tissues are composed of a unique combination of extracellular matrix components that gives each tissue its particular structural characteristics. The high concentration of collagen and the dense, highly ordered arrangement of fibrils parallel to the long axis of the tendon, endows the tendon with much of its mechanical properties, enabling the transmission of potentially huge tensile forces between muscle and bone (Evans and Barbenel, 1975; Davison, 1992).

Normal adult flexor tendon is composed predominantly of type I collagen which constitutes between 50% and 85% of the tendon dry weight depending on the tendon, species and location (Elliott, 1965). A number of other collagens have also been identified in tendon, and these include collagen types III, V, VI, XII and XIV, although together they comprise less than 5% of the typical flexor tendon (von der Mark, 1981).

In a recently published biochemical study (Riley *et al.*, 1994a), we have shown that the collagen content of the normal (cadaver) supraspinatus tendon averaged 67% of the tendon dry weight, and did not change significantly with age, although there was considerable variation within the sample (range 55% to 79%, $n = 60$). This was not significantly different from the tendon at the insertion of biceps.

In degenerate tendons, the amount of collagen was significantly reduced, although many specimens were within the (lower) limits of the normal range. This data is consistent with an increase in collagen turnover in degenerative tendinitis, possibly mediated by interstitial collagenase (MMP-1), an enzyme which is known to be produced by tendon explants in culture (Riley *et al.*, 1994b; Dalton *et al.*, 1995) and has recently been immunolocalised to tenocytes throughout the degenerate tendon matrix (Riley, G.P., unpublished observations).

Much of the collagen was extremely insoluble, limiting our ability to estimate the proportion of different collagen types in the tendon matrix, although Western blotting of pepsin-soluble collagen showed type III collagen was present in many degenerate and ruptured tendons, but not abundant in normal tendon. Chemical digestion with cyanogen bromide, cleaving collagens into large peptides at methionine residues, was able to release substantially more collagen for analysis. Using SDS-PAGE and scanning densitometry of Coomasie blue-stained peptides, we were able to show that nearly 90% of ruptured tendons contained more type III collagen, averaging almost 10% of the total collagen, compared to less than 3% [type III collagen] in normal tendons (Riley *et al.*, 1994a). No other collagen types were identified, although the technique is relatively insensitive for low levels of collagen expression. Interestingly, we found that 17% (10/60) of non-ruptured cadaver tendons also contained greater than 5% (up to 15%) type III collagen, suggesting that changes in collagen expression might weaken the tendon and predispose to tendon rupture.

In immunolocalisation studies, we found that type III collagen was distributed throughout the tendon matrix in degenerate tendons, co-localised with type I collagen, where it may be intercalated into the fibrillar structure. Type VI collagen was found distributed throughout the tendon matrix in regions in normal tendons with an organised fibril structure. However, in regions where the tendon matrix was fibrocartilaginous, type VI collagen was distributed pericellularly, associated with the rounded cells, much as it is in cartilage. We looked for the expression of type II collagen, a collagen usually restricted to cartilage or fibrocartilage at tendon and ligament insertions (Benjamin and Ralphs, 1995). Positive staining was found in only one out of twenty four supraspinatus tendons examined. Either Type II collagen expression is not a general feature of fibrocartilaginous change in the supraspinatus, or alternatively low levels of type II collagen expression might not be revealed by immunostaining.

CHANGES IN PROTEOGLYCAN COMPOSITION

Proteoglycans (PGs) and GAGs typically constitute less than 0.5% of the normal flexor tendon dry weight, although higher levels – approaching 3.5% of the dry weight – are found in fibrocartilaginous regions of animal flexor digitorum profundus (FDP) tendons (Merrilees and Flint, 1980). In these fibrocartilaginous regions, the tendon is weight bearing and subject to compressive loading. The small dermatan sulphate PG decorin is the principal PG in the typical flexor tendon, where it is associated with specific regions of the collagen molecule and may have some role in determining the collagen fibre diameter (Scott and Orford, 1981). Fibromodulin, a keratan sulphate-containing PG, is also found associated with collagen fibres, where it may have a similar role to decorin (Hardingham and Fosang, 1992). Biglycan and the large, aggregating PG aggrecan are also found in tendon, but restricted to the specialised region of fibrocartilage in the bovine and other FDP tendons (Vogel and Koob, 1989). Aggrecan and other large proteoglycans are hydrophilic, acting to maintain tissue turgor and resist compressive forces; the function of biglycan is unknown (Hardingham and Fosang, 1992).

Supraspinatus tendons have a very different PG composition compared to a normal flexor tendon (Riley *et al.*, 1994c; Berenson *et al.*, 1996). Normal tendons have between 3 and 10 fold as much GAG compared to the biceps tendon, with a greater concentration toward the bone insertion, where the tendons wrap around the head of humerus (Riley *et al.*, 1994c). Chondroitin sulphate was the most abundant GAG, with a smaller proportion of dermatan sulphate (56% and 20% of the total respectively), whereas the major GAG in biceps was dermatan sulphate (80%) with only a small proportion of chondroitin sulphate (20%). The supraspinatus was also shown to contain a large PG similar to aggrecan, as demonstrated by SDS PAGE, elution from sepharose CL-4B, and the presence of chondroitin sulphate and keratan sulphate chains (Riley *et al.*, 1994c; Berenson *et al.*, 1996). Decorin and biglycan were both present, as demonstrated by SDS PAGE and core protein immunoreactivity. In contrast, only the small dermatan sulphate PG decorin was found in the biceps tendon (Riley *et al.*, 1994c).

In degenerative supraspinatus tendinitis there was a significant increase in hyaluronan ($p < 0.001$), chondroitin sulphate ($p < 0.05$) and dermatan sulphate ($p < 0.001$) compared to age matched normal tendons (Riley *et al.*, 1994c). Together with the increase in type III collagen, these changes are consistent with a wound healing response and the production of fibrous scar tissue. This is consistent with an abortive attempt to repair, occurring either before or after the tendon rupture, and suggests that the supraspinatus tenocytes have only a limited repair potential.

In summary, the PG content of the supraspinatus is similar to fibrocartilage of tendons that have been subjected to compressive loads. We have previously shown that fibrocartilage metaplasia is relatively common in the supraspinatus tendon, presumably in response to the particular mechanical demands placed upon the rotator cuff tendons at the shoulder (Chard *et al.*, 1994). Not all supraspinatus tendons have the typical histological appearance of mature fibrocartilage however, as much of the GAG is found between collagen fibres, where it may act to separate and lubricate movement of collagen bundles during shoulder motion (Berenson *et al.*, 1996). Thus the importance of fibrocartilaginous metaplasia, and the relationship with supraspinatus tendon pathology, remain the matter of debate.

TENASCIN-C AND FIBROCARTILAGINOUS CHANGE

We have recently proposed that the cell rounding and fibrocartilaginous change, seen in many degenerate and ruptured tendons, has a major role in supraspinatus tendon pathology (Cawston *et al.*, 1996). Tendon fibrocartilage develops where tendons are compressed, involves changes in matrix synthesis and turnover, and the tissue has a number of different functional characteristics compared to normal, tension-bearing tendons. Fibrocartilage is potentially less strong under tension, is relatively avascular, has a reduced metabolic activity, and a differential ability to repair after injury (Vogel and Koob, 1989; Abrahamsson, 1991; Nessler *et al.*, 1992).

The changes in tendon cell phenotype found in fibrocartilage metaplasia may be directed by a number of mechanisms, including locally produced cytokines and growth factors, the direct effects of mechanical forces on the cytoskeleton, and interactions between the cell and matrix components. We became interested in the extracellular matrix glycoprotein tenascin-C, which was reported to be involved in chondrocyte differentiation, an effect which may be mediated by its ability to promote mesenchymal cell rounding (Mackie *et al.*, 1987; Choung *et al.*, 1993). Consequently we examined the hypothesis that tenascin-C has a role in fibrocartilaginous change and supraspinatus tendon pathology.

Tenascin-C (hereafter referred to as tenascin) is found in many connective tissues in association with tissue remodelling during embryogenesis, development and pathogenesis. The structure of tenascin is reviewed in detail elsewhere and is only briefly discussed here (Chiquet *et al.*, 1984; Gulcher *et al.*, 1989; Spring *et al.*, 1989). Tenascin is a hexameric protein with disulphide-linked subunits of between 200 kDa and 300 kDa in man, each consisting of a series of domains with structural homology to epidermal growth factor, fibronectin and fibrinogen (Chiquet and Fambrough, 1984). Alternative splicing of the tenascin gene results in up to eight different isoforms (in the human) with differing numbers of fibronectin type III repeats (Gulcher *et al.*, 1989; Spring *et al.*, 1989). Patterns of expression of splice variants are tissue-specific and can vary with pathology (Mackie and Tucker, 1992; Chuong and Chen, 1991). There is evidence that different variants have different functions (Chiquet-Ehrismann *et al.*, 1991; Murphy-Ullrich *et al.*, 1991). Functions of tenascin so far identified include regulation of cell proliferation and migration (Mackie, 1994). Tenascin is present in normal adult tendon, but its expression is markedly enhanced in healing chicken tendon wounds (Chuong and Chen, 1991).

We observed striking alterations in the distribution of tenascin in degenerate tendons (Figure 20.1, Riley *et al.*, 1996). In normal, fibrous regions of tendons, tenascin staining was associated with the collagen fibrils. In degenerate and ruptured tendons, tenascin staining was absent from the disorganised regions of matrix, but strong staining was found in the immediate pericellular region of cells demonstrating a fibrocartilaginous phenotype. Since tenascin is able to stimulate chondrogenesis in undifferentiated limb mesenchyme, these data suggest that tenascin may be involved in the induction and maintenance of the fibrocartilaginous change seen in these tendons.

Western blotting of tendon protein extracts showed differences in tenascin isoform expression between normal and degenerate tendons (Figure 20.2). In normal tendons, only a single 200 kDa isoform of tenascin was present. In degenerate and ruptured tendons there were at least two isoforms – of 200 kDa and 300 kDa – as well as a variety of smaller molecular weight fragments, which are thought to be proteolytic fragments of tenascin, which is susceptible to digestion by matrix metalloproteinase enzymes (Siri *et al.*, 1995). In tendons from patients with calcifying tendinitis there were also two isoforms, but with

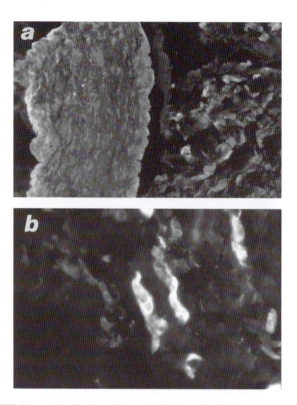

FIGURE 20.1   TRITC immunolocalisation of tenascin-C in ruptured human supraspinatus tendon from a 39 year old, showing two distinct patterns of tenascin expression: (a) Tenascin associated with organised collagen fibres, typical of the normal tendon structure. (b) Tenascin in the pericellular domain of rounded cells within a disorganised, 'fibrocartilaginous' region of the tendon.

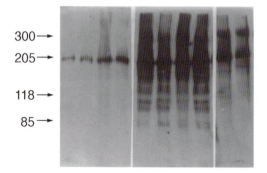

FIGURE 20.2   ECL immunoblot of tenascin-C in 4M guanidine extracts of human tendons, showing different patterns of tenascin isoform expression in normal and degenerate supraspinatus tendons. The left hand panel shows that only the 200 kDa isoform was expressed in four normal cadaver tendons (aged 76, 88, 88 and 74 years respectively). The centre panel shows that both 200 kDa and 300 kDa isoforms were expressed in four degenerate, ruptured tendons (cadavers aged 80, 55, 67 and 55 years respectively), in addition to a variety of lower molecular fragments. The right hand panel shows that both 200 kDa and 300 kDa tenascin isoforms were expressed in two calcifying tendinitis specimens (aged 50 and 63 years respectively), with a few minor, lower molecular weight fragments. A similar quantity of protein was loaded in each sample lane (approximately 10 μg/well). Molecular weights were estimated by comparison with Bio-rad pre-stained molecular weight markers, and a purified preparation of the 300 kDa tenascin isoform produced by SAOS cells, a human osteoblastic cell line.

less molecular weight fragments; this is consistent with a lower level of proteinase activity associated with tendon calcification. Thus it appears that the 200 kDa isoform of tenascin may have a role in normal tendon matrix organisation, and the 300 kDa isoform may be involved in the process of cell rounding and fibrocartilaginous metaplasia, although this hypothesis awaits confirmation using isoform specific antibodies which are currently in preparation.

SUMMARY

Fibrocartilaginous change, involving cell rounding and an altered pattern of collagen and GAG/PG synthesis, is one of the most common features of pathological change in degenerate tendons of the rotator cuff. Similar changes have been found in the common extensor tendons affected by lateral epicodylitis (tennis elbow), and in Achilles and patellar tendons affected by chronic tendinitis (Leadbetter, 1992). However, tendon fibrocartilage also develops in some normal tendons as a consequence of shear or compressive forces, and presumably represents an adaptation to prevent or limit tissue damage, with physical properties somewhere between those of typical tendon and articular cartilage. However caused, there is an altered pattern of matrix synthesis and remodelling of the existing tendon matrix, potentially resulting in a tissue less capable of resisting normal tensile loads.

If fibrocartilage metaplasia is an important stage in the development of degenerating tendon lesions, which our own recent results and those of others would suggest, then the mechanisms that control the activity of the tenocytes, and the altered synthesis and degradation of matrix components, would appear to be critical to our understanding of the disease mechanism and in establishing new therapeutic interventions. The synthesis and secretion of the 300 kDa isoform of tenascin appears to be closely associated with the formation of tendon fibrocartilage, though it remains to be determined whether the changes in tenascin isoform expression are part of the degenerative process, or secondary to the tendon rupture as part of the wound healing response.

ACKNOWLEDGEMENTS

The author is supported by grants from the Sir Halley Stewart Trust, the Sybil Eastwood Trust and the Cambridge Arthritis Research Endeavour. The author is also indebted to Mr Constant, consultant orthopaedic surgeon at Addenbrooke's Hospital, Cambridge, who provided the patient material used in this study. Acknowledgements are also due to Miss Rebecca Harrall, for technical assistance and to Professor Tim Cawston and Dr Brian Hazleman for their support and encouragement.

REFERENCES

Abrahamsson, S.O. (1991) Matrix metabolism and healing in the flexor tendon: Experimental studies on rabbit tendon. *Scand. J. Plast. Surg. Hand*, **25**, Suppl. 23, 1–51.

Bamji, A.N., Dieppe, P.A., Haslock, D.I. and Shipley, M.E. (1990) What do rheumatologists do? A pilot audit study. *Br. J. Rheum.*, **29**, 295–298.

Benjamin, M. and Ralphs, J.R. (1995) Developmental and functional anatomy of tendons and ligaments. In: *Repetitive Motion Disorders of the Upper Extremity* (Eds. Gordon, S.L., Blair, S.J. and Fine, L.J.) pp. 185–203. American Academy of Orthopaedic Surgeons, Rosemont.

Berenson, M.C., Blevins, F.T., Plaas, A.H.K. and Vogel, K.G. (1996) Proteoglycans of human rotator cuff tendons. *J. Orthop. Res.*, **14**, 518–525.

Berry, H., Fernandes, L., Bloom, B., Clarke, R.J. and Hamilton, E.D.B. (1980) Clinical study comparing acupuncture physiotherapy injection and oral anti-inflammatory therapy in shoulder cuff lesions. *Curr. Med. Res. Op.*, **7**, 121–126.

Binder, A.I. and Hazleman, B.L. (1983) Lateral humeral epicondylitis – a study of natural history and the effect of conservative therapy. *Br. J. Rheum.*, **22**, 73–76.

Binder, A.I., Bulgen, D.Y., Hazleman, B.L. and Roberts, S. (1984) Frozen shoulder: a long-term prospective study. *Ann. Rheum. Dis.*, **43**, 361–364.

Bjelle, A. (1989) Epidemiology of shoulder problems. In: *The Shoulder Joint*, (Eds. Hazleman, B.L. and Dieppe, P.A.) pp. 437–451, Balliere Tindall, London.

Brooks. C.H., Revell, W.J. and Heatley, F.W. (1992) A quantitative histological study of the vascularity of the rotator cuff tendon. *J. Bone Joint Surg.*, **74B**, 151–153.

Bulgen, D.Y., Binder, A.I., Hazleman, B.L., Dutton, J. and Roberts, S. (1984) Frozen shoulder: prospective clinical study with an evaluation of three treatment regimens. *Ann. Rheum. Dis.*, **43**, 353–360.

Bywaters, E.G.L. (1979) Lesions of bursae, tendons and tendon sheaths, *Clin. Rheum. Dis.*, **5**, 883–925.

Cawston, T.E., Riley, G.P. and Hazleman, B.L. (1996) Tendons and soft tissue rheumatism. Great outback or great opportunity? *Ann. Rheum. Dis.*, **55**, 1–3.

Chansky, H.A. and Iannotti, J.P. (1991) The vascularity of the rotator cuff. *Clinics in Sports Medicine*, **10**, 807–822.

Chard, M.D. and Hazleman, B.L. (1987) Shoulder disorders in the elderly (a hospital study). *Ann. Rheum. Dis.*, **46**, 684–487.

Chard, M.D., Cawston, T.E., Riley, G.P., Gresham, G.A. and Hazleman, B.L. (1994) Rotator cuff degeneration and lateral epicondylitis – a comparative histological study. *Ann. Rheum. Dis.*, **53**, 30–34.

Chiquet, M. and Fambrough, D.M. (1984) Chick myotendinous antigen. A novel extracellular glycoprotein consisting of large disulphide-linked subunits. *J. Cell Biol.*, **98**, 1937–1946.

Chiquet-Ehrismann, R., Matsuoka, Y., Hofer, U., Spring, J., Berlusconi, C. and Chiquet, M. (1991) Tenascin variants: differential binding to fibronectin and distinct distribution in cell cultures and tissues. *Cell Regulation*, **2**, 927–938.

Choung, C.-M., Widelitz, R.B., Jiang, T.-X., Abbott, U.K., Lee, Y.-S. and Chen, H.-M. (1993) Roles of the adhesion molecules NCAM and tenascin in limb skeletogenesis: analysis with antibody perturbation exogenous gene expression talpid mutants and activin stimulation. *Prog. Clin. Biol. Res.*, **383B**, 465–474.

Choung, C.-M. and Chen, H.-M. (1991) Enhanced expression of neural cell adhesion molecules and tenascin (cytotactin) during wound healing. *Am. J. Pathol.*, **138**, 427–440.

Codman, E.A. (1934) *The Shoulder*. Todd Co., Boston.

Cofield, R.H. (1985) Current concepts review: rotator cuff disease of the shoulder. *J. Bone Joint Surg.*, **67A**, 974–979.

Constant, C.R. (1989) Historical background, anatomy and shoulder function. In: *The Shoulder Joint* (Eds. Hazleman, B.L. and Dieppe, P.A.) pp. 429–435. Balliere Tindall , London.

Cotton, R.E. and Rideout, D.F. (1964) Tears of the humeral rotator cuff. *J. Bone Joint Surg.*, **46B**, 314–328.

Cronkite, A.E. (1936) The tensile strength of human tendons. *Anat. Record*, **18**, 921–940.

Dalton, S., Cawston, T.E., Riley, G.P., Bayley, I.J.L. and Hazleman, B.L. (1995) Human shoulder tendon biopsy samples in organ culture produce procollagenase and tissue inhibitor of metalloproteinases. *Ann. Rheum. Dis.*, **54**, 571–577.

Dalton, S.E. (1989) Clinical examination of the painful shoulder. In: *The Shoulder Joint* (Eds. Hazleman, B.L. and Dieppe, P.A.) pp. 453–474, Balliere Tindall, London.

Davison, P.F. (1992) Tendon. In: *Collagen in Health and Disease* (Eds. Weiss, J.B. and Jayson, M.I.V.) pp. 498–505, Churchill Livingstone, New York.

Day, B.H., Gorindasany, N. and Patnaik, R. (1978) Corticosteroid injections in the treatment of tennis elbow. *Practitioner*, **220**, 459–462.

De Palma, A.F. (1983) In: *Surgery of the Shoulder*. Lippincott, Philadelphia.

Elliott, D.H. (1965) Structure and function of mammalian tendon. *Biol. Rev.*, **40**, 392–421.

Evans, J.H. and Barbenel, J.C. (1975) Structural and mechanical properties of tendon related to function. *Eq. Vet. J.*, **7**, 1–8.

Fearnley, M.E. and Vadasz, I. (1969) Factors influencing the response of lesions of the rotator cuff of the shoulder to local steroid injections. *Ann. Phys. Med.*, **10**, 53–63.

Fukuda, H., Hamada, K. and Yamanaka, K. (1990) Pathology and pathogenesis of bursal-side rotator cuff tears viewed from en bloc histologic sections. *Clin. Orthop.*, **254**, 75–80.

Goddard, M.J., Riley, G.P., Cawston, T.E., Gresham, G.A., Hazleman, B.L. and Constant, C.R. (1992) Histological changes associated with rotator cuff lesions. *J. Pathol.*, **168**(S), A108.

Gulcher, J.R., Nies, D.E., Marton, L.S. and Stefansson, K. (1989) An alternatively spliced region of the human hexabrachion contains a repeat of potential N-glycosylation sites *PNAS*, **86**, 1588–1592.

Hardingham, T.E. and Fosang, A.J. (1992) Proteoglycans: many forms and many functions. *FASEB J.*, **6**, 861–870.

Hazleman, B.L. (1989) Editors foreword In: *The Shoulder Joint* (Eds. Hazleman, B.L. and Dieppe, P.A.) pp. ix–xii, Balliere Tindall, London.

Kessel, L. and Bayley, I. (1986) Clinical disorders of the shoulder. Churchill Livingstone, Edinburgh.

Kessel, L. and Watson, M. (1977) The painful arc syndrome. *J. Bone Joint Surg.*, **58**, 116–172.

Keyes, E.L. (1935) Anatomical observations on senile changes in the shoulder. *J. Bone Joint Surg.*, **17**, 953–960.

Leadbetter, W.B. (1992) Cell-matrix response in tendon injury. *Clinics in Sports Medicine*, **11**, 533–578.

Lindblom, K. (1939) On the pathogenesis of ruptures of the tendon aponeurosis of the supraspinatus tendon. *Acta Radiologica*, **20**, 563–577.

Lundborg, G., Hansson, H.-A., Rank, F. and Rydevik, B. (1980) Superficial repair of severed flexor tendons in synovial environment. *J. Hand Surg.*, **5**, 451–461.

Mackie, E.J. (1994) Tenascin in connective tissue development and pathogenesis. *Persp. Dev. Neurobiol.*, **2**, 125–132.

Mackie, E.J., Thesleff, I. and Chiquet-Ehrismann, R. (1987) Tenascin is associated with chondrogenic and osteogenic differentiation *in vivo* and promotes chondrogenesis *in vitro*. *J. Cell Biol.*, **105**, 2569–2579.

Mackie, E.J. and Tucker, R.P. (1992) Tenascin in bone morphogenesis: expression by osteoblasts and cell type-specific expression of splice variants. *J. Cell Sci.*, **103**, 765–771.

MacNab, I. (1973) Rotator cuff tendinitis. *Ann. Royal Coll. Surg. Eng.*, **52**, 271–287.

Merrilees, M.J. and Flint, M.H. (1980) Ultrastructural study of tension and pressure zones in a rabbit flexor tendon. *Amer. J. Anat.*, **157**, 87–106.

Moseley, H.F. and Goldie, I. (1963) The arterial pattern of the rotator cuff of the shoulder. *J. Bone Joint Surg.*, **45B**, 780–789.

Murphy-Ullrich, J.E., Lightner, V.A., Aukhil, I., Yan, Y.Z., Erickson, H.P. and Höök, M. (1991) Focal adhesion integrity is downregulated by the alternatively spliced domain of human tenascin. *J. Cell Biol.*, **115**, 1127–1136.

Neer, C.S. (1983) Impingement lesions. *Orthop.*, **173**, 70–77.

Nessler, J.P., Amadio, P.C., Berglund, L.J. and An, K.-N. (1992) Healing of canine tendon in zones subjected to different mechanical forces. *J. Hand Surg.*, **17B**, 561–568.

Nirschl, R.P. and Pettrone, F.A. (1973) Tennis elbow. *J. Bone Joint Surg.*, **61A**, 832–839.

Olson, O. (1953) Degenerative changes of the shoulder joint particularly of the cuff and biceps tendon. *Act. Chirg. Scand. Suppl.*, **181**, 35–125.

Ozaki, J., Fujimoto, S., Nakagawa, Y., Masuhar, K. and Tamai, S. (1988) Tears of the rotator cuff of the shoulder associated with pathological changes in the acromion. A study in cadavers. *J. Bone Joint Surg.*, **70A**, 1224–1230.

Rathbun, J.B. and MacNab, I. (1970) The microvascular pattern of rotator cuff. *J. Bone Joint Surg.*, **52A**, 540–553.

Riley, G.P., Harrall, R.L., Constant, C.R., Chard, M.D., Cawston, T.E. and Hazleman, B.L. (1994a) Tendon degeneration and chronic shoulder pain: changes in the collagen composition of the human rotator cuff tendons in rotator cuff tendinitis. *Ann. Rheum. Dis.*, **53**, 359–66.

Riley, G.P., Harrall, R.L., Cawston, T.E. and Hazleman, B.L. (1994b) Collagen degradation in tendon explants correlates with an excess of interstitial collagenase (MMP-1) secretion relative to TIMP-1. *Int. J. Exp. Pathol.*, **75**, A97.

Riley, G.P., Harrall, R.L., Constant, C.R., Chard, M.D., Cawston, T.E. and Hazleman, B.L. (1994c) Glycosaminoglycans of human rotator cuff tendons: changes with age and in chronic rotator cuff tendinitis. *Ann. Rheum. Dis.*, **53**, 367–76.

Riley, G.P., Harrall, R.L., Cawston, T.E., Hazleman, B.L. and Mackie, E.J. (1996) Tenascin-C and human tendon degeneration. *Am. J. Pathol.*, **149**, 933–943.

Rothman, R.H. and Parke, W.W. (1965) The vascular anatomy of the rotator cuff. *Clin. Orthop. Rel. Res.*, **41**, 176–186.

Scott, J.E. and Orford, C.R. (1981) Dermatan suphate-rich proteoglycan associates with rat tail-tendon collagen and the d band in the gap region. *Biochem. J.*, **197**, 213–216.

Simmonds, F.A. (1943) Shoulder pain with particular reference to the frozen shoulder. *J. Bone Joint Surg.*, **31B**, 426–432.

Siri, A., Knäuper, V., Veirana, N., Caocci, F., Murphy, G. and Zardi, L. (1995) Different susceptibility of small and large tenascin-C isoforms to degradation by matrix metalloproteinases. *J. Biol. Chem.*, **15**, 8650–8654.

Spring, J., Beck, K. and Chiquet-Ehrismann, R. (1989) Two contrary functions of tenascin: dissection of the active sites by recombinant tenascin fragments. *Cell*, **59**, 325–334.

Vogel, K.G. and Koob, T.J. (1989) Structural specialisation in tendons under compression. *Int. Rev. Cytol.*, **115**, 267–93.

von der Mark, K. (1981) Localization of collagen types in tissues. *Int. Rev. Conn. Tiss. Res.*, **9**, 265–324.

Webster, D.F. and Burry, H.C. (1982) The effects of hypoxia on human skin lung and tendon cells *in vitro*. *Br. J. Exp. Path.*, **63**, 50–55.

Wilson, C.L. and Duff, G.L. (1943) Pathological study of degeneration and rupture of the supraspinatus tendon. *Archiv. Surg.*, **47**, 121–135.

Wood, P.H.N., Sturrock, A.W. and Badley, E.M. (1979) Soft tissue rheumatism in the community. *Clin. Rheum. Dis.*, **5**, 743–753.

Section 5
Tissue Interfaces in Joints

21 Observations on the Tidemark and Calcified Layer of Articular Cartilage

Stan Havelka[1,*] and Vitezslav Horn[2]

[1]*Institute of Rheumatology, Prague;*
[2]*Tissue Bank, University Hospital, Brno, Czech Republic*

INTRODUCTION

The articular tidemark (TM) may, in general, be defined as an interface between calcified and noncalcified hyaline layers of articular cartilage. It is a thin (5–10 µm) band, basophilic in hematoxylin-eosin stained sections, appearing during early adolescence. The tidemark acts as a mineralisation front realising the steady creeping advancement of the calcified layer to the articular surface (Boskey *et al.*, 1981; Bullough and Jagannath, 1983; Dmitrovsky *et al.*, 1978; Green *et al.*, 1970; Havelka *et al.*, 1984; Haynes, 1981; Lane *et al.*, 1977; Lemperg, 1971; Oettmeier *et al.*, 1989; Revell *et al.*, 1990; Spinelli, 1976). However, a tidemark is also present between calcified and noncalcified fibrocartilage components in all types of insertion (tendon, ligament, joint capsule) (Havelka *et al.*, 1991; Niepel and Sitaj, 1979). Although the articular TM is a prominent feature, its variability in appearance at the light microscopical level, together with uncertainty both about its ultrastructural appearance and mechanical significance (Broom and Poole, 1982; Redler *et al.*, 1975) remain challenges for the future. Consequently, we aim to compare and contrast our own findings with those in the literature and to emphasise that we will incorporate the calcified cartilage layer as an integral and functional companion of the TM.

PROCEDURES

Osteochondral samples were collected from several mammal species and human specimens were from disease-free patients at surgery or post-mortem, together with samples

* Corresponding author.
Current address: Institute of Rheumatology, Na slupi 4, CZ-12850, Prague, Czech Republic.

from both osteoarthritic and rheumatoid arthritic joints. Our findings were gained from osteochondral samples (OCHS) of articular cartilage with adjacent sub-chondral bone of human and animal origin. All animals were healthy; both human and animal samples were from skeletally mature specimens. OCHS were maintained at $-20°C$ and then processed in several ways. After routine processing into paraffin, sections were stained with hematoxylin-eosin, Goldner stain or methylene blue and eosin, and studied by light microscopy.

Other OCHS were examined for cell enzyme activities. Demineralised sections were processed for alkaline phosphatase and lactic dehydrogenase histochemistry according to previously published methods (Havelka et al., 1984; Horn et al., 1988). Undemineralised tissue was also investigated by microradiography of 80 µm thick sections and stained with eosin/methylene blue.

Other samples were fractured in a plan perpendicular to the articular surface, fixed in 10% formaldehyde, dehydrated, sputter coated and examined in a scanning electron microscopy (SEM). Both mineralised and decalcified OCHS were used.

Lastly, some OCHS were fixed in 10% formaldehyde and embedded in methylmethacrylate and 150–200 µm sections cut on a Buehler rotation saw. These mineralised sections were evaluated by light microscopy without staining, for which we proposed the term 'native microscopy of OCHS' (Havelka et al., 1991a; Havelka and Neuzil, 1990). Because of the thickness of sections, stereomicroscopy was also achievable.

RESULTS

At the light microscopical level, two and sometimes more TM lines were apparent in healthy young humans (Figures 21.1 and 21.2). Examining OCHS for activity of alkaline phosphatase and lactic dehydrogenase we found positively-labelled chondrocytes in both calcified and non-calcified cartilage layers, confirming viability of the calcified zone. Lactic dehydrogenase positivity was diffuse (highest closer to articular surface); alkaline phosphatase appeared on both sides of TM and, to a lesser degree, to the bottom of calcified layer. This enzyme was also present in walls of vascular vessels within bone (Figures 21.3 and 21.4).

Detailed observation of the fate of the TM at the marginal zone of joints led to the recognition that it usually continues into the periosteum. By observing alkaline phosphatase activity, positive TM-bound chondrocytes interface with positive periosteal osteoblasts, thus forming a functional unit, an envelope with osteoblastic properties (Figures 21.4–21.6). The tidemark itself never stains for alkaline phosphatase activity, which is in contrast to its rapid mineral turnover demonstrated by tetracycline labelling (Revell et al., 1990; Havelka et al., 1991b; Havelka and Neuzil, 1990).

In relation to arthritic disorders, most of the attention has focused on osteoarthrosis (osteoarthritis). Figure 21.7 shows cartilage from a femoral head removed during arthroplasty. The outpost location of the freshest TM line is characteristic for reactive progression of calcification upwards through the tissue depth. Generally, other TMs appear

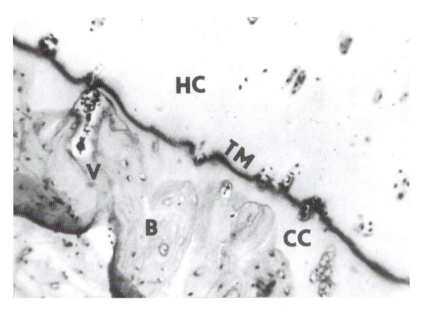

FIGURE 21.1   OCHS from femoral head, healthy male, 21 yrs. A textbook appearance of the osteochondral junction. 150×. Hem.-eos.

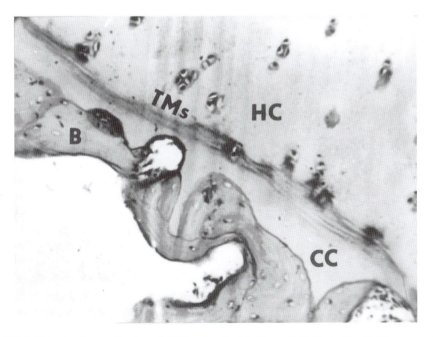

FIGURE 21.2   Another section from OCHS as described in Figure 21.1. Up to five TM lines present. 150×. Hem.-eos.

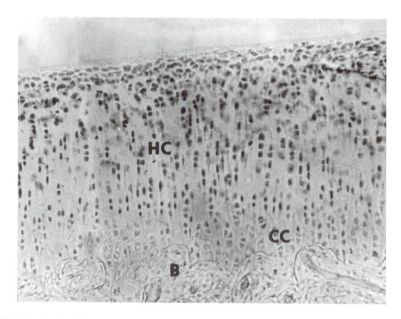

FIGURE 21.3 Lactic dehydrogenase activity in chondrocytes of hyaline and calcified cartilage layer diffusely, but mainly in more superficial portions of hyaline cartilage. Knee joint, healthy rabbit. 200×.

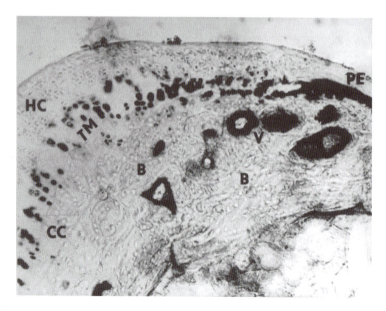

FIGURE 21.4 Activity of alkaline phosphatase, OCHS from knee joint, healthy rabbit. Highly positive broad band of chondrocytes accompanying the TM on both sides and diminishing activity to the base of calcified layer. This micrograph also demonstrates smooth transition of this TM cellular belt into positive periosteal cells. 200×.

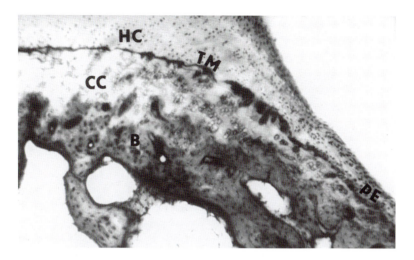

FIGURE 21.5 OCHS from rabbit knee joint. Smooth transition of TM into periosteum. Hem.-eos. stain. 200×.

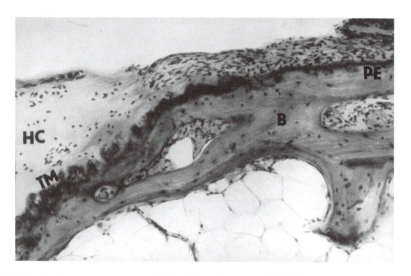

FIGURE 21.6 Continuous connection of TM with periosteum in OCHS from a female with ochronosis, 70 yrs, knee joint. 200×. Hem.-eos.

normal even under heavily damaged hyaline cartilage (data not shown). On a rare occasion, in a severely eroded specimen, the TM appeared as a ribbon-like structure even passing through cavities in the tissue (Figure 21.8).

In undecalcified samples from a rheumatoid metatarsophalangeal joint, 3 well defined TMs can be resolved (Figure 21.10). Microradiographic analysis shows that the density of the calcified cartilage is close to that of bone, with the TMs showing high density (Figure 21.11).

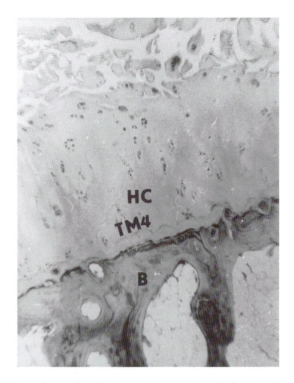

FIGURE 21.7   OCHS from femoral head in advanced human osteoarthritis. Up to four TMs under a heavily severed hyaline zone. 20×. Hem.-eos.

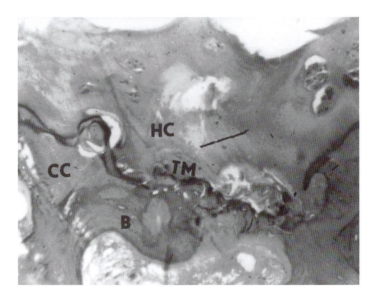

FIGURE 21.8   OCHS with extremely damaged structures, human osteoarthritis of the hip. Doubled ribbon-like TM running through a cavitation (left). 150×. Hem.-eos.

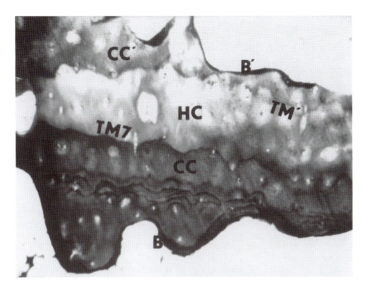

FIGURE 21.9   Osteophyte, femoral head, human osteoarthritis. Up to seven TM lines in the original cartilage (lower half). Additional bone layer (B') with its own calcified cartilage (CC') and one TM' (above). 100×. Goldner stain.

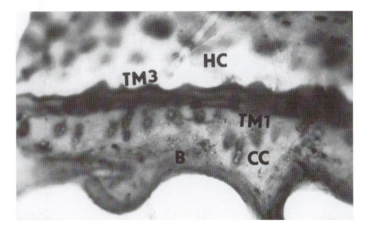

FIGURE 21.10   Metatarsophalangeal joint, female with rheumatoid arthritis. Three distinct TMs. Undecalcified OCHS, resin-embedded. 130×. Eosin and methylene blue stain.

Moving from light microscopy to SEM, figures 21.12 and 21.13 demonstrate the TM as a narrow ridge between both cartilage layers in normal rabbit knees. In these and the following electron micrographs the calcified layer appears darker and more compact in fully mineralised specimens. In other rabbit specimen, the TM can only be identified as a boundary between hyaline and calcified cartilage which are bridged by collagen fibrils (Figure 21.14). The origin of the TM can be seen at the marginal transition zone again in a rabbit specimen (Figure 21.15). At high magnification under the SEM, the TM can

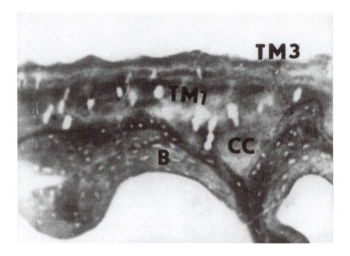

FIGURE 21.11 Microradiographic counterpart to Figure 21.10. Dense lines correspond to TMs. Calcified layer density is, on average, equal to that of subchondral bone. 150×.

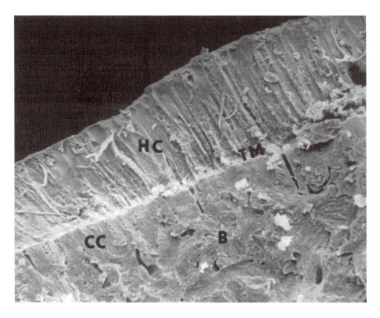

FIGURE 21.12 OCHS from healthy rabbit knee joint. The tidemark is clearly visible beneath the perpendicularly arranged hyline cartilage. Undecalcified. 130×. SEM.

appear as a prominent granular ridge (Figure 21.16) although in other normal specimens, the structure is more fibrillar (Figure 21.17). In the diseased condition, by contrast, the TM can be very ill-defined (Figure 21.18).

Lastly, a novel method was utilised to obtain minimally processed OCHSs for 'native microscopy' (Havelka et al., 1991b; Havelka and Neuzil, 1990). Thick sections have the

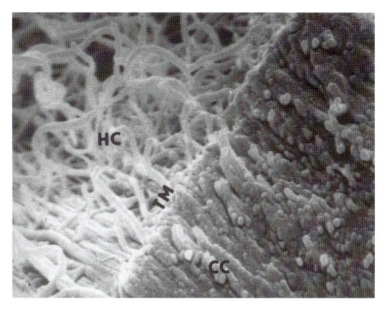

FIGURE 21.13   Detail of Figure 21.12. Under high-magnification, TM forms a dividing ridge between hyaline and calcified layers. Undecalcified. 6000×. SEM.

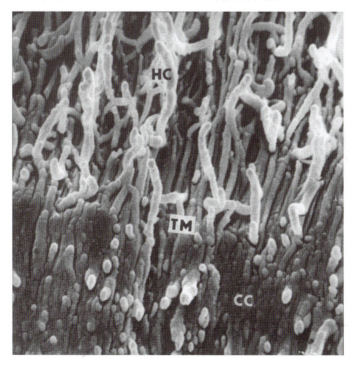

FIGURE 21.14   OCHS from a healthy rabbit knee joint. Under high magnification, the TM is visible only as an interface dividing brighter hyaline from darker and denser calcified cartilage. Interconnecting collagen fibers. Undecalcified. 6000×. SEM.

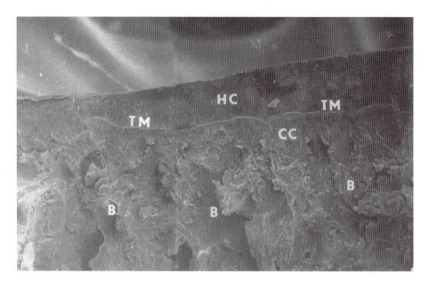

FIGURE 21.15   Knee joint of another healthy rabbit. The origin of the TM can be seen on the left side at the marginal transitional zone. Undecalcified. 60×. SEM.

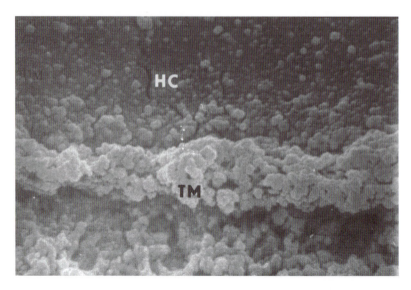

FIGURE 21.16   Higher power detail of Figure 21.15. Note at higher magnification the granular appearance of the TM. Undecalcified. 6000×. SEM.

additional advantage of permitting stereo-like images of tissues. However, limited magnification is a restricting factor. Figure 21.19 demonstrates good visibility of the TM, dark columns of chondrocytes in calcified cartilage, oriented perpendicularly to articular surface, and the vascular network penetrating from the marrow cavity through the calcified cartilage zone and terminating beneath the TM frontier under normal healthy

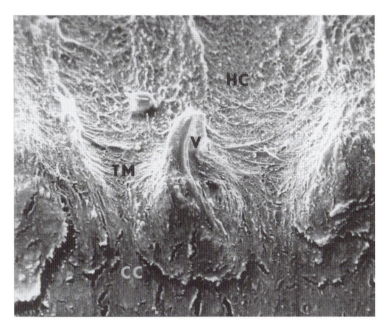

FIGURE 21.17 OCHS from femoral head. Healthy male, 50 yrs. The fibrillar nature of the TM can be resolved together with penetrating vessels (V). Undecalcified. 1500×. SEM.

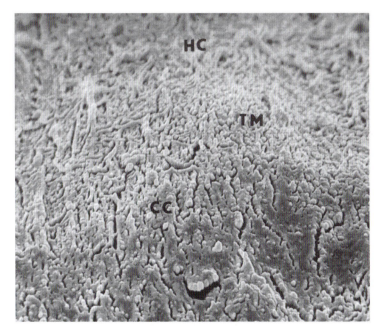

FIGURE 21.18 OCHS from an osteoarthritic 1st metatarsophalangeal joint. Female, 46 yrs. The TM can only be estimated between brighter and more fibrillar hyaline cartilage and the darker, particulate calcified cartilage zones. Undecalcified. 2200×. SEM.

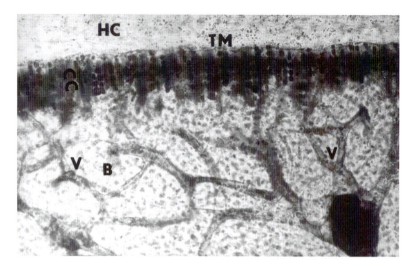

FIGURE 21.19 Distal femur from healthy rabbit hip joint. The micrograph shows the TM, dark chondrocyte columns and vascular network in the calcified cartilage layer. Undecalcified. 140×. No staining.

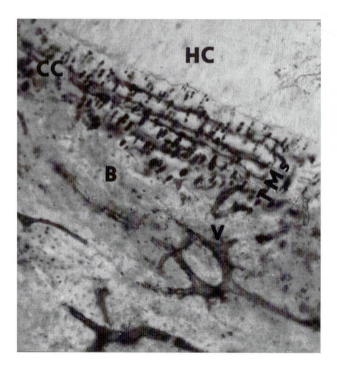

FIGURE 21.20 OCHS from proximal tibia. Healthy bison, 9 yrs, approx. 400 kg bodyweight. Up to six TMs can be detected together with, dark appearing chondrocytes arranged perpendicularly to the surface in the calcified layer. Note also, underlying blood vessels. Undecalcified, unstained. 50×.

conditions. Using similar thick sections, a register of systematic remodelling is presented by Figure 21.20 showing six TM lines and residual columnar chondrocyte formations in calcified cartilage of a weight-loaded articulation (healthy bison cow, 400 kg bodyweight).

DISCUSSION

In arthritic cartilage, reduplication of the tidemark is commonplace and probably represents an expression of imbalance between load and tissue quality (Revell et al., 1990; Havelka et al., 1982; Hough et al., 1975; Lane and Bullough, 1980; Luck, 1982; Macys et al., 1980; Meachim and Allibone, 1984). They are also common in specimens from individuals after the age of 70. The original and earlier TMs become subsumed within the calcified cartilage but still retain their basophilia and increased mineral content (Figure 21.11). However, we have also observed TM reduplication in healthy young adult humans as young as 21 (Figure 21.2) although the significance of this is unknown. Since it appears that the TM is associated with the calcified layer progression, reduplication might accompany thickening of calcified cartilage after loading (Muller-Gerbl et al., 1978). Conversely, TM reduplication is also a characteristic outside pressure zone in osteoarthritis (Macys et al., 1980). Additionally, there appears to be no correlation between age and thickness of the calcified cartilage (Haynes, 1981; Lane and Bullough, 1980).

Recent detailed observations (Brauer, 1991; Numssen, 1992) underline the high degree of individual variability in morphological parameters of this region both in health and in disease. It will be necessary to collect further data separately for large and small joints of humans and large and small animals, young and old, in both health and disease. In relation to reduplicated TMs, a plausible explanation of some of them could be marginal overlapping of two TM sheets in our perpendicular sections.

According to opinion based on the paper of Redler et al. (1975), the TM has a structure with a protective role for collagen fibrils connecting hyaline and calcified cartilage. Three types of fibrils were described: random, vertical and horizontal. The question becomes whether such a complex structure can be present in all TMs? Probably not, since Broom and Poole (1982) report the high variability of TM ultrastructure and they do not recognise the role of the TM and calcified cartilage as an intermediate layer between rigid subchondral bone and compliant hyaline cartilage. It is also surprising of the lack of reports on more than one TM in SEM micrographs. In our material using the SEM (Figures 21.12–21.18), there were different structural types of TM, varying from apparently structureless boundaries to granular ridges.

We believe that a permanent structure, as substantiated by Redler et al.'s (1975) descriptions, by our observations or other reports (Gilmore and Palfrey, 1987), can be present in a minor part of TMs only. The arrangement of collagen fibrils, as demonstrated by Redler et al. (1975), can certainly not be a priori formation but would represent a response to biomechanical loading, a response necessitating a substantial amount of time to emerge. A TM with permanent structure would, as a mature TM, correspond to mature calcified cartilage which can be recognised by its high mineral content (Green et al.,

1970). A marker of the 'genuineness' of a calcified cartilage layer is the arrangement of chondrocytes in columns (Figure 21.19) reflecting previous intense growth of this epiphyseal region before the stop of growth (Johnson, 1987). Confirming the identity of such genuine calcified cartilage is its content of type X collagen, a specific collagen of hypertrophic chondrocytes in the growth plate, but in adulthood to be found only in calcified cartilage (Eyre, 1991). TMs should be further classified according to their mineral turnover by tetracycline labelling (Lemperg, 1971; Revell *et al.*, 1990; Havelka *et al.*, 1991b), this being possible in combination with assessment of alkaline phosphatase activity in adjacent chondrocytes (Figure 21.4). Complex evaluation including SEM and EM, should then be applied to differentiate immature, mature and aged TMs and calcified cartilages. It would also be useful to know how long it takes for a TM to develop and mature.

We further presented the concept of an osteoplastic envelope (Havelka and Horn, 1986) composed of periosteum with its associated osteoblasts and of TM with its accompanying chondrocytes. We confirmed the viability of calcified cartilage reported by others (Hunziker, 1989; Meachim and Stockwell, 1979). By introducing a novel procedure, the so-called native microscopy of OCHS (Havelka *et al.*, 1991b; Havelka and Neuzil, 1990) we gained new knowledge (Lane *et al.*, 1977; Clark and Huber, 1990; Duncan *et al.*, 1987) on vascular supply of the subchondral bone and calcified cartilage (Figures 21.19, 21.20). At the same time, we confirmed the general barrier role of TM preventing blood vessels from invading healthy hyaline articular cartilage. Last but not least, we contributed to the idea that there exists an additional subchondral supplying route for articular cartilage in adulthood, by means of intravenous tetracycline labelling (Havelka *et al.*, 1991b; Havelka and Neuzil, 1990; Havelka *et al.*, 1990).

Interest in the structure and role of the tidemark and calcified zone of joint cartilage is being documented by further publications (Sokoloff, 1993; Archer, 1994). There is still much to be done in unravelling the secrets of this region.

SUMMARY

Data are presented on long term studies of human and animal articular osteochondral samples by light microscopy, scanning electron microscopy and 'native' microscopy in health and disease. Both mineralised and decalcified material were studied. Results are compared with published data. There exists a whole spectrum of 'tidemarks' which are functionally and structurally not equivalent. Further differentiation in this respect is necessary for separating immature, mature, aged and pathological tidemarks together with the associated calcified cartilages. Evidence is presented for subchondral blood supply of the calcified cartilage and for its viability. The authors propose that the periosteal and articular tidemark systems together form one osteoplastic envelope. Novel techniques will be required to assist in elucidating many persisting problems of the osteochondral junction.

ABBREVIATIONS TO MICROGRAPHS

OCHS – osteochondral sample
TM – tidemark
CC – calcified cartilage
HC – hyaline cartilage
B – bone
V – vessel
IN – insertion
PE – periosteum

ACKNOWLEDGEMENTS

The authors are indebted to Prof. C.W. Archer for the final English adaptation of this manuscript. S. Havelka thanks Profs. R. Amprino, G. Dominok, and L. Módis for introducing him into skeletal morphology.

REFERENCES

Archer, C.W. (1994) Skeletal development and osteoarthritis. *Ann. Rheum. Dis.*, **53**, 624–630.

Boskey, A.L., Bullough, P.G. and Dmitrovsky, E. (1981) The biochemistry of the mineralisation front. In: *Bone Histomorphometrey* (Eds Jee, W.S.S. and Parfitt, A.M.). Soc. Nouvelle Public Med. Dent., Paris, pp. 61–67.

Brauer, F.U. (1991) Untersuchungen zur flachenhaften Verteilung histomorphometrisch erfassbarer Parameter im Gelenkknorpel von adulten Hunden unter besonderer Berucksichtigung der Tidemark-Auspragung. Inaugural Dissertation. University of Greifswald, pp. 90.

Broom, N.D. and Poole, C.A. (1982) A functional–morphological study of the tidemark region of articular cartilage maintained in a non-viable physiological condition. *J. Anat.*, **135**, 65–82.

Bullough, P. and Jagannath, A. (1983) The morphology of the calcification front in articular cartilage. *J. Bone Jt. Surg.*, **65**(B), 72–78.

Clark, J.M. and Huber, J.D. (1990) The structure of the human subchondral plate. *J. Bone Jt. Surg.*, **72**(B), 866–873.

Dhem, A. and Vincent, A. (1965) Analyse microradiographique du squelette. *Recipe*, **10**, 515–536.

Dmitrovsky, E., Lane, L.B. and Bullough, P.G. (1978) The characterization of the tidemark in human articular cartilage. *Metab. Bone Dis. Rel. Res.*, **1**, 115–118.

Duncan, H., Jundt, J., Riddle, J.M., Pitchford, W. and Christophersen, T. (1987) The tibial subchondral plateau. *J. Bone Jt. Surg.*, **69**(A), 1212–1220.

Eyre, D.R. (1991) The collagens of articular cartilage. *Semin. Arthritis Rheum.*, **21**(2), 2–11.

Gilmore, R.S.T.C. and Palfrey, A.J. (1987) A histological study of human femoral condylar articular cartilage. *J. Anat.*, **155**, 77–85.

Green, W.T., Martin, G.N., Eanes, E.D. and Sokoloff, L. (1970) Microradiographic study of the calcified layer of articular cartilage. *Arch. Pathol.*, **90**, 151–158.

Havelka, S. and Horn, V. (1986) Joint cartilage tidemark and periosteum: two components of one envelope. *Acta Univ. Carol Med. Prague*, **32**, 311–318.

Havelka, S., Horn, V. and Neuzil, A. (1991a) Die Kalkschicht des Sehnenansatzes und das Ruptur-Risiko bei Enthesopathie. In: *Osteologie – Interdisziplinar* (Eds Werner, E. and Matthiass, H.H.). Springer-Verlag, Berlin, Heidelberg, pp. 412–415.

Havelka, S., Horn, V., Spohrova, D. and Valouch, P. (1984) The calcified–noncalcified cartilage interface: the tidemark. *Acta. Biol. Hungar.*, **35**, 271–279.

Havelka, S., Motl, V., Hess, L. and Neuzil, A. (1991b) Nachweis der subchondralen Ernahrungsroute im erwachsenen Gelenkknorpel. *Akt. Rheumatol.*, **16**, 10–12.

Havelka, S. and Neuzil, A. (1990) Vascularization of osteochondral junctions of joints and spine. In: *Bone Circulation and Bone Necrosis* (Eds Arlet, J. and Mazieres, B.). Springer-Verlag, Berlin, Heidelberg, New York, London, Paris, Tokyo, Hong Kong, pp. 11–15.

Havelka, S., Neuzil, A., Motl, V. and Hess, L. (1990) Subchondral nutritional route of adult articular cartilage does exist. *Periodicum Biologorum*, **92**(1), 12.

Havelka, S., Valouch, P. and Modis, L. (1982) Zur Remodelation der Knorpel-Knochengrenze bei Gelenkerkrankungen. *Wissensch. Beitr. F-Schiller Univ. Jena*, **19**, 74–82.

Haynes, D.W. (1981) The mineralization front of articular cartilage. In: *Bone Histomorphometry* (Eds Jee, W.S.S. and Parfitt, A.M.). Soc. Nouvelle Public Med. Dent., Paris, pp. 55–59.

Horn, V., Papousek, F. and Havelka, S. (1988) Die experimentelle Arthrose durch chemische Knorpelbeschadigung. *Z. Orthop.*, **126**, 71–75.

Hough, A.J., Banfield, W.G., Mottram, F.C. and Sokoloff, L. (1975) The osteochondral junction of mammalian joints. *Lab. Invest.*, **31**, 685–695.

Hunziker, E.B. (1989) Ultrastructure of the calcified zone in articular cartilage. *Calc. Tiss. Int.*, **44**, S-75/M6.

Johnson, D.R. (1987) Genetic and mechanical features governing the growth of epiphyseal cartilage. In: *Joint Loading. Biology and Health of Articular Structures* (Eds Helminen, J.H. *et al.*). Wright, Bristol, pp. 227–258.

Lane, L.B. and Bullough, P.G. (1980) Age-related changes in the thickness of the calcified zone and the number of tidemarks in adult human articular cartilage. *J. Bone Jt. Surg.*, **62**(B), 372–375.

Lane, L.B., Villacin, A. and Bullough, P.G. (1977) The vascularity and remodelling of subchondral bone and calcified cartilage in adult human femoral and humeral heads. *J. Bone Jt. Surg.*, **59**(B), 272–278.

Lemperg, R. (1971) The subchondral boneplate of the femoral head in adult rabbits. I. Spontaneous remodelling studied by microradiography and tetracycline labelling. *Virchows Arch. Path. Anat.*, **352**, 1–13.

Luck, G. (1982) Die Gelenkknorpelknochengrenze und ihr altersgemasses Verhalten. Candidate Thesis, Cottbus.

Macys, J.R., Bullough, P.G. and Wilson, P.D. (1980) Coxarthrosis: a study of the natural history based on a correlation of clinical radiographic and pathologic findings. *Semin. Arthritis Rheum.*, **10**, 66–88.

Meachim, G. and Allibone, R. (1984) Topographical variation in the calcified zone of upper femoral articular cartilage. *J. Anat.*, **193**, 341–352.

Meachim, G. and Stockwell, R.A. (1979) The matrix. In: *Adult Articular Cartilage* (Ed. Freeman, M.A.R.). 2nd Edit. Pitman Medical, Tunbridge Wells, pp. 1–67.

Muller-Gerbl, M., Schulte, E. and Putz, R. (1978) The thickness of the calcified layer of articular cartilage: a function of the load supported? *J. Anat.*, **154**, 103–111.

Niepel, G.A. and Sitaj, S. (1979) Enthesopathy. *Clin. Rheumatic Dis.*, **5**, 857–872.

Numssen, U. (1992) Untersuchungen zur flachenhaften Verteilung histomorphologischer und histomorphometrischer Parameter im Gelenkknorpel primar arthrotischer Femurkopfe adulter Hunde. Inaugural Dissertation. University of Greifswald, pp. 115.

Oettmeier, R., Oettmeier, S. and Abendroth, K. (1989) Tidemark-analysen am menschlichen Femurkopf. In: *Neuere Ergbnisse in der Osteologie* (Eds Willert, H.G. and Heuck, F.H.W.). Springer-Verlag, Berlin, Heidelberg, New York, London, Paris, Tokyo, Hong Kong, pp. 639–644.

Redler, I., Mow, V.C., Zimny, M.L. and Mansell, J. (1975) The ultrastructure and biomechanical significance of the tidemark of articular cartilage. *Clin. Orthop.*, **112**, 357–362.

Revell, P.A., Pirie, C., Amir, G., Rashad, S. and Walker, F. (1990) Metabolic activity in the calcified zone of cartilage in human osteoarthritis hips. *Rheumatol. Int.*, **10**, 143–147.

Sokoloff, L. (1993) Microcracks in the calcified layer of articular cartilage. *Arch. Pathol. Lab. Med.*, **117**, 191–195.

Spinelli, R. (1976) New aspects of the structure of articular cartilage. The tidemark seen on the scanning electron microscope. *Ital. J. Orthop. Traumatol.*, **2/3**, 393–401.

22 Tissue Interfaces in the Synovial Joint: Changes during the Development of Arthritic Disease

M.E.J. Billingham*

*Rheumatology Unit, Department of Medicine,
University of Bristol, Bristol, BS2 8HW*

INTRODUCTION

The interface between articular cartilage, calcified cartilage and subchondral bone has a precise and important role for the integrity of the joint during motion. Mechanical forces generated during motion need to be transmitted, dissipated and absorbed within these tissues in a manner that does not compromise the deeper tissues. Such structural issues have been honed by evolutionary pressure but many questions remain on the control of the proportions of these tissues during organogenesis and what mechanisms and molecules are involved in maintaining the precise dimensions of the joint during growth and throughout adult life. Some of the developmental issues are addressed within this volume and will not be covered here. The changes which occur at tissue interfaces during the development of arthritic diseases, osteoarthritis (OA) and rheumatoid arthritis (RA) will form the basis of this discussion.

Most joints maintain their structural integrity throughout life, but arthritic disease can cause joint destruction and failure through loss of articular cartilage during OA or through invasion of both cartilage and bone, as is seen in RA. Both these diseases are associated with extensive alteration and remodelling of all the joint structures, but particularly at the cartilage, calcified cartilage and subchondral interfaces. OA develops when the mechanics of the joint are altered, seen dramatically following sports injuries such as cruciate ligament rupture or meniscal damage, but more subtle changes occur during the development

*Current address: Rheumatology Laboratories, OSCOR Facility, University Veterinary School, Southwell Street, Bristol, BS2 8EJ.

of spontaneous disease. Spontaneous OA of the medial compartment of the knee occurs in several mammalian species, including certain strains of mice, guinea pigs, Rhesus and Cynomolgus macaques and also man (Billingham, 1998 for recent review in relation to drug discovery). The disease that occurs in the guinea pig and the macaques is interesting in that changes to the subchondral bone appear to precede the response of the articular cartilage; how this may relate to the human situation is unclear at present as is the possibility that ligament change may also accompany or precipitate the subchondral bone change. The concept that change in one connective tissue of the joint will precipitate changes in other connective tissues will be developed further below.

For RA, the cartilage/subchondral bone region is the site of attack by invasive pannus, a tissue formed from the synovium and periosteum, particularly in regions where the periosteum meets articular cartilage at ligament insertion sites within the synovial cavity. It is probable that an insult to the synovium, inflammatory or immune, stimulates proliferation, overgrowth and invasion of cartilage and bone, but it is unclear why some patients have erosive RA and others do not, nor is it known why these particular sites are so vulnerable to erosive attack, particularly in the small joints of the hands and feet. The nature of the erosive process is becoming clearer, however, as is the identity of the cells responsible for bone and cartilage destruction. Recent evidence points to bone and cartilage erosion being a separate and unconnected process to the inflammatory signs and symptoms. The influence of the T-lymphocyte in tissue erosion is also questionable and the role of inflammatory cytokines in cartilage and bone destruction during erosion remains to be completely clarified.

It is timely to readdress how these interface regions are involved in arthritic disease. In the past, there has been concentration on certain connective tissues to the relative neglect of others; all the connective tissues of the joint subserve the the need for stability, so change within one will have a 'knock-on' effect on the other tissues and ultimately lead to the joint failure seen in OA if uncorrected. Inflammatory arthritis, typified by RA, needs redefining in terms of therapeutic strategy if the inflammatory immune events are a separate phenomenon to the erosive progression.

TISSUE INTERFACE CHANGES
DURING THE DEVELOPMENT OF OA

It is inappropriate here to give detailed descriptions of the types, sites, prevalence, genetics and predisposing factors of OA; these will be found partly in this volume and in new textbooks on OA, as will descriptions of the tissues and matrix macromolecules involved. However, for any overview of OA a few salient points need to be made. Some researchers refer to "osteoarthritic diseases" to indicate that OA is not all the same problem (Dieppe, 1995) at each site where it occurs, though the scientist with responsibility for finding a disease modifying drug for OA hopes for a single pathway leading to failure at all sites and in all circumstances. Also, the joint must be viewed as an organ with all the constituent tissues subserving the need for biomechanical stability (Radin et al., 1995); change within one tissue e.g. ligament or bone could alter the mechanical environment such that cartilage eventually fails, or vice versa; in fact, adaptation and joint remodelling have been considered as the basis of osteoarthritis since 1962 (Johnson, 1962). A suitable disease paradigm for study of initiation and progression of OA would be a spontaneous form of the disease that occurs across the mammalian species, so that early events can be elucidated in animals for contrast and comparison with the human disease.

Spontaneous OA of the medial compartment of the knee occurs in several species including man, but the early events are only readily studied in the rodent species and primates such as Rhesus and Cynomolgus macaques. In fact, comprehensive studies are available in the guinea pig (Bendele and Hulman, 1988; Bendele et al., 1989; Meacock et al., 1990) and Cynomolgus macaque (Carlson et al., 1994, 1995, 1996) and to a lesser degree in certain mouse strains, though this is not entirely medial compartment disease (Evans et al., 1994; Collins et al., 1994; Walton, 1977). The real question here is why does this particular form of OA reside in so many species, and what causes it? The eminent dermatologist, Sam Schuster, had some advice on this when he pointed out to the Heberden Society in Newcastle, England in 1981, that for any medical scientific problem "the facts will not be discovered until you first guess the answer".

So, what is the answer? Probably stability, as mechanical stability requires that all the tissues involved in articulation should be in balance, in terms of tissue mass, composition and strength, to resist the forces transmitted through them. An example of such a balance comes from elegant studies by Simon Rodbard, not in osteoarthrology, but from the control of vascular wall calibre and strength (Rodbard, 1970, 1974). Such principles apply equally to other connective tissues. Rodbard's thesis is that mesenchymal cells will respond to mechanical stress by producing materials (elastin, collagen, proteoglycan etc.) to counter such stress, or will remove these if the stress is diminished; this is under local control but influenced by hormonal and other systemic factors. He noted that there is little elastin in arteries within bone fossae as there is no stretching at such sites with each pulse of blood and, therefore, no need for the recoil properties of elastin. Placement of a suture in the descending aorta of the dog increased pressure upstream and was associated with a loss of elastin upstream as the vessel wall increased in muscle and collagen to resist the pressure change, yet downstream the wall thinned as seen in post-stenotic dilatation. The suture involved an area of a few hundred microns but the connective tissues were remodelled over several centimetres; this is relevant to the remodelling of the knee joint seen during the development of spontaneous OA in animals (detailed below). The most poignant observation of Rodbard in relation to OA, however, was the reaction to a steel wire placed through the intimal layers of the descending aorta (Rodbard, 1974); here the intimal mesenchymal cells were being compressed against a solid material so they changed phenotype to chondrocytes and secreted cartilage around the wire to counter the compressive stress. This emphasises the local nature of the control of tissue structure, and the facility to put down any component structure anywhere in the body depending on the mechanics.

From the perspective of the joint, consisting of an outer capsule, a variety of stabilising ligaments, subchondral bone, synovium, menisci, calcified and articular hyaline cartilage, all of which contribute to mechanical stability, any change within any component tissue will influence the synthetic and/or degradative activity of cells in the other tissues as they strive to maintain mechanical stability. Surgical models of OA, or those involving intra-articular injection of degradative enzymes, destabilise the joint through the gross disruption of one or a number of tissues, but are more relevant to the sports injuries in man which lead on to OA, e.g. cruciate ligament rupture and meniscal tears. The recent publications on spontaneous OA in the knees of animals (Bendele and Hulman, 1988; Bendele *et al.*, 1989; Meacock *et al.*, 1990; Evans *et al.*, 1994; Collins *et al.*, 1994; Carlson *et al.*, 1994, 1995, 1996) will provide information on tissue change, but no model can perfectly mimic the human situation. However, a thorough understanding of the way spontaneous OA of animals initiates, what the macromolecular changes comprise and how the balance of synthetic and degradative processes influence disease progression, will provide valuable information on tissue interplay, and may also provide the strategies for discovery of therapeutic measures to control OA. This is the real advantage of animal models as it is difficult to obtain sequential diseased tissue from the human species.

SPONTANEOUS OSTEOARTHRITIS IN ANIMALS

Natural OA in animal species represent a model system for idiopathic human disease and should be considered separately from those induced models of arthritis involving surgical manipulation or enzymatic destruction of component structures. Comprehensive descriptions of medial compartment knee OA have been presented for mouse strains, the Dunkin Hartley guinea pig and Rhesus and Cynomolgus macaque monkeys (Bendele and Hulman, 1988; Bendele *et al.*, 1989; Meacock *et al.*, 1990; Evans *et al.*, 1994; Collins *et al.*, 1994; Carlson *et al.*, 1994, 1995, 1996). Recently, spontaneous OA in the knee of Lewis and Fischer 344 strains of rat has been described (Smale *et al.*, 1995). Their importance lies in their similarities with idiopathic, human medial compartment knee OA and the likelihood that mechanisms of initiation and progression will be discovered which are more relevant to human disease than the induced models. This will enable drug discovery to proceed rationally and remove inaccurate guesswork from mechanistic approaches.

SPONTANEOUS OSTEOARTHRITIS IN MICE

Nearly all inbred strains of mice develop some degree of OA, although the incidence, severity and localisation of the articular lesion varies between strains. The highest incidence and most severe form of the disease occurs in mice of the STR strains (Sokoloff, 1956), STR/ORT and STR/IN. There have been several studies of these mice over the years but these have been mainly subjective and descriptive and very few drug studies have been reported. It is generally agreed that the initial cartilage lesion is in the medial tibial plateau but there is debate as to whether patella displacement precedes and thus causes cartilage degeneration. Radiographic assessment of the lesions in the knee (Evans *et al.*, 1994) has demonstrated that male mice of the STR/ORT strain get more severe disease than female mice and a higher incidence. The conclusions reached by Evans *et al.* (1994) and Collins *et al.* (1994) were that patella displacement was not the predisposing factor, since by eleven months of age all mice had arthritis but not all had patella displacement. Secondly, and particularly in male mice, they observed chondro-osseous metaplasia in the tendinous structures around the joint and the major ligament entheses such as the patella ligament insertions. These had occurred by three months of age, preceding articular changes by at least a month, leading the authors to propose that this was the primary event in the development of OA in these strains of mice. Subsequently, as others had previously described (Walton, 1977; Schunke et al., 1988), articular lesions appeared in the medial tibial plateau, initially as superficial fibrillation which eventually progressed to complete cartilage erosion with accompanying osteophyte formation. Interestingly, they noted that subchondral bone sclerosis was only seen in late disease and in this respect OA in mice differs from that seen in the knees of guinea pigs and macaques where subchondral bone changes, particularly sclerosis, precede the development of cartilage degeneration. Whether this disease can be considered a model of primary or idiopathic OA, since it is associated with early calcification of ligaments and tendons, was questioned by the authors (Collins et al., 1994). Nonetheless, it does have striking similarities with human knee OA. It also illustrates that change in one tissue or tissues, i.e. calcification of ligaments and tendons, will lead to changes in others, in this case the development of the cartilage degeneration and osteophyte formation typical of OA. Calcification of key ligaments will alter the mechanical stresses within the joint structures and the ensuing tissue alterations can be viewed as an attempt, and failure, to maintain mechanical stability.

SPONTANEOUS OA IN THE GUINEA PIG

The original observation of OA in the guinea pig was made by Silverstein and Sokoloff (1958) but the model has come to prominence following the studies of Bendele and her colleagues (1988, 1989) and those of Meacock et al. (1990) during the late 1980's. These fully described the natural history of the disease and male to female prevalence. Attention was focussed initially on the cartilage changes, reflecting the general view that these are the initiating events. It is now apparent that all male guinea pigs of the Dunkin Hartley strain begin to show cartilage degeneration after three months of age (Bendele and Hulman, 1988; Meacock et al., 1990). The time that the lesion initiates is variable from animal to animal, but all will be involved by five months of age. Females show similar changes but these initiate around six months of age, essentially mirroring the development of OA seen in males though the final outcome is not so severe as in the males. Initially there is loss of proteoglycan and cell death in the centre of the medial tibial plateau that is not covered by the meniscus. Loss of proteoglycan and cell death then progress to cover larger areas of the tibial plateau, fibrillation is significant by six months of age together with osteophyte formation and the medial meniscus and femoral condyle are involved by nine months of age. At one year of age there can be complete loss of cartilage with exposure of bone in the medial femoral condyle and tibial plateau. Body weight can increase disease severity and diet restriction to keep the animals less than 900 gms can essentially halve the rate of progression.

In studies involving MRI to follow progression non-invasively (Watson *et al.*, 1996) it was observed that a change within the subchondral bone was present at least as early as eight weeks of age, prior to any obvious change in the articular cartilage. X-radiography of thick, 1.5 mm, slices of undecalcified knee in plastic revealed that, even prior to four weeks of age, considerable remodelling of the subchondral trabeculae in the tibial and femoral compartments was underway, particularly at the cruciate ligament insertion sites. This is illustrated in figure 22.1(a–b) where it can also be seen that the medial subchondral plate increases in thickness to compensate for the loss of trabeculae and to maintain mechanical stability. This loss of trabecular bone was associated with high levels of cathepsin B activity (Meijers *et al.*, 1994). As with OA in mice, cartilage degeneration in the guinea pig is associated with, and preceded by, change in another tissue, in this case subchondral bone. Change within the cruciate ligaments also occurs at the same time, 4/5 weeks of age, as the bone remodelling, with a progressive production of type II collagen within these ligaments before the cartilage begins to fibrillate (Young *et al.*, 1997). This provides a further illustration of Rodbard's thesis that a structure will alter if the mechanics change. Loss of trabecular bone initiates a series of structural changes that essentially

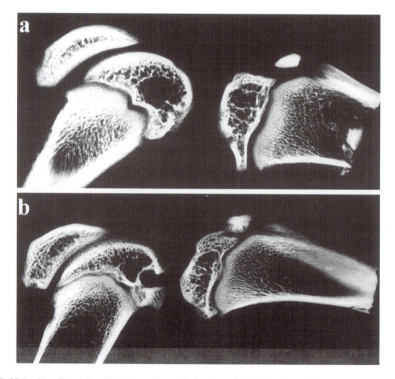

FIGURE 22.1 X-radiography of 1.5 mm slices of plastic embedded guinea pig knee, demonstrating bone remodelling prior to histological evidence of cartilage degeneration. Sagittal sections from the middle of the joint taken in the region of the cruciate ligament insertions. (a) shows the loss of trabecular bone at 4 weeks of age and beginning of subchondral plate thickening (× 5.5). (b) is at 10 weeks of age and demonstrates the progression of bone loss and remodelling of bone at the ligament insertion site (× 4.5).

place the cartilage between a 'rock and a hard place', leading to eventual failure. It is not possible at present to rule out that a change in articular cartilage precipitates the subchondral bone remodelling and that this model of OA is driven by such cartilage change. Osborne and his colleagues (1994) have demonstrated that the ratio of 6-sulphated chondroitin to the 4-sulphated isomer on the glycosaminoglycan chains of cartilage proteoglycan is changing dramatically by eight weeks of age, but the appearance of the 3-B-3 minus mimitope, typical of the osteoarthritic proteoglycan phenotype, is not present before nine weeks of age (Caterson *et al.*, 1996). Debate on what changes first, hence initiating OA, may be considered academic but is, in fact, important when defining strategies for rational treatment of the disease. If bone change initiates and promulgates OA then bone may be a worthwhile target for intervention. Progression to failure of the knee joint in human OA may be predicted by a positive scintigraph (Dieppe *et al.*, 1993), using a technetium labelled bone seeking bisphosphonate; remodelling of bone in late stage OA is a prerequisite for final failure.

SPONTANEOUS OA IN RHESUS AND CYNOMOLGUS MACAQUES

OA in rhesus monkeys has been described by DeRousseau (1985) and by Kessler *et al.* (1986) and Pritzker and his colleagues (1989). However, the availability of this species for comprehensive study is limited, so the development of a similar disease pattern in the more prevalent Cynomolgus species has enabled detailed study of a model of naturally occurring medial compartment knee OA in a primate species (Carlson *et al.*, 1994, 1995, 1996). The value of this model is that it occurs in middle-aged to elderly animals which are bipedal, unlike mice and guinea pigs. Yet there are considerable similarities between the OA initiation and progression in guinea pigs and monkeys which resemble the human disease. Carlson and her colleagues (1995) have pointed out the value of a model that develops insidiously and which simulates the human condition more closely than chemical, mechanical and surgical manipulations, where extrapolation to the human condition should be done with caution. The earliest change they observed histologically was thickening of the subchondral plate and this was followed by fibrillation and clefting of cartilage. This occurred initially in the medial plateau but with severe disease the lateral compartment became involved; a similar situation exists with involvement of the lateral compartment in guinea pig OA. In their latest study (Carlson *et al.*, 1996) it was apparent that degeneration of cartilage did not occur until the subchondral bone had thickened to a significant degree. In fact, it had to reach 400 mm before the cartilage became involved. As with the guinea pig, the appearance of the 3-B-3 minus mimitope seen on the osteoarthritic phenotype of proteoglycans occurred after the subchondral bone had increased in thickness (Carlson *et al.*, 1995). It was also established that prevalence and severity of OA increased with age but these were not affected by gender or weight, providing some contrast with human OA of the knee. They concluded that thickening of the subchondral plate may be more important than the volume of epiphyseal/metaphyseal bone in determining the mechanical stresses in the joint and in influencing the development of articular cartilage lesions.

Cynomolgus macaque OA provides another example of change in one tissue influencing change in other structures to maintain stability, yet ultimately failing to do so thereby leading to OA and joint failure. Why the subchondral bone becomes thickened is unknown but perhaps ligament changes may be precipitative in this species; this is a speculation, however, and needs to addressed in macaques.

TISSUE INTERFACE CHANGES DURING THE DEVELOPMENT OF RA

Rheumatoid arthritis affects approximately 2% of the world population and of these about half have the crippling form of the disease that results in cartilage and bone destruction. Tissue loss occurs through the activity of a tissue arising from the synovium/periosteum interface called pannus. It is not totally clear what initiates pannus formation in RA though the initial inflammatory and immune reactivity within the synovial cavity would result in the generation of cell proliferative cytokines and growth factors. Reactivity to self antigens with similar epitopes on common bacteria, e.g. the QKRAA epitope on Escherishia coli (Albani et al., 1995) is cited as one of the initiating immune events. Evidence is accumulating, however, that the continuing immunity and inflammation of RA are not required for the progressive erosion of cartilage and bone (Kirwan et al., 1995; Mulherin et al., 1996).

Not everyone who has the symmetrical inflammation of RA, particularly in the carpal and tarsal joints, experiences tissue destruction so there must be other factors that initiate the invasive process. When erosion does occur, it is interesting to note that the process is relatively slow, taking years to erode the cartilage and bone in the small joints of the hands and feet. The question arises as to why this erosive process is so slow; is there a process that can account for this slow erosive progression? It is also important to recognise that though pannus can grow to proportions that occupy much of the joint space, the erosion of cartilage and bone occurs through a small population of cells tightly apposed to the cartilage and bone pannus interfaces. The nature of these cells and the mechanisms of destruction they employ will be the subject of this review. The cellular nature of the bulk of pannus has been described many times in many textbooks and need not be included here.

THE EROSION INTERFACE

The overgrowth of cartilage by pannus during the erosive development of RA in man has been elegantly reviewed by Fassbender in 1994. In his review Fassbender describes, and illustrates, the development of pannus at the synovial/periosteal interface just adjacent to where the cartilage and bone meet. Two types of erosive attack can be delineated in the small joints of the hands and feet. Pannus may directly move into the subchondral bone and then move up into the overlying cartilage, or grow over the surface of cartilage before attacking that tissue. Buckland-Wright (1984) has also shown that for the small joints of the wrist and the metacarpal-interphalangeal joints the erosive process is first detected at the sites of intrasynovial ligament insertions. Erosion then proceeds through the subchondral bone and into the articular cartilage after the pannus has grown over the surface (Fassbender, 1994). As mentioned above, the process is considered to be initiated by the immune/inflammatory events associated with some foreign or perhaps host antigen (Albani *et al.*, 1995). However, in the experience of the author, surgical trauma to the joint, in the absence of any immune complications, can be sufficient to initiate a process of synovial outgrowth over cartilage with limited invasion. This is shown in figure 22.2(a–c),

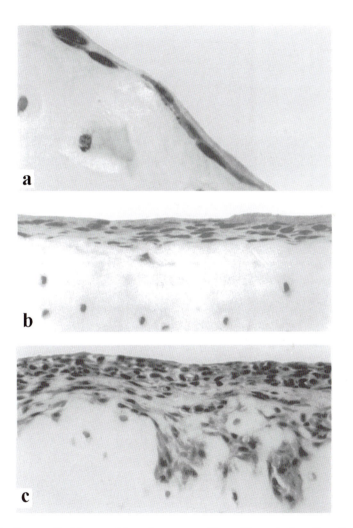

FIGURE 22.2   Overgrowth of the synovial membrane over cartilage of the canine knee 6 months after surgery for cruciate ligament transection. The pannus-like tissue increases in thickness with time and invades cartilage when it reaches 5–10 cells in thickness; this is accompanied by a change in cell shape, reminiscent of the 'trans-formed' phenotype described by Fassbender and Gay's group. (a) shows the tissue at 1–2 cells in thickess; (b) shows the tissue at the 5 cell stage, note the flattened fibroblastic shape and (c) demonstrates the shape change and reorganisation of the tissue as it begins to invade the cartilage matrix.

where the synovium in the knee joint of a dog has grown over and started to penetrate cartilage in the six month period following surgery for cruciate ligament transection.

The tissue found overlying the dog cartilage, after injury to the synovium, was just one cell thick at the leading edge. What initially attracted the cells to grow over the cartilage is unclear, though Muller-Ladner *et al.* (1996) suggest this may be due to expression of vascular cell adhesion molecule (VCAM-1). This cell layer increased in thickness with time, becoming multilayered until a point was reached at 6–10 cells in thickness, when the cells began to change shape to a rounded appearance and then moved into the subjacent cartilage. This is very similar to the process of cellular invasion of cartilage described by Fassbender (1994) and by Muller-Ladner *et al.* (1996) where they have modelled erosion of human cartilage by rheumatoid synovial fibroblasts in SCID mice, see figure 22.3. Invasive fibroblastic cells change shape to a rounded appearance prior to invasion of cartilage and they can maintain this phenotype in culture in the absence of T-lymphocytes. Most interestingly, other studies by Gay and his group (Muller-Ladner *et al.*, 1995) have shown that invasion of cartilage and bone continues in RA patients with terminal AIDS when the lymphocyte count has dropped dramatically and the inflammatory symptoms have disappeared. These studies suggest that the change in phenotype of the synovial fibroblasts to an aggressive, erosive form is not dependent upon the inflammatory and immune processes that accompany RA. It is also reminiscent of the observations on the tissue invading cartilage in the knee of the dog following surgery for cruciate ligament transection. Here, erosion of cartilage continued long after the initial

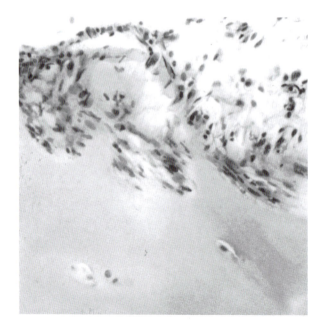

FIGURE 22.3   Invasion by RA synovial tissue into human cartilage following co-implantation under the kidney capsule of the SCID mouse. The appearance is similar to that of 22.2c, with invasion of the cartilage by rounded mesenchymal cells (Courtesy of Professor Steffen Gay, Zurich).

inflammation had subsided, and in the absence of obvious immune complications. In all these circumstances, it was striking that the eroding fibroblastic cells were, relatively, at a considerable distance from any blood vessels (Fassbender, 1994; Muller-Ladner et al., 1996) and essentially unassociated with other cell types, e.g. macrophages.

THE EROSIVE CELL

Fassbender (1994) has likened the invasive fibroblastic cells to 'transformed' cells and has termed the small clusters of cells which attack cartilage 'tumour-like proliferative' cell masses (TLP). Gay's group also refer to such cells as having a 'transformed' appearance (Muller-Ladner et al., 1996) and these invasive fibroblast-like synoviocytes have been the subject of a recent review by Firestein (1996). The term 'transformed' does not imply uncontrolled proliferation as in malignancy, but describes a state of cellular activation combined with a transformed-appearing cellular phenotype. Fassbender (1994), in fact, regards such cells as having a limited life-span in view of the lack of nutrients available, since this tissue is avascular. All authors refer to the expression of VCAM-1 as being of considerable significance in the attachment of the invasive cells to cartilage, though this is uncertain for bone invasion. All reports emphasise the expression of proto-oncogenes such as c-myc, fos and ras which could be important for the alteration of cell structure and phenotype (Muller-Ladner et al., 1996). Studies at the molecular level have shown the expression of the cysteine proteinases at the invading edge, particularly cathepsins B and L (Muller-Ladner et al., 1996) though it is evident that members of the MMP family of degradative enzymes are also released by these cells (Firestein, 1996). The activation of these cells is uncertain, apart from the notion that oncogene activation has a role. However, it appears that cytokines such as IL1 are not necessary for the continued erosion through cartilage by these cells (Muller-Ladner et al., 1997). Transfection of the invading cells with the IL1 receptor antagonist protein (IRAP), so that this was overexpressed at the site of invasion in the SCID mouse model system, did not slow down the rate of erosive progression through cartilage, but the overexpressed IRAP did prevent the chondrocytic chondrolysis induced by the control, invasive fibroblastic cells transfected with an irrelevant transgene. This appears to be true also for TNFa (Steffan Gay, personnel communication).

So what does switch the fibroblastic cells to the 'transformed' invasive phenotype? The answer may lie partially in the nature of fibroblasts when confronted with the need to clean up debris in the normal process of wound repair, wound debridement as it was originally termed. Anderson and Stoler (review 1993) have described a phenomenon that they call the 'anoxic response system', which occurs when fibroblasts enter the clot formed at a site of trauma or wounding. At such a site the vasculature has been disrupted and there is essentially no oxygen available for normal metabolism. Fibroblasts have the ability to change to anaerobic metabolism, expressing a novel LDHk isoenzyme and subsequently secreting the cysteine proteinases cathepsins B and L (Anderson and Stoler, 1993). This proteolytic activity, together with MMP activation, clears the clot away and allows for angiogenesis through the secretion of the necessary factors from these wound fibroblast cells and accompanying macrophages. Once new blood vessels enter the site, the oxygen tension rises and the anoxic response system switches off, allowing new matrix to be secreted and final repair of the wound. Anderson and Stoler (1993) suggest that the anoxic response system has been 'borrowed' by invasive tumours since experiments in rats have shown that certain tumours cause expression of retrotransposons at the invasion sites; these are of viral origin but have become part of the genome of certain rodents. The function of the retrotransposons is unknown, but they are only up-regulated at sites of tumour invasion and during wound repair in the rodent species which have copies of these genes in their mesenchymal cells (Estes *et al.*, 1995).

It is intriguing to speculate that at the site of invasion of cartilage during RA erosion, the anoxic response system may be active and driving the destructive process. Lack of oxygen could activate the cells to the invasive phenotype and the eventual appearance of blood vessels would cause the system to revert to quiescence. This may account for the slow, sporadic loss of tissue in microenvironments at the cartilage pannus interface, so characteristic of the tissue loss in RA. This needs experimental validation, however, and the anoxic response system may not explain the erosion of bone which is much more vascular. Whatever the answer, the activation of the 'transformed' phenotype is of crucial significance to the loss of cartilage and bone during the erosive progression of RA.

CONCLUDING COMMENTS

It is clear that the interface zones between cartilage, calcified cartilage and subchondral bone are highly involved in the remodelling of the articular joint during the development of osteoarthritis, and that the cruciate ligament insertion sites into subchondral bone are interfaces of great mechanical sensitivity in at least one species, the guinea pig. Rodbard's (1974) thesis that change in the mechanics of one tissue will cause changes to the structure of other dependent tissues is well illustrated by the development of spontaneous OA of the knee of several mammalian species. There are still many details to fill in for knee OA and the situation may not be the same for all joints, though it appears likely that the same may pertain for hip OA. OA can thus be viewed as a biomechanically driven but biochemically mediated disorder, dependent upon the fact that different forms of stress result in different connective tissue types. The animal models are thus proving invaluable for elucidating early events which cannot be addressed in the human disease. Only time will tell if the animal events mimic the human initiation and progression of OA.

Ligament insertion sites at the interface between the peristeum and synovium, within articular joints, become intimately involved in the process of erosive destruction of cartilage and bone during the progression of rheumatoid arthritis. A particular variant of the synovial fibroblast appears to responsible for the destruction of the connective tissues when it changes to a so-called 'transformed' phenotype. The reason for this change remains to be fully elucidated but one speculation is that it is related to the phenotype seen during wound repair, which involves the 'anoxic response system' (Anderson and Stoler, 1993). There is still much to be done to establish this but the articular joint has to viewed as a dynamic organ that can respond in a subtle manner or dramatically to mechanical change and proliferative injury to the synovium. Tissue interfaces bear the brunt of all this.

REFERENCES

Albani, S., Keystone, E.C., Nelson, J.L., Ollier, W.E.R., La Cava, A.L., Montemayor, A.C., Weber, D.A., Montecucco, C., Martini, A. and Carson, D.A. (1995) Positive selection in autoimmunity: abnormal responses to a bacterial dnaJ antigenic determinant in patients with early rheumatoid arthritis. *Nature Medicine*, **1**, 448–452.

Anderson, G.R. and Stoler, D.L. (1993) Anoxia, wound healing, VL30 elements and the molecular basis of malignant conversion. *Bioessays*, **15**, 265–271.

Bendele, A.M. and Hulman, J.F. (1988) Spontaneous cartilage degeneration in guinea pigs. *Arthritis Rheum.*, **31**, 561–565.

Bendele, A.M., White, S.L. and Hulman, J.F. (1989) Osteoarthritis in guinea pigs: histopathologic and scanning electron microscopic features. *Lab. An. Sci.*, **39**, 115–121.

Billingham, M.E.J. (1998) Advantages afforded by the use of animal models for the evaluation of potential DMOADS. In: *Textbook of Osteoarthritis*. (Ed. Doherty, M., Brandt, K.D. and Lohmander, S.) Oxford University Press. In Press.

Buckland-Wright, J.C. (1984) Microfocal radiographic examination of erosions in the wrist and hand of patients with rheumatoid arthritis. *Ann. Rheum. Dis.*, **43**, 160–171.

Carlson, C.S., Loeser, R.F., Jayo, M.J., Weaver, D.S., Adams, M.R. and Jerome, C.P. (1994) Osteoarthritis in Cynomolgus macaques: a primate model on naturally occurring disease. *J. Orth. Res.*, **12**, 331–339.

Carlson, C.S., Loeser, R.F., Johnstone, B., Tulli, H.M., Dodson, D.B. and Caterson, B. (1995) Osteoarthritis in Cynomolgus macaques II. Detection of modulated proteoglycan epitopes in cartilage and synovial fluid. *J. Orthop. Res.*, **13**, 399–409.

Carlson, C.S., Loeser, R.F., Purser, C.B., Gardin, J.F. and Jerome, C.P. (1996) Osteoarthritis in Cynomolgus macaques III. Effects of age, gender, and subchondral bone thickness on the severity of disease. *J. Bone Min. Res.*, **46**, 36–41.

Caterson, B., Slater, R.R., Blankenship-Paris, T., Carney, S.L., Bendele, A.M. and Chandrasekar, S. (1996) Natural osteoarthritis in guinea pigs 1: expression of 3-B-3 (−) epitope in cartilage proteoglycans as a biochemical marker for the development of osteoarthritis. *Arthritis Rheum.*, (In revision).

Collins, C., Evans, R.G., Ponsford, F., Miller, P. and Elson, C.J. (1994) Chondro-osseous metaplasia, bone density and patella cartilage proteoglycan content in the osteoarthritis of STR/ORT mice. *Osteoarthritis Cart.*, **2**, 111–118.

DeRousseau, C.J. (1985) Aging in the musculoskeletal system of rhesus monkeys. II. Degenerative joint disease. *Am. J. Phys. Anthropol.*, **67**, 177–184.

Dieppe, P.A., Cushnaghan, J., Young, P. and Kirwan, J.R. (1993) Prediction of the progression of joint space narrowing in osteoarthritis of the knee by bone scintigraphy. *Ann. Rheum. Dis.*, **52**, 557–563.

Dieppe, P.A. (1995) The classification and diagnosis of osteoarthritis. In: *Osteoarthritic disorders*. (Eds. Kuettner, K. and Goldberg, V.M.) American Academy of Orthopaedic Surgeons, Rosemont IL, pp. 5–12.

Estes, S.D., Stoler, D.L. and Anderson, G.R. (1995) Anoxic induction of a sarcoma virus-related VL30 retro-transposon is mediated by a cis-acting element which binds hypoxia-inducible factor 1 and an anoxia-inducible factor. *J. Virol.*, **69**, 6335–6341.

Evans, R.G., Collins, C., Miller, P., Ponsford, P.M. and Elson, C.J. (1994) Radiological scoring of osteoarthritis progression in STR/ORT mice. *Osteoarthritis Cart.*, **2**, 103–109.

Fassbender, H.G. (1994) Inflammatory reactions in arthritis. In *Immunopharmacology of joints and connective tissues*. (Eds. Davies, E. and Dingle, J.T.) Academic Press, London, pp. 165–198.

Firestein, G.S. (1996) Invasive fibroblast-like synoviocytes in rheumatoid arthritis. Passive responders or trans-formed aggressors. *Arth. Rheum.*, **39**, 1781–1790.

Johnson, L.C. (1962) Joint remodelling as a basis for osteoarthritis. *J. Am. Vet. Med. Assoc.*, **141**, 1237–1241.

Kessler, M.J., Turnquist, J.E., Pritzker, K.P.H. and London, W.T. (1986) Reduction of passive extension and radiographic evidence of degenerative knee joint diseases in cage-raised and free-ranging aged rhesus monkeys (Maccaca mulatta). *J. Med. Primatol.*, **15**, 1–9.

Kirwan, J.R. and the ARC low-dose corticosteroid study group (1995) The effect of glucocorticoids on joint destruction in rheum arthritis. *NEJM*, **333**, 142–146.

Meacock, S.C.R., Bodmer, J.L. and Billingham, M.E.J. (1990) Experimental osteoarthritis in guinea pigs. *J. Exp. Path.*, **71**, 279–293.

Meijers, M.H.M., Bunning, R.A.D., Russell, R.G.G. and Billingham, M.E.J. (1994) Evidence for cathepsin B involvement in subchondral bone changes during early natural osteoarthritis in the guinea pig. *Brit. J. Rhem.*, **33** (Suppl. 1), 90.

Mulherin, D., Fitzgerald, O. and Bresnihan, B. (1996) Clinical improvement and radiological deterioration in rheumatoid arthritis: evidence that the pathogenesis of synovial inflammation and articular erosion may differ. *Brit. J. Rheum.*, **35**, 1263–1268.

Muller-Ladner, U., Kriegsmann, J., Gay, R.E., Koopman, W.J., Gay, S. and Chatham, W.W. (1995) Progressive joint disease in a human immunodeficiency virus-infected patient with rheumatoid arthritis. *Arth. Rheum.*, **38**, 1328–1332.

Muller-Ladner, U., Kriegsmann, J., Franklin, B.N., Matsumoto, S., Geiler, T., Gay, R.E. and Gay, S. (1996) Synovial fibroblasts of patients with rheumatoid arthritis attach to and invade normal cartilage when engrafted into SCID mice. *Am. J. Path.*, **149**, 1607–1615.

Muller-Ladner, U., Roberts, C.R., Franklin, B.N., Gay, R.E., Robbins, P.D. Evans, C.H. and Gay, S. (1997) Human IL1ra gene transfer into human synovial fibroblasts is chondroprotective. *J. Immunol.* **158**, 3492–3498.

Osborne, D.J., Woodhouse, S. and Meacock, S.C.R. (1994) Early changes in the sulfation of chondroitin in guinea-pig articular cartilage, a possible predictor of osteoarthritis. *Osteoarthritis Cart.*, **2**, 215–223.

Pritzker, K.P.H., Chateauvert, J., Grynpas, M.D., Renlund, R.C., Turnquist, J. and Kessler, M.J. (1989) Rhesus macaques as an experimental model for degenerative arthritis. *P. R. Health Sci. J.*, **8**, 99–102.

Radin, E.L., Schaffler, M., Gibson, G. and Tashman, S. (1995) Osteoarthrosis as a result of repetitive trauma. In: Osteoarthritic disorders (Ed. K.E. Kuettner and V.M. Goldberg). American Academy of Orthopaedic Surgeons, Rosemont IL, pp. 197–203.

Rodbard, S. (1970) Negative feedback mechanisms in the architecture and function of the connective and cardiovascular tissues. *Perspectives Biol. Med.*, **13**, 507–527.

Rodbard, S. (1974): Biophysical factors in vascular structure and caliber. In: *Atherosclerosis III.* (Ed. G. Schettlar, A. Weizel) Springer-Verlag, Berlin, pp. 46–63.

Smale, G., Bendele, A.M. and Horton, W.E. (1995) Comparison of age-associated degeneration of articular cartilage in Wistar and Fischer 344 rats. *Lab. An. Sci.*, **45**, 191–194.

Schunke, M., Tillman, B., Bruck, M. and Muller-Ruchholtz, W. (1988) Morphologic characteristics of developing osteoarthrotic lesions in the knee cartilage of STR/IN mice. *Arthritis Rheum.*, **31**, 898–905.

Silverstein, E. and Sokoloff, L. (1958) Natural history of degenerative joint disease in small laboratory animals. 5. Osteoarthritis in guinea pigs. *Arthritis Rheum.*, **1**, 82–86.

Sokoloff, L. (1956) Natural history of degenerative joint disease in small laboratory animals. 1. Pathological anatomy of degenerative joint disease in mice. *Arch. Pathol.*, **62**, 118–128.

Walton, M. (1977) Studies of degenerative joint disease in the mouse knee joint: histological observations. *J. Pathol.*, **123**, 109–122.

Watson, P.J., Hall, L.D., Malcolm, A. and Tyler, J.A. (1996) Degenerative joint disease in the guinea pig. Use of magnetic resonance imaging to monitor progression of bone pathology. *Arthritis Rheum.*, **39**, 1327–1337.

Young, R.D., Vaughan-Thomas, A., Wardale, J., Mason, D. and Duance, V.C. (1997) Cartilage collagen expression in cruciate ligaments in the early stages of osteoarthritis. *Trans. Orthop. Res. Soc.*, **22**, 500.

23 The Attachment of Tendons and Ligaments to Bone

M. Benjamin* and J.R. Ralphs

*Connective Tissue Biology Labs, Cardiff School of Biosciences,
University of Wales Cardiff, PO Box 911,
Museum Avenue, Cardiff CF1 3US*

Both ligaments and tendons form an important part of joint capsules and thus the strength of their junction with bone (the 'enthesis') is of critical importance for the integrity of synovial joints. The current review concentrates on the cell and matrix biology of entheses and the reader is referred to Woo *et al.* (1988) for an earlier and more biomechanical treatment.

ENTHESIS STRUCTURE

It has been known for many years – largely through the work of German histologists (Dolgo-Saburoff, 1929; Petersen, 1930; Schneider, 1956; Biermann, 1957; Knese and Biermann, 1958) that there are two fundamentally distinct forms of enthesis. Typically, those near the ends of long bones (above the growth plate and near the joint cavity) or on the short bones of the hand and foot, attach to bone via a region of fibrocartilage. Those attaching to the shafts of long bones are purely fibrous. Because most ligaments and tendons attach near synovial joints, fibrocartilaginous attachments are the most common and by far the most widely studied. They are the 'chondral insertions' of Knese (1979) and the 'direct insertions' of Woo *et al.* (1988). Although the term 'direct insertion' has been widely adopted (e.g. by Kang *et al.*, 1996; Liu *et al.*, 1995; Ma *et al.*, 1996), it could be argued that such tendons or ligaments actually attach *indirectly* to bone – i.e. via a transitional zone of fibrocartilage. Furthermore, as Woo *et al.* (1988) themselves point out, the superficial fibres of a 'direct' insertion can attach 'indirectly' to the periosteum. It is for

* Corresponding author.

these reasons that we prefer to call entheses simply 'fibrocartilaginous' or 'fibrous' (Benjamin and Ralphs, 1995).

FIBROCARTILAGINOUS ENTHESES

A typical example of a fibrocartilaginous enthesis is the attachment of supraspinatus to the head of the humerus (see Figure 1 in Benjamin et al., 1986). The fibrocartilage is part of a sequence of 4 tissues – dense regular connective tissue of the tendon or ligament, uncalcified fibrocartilage, calcified fibrocartilage and bone (Dolgo-Saburoff, 1929; Cooper and Misol, 1970). The uncalcified fibrocartilage consists of rows of large rounded cells, surrounded by a small amount of pericellular matrix and lying between bundles of collagen fibres. Commonly, the fibres splay out near their insertion so that tension is distributed over a wide area and in all positions of the neighbouring joint (Clark and Sidles, 1990; Clark and Harryman, 1992). Thus, the area of the enthesis is often much larger than that of the ligament or tendon midsubstance (e.g. Harner et al., 1993). In most tendons and ligaments, the fibrocartilage is not evenly distributed over the entire insertion site. It is more conspicuous in the deep (inner) parts nearer to the joint that the tendon or ligament crosses (Benjamin et al., 1986; Evans et al., 1990; Matyas et al., 1995). This is the part of the attachment site that is subject to the greatest compression (Matyas et al., 1995).

The regions of calcified and uncalcified fibrocartilage are separated by a calcification front called the tidemark. It appears as a basophilic line in routine light microscopy sections (Benjamin et al., 1986) and an electron dense line in ultrastructural studies (Cooper and Misol, 1970; Rufai et al., 1996). Occasional fibrocartilage cells can straddle the tidemark and multiple tidemarks probably represent successive periods of calcification (Rufai et al., 1996). In local parts of an enthesis, either the zone of calcified or uncalcified fibrocartilage can be missing (Benjamin and Ralphs, unpublished observations). Thus in Woo et al.'s (1988) illustration of the femoral attachment of the medial collateral ligament (MCL) of the rabbit, the tidemark occurs at the junction of the ligament with the zone of calcified fibrocartilage. The calcified fibrocartilage has an irregular interface with the underlying bone that increases the contact surface area and provides resistance to shear in a manner analogous to that at the dermal–epidermal junction of the skin. By contrast, tidemarks are relatively straight and it is at the outermost tidemark that the soft tissues fall away in a macerated skeleton (Benjamin et al., 1986). Because enthesis fibrocartilage is commonly avascular (Benjamin et al., 1986; Weiss et al., 1995), blood vessels do not cross the tidemark passing between tendon/ligament and bone. Hence, tendons and ligaments with significant quantities of fibrocartilage at their entheses leave smooth, circumscribed markings on bones that resemble those on adjacent articular surfaces (Benjamin et al., 1986).

FIBROUS ENTHESES

Purely fibrous entheses correspond to the periosteal insertions of Knese (1979) and the indirect insertions of Woo et al. (1988). No fibrocartilage is present and the tendon or ligament either attaches directly to the bone (in adults) or indirectly to the periosteum (during the growing period). Characteristically, the collagen fibres of the tendon or ligament run almost parallel to the long axis of the bone and approach the enthesis at an oblique angle (see Figure 4 in Benjamin *et al.*, 1986 and Figure 172 in Knese 1979). Typically, tendons and ligaments with fibrous entheses have broader areas of attachment to bone than do those with fibrocartilaginous entheses.

FUNCTIONAL SIGNIFICANCE OF ENTHESIS FIBROCARTILAGE

It is widely considered that enthesis fibrocartilage reduces stress concentration at bony interfaces where hard and soft tissues meet (see reviews Woo *et al.*, 1988; Benjamin and Ralphs, 1995, 1996). The uncalcified fibrocartilage probably has a role rather like that of a plastic grommet where an electric cable joins a plug – the grommet ensures that cable bending occurs away from the electrical connections (Schneider, 1956). As the collagen fibres approach the bone, they change direction through the uncalcified fibrocartilage and eventually meet the tidemark approximately at right angles (Benjamin *et al.*, 1986; Clark and Sidles, 1990).

There is an important mechanical difference to appreciate between tendons or ligaments that attach close to a joint and those that attach far away, that helps in understanding why epiphyseal attachment sites are fibrocartilaginous and diaphyseal ones are fibrous (Benjamin *et al.*, 1986). Compare the attachment of deltoid half way down the arm (i.e. to the diaphysis), with that of supraspinatus near the shoulder joint on the humeral head (i.e. to the epiphysis). As the arm is abducted at the shoulder, the angle between the tendon of supraspinatus and the humerus increases, whereas that between the tendon of deltoid and the humerus changes very little (Figure 23.1). This means that there is an increased

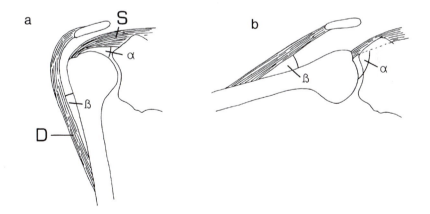

FIGURE 23.1   A tendon attaching to the end of a long bone (supraspinatus, S) is subject to a greater risk of fraying at its enthesis during joint movement than one attached to the diaphysis (deltoid, D). There is a marked change in angle (α) between the tendon of supraspinatus and the humerus when the arm is moved away from the side (a) to the abducted position (b). In contrast, there is little change in the angle (β) between the tendon of deltoid and the humerus.

risk of fibre-fraying at sites where tendons and ligaments attach to the ends of long bones. The fibrocartilage at epiphyseal attachment sites probably controls the bending of the fibres and ensures that it does not occur at the hard tissue interface, but is displaced gradually through the fibrocartilage and into the tendon/ligament itself. The presence of fibrocartilage indicates that compressive stresses are greater nearer the bone than in the midsubstance. Conversely, tensile stresses must be greater in the midsubstance. These concepts are supported by the work of Matyas *et al.* (1995) who correlated cell shape with a finite element analysis of the mechanical stresses and strains at the femoral attachment of the rabbit MCL.

There is a good correlation between the amount of uncalcified fibrocartilage at an enthesis and the degree of bending that occurs near the bony interface. In our laboratory, we have compared the thickness of the fibrocartilage at a number of sites in the body (Evans *et al.*, 1990; Benjamin *et al.*, 1991, 1992). In the quadriceps and patellar tendons for example, there is more fibrocartilage at the insertion of the quadriceps and patellar tendons than at the origin of the patellar tendon (Evans *et al.*, 1990). The radiographic studies of Eijden *et al.* (1985, 1986) have shown that there is a 30° change in angle between the tendon and bone at the insertions of the quadriceps and patellar tendons during flexion and extension of the knee, but virtually no change in angle at the origin of the patellar tendon. Hence the fibrocartilage zone is thickest where there is the most movement. Comparable differences exist at the insertions of biceps brachii, brachialis and triceps (Benjamin *et al.*, 1992). Biceps is the most 'mobile' as it were, for it alone both supinates the forearm and flexes the elbow, whereas the others act in one plane only, either flexing or extending the elbow. The biceps tendon has more enthesis fibrocartilage than either of the other two, even though it is the smallest tendon. Finally, at the knee, the lateral meniscus is more mobile than the medial, and its horns have significantly more enthesis fibrocartilage (Benjamin *et al.*, 1991).

Enthesis fibrocartilage probably has other functions besides that of controlling the bending of collagen fibres near the bony interface. Both tendons and ligaments can stretch to some degree and as a consequence they must narrow slightly under load. It is possible that fibrocartilage at an enthesis could prevent the narrowing from occurring just at the bony junction. This 'stretching-brake' hypothesis of Knese and Biermann (1958) is supported by the finding that elastic fibres largely disappear from the entheses of elastic ligaments (Hotta, 1985). Knese and Biermann (1958) have also suggested that enthesis fibrocartilage can act as a growth plate for epiphyses and this has been supported by the developmental studies of Gao *et al.* (1996a) which are reviewed below.

Less attention has been paid to the zone of calcified fibrocartilage at entheses, though Gao and Messner (1996) have proposed that it is capable of two types of physiological adaptation. From their study of rabbit knee ligaments, they suggest that the extent of the interdigitations between calcified fibrocartilage and bone are established at puberty according to tensile loads in the ligaments, but that the size of the calcified fibrocartilage region continues to develop beyond puberty, wherever there is considerable motion at the hard–soft tissue interface.

Evans *et al.* (1991) considered the zone of calcified fibrocartilage and the underlying bone as a single unit and found that the thickness of the region was related to the tensile load transmitted through the tendon or ligament. Ikeda *et al.* (1996) have used this association to predict which regions of the acromion transmit the major tensile forces generated by the contraction of deltoid and thus which parts of the bone should be preserved during shoulder surgery if deltoid muscle weakness is to be avoided.

In an earlier chapter of this book, Ralphs and Benjamin (1997) highlighted the extensive network of cell–cell communication in tendons and ligaments where the fibroblasts are linked to each other by gap junctions. The immunolabeling for connexins is reduced in the zone of uncalcified fibrocartilage and virtually absent in the calcified zone (Gao et al., 1997). The reduction in labeling at the enthesis compared with the midsubstance is probably associated with the retraction of cell processes by fibroblasts that have metaplased into fibrocartilage cells. The findings suggest that in addition to acting as a vascular barrier between tendon and bone, enthesis fibrocartilage also restricts communication between their respective cells. Furthermore, calcified fibrocartilage in particular could act as a diffusion barrier between bone and ligament/tendon preventing the spread of e.g. growth factors between the two regions.

It is important to appreciate that enthesis fibrocartilage is just one of a series of protective devices to reduce wear and tear at entheses. At many attachment sites, there is also a small bursa that allows the tendon/ligament to move freely relative to the bone, a sesamoid fibrocartilage (SF) on the deep surface of the tendon/ligament and a periosteal fibrocartilage (PF) on the bone. The SF and PF protect the bone and the tendon/ligament where they rub against each other. This complex insertional region is well developed in the human Achilles tendon and is illustrated in Figure 1 of Rufai et al. (1995). SF adjacent to the enthesis is a prominent feature of the central slip of the extensor tendon in both the fingers and toes (Benjamin et al., 1993; Milz et al., 1996). Here, the fibrocartilage provides an articular surface for the proximal phalanx when the proximal interphalangeal joints are flexed.

ENTHESOPATHIES

The term 'enthesopathy' is widely used in rheumatology to denote any disorder of an enthesis (Niepel and Sitaj, 1979; Resnick and Niwayama, 1983). Tendon, ligament and joint capsule insertions can be the site of degenerative, traumatic or inflammatory change and are implicated in many cases of soft tissue rheumatism. Enthesopathies include such common conditions as tennis elbow, jumper's knee and calcaneal spurs and are among the most characteristic changes that occur in diffuse idiopathic skeletal hyperostosis (DISH) and ankylosing spondylitis. Simple mechanical damage at entheses e.g. partial tears, is often difficult to repair. Experimental studies of the rabbit MCL injured at its proximal and distal attachments have shown that injury at either end is slower to heal than are tears in midsubstance (Frank et al., 1995). Waggy et al. (1994) used poor healing in a model of partial tears at the patellar tendon insertion to suggest that such enthesopathies heal poorly because the damaged parts of the tendon are not load-bearing. They made the interesting suggestion that partial tears at tendon entheses are the soft tissue equivalent of painful bony non-union.

In a study of rabbit knee ligaments and tendons, Gao et al. (1996b) found that at low strain velocity, traumatic failures often occurred at two sites simultaneously, but that the principal mode of failure of the cruciate and MCL ligaments was by bony avulsion below the enthesis. Although failures did occur at the cement line (i.e. the junction between calcified fibrocartilage and bone) and in the fibrocartilage regions, as a general rule the enthesis itself seemed to protect the tendon or ligament against failure. The orientation of enthesis fibrocartilage relative to the bone as a whole is probably important in determining the site of failure. Ma *et al.* (1996) loaded dog patellar tendons at different angles with respect to the position of the enthesis fibrocartilage and found that the loading direction determined whether failures occurred by bony avulsion or by tears in the tendon midsubstance. They thought that the orientation of the fibrocartilage with respect to the tibial plateau represents the cut-off between the two failure mechanisms.

Rufai *et al.* (1995) have recently described a number of pathological changes that are common at the attachment of the Achilles tendon, though the cause of the changes is obscure. The changes include fissuring, fragmentation and degeneration of the SF and PF fibrocartilages that directly form the boundaries of the retrocalcaneal bursa. The enthesis fibrocartilage itself can develop bony spurs that grow by endochondral ossification and longitudinal fissures that are similar to those developing in articular cartilage in the early stages of osteoarthritis (Rothwell and Bentley, 1973). In both tendon and articular cartilage, there are large clusters of hypertrophied cells at the edges of the fissures. In the tendon, the clusters are restricted to the fibrocartilage region, but where the fissures extend more proximally, there is no cartilage cell response. The obvious difference between Achilles tendon fissures and those in articular cartilage is that the former are often calcified and filled with amorphous metachromatic material or poorly organised fibrous extracellular matrix (ECM). It seems likely that the contents of the fissures indicate an attempted repair response. It could be that similar material is absent from cartilage fissures because these open onto a joint cavity and are leached out. Transverse tears are completely different (Rufai *et al.*, 1995). They are small, lie at the junction of calcified and uncalcified regions of fibrocartilage and are filled with loose vascular connective tissue. There is no obvious cell response.

BIOCHEMICAL COMPOSITION

The relatively small quantities of fibrocartilage present at entheses makes biochemical analyses difficult. Recently however Visconti *et al.* (1996) and Waggett *et al.* (1997) have taken advantage of the large size of the human Achilles tendon and the steer anterior cruciate ligament (ACL) and MCL to analyse qualitatively the ECM macromolecules present at the enthesis by RT-PCR and Western blotting. Visconti *et al.* (1996) have found types I, II, IX and XI collagens in the fibrocartilage, while Waggett *et al.* (1997) report types I, II, III, V and VI collagens. Although no quantitative data is available from either study, Visconti *et al.* (1996) have suggested that type II collagen represents a significant proportion of the total collagens. Only Waggett *et al.* (1997) have analysed the proteoglycan (PG) and glycosaminoglycan (GAG) composition of enthesis fibrocartilage and of a neighbouring SF on the deep surface of the Achilles tendon. They report the presence of decorin, biglycan, fibromodulin, and lumican in both fibrocartilages as well as in the midtendon. Versican mRNA was only found in the mid tendon, although the protein itself was present in the sesamoid fibrocartilage. Aggrecan was detected in both the tendon and its fibrocartilages although the role that it performs in the tendon is unclear.

In contrast, there have been a much larger number of immunohistochemical studies dealing with the distribution of collagens, GAGs and PGs. These have been performed on a wide variety of tendons and ligaments in both Man and other animals. The tendons and ligaments include the extensor tendon and collateral ligaments of the fingers and toes (Benjamin et al., 1993; Lewis, 1996; Milz et al., 1996) the tendon of supraspinatus (Kumagai et al., 1994a,b), the quadriceps tendon (Ralphs et al., 1991, 1992), patellar tendon (Liu et al., 1996), MCL (Visconti et al., 1996; Niyibizi et al., 1995, 1996), ACL (Visconti et al., 1996; Liu et al., 1996) and Achilles tendon (Rufai et al., 1992; Waggett et al., 1997). A wide variety of GAGs (chondroitin 4 and 6 sulphate, keratan sulphate and dermatan sulphate), PGs (biglycan, decorin, lumican and aggrecan) and collagens (types I, II, III, V, VI, IX, X, XI and XIV) have been reported. Type II collagen is constantly present in the fibrocartilage of all entheses, though the extent of labeling is greatly reduced in the extensor tendons of rheumatoid fingers (Benjamin et al., 1993). Immunolabeling is generally stronger in the uncalcified fibrocartilage, but the calcified tissue labels as well. According to Visconti et al. (1996), the type II collagen differs from that of articular cartilage from the same animal in containing half hydroxypyridinium cross linking residues. The poor labeling of enthesis fibrocartilage for type I collagen reported by Kumagai et al. (1994a,b) is puzzling, but could be a technical problem. Certainly, one would anticipate the presence of type I collagen in the fibrocartilage in view of the metaplastic development of enthesis fibrocartilage from tendon itself (see below).

DEVELOPMENT

FIBROCARTILAGINOUS ENTHESES

Enthesis fibrocartilage initially represents cartilage that remains uneroded after endochondral ossification has commenced (Ralphs et al., 1992). However, as growth continues and the bones enlarge, the original cartilage rudiment is completely removed and new fibrocartilage develops by metaplasia of fibrous connective tissue in the tendon or ligament (Gao et al., 1996a). This fibrocartilage probably develops in response to mechanical stimulation and its metaplastic origin explains why there are different quantities of fibrocartilage at different entheses (see above) and how fibrocartilage can re-appear at new insertions created during surgical repairs (Jones et al., 1987; Schiavone Panni et al., 1993a,b; Jackson et al., 1996; Kang et al., 1996). The key evidence to support the idea that the origin of enthesis fibrocartilage changes with age, relates to differences in immunolabeling for types I and II collagen at the femoral attachment of the medial collateral ligament (MCL) in the rat, at different stages of development (Gao et al., 1996a). The evidence is summarised diagrammatically in Figure 23.2. New fibrocartilage develops by metaplasia on the ligament side of the enthesis and old fibrocartilage is removed

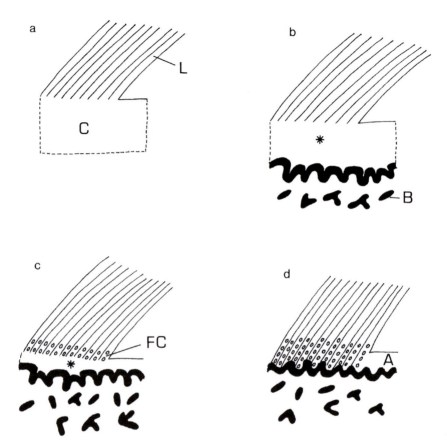

FIGURE 23.2 A simplified and diagrammatic representation of the development of the femoral attachment of the medial collateral ligament, based on the work of Gao *et al.* (1996). (a) The ligament (L) initially attaches to the cartilage (C) rudiment of the femur. (b) Endochondral ossification commences beneath the attachment site and bone (B) begins to replace the cartilage but initially leaves a band uneroded at the enthesis (*). (c) As the epiphysis continues to enlarge, ossification spreads towards the ligament and the band of original cartilage (*) becomes smaller. At the same time, fibrocartilage (FC) appears in the ligament by metaplasia of ligament fibroblasts. (d) The original cartilage rudiment has now disappeared completely and fibrocartilage continues to develop in the ligament by metaplasia.

on the bone side by osteoclastic erosion. Thus, enthesis fibrocartilage does indeed act as a growth plate as suggested by Knese and Biermann (1958). It allows for the growth of an epiphysis at the site of a tendon or ligament attachment. In contrast however, the enthesis does not seem to be a site where tendons grow greatly in length (Nishijima *et al.*, 1994). Perhaps active growth at a tendon-bone junction would reduce the strength of the union.

FIBROUS ENTHESES

The development of entheses in tendons or ligaments that attach to the metaphysis of long bones is governed by the need for such attachment sites to migrate towards the end of the growing bone and maintain the same relative position with respect to the joint cavity (Videman, 1970; Dörfl, 1980a,b). Thus, the development of the tibial end of the rat MCL (below the growth plate) is fundamentally different from the development of the femoral end (above the growth plate). In order for the ligament to migrate and thus avoid becoming increasingly diaphyseal in position, it attaches indirectly to the periosteum during the growing period and only links directly to the bone when growth is over (Matyas et al., 1990; Wei and Messner, 1995; Gao et al., 1996a). If the periosteum on the tibia is cut proximal to the attachment of the MCL, the ligament fails to migrate normally during development (Muhl and Gedak, 1986). The MCL maintains its metaphyseal position because of interstitial growth in the periosteum, erosion of bone at the leading edge of the enthesis and deposition of bone at the trailing edge (Wei and Messner, 1995). A direct link of the MCL to bone (which cannot grow interstitially) at an early stage of development would prevent the ligament from migrating. Thus, the absence of fibrocartilage at the attachment of metaphyseal or diaphyseal tendons and ligaments is a direct consequence of how they develop.

REFERENCES

Benjamin, M., Evans, E.J. and Copp, L. (1986) The histology of tendon attachments in man. *J. Anat.*, **149**, 89–100.

Benjamin, M., Evans, E.J., Donthineni Rao, R., Findlay, J.A. and Pemberton, D.J. (1991) Quantitative differences in the histology of the attachment zones of the meniscal horns in the knee joint of Man. *J. Anat.*, **177**, 127–134.

Benjamin, M., Newell, R.L.M., Evans, E.J., Ralphs, J.R. and Pemberton, D.J. (1992) The structure of the insertions of the tendons of biceps brachii, triceps and brachialis in elderly dissecting room cadavers. *J. Anat.*, **180**, 327–332.

Benjamin, M., Ralphs, J.R., Shibu, M. and Irwin, M. (1993) Capsular tissues of the proximal interphalangeal joint: normal composition and effects of Dupuytren's disease and rheumatoid arthritis. *J. Hand Surg.*, **18B**, 371–376.

Benjamin, M. and Ralphs, J.R. (1995) Developmental and functional anatomy of tendons and ligaments. In: *Repetitive Motion Disorders of the Upper Extremity* (Eds. Gordon, S.L., Blair, S.J. and Fine, L.J.) pp. 185–203. American Academy of Orthopaedic Surgeons, Rosemont.

Benjamin, M. and Ralphs, J.R. (1996) Tendons and ligaments in health and disease. *Manual Therapy*, **1**, 186–191.

Biermann, H. (1957) Die Knochenbildung im Bereich periostaler-diaphysärer Sehnen- und Bandansätze. *Z. Zellforsch*, **46**, 635–671.

Clark, J.M. and Sidles, J.A. (1990) The interrelation of fiber-bundles in the anterior cruciate ligament. *J. Orthop. Res.*, **8**, 180–188.

Clark, J.M. and Harryman, D.T. (1992) Tendons, ligaments, and capsule of the rotator cuff. *J. Bone Joint Surg.*, **74A**, 713–725.

Cooper, R. and Misol, S. (1970) Tendon and ligament insertion. *J. Bone and Joint Surg.*, **52A**, 1–20.

Dolgo-Saburoff, B. (1929) Über Ursprung und Insertion der Skeletmuskeln. *Anat. Anz.*, **68**, 80–87.

Dörfl, J. (1980a) Migration of tendinous insertions. I. Cause and mechanism. *J. Anat.*, **131**, 179–195.

Dörfl, J. (1980b) Migration of tendinous insertions. II. Experimental modifications. *J. Anat.*, **131**, 229–237.

Eijden, T.M.G.J. van, Boer, W. de and Weijs, W.A. (1985) The orientation of the distal part of the quadriceps femoris muscle as a function of the knee flexion-extension angle. *J. Biomech.*, **18**, 803–809.

Eijden, T.M.G.J. van, Kouwenhoven, E., Verburg, J. and Weijs, W.A. (1986) A mathematical model of the patellofemoral joint. *J. Biomechan.*, **19**, 219–229.

Evans, E.J., Benjamin, M. and Pemberton, D.J. (1990) Fibrocartilage in the attachment zones of the quadriceps tendon and patellar ligament of man. *J. Anat.*, **171**, 155–162.

Evans, E.J., Benjamin, M. and Pemberton, D.J. (1991) Variations in the amount of calcified tissue at the attachments of the quadriceps tendon and patellar ligament in man. *J. Anat.*, **174**, 145–151.

Frank, C.B., Loitz, B.J. and Shrive, N.G. (1995) Injury location affects ligament healing: A morphologic and mechanical study of the healing rabbit medial collateral ligament. *Acta Orthop. Scand.*, **66**, 455–462.

Gao, J. and Messner, K. (1996) Quantitative comparison of soft tissue-bone interface at chondral ligament insertions in the rabbit knee joint. *J. Anat.*, **188**, 367–374.

Gao, J., Messner, K., Ralphs, J.R. and Benjamin, M. (1996a) An immunohistochemical study of the development of the medial collateral ligament of the rat knee joint. *Anat. Embryol.*, **194**, 399–406.

Gao, J., Räsänen, T., Persliden, J. and Messner, K. (1996b) The morphology of ligament insertions after failure at low strain velocity: an evaluation of ligament entheses in the rabbit knee. *J. Anat.*, **189**, 127–133.

Gao, J., Benjamin, M., Banes, A.J., Hill, B., Messner, K. and Ralphs, J.R. (1997) Regional differences in cell shape and gap junction expression in the Achilles tendon relate to fibrocartilage differentiation. *Trans. Orthop. Res. Soc.*, **22**, 449.

Harner, C.D., Kashiwaguchi, S., Livesay, G.A. and Fujie, H. (1993) Insertion site anatomy of the human anterior and posterior cruciate ligaments. *Trans. Orthop. Res. Soc.*, **18**, 341.

Hotta, Y. (1985) Anatomical study of the yellow ligament of spine with special reference to its ossification. *J. Jap. Orthop. Assoc.*, **59**, 311–325.

Ikeda, K., McFarland, E.G., Torpey, B.M., Inoue, N. and Chao, E.Y.S. (1996) Histomorphometric analysis of the deltoid muscle attachment to the acromion. *Trans. Orthop. Res. Soc.*, **21**, 706.

Jackson, D.W., Simon, T.M., Lowery, W. and Gendler, E. (1996) Biologic remodeling after anterior cruciate ligament reconstruction using a collagen matrix derived from demineralized bone. An experimental study in the goat model. *Amer. J. Sports Med.*, **24**, 405–414.

Jones, J.R., Smibert, J.G., McCullough, C.J., Price, A.B. and Hutton, W.C. (1987) Tendon implantation into bone: an experimental study. *J. Hand Surg.*, **12B**, 306–312.

Kang, Y.-K., Kim, I., Kim, J.-M., Woo, Y.-K., Rhee, S.-K., Kim, H.-M., Song, S.-W. and Bahk, W.-J. (1996) The role of fibrocartilage of insertion sites in tendon to bone healing. An experimental study of rabbits. *Trans. Orthop. Res. Soc.*, **21**, 367.

Knese, K.-H. (1979) Stützgewebe und Skelettsystem. In: *Handbuch der mikroskopischen Anatomie des Menschen*, Band 2, Teil 5 (Eds. Möllendorff, W. von, and Bargmann, W.) Springer-Verlag, Berlin.

Knese, K.-H. and Biermann, H. (1958) Die Knochenbildung an Sehnen- und Bandsätzen im Bereich ursprünglich chondraler Apophysen. *Z. Zellforsch*, **49**, 142–187.

Kumagai, J., Sarkar, K. and Uhthoff, H.K. (1994a) The collagen types in the attachment zone of rotator cuff tendons in the elderly: an immunohistochemical study. *J. Rheumatol.*, **21**, 2096–2100.

Kumagai, J., Sarkar, K., Uhthoff, H.K., Okawara, Y. and Ooshima, A. (1994b) Immunohistochemical distribution of type I, II and III collagens in the rabbit supraspinatus tendon insertion. *J. Anat.*, **185**, 279–284.

Lewis, A.R. (1996) The proximal interphalangeal joint of the human finger. *PhD Thesis*. University of Wales.

Liu, S.H., Yang, R.-S., Al-Shaikh, R. and Lane, J.M. (1995) Collagen in tendon, ligament, and bone healing. A current review. *Clin. Orthop. Rel. Res.*, **318**, 265–278.

Liu, S.H., Panossian, V., Al-Shaikh, R. and Yang, R.S. (1996) Immunolocalization of collagen types I, II and III in the rabbit anterior cruciate ligament and patellar tendon insertions. *Trans. Orthop. Res. Soc.*, **21**, 781.

Ma, C.B., Ikeda, K., Inoue, N., McFarland, E.G. and Chao, E.Y.S. (1996) Biomechanical analysis of the effect of loading angle on the failure mechanism of canine patellar tendon-tibia unit. *Trans. Orthop. Res. Soc.*, **21**, 30.

Matyas, J.R., Bodie, D., Andersen, M. and Frank, C.B. (1990) The developmental morphology of a "periosteal" ligament insertion: growth and maturation of the tibial insertion of the rabbit medial collateral ligament. *J. Orthop. Res.*, **8**, 412–424.

Matyas, J.R., Anton, M.G., Shrive, N.G. and Frank, C.B. (1995) Stress governs tissue phenotype at the femoral insertion of the rabbit MCL. *J. Biomechan.*, **28**, 147–157.

Milz, S., McNeilly, C., Ralphs, J.R. and Benjamin, M. (1996) Fibrocartilage in the extensor tendons of the interphalangeal joints of the toes. *Ann. Anat. Suppl.*, **178**, 28–29.

Muhl, Z.F. and Gedak, G.K. (1986) The influence of periosteum on tendon and ligament migration. *J. Anat.*, **145**, 161–171.

Niepel, G.A. and Sitaj, S. (1979) Enthesopathy. *Clin. Rheum. Dis.*, **5**, 857–872.

Nishijima, N., Yamamuro, T. and Ueba, Y. (1994) Flexor tendon growth in chickens. *J. Orthop. Res.*, **12**, 576–581.

Niyibizi, C., Visconti, C.S., Kavalkovich, K. and Woo, S.L.Y. (1995) Collagens in an adult bovine medial collateral ligament: Immunofluorescence localization by confocal microscopy reveals that type XIV collagen predominates at the ligament-bone junction. *Matrix Biol.*, **14**, 743–751.

Niyibizi, C., Visconti, C.S., Gibson, G. and Kavalkovich, K. (1996) Identification and immunolocalization of type X collagen at the ligament-bone interface. *Biochem. Biophys. Res. Commun.*, **222**, 584–589.

Petersen, H. (1930) Die Organe des Skeletsystems. Handbuch der mikroskopischen Anatomie des Menschen. Band 2, Teil 2 (Eds. von Möllendorff, W. and Bargmann, W.)

Ralphs, J.R. and Benjamin, M. (1997) Cell and matrix organisation in tendons and ligaments. In: *Biology of the Synovial Joint* (Eds. Archer, C.W., Benjamin, M., Caterson, B. and Ralphs, J.R.). Harwood Academic Press.

Ralphs, J.R., Benjamin, M. and Thornett, A. (1991) Cell and matrix biology of the suprapatella in the rat: a structural and immunocytochemical study of fibrocartilage in a tendon subject to compression. *Anat. Rec.*, **231**, 167–177.

Ralphs, J.R., Tyers, R.N.S. and Benjamin, M. (1992) Development of functionally distinct fibrocartilages at two sites in the quadriceps tendon of the rat: the suprapatella and the attachment of the tendon to the patella. *Anat. Embryol.*, **185**, 181–187.

Resnick, D. and Niwayama, G. (1983) Entheses and enthesopathy. *Radiology*, **146**, 1–9.

Rothwell, A.G. and Bentley, G. (1973) Chondrocyte multiplication in osteoarthritic articular cartilage. *J. Bone Joint Surg.*, **55B**, 588–594.

Rufai, A., Benjamin, M. and Ralphs, J.R. (1992) Development and ageing of phenotypically distinct fibrocartilages associated with the rat Achilles tendon. *Anat. Embryol.*, **186**, 611–618.

Rufai, A., Ralphs, J.R. and Benjamin, M. (1995) The structure and histopathology of the insertional region of the human Achilles tendon. *J. Orthop. Res.*, **13**, 585–593.

Rufai, A., Ralphs, J.R. and Benjamin, M. (1996) The ultrastructure of fibrocartilages associated with the insertion of the Achilles tendon of the rat. *J. Anat.*, **189**, 185–191.

Schiavone Panni, A., Fabbriciani, C., Delcogliano, C. and Franzese, S. (1993a) Bone–ligament interaction in patellar tendon reconstruction of the ACL. *Knee Surg. Sports Traumatol. Arthrosc.*, **1**, 4–8.

Schiavone Panni, A., Denti, M., Franzese, S. and Monteleone, M. (1993b) The bone–ligament junction: a comparison between biological and artificial ACL reconstruction. *Knee Surg. Sports Traumatol. Arthros.*, **1**, 9–12.

Schneider, H. (1956) Zur Struktur der Sehnenansatzzonen. *Z. Anat. Entwickl. Gesch.*, **119**, 431–456.

Videman, T. (1970) An experimental study of the effects of growth on the relationship of tendons and ligaments to bone at the site of diaphyseal insertion. *Ann. Chir. Gynaecol.*, **59**, 22–34.

Visconti, C.S., Kavalkovich, K., Wu, J.-J. and Niyibizi, C. (1996) Biochemical analysis of collagens at the ligament-bone interface reveals presence of cartilage-specific collagens. *Arch. Biochem. Biophys.*, **328**, 135–142.

Waggett, A.D., Kwan, A.P.L., Woodnutt, D., Ralphs, J.R. and Benjamin, M. (1997) Characterisation of collagens and proteoglycans at the insertion of the human Achilles tendon. (In preparation)

Waggy, C.A., Blaha, J.D., Labosky, D.A., Beresford, W.A., Clovis, N.B. and Smith, E.S. (1994) Healing of tendon insertion site in rabbits: a model of the effect of partial disruption. *Trans. Orthop. Res. Soc.*, **19**, 39.

Wei, X. and Messner, K. (1995) The postnatal development of the insertions of the medial collateral ligament in the rat knee. *Anat. Embryol.*, **193**, 53–59.

Weiss, J.A., Beck, C.L. and Greenwald, R.M. (1995) Microvasculature of the normal and healing medial collateral ligament. *Trans. Orthop. Res. Soc.*, **20**, 162.

Woo, S., Maynard, J., Butler, D., Lyon, R., Torzilli, P., Akeson, W., Cooper, R. and Oakes, B. (1988) Ligament, tendon, and joint capsule insertions to bone. In: *Injury and repair of the musculoskeletal soft tissues* (Eds. Woo, S.L.-Y. and Buckwalter, J.A.), pp. 133–166. Park Ridge, American Academy of Orthopaedic Surgeons.

24　Principles of Joint Biomechanics

J.J. O'Connor*, T.-W. Lu, A. Leardini, D.R. Wilson,
J. Feikes, H.S. Gill and A.B. Zavatsky

University of Oxford, Parks Road, Oxford, OX1 3PJ, UK

INTRODUCTION

The interest of the authors of most of the chapters of this book in the biology of the synovial joint stems from the need to understand various forms of joint disease. Osteoarthritis is very common. It is usual to assume that mechanical factors play some role but that role has not been defined unequivocally. To motivate the biologist to read a chapter called "principles of joint biomechanics", we will start by describing anteromedial gonarthrosis. Having then dealt with the subject matter of the chapter, we will describe in detail the mechanical circumstances which may contribute to the aetiology of anteromedial gonarthrosis, a consistent localised lesion on the anterior tibial plateau and the distal femoral condyle of the medial compartment of the knee.

ANTEROMEDIAL GONARTHROSIS

White *et al.* (1991) described the appearance of a group of medial tibial plateaux removed during medial compartment arthroplasty for arthrosis. They found that the lesion was confined to the anterior portion of the plateau in all cases, with full thickness loss of cartilage and some erosion of the underlying bone. A similar kissing lesion was found on the distal medial femoral condyle. The cartilage on the posterior tibial plateau and posterior femoral condyle of the medial compartment and that of the lateral compartment and patellofemoral joint remained full thickness, although there was occasionally some local fibrillation. All the ligaments of the joint remained intact, the varus deformity and flexion

*Corresponding author. University of Oxford, Department of Engineering Science and Oxford Orthopaedic Engineering Centre at the Nuffield Orthopaedic Centre, Oxford OX3 7LD. E-mail: john.oconnor@eng.ox.ac.uk.

deformity were both limited to less than 10°. The varus deformity was correctable but not overcorrectable under an abducting load. At this stage, unicompartmental replacement can hold back the progression of the disease with pain-free function in over 90% of patients at 10 years and no need for further surgery in over 97% of patients at 10 years (Murray *et al.*, 1997). Medial arthrosis may be twenty times more common than lateral.

The questions arise: why is the lesion most often found medially? Why on the anterior tibial plateau and the distal femoral condyle? Why do the lesions not progress to other parts of the joint? In particular, what are the mechanical circumstances of those areas of the knee joint? We will return to these questions at the end of the chapter.

MOBILITY AND STABILITY OF JOINTS

The joints give the skeleton its mobility. Although the joints of the lower limb all have surfaces covered with articular cartilage which hold the bones apart and ligaments which hold the bones together, their ranges of motion differ widely. The hip allows a wide range of unresisted multi-axial motion, about 150° of flexion/extension, about 80° of abduction/adduction and 100° of axial rotation (Kpandji, 1970). Passive displacement of the bones from one position to another within that range is not resisted by the tissues of the joint. The knee and the ankle allow a more restricted range of motion while movement at the sub-talar and some of the more distal joints of the foot is more limited still. These differences in mobility arise not because of differences in the mechanical properties of the tissues but because of differences in the geometry of the articular surfaces and differences in the geometric arrangements of the ligaments and capsule.

As well as allowing mobility, the joints also have to transmit load. In the presence of external loads due mainly to gravity, muscle forces are required to stabilise the skeleton by suppressing movement at the joints. During activity, muscle forces also initiate and maintain movement and can, when required, achieve precise control of limb position and velocity. The passive structures of each of the joints contribute to load transfer and joint stabilisation through the transmission of compressive stress between the articular surfaces and the transmission of the tensile stress along the fibres of the ligaments and capsules.

It has been known for centuries that it is the levels of force transmitted by the muscles which determine the loading of bones and joints. Borelli (1679) performed extensive experiments with post-mortem specimens and demonstrated that the forces transmitted by muscle tendons as they span the joints can be much larger than the loads applied by hanging weights on the ends of the limbs. He explained these results using the principle of the lever:

$$M \cdot r = W \cdot \ell \tag{1}$$

or

$$M = W \cdot \ell / r. \tag{2}$$

The muscle force M balances a load W. As equation 2 suggests, the muscle force may be many times larger than the applied load because its lever arm r may be only a fraction of the length of the lever arm ℓ of the load and ℓ/r may be much greater than unity.

Figure 24.1a shows a much simplified diagram of the lower limb during single leg stance when the ground reaction vector W balances the weight of the body and passes medial to the hip joint through the centre of gravity of the body. Equilibrium at the hip is achieved because of tension M in the hip abductors. The lever arm available to the external load at the hip in these circumstances is about three times that available to the muscle tendon so that the muscle force is about three times the external load, three times body weight. Figure 24.1b shows an elementary triangle of forces which determines the value

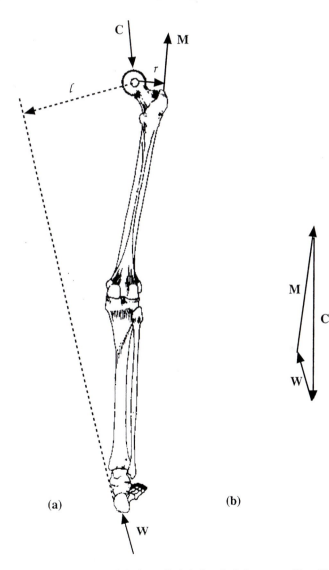

FIGURE 24.1   (a) Free body diagram of the lower limb during single leg stance. The adducting moment due to the ground reaction force W supporting the weight of the body is balanced by tension M in the hip abductors and by the hip contact force C. (b) The triangle of forces relating the values of the three forces in (a).

of the contact force C at the hip required to balance the combined upthrusts due to ground reaction vector and the muscle tendon force. The hip contact force is about four times the value of the external load, four times body weight. The contact forces transmitted by the joints can therefore be large because the muscle forces are large and the muscle forces are large because of the imbalance of lever arm lengths.

This very simple analysis explains in general terms the large levels of hip contact forces calculated by Paul (1965) and measured with instrumented prostheses by Rydell (1966), English and Kilvington (1979), Davy *et al.* (1988) and Bergmann *et al.* (1993). Similar measurements (Taylor and Donaldson, 1990; Taylor *et al.*, 1997) of the axial force in the shaft of a massive proximal femoral prosthesis show that equally large forces are transmitted along the shafts of the bones. Analysis of the results of these experiments (Lu *et al.*, 1996, 1997) has vindicated Pauwels's arguments that bi-articular muscles, acting as tension bands, play an important role in the transmission of bending moment along the limbs (Pauwels, 1950). Pauwels used simple bending theory to demonstrate that the action of bi-articular muscles can have profound effects on the distribution of stress within the bones.

The simple lever equations (1) and (2) have been displayed to emphasise the point that the geometric factors which control the lengths of the lever arms of the muscle tendons at the joints are prime determinants of the levels of force transmitted by the muscles and therefore, according to Pauwels, of the distributions of stress in the bones. The values of W, ℓ and r in equations (1) and (2) all vary during activity. The values of W and ℓ can be measured in the gait laboratory. The lengths of the muscle lever-arms are determined by the positions of their tendons relative to the articular surfaces and ligaments of the joints, so that understanding the kinematics, the changing geometry, of joints is key to understanding load transmission through the musculoskeletal system. It is instructive to distinguish between those features of joint behaviour which control mobility and those which contribute to stability and load transfer. It will be shown that the features which control mobility can be deduced mainly from geometric analysis while the study of stability and load transfer obviously also requires mechanics. In the following, the knee joint will be used as a paradigm. The geometry and mechanics of the joint will be explained through computer-based mathematical models.

MOBILITY OF THE KNEE

THE TIBIOFEMORAL JOINT

The human knee joint is not a simple hinge, with an axis of rotation fixed relative to both the femur and the tibia. Weber and Weber (1836) first described how the femur rolls backwards on the tibia during flexion and forwards during extension. Strasser (1917) explained these movements by describing the knee as a mechanism, the femur, the tibia and the two cruciate ligaments forming a four-bar linkage. Kapandji (1970), Menschik (1974) and Huson (1974) developed the model further and Goodfellow and O'Connor (1978) used it to explain the movements of the meniscal bearings in their knee prosthesis.

The computer-drawn mathematical model of the knee in the sagittal plane shown in Figure 24.2 demonstrates the action of the linkage. The lines *AB* and *CD* represent fibres within the anterior and posterior cruciate ligaments which remain isometric during passive flexion. As the joint flexes, the ACL fibre *AB* rotates isometrically towards the tibial plateau about its tibial insertion *A* while the PCL fibre *CD* rotates isometrically away from the tibial plateau about its tibial insertion *D*. The femoral origins of the two fibres rotate on circular arcs about their tibial insertions.

This simple model shows why the passive movement of flexion/extension of the bones upon each other is not resisted. The ligament fibres rotate but do not stretch and the articular surfaces slide upon each other but do not indent so that movement can be accomplished without tissue deformation. The simple four-bar linkage is therefore a model of unresisted passive flexion–extension.

An important feature of the linkage is that its instant centre (*I*) lies at the point at which the two cruciate fibres cross (O'Connor *et al.*, 1989). The model femur flexes and extends about an axis passing through the instant centre. Because the geometry of the linkage changes, the instant centre moves backwards during flexion and forwards during extension.

A second feature of the linkage is that the normal to the articular surfaces at their point of contact must pass through the instant centre (O'Connor *et al.*, 1989). This is necessary to avoid separation or interpenetration of the surfaces and stretching or slackening of the ligament fibres. To satisfy this condition, the contact point moves from the front of the tibial plateau in extension (X_1, Figure 24.2a) to the back in flexion (X_3, Figure 24.2c) so that the model femur rolls backwards on the tibia during flexion and forwards during extension. The model both reproduces and explains the observations of Weber and

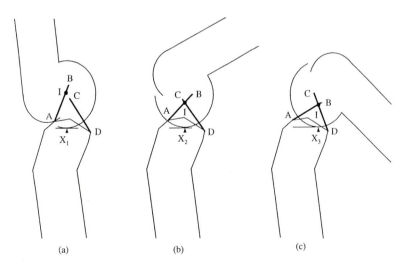

(a)   (b)   (c)

FIGURE 24.2   Computer drawn model of the knee joint. The linkage formed by the femur, the tibia, the anterior cruciate ligament *AB* and the posterior cruciate ligament *CD* control the movements of the bones upon each other. The instant centre of the linkage, *I*, lies at the intersection of the ligaments and moves backwards during flexion. As a consequence, the contact point between the femur and the tibia moves backwards from X_1 in extension (a) to X_3 in flexion (c).

Weber, 1836. The common normal theorem allows the calculation of surface shapes and a movement path compatible with an absence of tissue deformation. The coupling between flexion and rolling is characteristic of a single degree of freedom system in which specification of the value of one quantity – flexion angle – completely determines the relative positions of the bones.

THE PATELLOFEMORAL JOINT

The model in Figure 24.2 shows a discontinuity between the anterior facet of the femur which makes contact with the patella and the distal facet which makes contact with the tibia. This discontinuity is based on the observation (Elias *et al.*, 1990; O'Connor *et al.*, 1989) that the femoral surfaces which guide the patella and those which guide the tibia over the femur are both circular in the sagittal plane but have different centres. Figure 24.3 shows the model knee with the addition of the flexor muscles and the extensor mechanism, including the patella (Gill and O'Connor, 1996a).

The muscles and their tendons are represented as straight lines. Figure 24.3 shows how the muscle tendons rotate about their points of origin and insertion on the bones during movement. It shows that the patellofemoral contact point moves from the distal pole of the patella in extension, Y_1 towards the proximal pole in flexion, Y_2, Y_3. The patella, therefore, rolls as well as slides upon the femur. The rolling movement is necessary because, with no friction, the patellofemoral contact force must lie on the perpendicular to the two articular surfaces at their point of contact and must pass through the point of intersection of the two tendons (Gill and O'Connor, 1996a).* As the joint flexes, the point of intersection of the two tendons moves proximally and the point of contact between the patella and the femur has to follow.

Figure 24.3 also demonstrates how the patellofemoral contact point moves from the trochlea, Figure 24.3a,b, onto the condyles of the femur in the highly flexed joint, Figure 24.3c. Dye exclusion studies showed that the contact area on the human patella moves proximally during flexion, and separates into medial and lateral areas as the patella passes off the trochlea onto the condyles (Goodfellow *et al.*, 1976). Miller *et al.* (1997) confirmed these patterns of contact using a different experimental technique.

STRAIN PATTERNS IN THE LIGAMENTS

The cruciate ligaments of the human knee do not consist each of a single fibre, as in the models in Figure 24.2 and 24.3. Figure 24.4 shows the same model but with the cruciate ligaments represented in a more lifelike way as continuous arrays of fibres (Lu and O'Connor, 1996a; Wilson *et al.*, 1996). Tight fibres are shown straight, slack fibres are shown buckled. The anterior fibre of the ACL and the central fibre of the PCL are the fibres in Figures 24.2 and 24.3 which remain isometric, staying just tight over the whole range of flexion of the unloaded joint. The reference lengths of the fibres in each ligament have to be defined in some position of the joint. All the fibres of the ACL and the posterior fibres of the PCL are just tight in extension where they are more or less parallel. The anterior fibres of the PCL are slack in extension but just tight at 120°.

---

* The concurrence of the tendons and patellofemoral normal, necessary for equilibrium of the patella, is the only contribution of mechanics to the formulation of the geometric model.

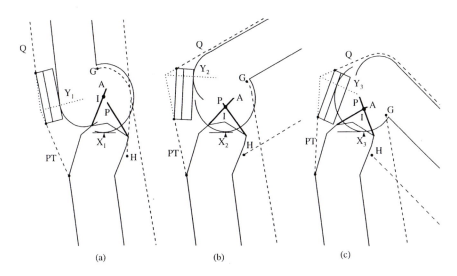

FIGURE 24.3 The knee model with lines representing the extensor and flexor muscles. The patellar tendon *PT* and the quadriceps tendon *Q* are connected to the proximal and distal poles of the patella which makes contact with the anterior femur at Y_1 in extension (a) and Y_3 in flexion (c). Contact on the patella occurs on the more posterior articular surface, representing the median ridge, near extension (a, b) and on the more anterior articular surface, representing the medial and lateral facets of the patella, in flexion (c). The quadriceps tendon wraps around the anterior femur in flexion (c). The gastrocnemius muscles arise at *G* on the posterior femur. They wrap around the femoral condyle near extension (a, b). They insert into the Achilles tendon, not shown. The hamstrings insert at *H*. They wrap around the posterior femoral condyle near extension (a). The lines *A* and *P* represent the anterior and posterior cruciate ligaments, the instant centre of the knee linkage lies at *I*.

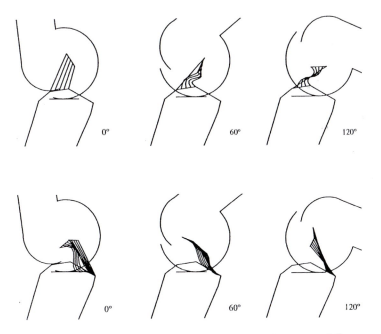

FIGURE 24.4 The anterior and posterior cruciate ligaments represented as arrays of fibres connecting the model femur to the model tibia. Tight fibres are shown straight, slack fibres buckled. Fibres slacken and tighten as their attachment areas on the two bones rotate relative to each other during extension and flexion.

As their attachment areas rotate relative to each other during flexion and extension, the apparent shapes of the ligaments change as fibres in both ligaments cross and uncross. The changes in apparent shapes of the ligaments are consistent with observations reported by Girgis *et al.* (1975) and Friederich *et al.* (1992). In the human knee, ligaments twist as well as bend because their attachment areas are not parallel to the axis of rotation of the joint, the axis having components parallel as well as perpendicular to the ligaments (Zavatsky and O'Connor, 1994).

As the joint flexes, all fibres slacken and buckle while they lie behind the instant centre and tighten again and straighten while they come to lie in front of the instant centre; vice versa during extension. Similar patterns of slackening and tightening of individual fibres have also been demonstrated in models of the collateral ligaments (Lu and O'Connor, 1996a), Figure 24.5. The patterns of fibre length change predicted by the model agree well (Zavatsky and O'Connor, 1992a) with those observed by Fuss (1989) and Sapega *et al.* (1990). The changes in direction of the model ligament fibres agree well (Lu and O'Connor, 1996b) with the measurements of Herzog and Read (1993). The changes in strain distributions within the ligaments are compatible with the movements of the bones on each other.

The diagrams in Figures 24.4 and 24.5 demonstrate that specification of the ligament architecture and fibre lengths in one position allows calculation of the strains (mainly negative) in the fibres in the unloaded state in any other position, providing a starting point for mechanical analysis.

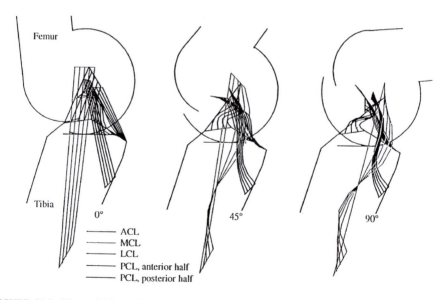

FIGURE 24.5   The model knee with arrays of fibres representing the anterior cruciate and posterior cruciate ligaments and the medial and lateral collateral ligaments. The patterns of fibres slackening and tightening during the extension and flexion in all ligaments are compatible with each other and are determined by the relative movements of their attachment areas.

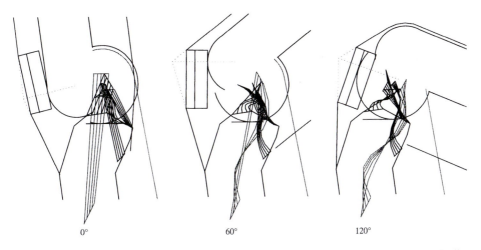

FIGURE 24.6   The model knee during passive flexion and extension with fibre arrays representing the ligaments and straight lines and circles representing the muscles.

THE COMPLETE TWO-DIMENSIONAL MODEL

Figure 24.6 shows the model with ligament arrays and muscle tendons, illustrating the simultaneous related changes in the geometry of bone contacts, ligament shapes and muscle tendon directions which occur during passive flexion. This model has been constructed on purely geometric principles and serves as the starting point for subsequent mechanical analysis. As a single degree of freedom system, specification of the flexion angle completely determines the configurations of the bones, the ligaments and the muscle tendons in the unloaded state. These configurations change when load is applied and tissues deform.

STABILITY OF THE KNEE

By *stability,* we mean the resistance that a joint offers to movement. *Passive stability* is provided by mechanical interactions between the articular surfaces and the ligaments and is measured by such clinical tests as the Lachman or Drawer tests. *Active stability* is provided by the added effects of myogenic forces when muscles are used to suppress or control movement at the joint in the presence of external loads.

PASSIVE STABILITY

PASSIVE RESISTANCE TO ANTERO-POSTERIOR TRANSLATION

The model joint can be used (Figure 24.7) to simulate the Lachman Test (Lu and O'Connor, 1996a; Zavatsky and O'Connor, 1992a). In Figures 24.7a and 24.7d, the ACL

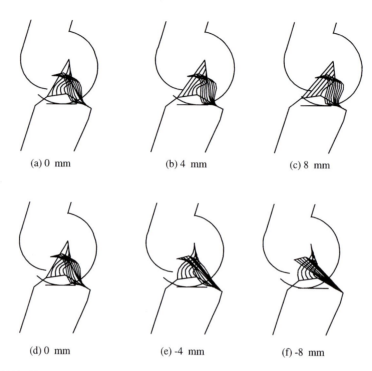

(a) 0 mm   (b) 4 mm   (c) 8 mm

(d) 0 mm   (e) -4 mm   (f) -8 mm

FIGURE 24.7   The model knee at 25° during the anterior (a, b, c) and posterior (d, e, f) translation of the tibia relative to the femur. During anterior translation (a, b, c), fibres in the anterior cruciate ligament are progressively tightened and recruited to bear load while fibres in the posterior cruciate ligament slacken. The reverse is true during posterior translation (d, e, f).

and PCL are shown in the unloaded state (0 mm) at 25° flexion, similar to Figure 24.4. The anterior fibre of the ACL and the central fibre of the PCL are just tight and are shown straight; all other fibres are slack and are shown buckled. When the tibia is pulled forwards 4 and then 8 mm, Figures 24.7b and c, the fibres of the ACL straighten and tighten progressively as they are recruited to bear load. There is a similar progressive tightening and recruitment of the fibres of the PCL when the tibia is moved backwards (4 and 8 mm) from its position in the unloaded state, Figures 24.7e and f. As one ligament tightens, the other slackens.

Figure 24.8 shows similar diagrams but with the collateral ligaments included. It demonstrates how the ACL and MCL tighten together to resist anterior translation of the tibia while the PCL and LCL share resistance to posterior translation. The developing patterns of strain in the pairs of ligaments are compatible with shared translations of their attachment areas relative to each other. The contributions of the various ligaments to the passive stability of the knee has been the subject of a considerable body of often contradictory experimental work, recently summarised by Shoemaker and Daniel (1990).

The diagrams in Figures 24.7 and 24.8 are based on purely geometric analysis. Having determined the distributions of strains within the ligaments for a specified translation of the tibia from geometry, mechanics is needed to determine the values of the external

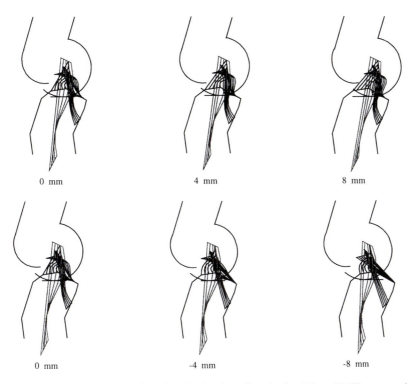

0 mm   4 mm   8 mm

0 mm   -4 mm   -8 mm

FIGURE 24.8   The model knee at 25° flexion showing how fibres in the ACL and MCL are recruited during anterior translation (4, 8 mm) and fibres of the PCL and LCL are recruited during posterior translation
(−4, −8 mm) of the tibia relative to the femur.

forces required to produce that translation. With the patterns of strain within the ligaments defined, constitutive equations can be used to calculate distributions of stress
within the ligaments and then ligament forces (Zavatsky and O'Connor, 1992b; Zavatsky
and O'Connor, 1993). The external forces which have to be applied to balance the ligament and contact forces resulting from any assumed tibial translation can then be calculated. In Figure 24.9, the horizontal force applied to the tibia is plotted against the
horizontal displacement of the tibia at five angles of flexion. These antero-posterior laxity
curves, calculated from the model, are similar in shape to those obtained experimentally
by Markolf et al. (1976).

The curves demonstrate that there is little resistance to the first 2 mm of antero-posterior
movements of the tibia in either direction but resistance increases rapidly as more fibres
within the ligaments tighten and are recruited to bear load (Figures 24.7 and 24.8).

The relationships between applied force and tibial displacement in Figure 24.9 are non-
linear because (Zavatsky and O'Connor, 1992b, 1993) the relationship between tibial displacement and fibre length is non-linear (the cosine rule), and because the relationship
between fibre strain and fibre stress is non-linear but mainly because the effective cross-
sectional area of a ligament increases as more fibres are recruited to bear load, Figures 24.7
and 24.8. The relationships between the tension and compressive forces vary over the

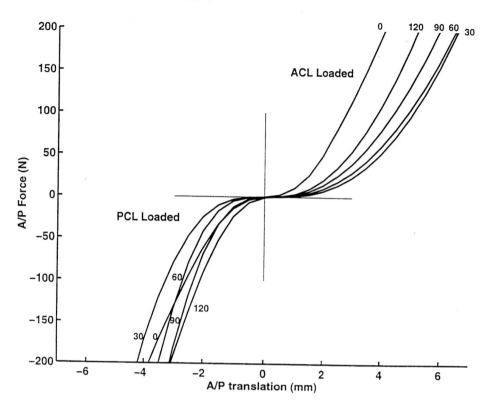

FIGURE 24.9   Calculated values of the anterior or posterior forces needed to translate the tibia relative to the femur at five different flexion angles.

range of flexion because the directions of the ligaments alter. These changes in the directions of the ligaments as well as the altering slackness of their fibres in various positions account for the differences in the force – displacement laxity curves in Figure 24.9 at different flexion angles.

When tension forces are developed in the ligaments, they force the articular surfaces against each other, loading the cartilage in compression. If the consequent indentation of the articular surfaces is also taken into account, the joint is more compliant and a preliminary analysis suggests that the force required to achieve any given antero-posterior displacement is reduced by about 20% compared to Figure 24.9.

Figures 24.7, 24.8 and 24.9 account for resisted deviations from the unloaded neutral track in the sagittal plane.

ACTIVE STABILITY

The passive structures of the knee (the ligaments, capsule, menisci and articular surfaces) suppress most of the possible six degrees of freedom of the tibia relative to the femur, confining the movement to a relatively narrow range of flexion from 0° to 140° with a small range of axial rotation and an even smaller range of abduction/adduction. To be able to stand vertically in the presence of gravity requires muscle forces, to suppress the remaining freedoms of movement at the joints. Additionally, muscles are used to initiate and maintain movement.

LEVER ARMS LENGTHS

As the knee moves, the lever arms of its muscles vary in length. Figure 24.3 illustrates how the tendons rotate about their origins and insertions during flexion and extension. At the same time, the flexion axis of the joint, the instant centre in Figures 24.2 and 24.3, moves backwards and forwards relative to the tibia. The lever arms of the muscles, the perpendicular distances from the instant centre to the tendons, therefore vary during flexion. Figure 24.10 shows the lengths of the lever arms of the patellar, hamstrings and gastrocnemius tendons plotted against flexion angle of the knee (O'Connor et al., 1990a; O'Connor, 1993). They were calculated from the geometry of the model in Figure 24.3.

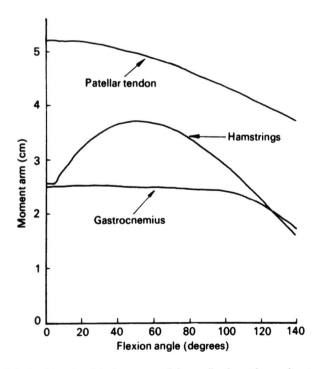

FIGURE 24.10   Calculated lengths of the lever arms of the patellar, hamstrings and gastrocnemius tendons, plotted against flexion angle. The lever arm length is the distance from the instant centre I to each of the muscle tendons in Figure 24.3.

MUSCLE FORCES

Figures 24.11a and b show the arrangements of experiments on the human knee, similar to those performed by Borelli (1679). The femur was held at 45° to the horizontal and a weight hung on the end of the tibia was balanced by tension in a wire sewn either to the quadriceps (Figure 24.11a) or the hamstrings tendons (Figure 24.11b) (O'Connor *et al.*, 1990c). The length of the wire was adjusted to hold the tibia stationary at different flexion angles and the force in the wire necessary to suppress movement was measured in each position.

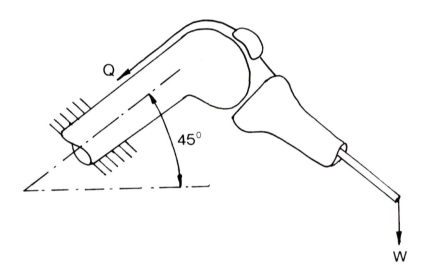

FIGURE 24.11a

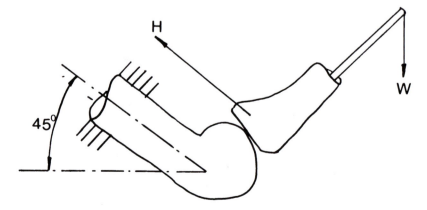

FIGURE 24.11b

Figures 24.11c and d show the measured tendon forces divided by the applied weight and plotted against flexion angle. The points represent the measurements for different applied loads on a single specimen and the solid lines represent calculations from the computer model in Figure 24.3 using model parameters derived from the same specimen (O'Connor *et al.*, 1990b,c). These results reflect the changes in the lengths of the lever arms both of the external loads and of the muscle tendons over the flexion range. The quadriceps force up to 16 times the applied load (Figure 24.11c) and the hamstrings force up to 12 times the applied load (Figure 24.11d) demonstrate that the levels of muscle force needed to suppress movement at the joints can be much larger than the external loads. The similarity of the measurements and calculations validate the mathematical model and the calculated muscle lever-arm lengths (Figure 24.10). The large muscle forces give rise to even larger tibio-femoral contact forces.

The sharp rise in the measured and calculated quadriceps force and the sharp fall in the measured and calculated hamstrings force as extension is approached occur because of

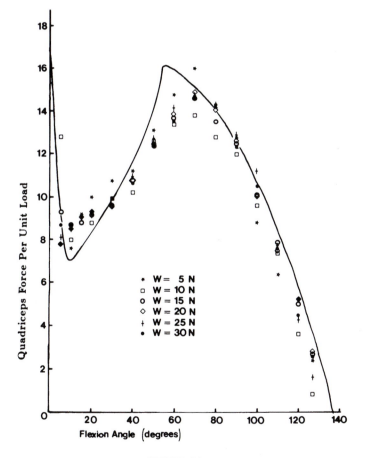

FIGURE 24.11c

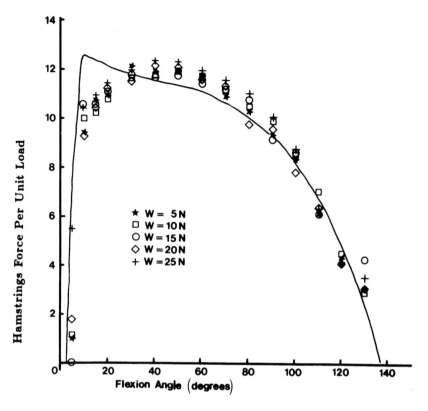

FIGURE 24.11d

FIGURE 24.11   Experiments in which weight W hung from the end of the tibia is balanced by tension force in the (a) quadriceps and (b) hamstrings tendons. The measured forces per unit applied load in the (c) quadriceps tendon, Q/W, and (d) in the hamstrings tendons, H/W, are plotted against flexion angle. The solid line was calculated from the geometry of the knee model, Figure 24.3, and the lever arm lengths, Figure 24.10. Near extension, a simulated posterior capsule (not shown in Figure 24.3) tightens, the quadriceps force increases (c) and the hamstrings forces decrease (d) as extension is approached.

the tightening of the posterior capsule (O'Connor *et al.*, 1990b,c). The capsule is slack when the knee is flexed beyond 15° and tightens progressively as extension is approached, adding another link to the knee mechanism, removing its single degree of freedom and converting it into a structure. Movement into hyper-extension can be accomplished only by deforming the tissues.

LIGAMENT FORCES

Forces in muscle tendons can be measured more easily than forces in the ligaments *in vitro*. Although buckle transducers have been used to measure ligament forces (Lewis *et al.*, 1982), they must necessarily disturb the patterns of fibre crossing and twisting suggested by Figures 24.4–24.6 and the patterns of fibre recruitment suggested by Figures 24.7 and 24.8. To evaluate ligament forces, it is generally necessary to resort to calculation. Morrison (1968) studied the gait of three subjects in the laboratory and used a mathematical model to calculate the forces transmitted by the ligaments. He found that the anterior cruciate ligament and the posterior cruciate ligament are each loaded at different phases of the gait cycle, as are the two collateral ligaments.

Figures 24.3 show that the tendons do not pass vertically across the knee joint cleft but are usually inclined to the tibial plateau. The forces they exert have components parallel to the tibial plateau. The primary function of a muscle is to balance the flexing or extending effect of an applied load and it is this requirement which mainly determines the magnitude of the muscle force. Any resultant of the muscle force and the load parallel to the tibial plateau is balanced by the ligaments. When the resultant tends to pull the tibia forwards, the ACL is loaded. When the resultant tends to pull the tibia backwards, the PCL is loaded. The collateral ligaments share these loads, Figure 24.8.

Some features of the complementary actions of the two cruciate ligaments can be demonstrated during a simulation of isometric quadriceps exercises, when the quadriceps act against a resisting force applied perpendicular to the tibia (Zavatsky and O'Connor, 1993). The ACL is loaded when the joint is flexed less than about 80° with the resistance placed distally on the tibia. The PCL is loaded when the joint is flexed more than 80° or when the resistance is placed proximally on the tibia. In Figure 24.12, the distance of the resistance from the tibial plateau is plotted against flexion angle. The curve defines the combination of resistance placement and flexion angle at which neither the ACL or

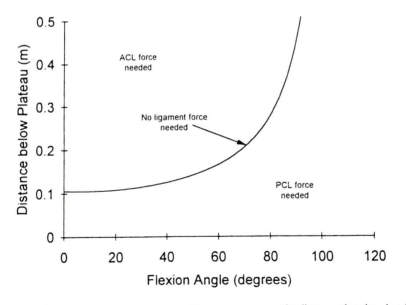

FIGURE 24.12   Isometric quadriceps contraction. The curve represents the distance, plotted against flexion angle, below the tibial plateau at which a resisting force can be balanced by quadriceps action without loading the ligaments. Below 90° of flexion, more distal placement of the resistance loads the anterior cruciate ligament. More proximal placement loads the posterior cruciate ligament.

the PCL is loaded. In these circumstances, the forward pull of the patellar tendon force is exactly balanced by the backwards thrust of the resisting force. If the resistance is placed more distally, the quadriceps force is larger than the resisting load. Near extension, the patella tendon pulls the tibia forwards (Figure 24.3a), loading the ACL. In the highly flexed joint, the patellar tendon pulls the tibia backwards (Figure 24.3c), loading the PCL. For more proximal placement of the resistance, the quadriceps force is relatively small and the PCL is loaded by the backwards thrust of the resisting force.

Figure 24.12 implies that ligament loading depends on the line of action of the external forces and on the values of the muscle forces, which in turn depend on the lengths of the lever-arms of the muscle tendons.

COMMENT

The results in Figure 24.12 show that evaluation of the forces transmitted by ligaments in activity requires prior knowledge of the directions of the muscle tendons and ligaments, obtained from a geometric model. They were calculated assuming the ligaments to be inextensible. When account is taken of tissue deformation, Figures 24.7–24.9, incremental loading must be considered, requiring iterative numerical solution of the non-linear equations at each increment (Zavatsky and O'Connor, 1993), with sequential geometrical and mechanical analysis during each iteration. The muscle, ligament and contact forces are then no longer proportional to the external load, as assumed for the calculated curves in Figures 24.11c and 24.11d.

CORONAL AND TRANSVERSE PLANES

EXPERIMENTAL

Although analysis of the behaviour of the knee joint in the sagittal plane has been instructive, it cannot account for events in the coronal plane and the effects of axial rotations.

Figure 24.13a shows curves of internal tibial rotation and abduction/adduction plotted against flexion angle for a knee specimen which was flexed and extended repeatedly under very small loads (the weight of about 15 cm of distal femur, about 5 N) (Wilson et al., 1993, 1996; Wilson, 1996). The curves demonstrate that, when unloaded, the bones followed a single unique track, the neutral track of passive flexion. Displacement of the bones along the track was not resisted. There was no elastic spring-back.

The curves also demonstrate that, in the unloaded state, axial rotation and abduction/adduction are uniquely coupled to flexion and the unloaded knee has a single degree of unresisted freedom. Meyer (1853) described the coupling of axial rotation to flexion, commonly called the "screw home mechanism".

Figure 24.13b shows the results of a similar experiment (Wilson et al., 1993, 1996; Wilson 1996). At three positions, the flexion movement of the specimen was stopped, the tibia was displaced from its position in the unloaded state and was then released.

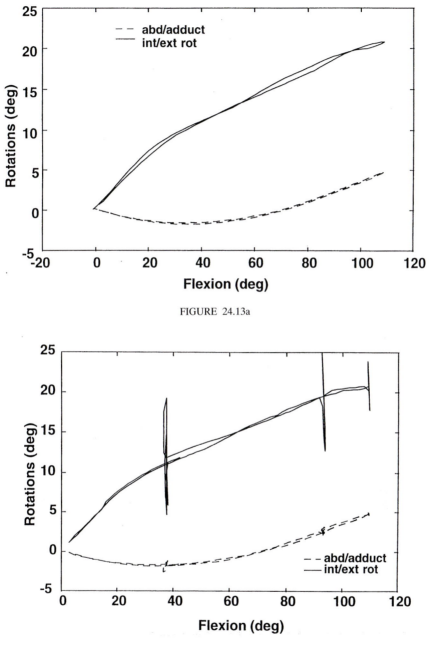

FIGURE 24.13a

FIGURE 24.13b

FIGURE 24.13   (a) Internal/external rotation and abduction/adduction plotted against flexion angle when an unloaded specimen is taken over its flexion range. The neutral paths traced out during extension and flexion are virtually identical. (b) Deviations from the neutral tracks of (a) induced by applying load are completely recovered, with elastic spring-back, when the load is removed.

It can be seen that the tibia could be rotated or abducted by the application of external load but, when that load was removed, it returned to its original track (elastic spring-back).

The experiment is a demonstration of the fact that the femur and the tibia follow a unique track relative to each other over the range of movement only in the unloaded state and that the unloaded human knee is a single degree of freedom system. Displacement of the bones from one position to another along that track is not resisted. Deviation from that track is resisted, requiring the application of external force and deformation of the tissues. The deviation is almost completely recovered when the applied force is quickly removed. Each combination of loads results in its own track.

THEORETICAL

Although many of their geometric predictions agree well with experiment, the models in Figures 24.2–24.5 are all two-dimensional. We have begun development of a 3-dimensional analogue of the four-bar linkage, a parallel spatial mechanism like an aircraft cockpit simulator (Wilson et al., 1993, 1996; Wilson, 1996). In this model, three lines represent isometric fibres in the ACL, PCL and MCL, holding together two pairs of articular surfaces to represent the medial and lateral compartments. A diagram of the mechanism is shown in Figure 24.14a. The five constraints represented by three ligaments and two pairs of surfaces in contact reduce the number of degrees of freedom of the mechanism to unity, coupling axial rotation and abduction/adduction to flexion. The kinematics of the mechanism were analysed (Wilson et al., 1993; Wilson 1996) using the method devised by Uicker et al. (1964). The analysis finds the path of unresisted motion which satisfies the geometric constraints that the ligament fibres do not stretch or slacken and that the articular surfaces do not separate or interpenetrate. When it is flexed and extended, the model exhibits the obligatory tibial rotation which is observed in the human knee

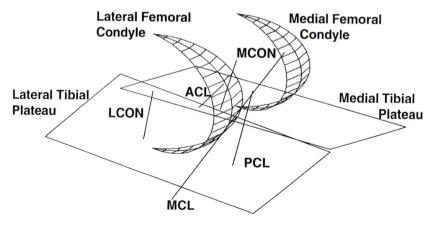

FIGURE 24.14a

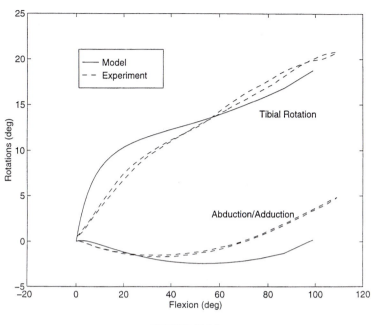

FIGURE 24.14b

FIGURE 24.14   (a) Diagram of the three-dimensional parallel spatial mechanism model of the knee, with two planar tibial plateaux and two spherical femoral condyles. The normals to the articular surfaces at the contact points are labelled LCOM and MCOM. The three ligament fibres are labelled ACL, PCL, and MCL. (b) Internal/external tibial rotation and abduction/adduction plotted against flexion angle. The solid lines were calculated, using the model (a) with parameters measured from a single specimen. The dashed lines were the measured rotations from the same specimen.

(the "screw-home mechanism") (Figure 24.14b). During flexion, the tibia rotates internally on the femur and during extension it rotates externally, as described first by Meyer (1853).

The similarity between the calculated and measured tracks of the bones upon each other (Figure 24.14b) confirms the hypotheses underlying the model, that the geometrical constraints offered by the three ligaments and the two pairs of articular surfaces can be satisfied by a precise coupling of rotation to flexion and that passive movement can occur without tissue deformation or surface separation.

The movement path and the range of movement of the model joint, Figure 24.14b, can be altered by changing the shapes of the articular surfaces or their positions on the bones or by altering the origins or insertions of the ligaments. The model can, therefore, provide a theoretical basis for prosthesis design or ligament reconstruction.

TORSIONAL STABILITY

Figures 24.13 and 24.14b above showed the automatic coupling of internal tibial rotation to flexion in the unloaded joint. This relationship is changed when applied load is balanced by muscle force.

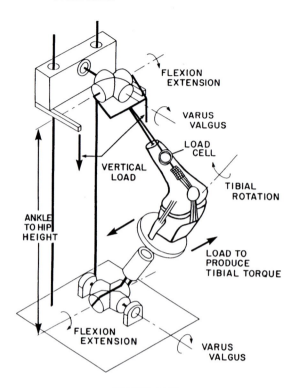

FIGURE 24.15a

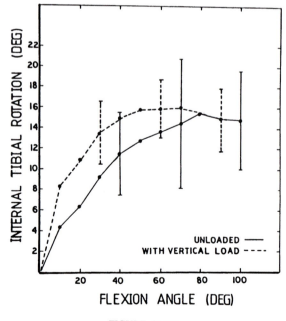

FIGURE 24.15b

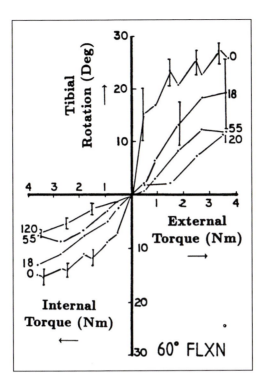

FIGURE 24.15c

FIGURE 24.15 (a) A six-degree-of-freedom apparatus used to simulate flexed knee stance. The specimen tibia is attached to an arm containing three sets of bearings allowing flexion/extension, abduction/adduction (labelled varus valgus) and tibial rotation. The specimen femur is attached to an arm allowing flexion/extension, abduction/adduction and vertical translation relative to the base plate. A pure axial torque can be applied about the tibia. Vertical load, balanced by tension in the quadriceps tendon, can be applied. The quadriceps tendon force is measured with a load cell. (b) Internal tibial rotation plotted against flexion angle for seven specimens tested in the flexed knee stance rig (a). The error bars show ±1 standard deviation from the mean. Curves are shown for the unloaded specimens and for specimens subjected to a vertical load, balanced by tension in the quadriceps tendon. (c) Tibial rotation plotted against applied torque for the seven specimens tested in the flexed knee stance rig (a). Curves are shown for the specimen with zero vertical load and with vertical loads of 18, 55, and 120 N, balanced by tension in the quadriceps tendon.

The apparatus in Figure 24.15a was used to test the torsional stability of knee specimens in a simulation of flexed knee stance (O'Connor et al., 1990c). Figure 24.15b gives the relationship between internal rotation and flexion for the unloaded joint and when a vertical load of 20 Newtons was applied along the hip/ankle axis, balanced by tension force in the quadriceps tendon (O'Connor et al., 1990c). The curve for the unloaded specimens is similar to those in Figures 24.13 and 24.14b above but, when load and muscle force are applied, the femur follows a different track on the tibia, most of the internal rotation occurring between 0° and 50° of flexion.

Tibial rotation is further altered by the application of torque about the axis of the tibia (O'Connor et al., 1990c). Curves are shown for the otherwise unloaded joint and for vertical loads of 18, 55 and 120 Newtons applied on the hip/ankle axis and balanced by tension in the quadriceps tendon (Figure 24.15c). Increasing load and muscle force tighten the ligaments and develop compressive forces between the femoral and tibial surfaces, systematically increasing the resistance of the joint to torsional movement.

Figure 24.15c shows that a finite torque, however small, is required to rotate the tibia from its position in the unloaded state. It quantifies the deviations from the neutral path shown in Figure 24.13b. It shows that deviation is resisted even within the "paths of passive motion" defined by torques of ±3 Nm applied by Blankevoort *et al.* (1988) in their experiments. It shows that the torsional stability of the joint is significantly altered by muscle force. Current development of the mathematical model of Figure 24.13a is necessary to allow the prediction of the curves in Figures 24.14b and 24.15c and to quantify the relative contributions of muscles, ligaments and articular surfaces to the control of torsional stability.

THE REAR-FOOT COMPLEX

Preliminary experiments and analysis of the rear-foot joints between the tibia, the fibula, the talus and the calcaneus suggest that the approach just described for the study of the knee may prove fruitful in the study of other joints (Leardini *et al.*, 1996a,b). Figure 24.16

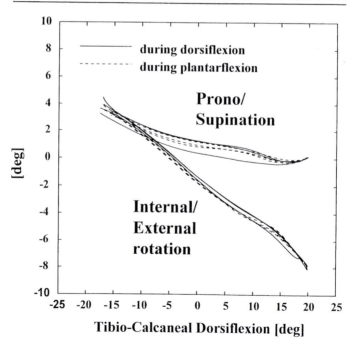

FIGURE 24.16   Pronation/supranation and internal/external rotation plotted against flexion angle for the rear foot complex. The motion of the calcaneus relative to the tibia was measured during three cycles of dorsi/plantar flexion.

shows internal/external rotation and pronation/supination of the calcaneus relative to the tibia plotted against dorsi/plantarflexion angle for one specimen moved under no load over its range of motion. The specimen exhibited a unique track characteristic of a single-degree of freedom system, with rotation and pronation coupled to flexion. Figure 24.17 shows the motion of the talus relative to the tibia and the calcaneus relative to the talus, demonstrating that most if not all passive motion of the rearfoot complex occurs at the ankle, with virtually no motion at the subtalar joints. Figure 24.17 also includes the effects of applying external force to the system, producing deviations from the neutral track of passive motion, similar to Figure 24.13b. The deviations were fully recovered when the external force was removed.

Figure 24.17 suggests that the ankle joint offers one degree of unresisted freedom in the unloaded state whereas the subtalar joints offer none. Motion could be induced at the subtalar joints only by the application of load, the bones returning to a single unique position when load was removed. During passive motion of the rearfoot complex, the fibular-calcaneal ligament and the central fibres of the deltoid ligament remained approximately isometric over the range of motion whereas all other ligament fibres joining the tibia to the calcaneus were slack except at the limits of dorsi- or plantarflexion. Fibres behind the isometric fibres were tight only in dorsiflexion and those in front of the isometric fibres

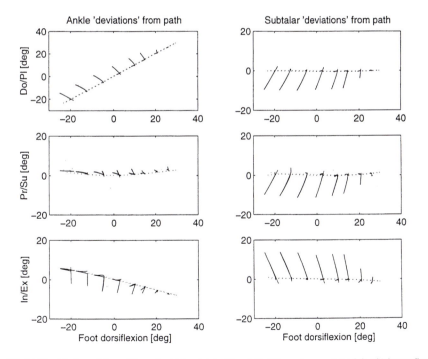

FIGURE 24.17   Motion of the ankle and subtalar joints. The dotted lines show paths of dorsi/plantar flexion, pronation/supranation and internal/external rotation plotted against foot dorsi-flexion for a single specimen. The solid lines show deviations from those paths when load was applied and removed.

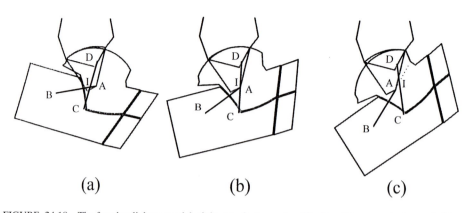

(a)   (b)   (c)

FIGURE 24.18   The four-bar linkage model of the rear foot complex. The line *AB* represents isometric fibres within the fibulo-calcaneal ligament, the line *CD* represents isometric fibres near the centre of the deltoid ligament. The tibia/fibula and the talus/calcaneus move relative to each other under the control of the ligament fibres *AB* and *CD*. The instant centre of the joint lies at *I*, where the ligament fibres intersect. The shape of the superior articular surface on the talus compatible with continuous contact on a circular tibial articular surface was calculated using the common normal theorem.

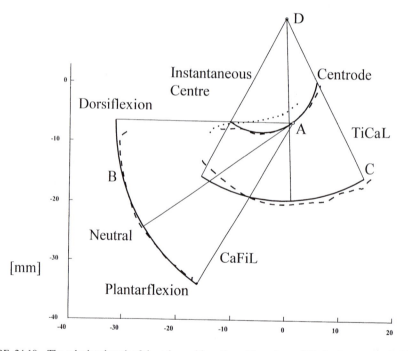

FIGURE 24.19   The calculated track of the calcaneal insertion of the calcaneal/fibular ligament and of the tibial/calcaneal ligament (solid lines labelled *B* and *C*) compared with the measurements (dashed lines) as the foot was moved from its limit of dorsi-flexion to its limit of plantar-flexion. The points *A* and *D* represent the origins of the ligaments on the fibula and tibia respectively. The calculated track of the point of intersection of the ligaments is the solid line marked *centrode*, compared with the measured position of the intersection, shown as a dashed line. The dotted line is the intersection of the screw axis of the rear foot complex with the sagittal plane through the centre of the angle.

were tight only in plantarflexion. The ligaments joining the talus to the calcaneus and the fibula to the tibia remained tight over the range of passive motion.

These experimental results imply that passive motion of the ankle-subtalar complex is controlled by a single degree of freedom mechanism, the isometric ligaments described above and the three sets of articular surfaces at the ankle serving as five constraints to motion. As a first step, we have modelled the complex as a four-bar linkage in the sagittal plane (Figure 24.18) with the tibia/fibula, the calcaneus/talus, the calcaneofibular ligament and the central fibres of the deltoid ligament acting as the four links in the mechanism (Leardini *et al.*, 1996b). As with the knee model, Figure 24.2, the instant centre of the linkage lies at the point at which the ligaments cross and the articular surfaces touch at the point where the common normal to the surfaces passes through the instant centre. As a consequence, the surfaces roll as well as slide upon each other, contact moving from the back of the tibial trochlea in plantarflexion, Figure 18a, to the front in dorsiflexion, Figure 24.18c. The calculated tracks of the ligament insertions on the calcaneus agree well with experiment (Figure 24.19).

A CLASSIFICATION OF JOINTS AND LIGAMENTS

Joints may be classified according to the number of degrees of unresisted passive motion they allow.

The hip allows three degrees of unresisted freedom, the articular surfaces providing the principal constraints to motion, the ligaments and capsule serving only to resist distraction and to define the limits to unresisted motion, being slack elsewhere (Kapandji, 1970). Ligaments are not involved in guiding the surfaces over each other. In the language of kinematics, the hip is a higher pair.

The knee and the ankle allow only one degree of unresisted freedom, the movements of abduction/adduction, axial rotation and all three components of translation being uniquely coupled to flexion/extension. These joints move as mechanisms, movement being controlled by interactions between certain isometric ligament fibres and sliding movements of the articular surfaces. Appropriate models for the study of the kinematic geometry (Hunt, 1978) of these joints can take the articular surfaces to be rigid and the isometric ligament fibres to be inextensible. The mobility of these joints does not, to a first approximation, depend on the mechanical properties of ligaments or cartilage. The kinematic analysis provides the configuration of the joint structures at any position in the unloaded state, serving as the starting point for subsequent mechanical analysis.

Joints such as the subtalar complex and tibio-fibular joint do not allow unresisted motion, force being required to deform the tissues and produce relative motion of the bones from a single unique configuration in the unloaded state. Such joints behave like flexible structures, their mobility depending critically on the mechanical properties of the tissues.

By the same token, there appear to be three classes of ligament. The ligaments of the hip tighten only at the limits of motion and play no part in the guidance of the articular surfaces on each other or in load transmission within the range of motion. Some ligaments (ACL, PCL, MCL) contain fibres which guide the movements of the bones on each other and other fibres which are slack in most positions but are recruited progressively to bear load. The configuration of these ligaments changes systematically over the range of passive movement. Some ligaments (the talar-calcaneal ligaments) hold the bones together and stretch or slacken to allow movement. These ligaments have a single configuration and remain uniformly tight in the unloaded state.

MECHANICAL FACTORS IN ANTEROMEDIAL GONARTHROSIS

We recall from the introduction to this chapter that the early lesion in osteoarthritis of the knee is found on the anterior aspects of the medial tibial plateau and the distal facets of the medial femoral condyle, the cartilage elsewhere remaining at full thickness. Inspection of Figure 24.2 shows that the sites of the lesions are the surfaces which make contact in extension and that the damaged tibial surface never makes contact with undamaged cartilage on the femur. This is consistent with Ahlbäch's observation (Ahlbäch, 1968) that medial unicompartmental disease can persist for many years without involving the other compartments of the knee.

What is unique about the mechanical circumstances of the surfaces of the knee which make contact in extension? They do not necessarily carry the largest loads; very large compressive forces are developed when climbing stairs when the knee is bent to 100°.

The leg is straight at the moment of heelstrike in level walking. Some subjects exhibit very high *loading rates* at heelstrike, the so-called heelstrike transient (Radin *et al.*, 1991). The early OA lesions therefore are found on surfaces which transmit the heelstrike transient. This deduction adds powerful clinical support to Radin's hypothesis (Radin and Paul, 1971) that repeated impulsive forces are necessary for osteoarthritic damage to cartilage. Recent work (Gill and O'Connor, 1996b) has shown that some subjects exhibit a medially-directed transient spike at heelstrike, possibly explaining why the OA lesion is found medially rather than laterally.

Recent work (Gill and O'Connor, 1997) has shown that the rate of loading at heelstrike is determined by the phasing of muscle activity in the lower limb during swing phase, subtle differences in phasing making significant differences to the downwards velocity of the foot just prior to heelstrike. This leaves open the possibility that subjects exhibiting high loading rates could be taught to alter the mechanics of swing phase to reduce loading rate and delay or prevent the onset of OA of the knee.

The systematic occurrence of anteromedial osteoarthrosis suggests that cartilage in this region should be a particularly rewarding subject for the study of the interactions between mechanical factors and biology.

REFERENCES

Ahlbäch, S. (1968) Osteoarthritis of the knee: A radiological investigation. *Acta. Radiol.*, **39**, Suppl. 227.
Bergmann, G., Graichen, F. and Rohlmann, A. (1993) Hip joint loading during walking and running, measured in two patients. *J. Biomech.*, **26**, 969–90.

Blankevoort, L., Huiskes, R. and de Lange, A. (1988) The envelope of passive knee joint motion. *J. Biomech.*, **21**, 705–20.

Borelli, G.A. (1679) *De motu animalium.* [English Translation: Maquet, P. (1989) *On the Movement of Animals.*] Springer-Verlag, Berlin.

Davy, D.T., Kotzar, G.M., Brown, R.H., Heiple, K.G. Sr., Goldberg, V.M., Heiple, K.G. Jr., Berilla, J. and Burstein, A.H. (1988) Telemetric force measurements across the hip after total arthroplasty. *J. Bone Jt. Surg.*, **70**-A, 45–50.

Elias, G.G., Freeman, M.A.R. and Gokçan, E.I. (1990) A correlative study of the geometry and anatomy of the distal femur. *Clin. Orthop.*, **260**, 98–103.

English, T.A. and Kilvington, M. (1979) *In vivo* records of hip loads using a femoral implant with telemetric output. *J. Biomed. Eng.*, **1**, 111–15.

Friederich, N.F., Muller, W. and O'Brien, W.R. (1992) Klinische anwendung biomechanischer und funktionell anatomischer daten am kniegelenk. *Orthopade.*, **21**, 41–50.

Fuss, F.K. (1989) Anatomy of the cruciate ligaments and their function in extension and flexion of the human knee joint. *Am. J. Anat.*, **184**, 165–76.

Gill, H.S. and O'Connor, J.J. (1996) A bi-articulating two-dimensional computer model of the human patellofemoral joint. *Clin. Biomech.*, **2**, 81–9.

Gill, H.S. and O'Connor, J.J. (1996) *The Pathomechanics of Anteromedial Gonarthrosis.* British Orthopaedic Research Society, September, Abstract 14.

Gill, H.S. and O'Connor, J.J. (1997) *Early Swing Phase Activity Determines the Loading at Heelstrike; Implications for Osteoarthritis.* European Orthopaedic Research Society Barcelona.

Girgis, F.G., Marshall, J.L and Monajem, A.R.S. (1975) The cruciate ligaments of the knee joint. *Clin. Orthop.*, **106**, 216–31.

Goodfellow, J.W., Hungerford, D. and Zindel, M. (1976) Patello-femoral joint mechanics and pathology: I. Functional anatomy of the patello-femoral joint. *J. Bone. Jt. Surg.*, [Br] **58**-B, 287–90.

Goodfellow, J. and O'Connor, J. (1978) The mechanics of the knee and prosthesis design. *J. Bone Jt. Surg.*, [Br] **60**-B, 358–69.

Herzog, W. and Read, L.J. (1993) Lines of action and moment arms of the major force-carrying structures crossing the human knee joint. *J. Anat.*, **182**, 213–30.

Hunt, K.H. (1978) *Kinematic Geometry of Mechanisms.* Oxford University Press, Oxford.

Huson, A. (1974) Biomechanische probleme des kniegelenks. *Orthopade.*, **3**, 119–26.

Kapandji, I. (1970) *The Physiology of the Joints, Vol 2: The Lower Limb* (2nd Ed) Churchill Livingstone, London, UK (Translated by L.H. Honore).

Leardini, A., Catani, F. and O'Connor, J.J. (1996a) *The One Degree of Freedom Nature of the Human Ankle Complex*, British Orthopaedic Research Society, September, Abstracts p. 41.

Leardini, A., Lu, T-W., Catani, F. and O'Connor, J.J. (1996b) *A Four-bar Linkage Model of the Ankle.* British Orthopaedic Research Society, September, Abstracts p. 16.

Lewis, J.L., Lew, W.D. and Schmidt, J. (1982) A note on the application and evaluation of the buckle transducer for knee ligament force measurement. *J. Biomech. Eng.*, **104**, 125–8.

Lu, T-W. and O'Connor, J.J. (1996a) Fibre recruitment and shape changes of knee ligaments during motion: as revealed by a computer graphics-based model. Proc. Instn. Mech. Engrs., Part H, *J. Eng. Med.*, **210**, 71–9.

Lu, T-W. and O'Connor, J.J. (1996b) Lines of action and moment arms of the major force-bearing structures crossing the human knee joint: comparison between theory and experiment. *J. Anat.*, **189**, 575–85.

Lu, T-W., O'Connor, J.J., Taylor, S.J.G. and Walker, P.S. (1996) *Interpretation of Isometric Tests on Patients with Instrumented Massive Prostheses.* European Society of Biomechanics, Abstracts p. 269 (Eds: J. Vander Sloten, G. Lowet, R. van Audekercke and G. van der Perre).

Lu, T-W., O'Connor, J.J., Taylor, S.J.G. and Walker, P.S. (1997) Comparison of femoral forces during double and single leg stance: application to knee replacement. European Orthopaedic Research Society (to be published).

Markolf, K.L., Mensch, J.S. and Amstutz, H.C. (1976) Stiffness and laxity of the knee – the contributions of the supporting structures. A quantitative *in vitro* study. *J. Bone Jt. Surg.* [Am], **58**-A, 583–93.

Menschik, A. (1974) Mechanik des kniegelenks – teil 1. *Z. Orthop.*, **112**, 481–95.

Meyer, H. (1853) Die mechanik des kniegelenks. *Archiv für Anatomie und Physiologie*, 497–547.

Miller, R.K., Murray, D.W., O'Connor J.J. and Goodfellow, J.W. (1997) *In vitro* patellofemoral joint force determined by a non-invasive technique. *Clin. Biomech.*, **12**(1),1–7.

Morrison, J.B. (1968) Bioengineering analysis of force actions transmitted by the knee joint. *Biomed. Eng.*, **90**, 164–70.

Murray, D.W., Goodfellow, J.W. and O'Connor, J.J. (1997) *10 Year Survival of the Oxford Unicompartmental Meniscal Knee Replacement.* EFORT, 3rd Congress, Barcelona.

O'Connor, J., Shercliff, T., Biden, E. and Goodfellow, J. (1989) The geometry of the knee in the sagittal plane. Proc. Inst. Mech. Eng. Part H, *J. Eng. Med.*, **203**, 223–33.

O'Connor, J.J., Shercliff, T., FitzPatrick, D., Bradley, J., Daniel, D., Biden, E. and Goodfellow, J. (1990a) Geometry of the knee. Chapter 10 In: *Knee Ligaments: Structure, Function, Injury and Repair*. (Eds: Daniel, D.M., Akeson, W.H. and O'Connor, J.J.) Raven Press, New York, 163–200.

O'Connor, J.J., Shercliff, T., FitzPatrick, D., Biden, E. and Goodfellow, J. (1990b) Mechanics of the Knee. Chapter 11 In: *Knee Ligaments: Structure, Function, Injury, and Repair*. (Eds: Daniel, D.M., Akeson, W.H. and O'Connor, J.J.) Raven Press, New York, pp. 201–38

O'Connor, J.J., Biden, E., Bradley, J., FitzPatrick, D., Young, S. Kershaw, C., Daniel, D. and Goodfellow, J. (1990c) The muscle-stabilized knee. Chapter 12 In: *Knee Ligaments: Structure, Function, Injury, and Repair*. (Eds: Daniel, D.M., Akeson, W.H. and O'Connor, J.J.) Raven Press, New York, 239–78.

O'Connor, J.J. (1993) Can muscle co-contraction protect knee ligaments after injury or repair? *J. Bone Jt. Surg.* [Br], **75-B**, 41–8.

Radin, E.L., Yang, K.A., Riegger, C., Kish, V.L. and O'Connor, J.J. (1991) Relationships between lower limb dynamics and knee joint pain. *J. Orthop. Res.*, **9**, 398–405.

Radin, E.L. and Paul, I.L. (1971) The response of joints to impact loading. I: *in vitro* wear. *Arthr. Rheum.*, **14**, 356–62.

Paul, J.P. (1965) Bio-engineering studies of the forces transmitted by joints: II. Engineering analysis. In: *Biomechanics and Related Bio-Engineering Topics* (Ed. Kenedi, R.M.) Pergamon Press, Oxford, 369–80.

Pauwels, F. (1950) Principles of construction of the lower extremity. Their significance for the stressing of the skeleton of the leg. Chapter 6 In: *Biomechanics of the Locomotor Apparatus*, Springer-Verlag, Berlin, 1980. (Original published in *Z. Anat. Entwickl. Gesch.* (1950) **114**, 525–38).

Rydell, N.W. (1966) Forces acting on the femoral head prosthesis. *Acta Orthop. Scand.* (Suppl) 88.

Sapega, A.A., Moyer, R.A., Schneck, C. and Komalahiranya, N. (1990) Testing for isometry during reconstruction of the anterior cruciate ligament. *J. Bone Jt. Surg.* [Am], **72-A**, 259–67.

Shoemaker, S.C. and Daniel, D.M. (1990) The limits of knee motion: *in vitro* studies. Chapter 9 In: *Knee Ligaments: Structure, Function, Injury and Repair* (Eds: Daniel, D.M., Akeson, W.H. and O'Connor, J.J.) Raven Press, New York, 153–62.

Strasser, H. (1917) *Lehrbuch der Muskel- und Gelenkmechanik*, Springer, Berlin, 1917.

Taylor, S.J. and Donaldson, N. (1990) Instrumenting Stanmore prostheses for long-term strain measurement *in vivo*. In: *Proc. of a Workshop on Implantable Telemetry in Orthopaedics* (Eds Bergmann, G., Graichen, F. and Rohlmann, A.) Freie Universitat, Berlin, 93–102.

Taylor, S.J.G., Perry, J.S., Meswania, J.M., Donaldson, N., Walker, P.S. and Cannon, S.R. (1997) Telemetry of forces from proximal femoral replacements and relevance to fixation. *J. Biomech.*, **30**, 225–34.

Uicker, J., Denavit, J. and Hartenberg, R. (1964) An iterative method for the displacement analysis of spatial mechanisms. Trans ASME, *J. Appl. Mech.*, **31**, 309–14.

Weber, W.E. and Weber, E.F.W. (1836) *Mechanik der menschlichen Gehwerkzeuge*. in der Dietrichschen Buchhandlung, Gottingen.

White, S.H., Ludkowski, P.F. and Goodfellow, J.W. (1991) Anteromedial osteoarthritis of the knee. *J. Bone. Jt. Surg.* [Br], **73B**, 582–6.

Wilson, D.R., Zavatsky, A.B. and O'Connor, J.J. (1993) Cruciate ligament forces at the knee in gait: parameter sensitivity and effects of ligament elasticity. In: *International Society of Biomechanics*, 1466–7.

Wilson, D. (1996) Three-dimensional kinematics of the knee. D. Phil thesis, University of Oxford, Oxford, UK.

Wilson, D., Feikes, J., Zavatsky, A., Bayona, F. and O'Connor, J.J. (1996) The one degree-of-freedom nature of the human knee joint – basis for a kinematic model. In: *Canadian Society of Biomechanics*, 194–5.

Zavatsky, A.B. and O'Connor, J.J. (1992a) A model of human knee ligaments in the sagittal plane. Part I: response to passive flexion. Proc. Instn. Mech. Engrs., Part H, *J. Eng. Med.*, **206**, 125–34.

Zavatsky, A.B. and O'Connor, J.J. (1992b) A model of human knee ligaments in the sagittal plane. Part II: fibre recruitment under load. Proc. Instn. Mech. Engrs., Part H, *J. Eng. Med.*, **206**, 135–45.

Zavatsky, A.B. and O'Connor, J.J. (1993) Ligament forces at the knee during isometric quadriceps contractions. Proc. Instn. Mech. Engrs., Part H, *J. Engng. Med.*, **207**, 7–18.

Zavatsky, A.B. and O'Connor, J.J. (1994) Three-dimensional geometrical models of human knee ligaments. Proc. Instn. Mech. Engrs., Part H, *J. Engng. Med.*, **208**, 229–40.

Section 6
Joint Innervation

25 The Innervation of Synovial Joints

Karola Messner

Sports Medicine, Faculty of Health Sciences,
University of Linköping, 581 85 Linköping, Sweden

KEY WORDS innervation, sensory innervation; autonomic innervation; nerve endings, mechanoreceptors; nociceptors; neurotransmitter substances, synovial joints, capsule; discs; ligaments; menisci; subchondral bone; synovium

BACKGROUND

Except for avascular cartilaginous tissues, most joint structures are richly innervated. Neuronal tissue in the anterior cruciate ligament (ACL) for example constitutes about 1.0–2.5% of the total tissue volume (Zimny *et al.*, 1986; Schutte *et al.*, 1987). The different nerve endings in articular tissue have primarily been classified on a structural and functional basis (Skoglund, 1956; Polacek, 1966; Freeman and Wyke, 1967; Halata, 1975). A distinction can be made between encapsulated and free nerve endings. In the former, the nerve endings are ensheathed by Schwann cells as a direct continuation of the perineurium (Polacek, 1966; Halata, 1975). Freeman and Wyke (1967) recognised 3 types of encapsulated nerve endings which also differ in their functional characteristics (Freeman and Wyke, 1967). These encapsulated nerve endings are mechanoreceptors and are also defined as Ruffini endings (type I), Pacinian corpuscles (type II), and Golgi tendon organs (type III) (Skoglund, 1956). Free nerve endings are pain receptors or have vasoregulatory functions (Freeman and Wyke, 1967). Both encapsulated and free sensory nerve endings have been found in joint capsules, articular discs, menisci, ligaments and tendons (Freeman and Wyke, 1967; Halata, 1977; Zimny and St. Onge, 1987) and similar types of nerve endings are found in other parts of the body e.g. the skin or mucous membranes (Halata, 1975; Halata and Munger, 1980a,b, 1983).

The different types of nerve endings, especially encapsulated mechanoreceptors, are usually demonstrated by silver or gold staining methods or general neuronal markers.

Immunohistochemical methods using antibodies against a variety of neuropeptides tend to label unmyelinated nerve fibres rather than nerve endings (Sharkey and Bray, 1990).

There is considerable support in the literature for the idea that the sensory innervation of joints plays a role in proprioception, muscle reflex activity, and the regulation of muscle and joint stiffness (Zimny, 1988; Johansson et al., 1991). Although the significance of innervation in joint development and remodeling under loading, ageing, and disease has been less extensively investigated, there is evidence that neurohormones may have a role in secondary ossification of joint epiphyses (Hedberg et al., 1995), and in regulating osteoblastic activity and bone remodeling (Hohmann et al., 1983; D'Sousa et al., 1986; Zaidi et al., 1987a,b; Bernhard and Shih, 1990; Bjurholm et al., 1992). Whether neuropeptides influence soft tissues such as cartilage, ligament, tendon and meniscus is unclear. An age-related loss (57%) of knee joint afferents has been described in certain strains of mice and particularly affected the larger mechanoreceptors. It is intriguing that the loss with age was approximately reciprocal to the increasing incidence of osteoarthritis in the mouse knee joint (Salo and Tatton, 1993). Besides this possible involvement in ageing and degenerative joint disease, neuropeptide activity may also play a role in inflammatory joint condition (Ahmed et al., 1995a,b).

The role and function of joint mechanoreceptors have to be considered together with that of receptors innervating skin, muscle and tendon (Edin and Abbs, 1991). For example, 72.5% of median and ulnar nerve sensory afferents of the hand are of cutaneous origin, and only 15% and 12.5% are joint and muscles afferents, respectively (Burke et al., 1988). Likewise, the dorsal spinocerebellar tract of the cat contains neurons excited by muscle spindles, Golgi tendon organs, and different types of cutaneous and joint mechanoreceptors (Lundberg and Oscarsson, 1960; Lindström and Takata, 1972).

TEMPORAL APPEARANCE OF NERVE FIBRES DURING BONE AND JOINT DEVELOPMENT

There is evidence that sensory nerves are involved in the process of secondary ossification of the epiphysis. During postnatal maturation, calcitonin gene-related peptide (CGRP)- and substance P (SP)-immunoreactive axons are present in cartilage canals and the perichondrium some days before the start of secondary ossification in the knee epiphysis (Hedberg et al., 1995). These canal-related axons disappear 13–15 days after birth. Tyrosine hydroxylase (TH)-like immunoreactivity appears at other sites in the developing knee joint (Hedberg et al., 1995). In addition, nerve fibres, immunoreactive to SP, CGRP, neuropeptide Y (NPY) and TH, have been seen among differentiating chondroblasts at an early stage of ectopic bone formation (Bjurholm, 1989), and CGRP-immunoreactive nerve fibres appear before the onset of mineralization of callus after tibial fracture (Hukkanen et al., 1993), presumably coinciding with angiogenesis. This temporal occurrence and distribution of different nerves during bone formation would seem to indicate that there is a neurogenic involvement in bone differentiation and development (Bjurholm, 1989), but the CGRP-immunoreactive fibres may also have a vasoregulatory function (Poyner, 1992).

MORPHOLOGY AND DISTRIBUTION

MECHANORECEPTORS

Any classification of encapsulated nerve endings into different morphological types is somewhat arbitrary (Boyd, 1954), but is nevertheless helpful for surveying the extensive literature. The different types of joint receptors vary in their morphological appearance, size, threshold to mechanical deformation, and anatomical location. The classification of Freeman and Wyke (1967) is used here.

Type I nerve endings

Type I nerve endings are encapsulated globular or ovoid corpuscles, 40–100 μm in diameter (Freeman and Wyke, 1967). Each has a delicate capsule enclosing a branching complex of unmyelinated nerve fibres embedded in a matrix. This nerve terminal is derived from a myelinated nerve axon 5–10 μm in diameter. A capillary approaches each corpuscle and breaks into arcades of vessels on the capsular surface. Type I endings are found in clusters of 3–6 corpuscles. They are low threshold, slowly-adapting mechanoreceptors. Type I endings are otherwise also called Ruffini endings, Golgi-Mazzoni endings, Meissner corpuscles, Spray type endings, Basket endings, Ball-of-tread endings or Bush-like endings (Figure 25.1, from Skoglund, 1956).

Type II nerve endings

Type II endings are elongated, cylindrical or conical corpuscles, often in clusters of 2–3, that have an average length of 280 μm and a diameter of 120 μm (Freeman and Wyke, 1967). A fibrous capsule 60–100 μm thick, and containing up to 12 cell layers surrounds

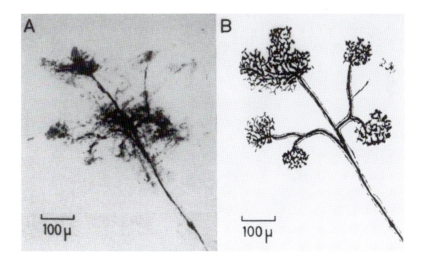

FIGURE 25.1   A sensory unit of the Ruffini type (type I ending) in the posterior part of the joint capsule. Five endings arising from the same axon. (A) Microphotograph (magnification ×132). Gold stain. (B) A drawing of the endings seen in A at the same magnification (from Skoglund, 1956 with permission).

the corpuscle and the whole structure is supplied by a capillary loop. A 8–12 µm thick myelinated nerve fibre leads to the encapsulated end organ, where it loses its myelin sheath. The axon finally terminates in the corpuscle tip by forming a bulbous expansion or a Y-shaped bifurcation. Type II nerve endings are low-threshold, rapidly-adapting mechanoreceptors and have numerous eponyms: Krause's Endkörperchen, Vater'schen Körper, Pacinian corpuscle, Vater-Pacinian corpuscle, modified Pacini(an) corpuscle, simple Pacinian corpuscle, Paciniform corpuscle, Golgi-Mazzoni body, Meissner corpuscle, Gelenknervenkörperchen, corpuscle of Krause, club-like ending, bulbous corpuscle and Corpuscula nervosa articularia (Freeman and Wyke, 1967; Figure 25.2, from Skoglund, 1956). Type-II endings are distinguishable from day 9 after birth in the mouse and initially consist of a central axon surrounded by irregular cytoplasmic processes of Schwann cells and their associated basal lamina (Takahashi, 1995). At 2 weeks, the inner core layers around the axon are formed, and thus the basic structure of the Pacinian corpuscle is established. By 3 weeks the structure resembles that in the adult, and by 5 weeks it is fully formed. The findings suggest that these nerve endings start functioning when the animal is about 3 weeks old (Takahashi, 1995).

Type III nerve endings

Type III nerve endings are large fusiform organs surrounded by a capsule that is 1–3 cells thick (Freeman and Wyke, 1967). They measure up to 600 µm in length and 100 µm in diameter and are supplied by a 13–17 µm diameter, afferent myelinated nerve fibre. This loses its myelin sheath as it enters the end-organ and breaks into diverging branches from which densely arborising filaments arise. The nerve filaments can have many fusiform or globular expansions along their length and may be solitary or arranged in clusters derived from a common parent axon. When the organs are clustered, the individual corpuscles are smaller. In contrast to type I and II endings, type III endings do not have any local relationship to blood vessels. They are high-threshold, slowly-adapting mechanoreceptors. They are also known as Golgi endings or Golgi Mazzoni corpuscles (Freeman and Wyke, 1967; Figure 25.3, from Skoglund 1956).

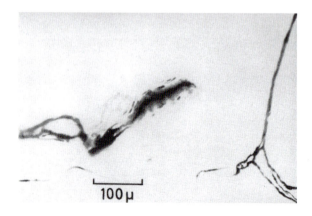

100 µ

FIGURE 25.2   Modified Vater-Pacini corpuscle (type II ending). Magnification ×185. Gold stain (from Skoglund, 1956 with permission).

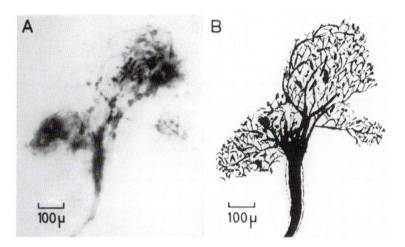

FIGURE 25.3   Golgi ending (type III ending) in the anterior cruciate ligament. (A) Microphotograph (magnification ×110). Gold stain. (B) Drawing of the ending seen in A at the same magnification (from Skoglund, 1956 with permission).

Free nerve endings (Type IV nerve endings)

Type IV endings include a variety of undifferentiated non-corpuscular terminals composed of unmyelinated nerve fibres. The term IVa endings has been used to describe plexuses or free nerve endings, and the term IVb endings for unmyelinated efferent terminals (Freeman and Wyke, 1967). Type IVa endings are present in 2 forms in articular tissue: (1) as unmyelinated 0.5–1.5 μm thick nerve fibres which form a close-meshed network throughout articular tissue. They are often associated with blood vessels and are derived from 2–5 μm thick, sparsely myelinated parent axons and (2) as unmyelinated free nerve terminals < 1 μm diameter, which branch out between collagen and elastic fibres of the articular connective tissue from unmyelinated, thin (1–2 μm) parent axons. Some groups of type IVa free nerve endings also arise as the terminal ramifications of thinly myelinated nerve fibres 2–4 μm thick. These unmyelinated or myelinated parent axons are intra-articular extensions of small diameter fibres in the articular nerves. Type IVb endings are confined to the articular blood vessels and are derived from unmyelinated parent axons < 2 μm in diameter. Type IVa endings are regarded as the pain-sensitive system of articular tissue, whereas type IVb endings represent vasomotor innervation (Freeman and Wyke, 1967).

DISTRIBUTION OF NERVE FIBRES AND ENDINGS

JOINT CAPSULE

In the cat knee, the fibrous joint capsule (excluding the synovium) contains in addition to free nerve endings mainly types I and II mechanoreceptors (Freeman and Wyke, 1967). The smaller type I receptors occur in the superficial layers of the joint capsule (Kennedy *et al.*,

1982), whereas type II receptors are located in deeper layers at fibro-adipose junctions near blood vessels (Freeman and Wyke, 1967) and adjacent to muscles and ligaments (Halata *et al.*, 1984). Type I receptors are arranged in clusters supplied by the same afferent nerve fibre. Type I receptors are more densely aggregated in anterior and posterior areas of the knee joint than in medial or lateral aspects, and are entirely absent from synovial or fat pad tissues (Freeman and Wyke, 1967). Type II nerve endings are less numerous than type I endings. Clusters of 2–4 corpuscles are more common on the medial and lateral sides of the knee joint than on its anterior and posterior aspects (Freeman and Wyke, 1967). More recently, Hashimoto *et al.* (1994) and Takahashi (1995) have confirmed the presence of type II receptors in the mouse knee joint capsule by immunolabelling with antibodies against S-100 protein. Type III nerve endings are absent from the knee joint capsule, but type IVa endings form a network throughout its fibrous parts (Freeman and Wyke, 1967). This network of fibres is often associated with the adventitial sheaths of small arteries and arterioles, but is completely absent from ligaments, menisci and synovial tissue. Type IVb endings are confined to small arteries and arterioles in the capsule where they terminate in the tunica media as fine plexuses on and around the smooth muscle cells (Freeman and Wyke, 1967).

In cat temporomandibular joint Type I receptors occur throughout the capsule but are more densely packed in its anterior and posterior regions (Zimny, 1988). The distribution of type II receptors is similar, but they are less numerous and are also present in the posterior articular fat pad. Type IVa endings are arranged as plexuses throughout the joint capsule (Zimny, 1988).

SYNOVIUM

Synovium has isolated single axons or larger nerve bundles, and joint fat pads are traversed by multiple fine fibres (Kennedy *et al.*, 1982). The stratum synoviale contains only autonomic fibres, running in the tunica adventitia of arteries and there are no free nerve endings (Halata and Groth, 1976; Halata *et al.*, 1984). Simple encapsulated type II nerve endings (Pacinian corpuscles) are occasionally observed at the border between the stratum synoviale and fibrosum (Halata and Groth, 1976). Sensory (SP, CGRP-immunoreactive nerve fibres), and autonomic innervation (NPY-immunoreactive fibres) of the synovial membrane has been described in the rat knee (Bjurholm *et al.*, 1988a) adjacent to or within blood vessel walls (Iwasaki *et al.*, 1995). Blood vessels in synovial membrane also contain interleukin-1 (IL-1)-immunoreactive nerves and varicose IL-1-positive fibres terminate amidst synoviocytes (Bjurholm *et al.*, 1994). IL-1-and NPY-immunoreactivity co-exist in synovial nerve fibres. NPY-positive fibres predominantly form a network around blood vessels in the subintima layer, and CGRP- and SP-immunoreactive fibres are especially numerous near the attachment of the meniscus to the synovium (Iwasaki *et al.*, 1995). In the synovium of the lumbar facet joint, SP- and CGRP-positive fibres are predominantly nonvascular (Ahmed *et al.*, 1993a). Autonomic innervation (e.g. NPY- and TH-positive fibres) occurs adjacent to or within blood vessel walls. Immunoreactivity to vasoactive intestinal polypeptide (VIP) is typical of varicose nerve terminals in the synoviocyte layer, and is mostly unrelated to blood vessels (Ahmed *et al.*, 1993a).

MENISCI

There is general agreement that the nerve supply to menisci is more extensive in the horns than the body (Day *et al.*, 1985), but reports vary as to whether any nerves at all are present in the latter. O'Connor and McConnaughey (1978) have demonstrated a rich neurovascular supply, including types I and II mechanoreceptors, in the meniscal horns in the cat, but could not find any nerves in the body. In a later paper, O'Connor (1984) described further 2 different type II receptors (a and b), and less commonly type III receptors at the transitional zone between the posterior horn of the lateral meniscus and its attachment in the dog. Similarly, Kennedy *et al.* (1982) found abundant axons, large nerve bundles, free nerve endings, and specialised receptors including complex end-bulbs and Golgi-type (type III endings) in perimeniscal capsular tissue, but not extending into the meniscal body. In contrast, Wilson *et al.* (1969) reported both myelinated and unmyelinated nerve fibres in the human medial meniscus that extended from a periarticular plexus onto the meniscus as far as its intermediate third of the body. These neural elements were not exclusively paravascular. Also Albright *et al.* (1987) showed nerves penetrating from the perimeniscal tissue into the outer and middle third of the meniscal fibrocartilage, especially near to the horns. They formed all 3 types of encapsulated end organs (types I–III) and free nerve endings (type IV). These somewhat controversial reports may be a consequence of different classifications of anatomical regions. However, it is evident that innervation predominates at capsular meniscal junctions, horns and attachments.

SP- and CGRP-positive nerve fibres have been seen near the attachment of the meniscus to the synovium (Iwasaki *et al.*, 1995). Meniscal insertions to bone are also innervated. Neuronal elements have been detected by immunohistochemistry in the uncalcified and calcified fibrocartilage and the subchondral bone at the meniscal attachments of the rabbit (Gao *et al.*, 1994).

ARTICULAR DISCS

Mechanoreceptors and free nerve endings are present in both the pericapsular tissue and the disc of the human tempomandibular joint (Zimny and St. Onge, 1987), and intervertebral discs contain NPY, TH and VIP-immunoreactive nerve fibres (Ahmed *et al.*, 1993b).

LIGAMENTS

The ACL has an extensive intraligamentous neural network (Zimny *et al.*, 1986). Nerves enter the ligament via neurovascular bundles in the subsynovial connective tissue and terminate in various receptors. A greater number of mechanoreceptors are found at the ligament insertions (especially the tibial) than in the ligament midsubstance. The ACL contains all types of nerve endings (Freeman and Wyke, 1967; Zimny *et al.*, 1986; Johansson *et al.*, 1991), but type III endings are the most numerous (Freeman and Wyke, 1967; Kennedy *et al.*, 1982; Andrew, 1954). These nerve endings have been identified in all ligaments of the knee, including the ligamentum patellae, and in the insertions of the lateral ligaments of the temporomandibular joint (Zimny, 1988). Ligaments and tendons also contain numerous type IVa endings (Freeman and Wyke, 1967; Biedert *et al.*, 1992). These spread in all directions between the collagen fibres, sometimes twining around them, but in contrast to those in the joint capsule, they do not form a network (Freeman and Wyke, 1967). Electron microscopical studies have shown that the connective tissue between the synovial membrane and the ACL contains type I nerve endings and lamellar corpuscles with several inner cores (Halata and Haus, 1989). The connective tissue septa between the individual fascicles of the cruciate ligaments contain of types I and IV nerve endings. The free endings (type IV) are innervated by C-fibres and myelinated A-delta fibres (Halata and Haus, 1989). SP- and CGRP-immunoreactive nerve fibres together mirror the pattern of unmyelinated fibres identified by silver staining and are mainly associated with blood vessels (Sharkey and Bray, 1990). Aune *et al.* (1996) have demonstrated nerve fibres in the human and rat ACL and patellar tendon that label for protein gene product 9.5 (general neural marker), growth associated protein 43/B-50 (neuronal regeneration), CGRP and SP. They occur in the dense collagenous tissue and at perivascular locations in the superficial part of the ligament near its insertion. The deltoid, talofibular and calcaneofibular ligaments of the human ankle joint are characterised by types II and III receptors (Michelson and Hutchins, 1995) and spinal ligaments and the dura mater have NPY, TH and VIP immunoreactive nerve fibres (Ahmed *et al.*, 1993b).

SUBCHONDRAL BONE

Reimann and Bach Christensen (1977) demonstrated unspecific, non-myelinated nerve fibres in subchondral bone marrow and reported an increase in the number of these nerves in osteoarthritis. Among 25 neuronal antibodies applied to bone, immunoreactivity to the neuropeptides SP, CGRP, VIP and NPY, IL-1 and TH has been reported in this tissue (Bjurholm, 1989; Ahmed *et al.*, 1993b). All are vasoactive except IL-1 which is primarily related to immune responses (Bjurholm, 1989). SP and CGRP are known to be involved in the mediation of sensory modalities, especially nociceptive stimuli.

Nerves are rare in cortical bone. Around the knee joint, SP-, CGRP- and NPY-immunoreactive fibres have been found in bone, bone marrow, periosteum, synovial membrane and adjacent soft tissues (Bjurholm *et al.*, 1988a; Iwasaki *et al.*, 1995). The distribution pattern of SP- and CGRP-positive nerve fibres is similar, although CGRP fibres are generally more numerous. Both types of nerves are particularly abundant near the epiphyseal plate, in the subchondral bone of the patella and in the epiphyses and periosteum (Bjurholm *et al.*, 1988a; Buma, 1994). Many SP- and CGRP-immunoreactive fibres are seen near blood vessels (Bjurholm *et al.*, 1988a), but give rarely off branches that directly supply blood vessel walls (Bjurholm, 1989). NPY, TH and IL-1 fibres are almost exclusively restricted to vessel walls mostly near the epiphyseal plate, but also in Volkmann canals (Bjurholm *et al.*, 1988c; Bjurholm, 1989). VIP nerve fibres are found in periosteal tissue and epiphysis (Bjurholm *et al.*, 1988c). Thus, bone has a rich supply of both noradrenergic (TH) and peptide-containing nerves. The differential distribution of these nerves may reflect specific roles in the local regulation of bone physiology, such as controlling blood flow, bone formation or resorption (Bjurholm *et al.*, 1988c).

PHYSIOLOGY OF NERVE FIBRES AND ENDINGS

SPECIFIC ACTIVATION PATTERN OF DIFFERENT MECHANORECEPTORS

Type I endings are low-threshold, slowly adapting receptors that respond to mechanical stresses (Freeman and Wyke, 1967). They appear to be stimulated by the displacement of collagen fibres with which they are intertwined. These fibres run axially in the core of the corpuscle and pass through both ends of it to merge with collagen in the surrounding tissue. The behavioral characteristics of the receptors characterise them as static and dynamic mechanoreceptors signalling static joint position, changes in intra-articular pressure, and the direction, amplitude and velocity of joint movements. They help to maintain muscle tone (Freeman and Wyke, 1967; Zimny, 1988). Type II endings are dynamic, rapidly-adapting low threshold mechanoreceptors (Freeman and Wyke, 1967). They are only active in a dynamic situation especially at the onset or cessation of motion, deceleration or acceleration, or a change in the stress or vibration patterns in a fat pad or joint capsule (Zimny, 1988). At the onset of mandibular movement, type II receptors in the capsule are stimulated suggesting a typical acceleration-deceleration response (Klineberg *et al.*, 1970). Type III nerve endings are high-threshold, very slowly-adapting mechanoreceptors (Freeman and Wyke, 1967). They become active at extreme ranges of movement or when considerable stresses are placed on ligaments (Zimny, 1988). Free nerve endings are high-threshold, non-adapting pain receptors (Freeman and Wyke, 1967; Zimny, 1988).

ACTIVATION OF JOINT RECEPTORS

MOTION, TENSION, VIBRATION, AND PRESSURE

There is evidence that joint position and motion activates joint receptors (Andrew and Dodt, 1953). In an experimental study it has been shown that slowly-adapting joint receptors in capsule and ligaments can adequately signal joint angle throughout the full range of motion and hence could make an important contribution to position sense (Ferrell, 1980). Andrew and Dodt (1953) postulated that these slowly-adapting receptors were arranged so that each has an arc of maximum sensitivity covering a few degrees of angular movement. During passive knee rotation, neurons mainly discharge at extreme angular displacements, and response to passive extension is linearly related to the torque applied to the knee (Grigg and Greenspan, 1977). In the absence of changes in joint angle active contractions of quadriceps, semimembranosus and gastrocnemius muscles activates joint afferents, but for quadriceps-activated neurons, rather high torques are required. These findings support the hypothesis that joint afferents function as capsular stretch receptors, responding to mechanical events which result in loading of the capsule (Grigg and Greenspan, 1977). Movement at the elbow joint has also been shown to activate joint afferents (Millar, 1975). The fibres respond to elbow extension with a phasic and graded, tonic or slowly-adapting response. All fibres have a maximum adapted discharge at full extension. Half of the units give a phasic or tonic response at full flexion, but this appears only at the extreme position of the arm. Slowly-adapting receptors in the capsule of the hip joint only discharge at the limits of the range of movement and have a low sensitivity to vibratory stimuli applied perpendicular to their receptive field (Aloisi *et al.*, 1988).

In a clinical experiment, Burke *et al.* (1988) have shown that joint afferents from the wrist are tonically active in the resting position of the hand and that most are also active during passive motion. The majority of the afferents only respond towards the limits of joint rotation. Receptors responding to passive motion do not necessarily also respond to active motion (Edin, 1990). In addition, joint afferents seem to have a limited capacity to signal direction of motion, as only part of them respond in 2 axes of angular displacement and very few in all 3 axes (Burke *et al.*, 1988). More afferents are activated in both directions of movement. Only a single afferent (associated with the interphalangeal joint of the thumb) responded unidirectionally throughout the physiological range of joint movement, and was thereby capable of encoding joint position and movement adequately. Thus it may be concluded that human joint afferents possess limited capacity to provide kinaesthetic information (Burke *et al.*, 1988).

The medial collateral and patellar ligaments are equipped with endings which signal tension, and alterations in tension or temperature changes under steady tension modulate discharge frequencies (Andrew and Dodt, 1953; Andrew, 1954). Local stimulation, such as that created by probing the knee joint with a glass rod or increasing the tension on the joint by applying pressure to the muscles which act on it, activates single or multiple spinal cord units (Schaible *et al.*, 1986). The receptive field of a single neuron investigated by Schaible *et al.* (1986) included the posterior capsule, lateral, medial and anterior aspects of the knee joint, but the neuron could also be activated by tension applied to the gastrocnemius-soleus muscle. A second spinal cord neuron investigated, had a receptive field which included the posterior capsule and the lateral aspect of the knee joint. This neuron was activated when the knee was extended, but the most prominent responses to joint movement occurred with forced extension, or medial/lateral rotation. Other units responded only to forced motions.

Direct measurement of afferent fibres from the ACL showed that local pressure near to the femoral attachment activated the nerves (Krauspe *et al.*, 1992). The afferents did not fire in the resting position of the knee joint (30°), but were activated with knee extension, flexion, or rotation. Activation was markedly increased with hyperextension and rotation.

Intra-articular pressure can also activate joint receptors. With increasing intra-articular volume, both intra-articular pressure and neural discharge from slowly-adapting mechanoreceptors initially increase of (Andrew and Dodt, 1953; Wood and Ferrell, 1984). This increase depends on the rate of fluid accumulation within the joint. However the joint nerve discharge levels out despite increasing intra-articular volume and pressure. This suggests that there is some limit on capsular distension in the posterior joint region beyond which fluid is diverted to other areas (Wood and Ferrell, 1984).

INTEGRATION OF INFORMATION

Schaibl *et al.* (1987) has demonstrated the coordination between sensory input of skin, deep tissue and joint receptors. In an experimental study using cats, neural responses were recorded from 160 ascending tract cells in segments L4-6 of the spinal cord. 32% of the neurons were activated just from receptors located in the skin, 11% by receptors from deep tissues, 10% had convergent input from receptors in skin and deep tissues, and 16% had convergent input from knee joint and either skin, deep tissues, or both. In the remaining 30% the receptive field could not be identified. Skin or combined skin–joint neurons were almost exclusively located in the dorsal horn of the spinal cord, whereas many neurons with deep receptive field combinations were in the ventral horn. All of the neurons that had a receptive field in the knee joint also had a convergent input from receptors in other tissues. Usually the corresponding cutaneous receptive field was near the knee joint, but sometimes was also remote (in the foot). The deep receptive fields coupled with joint areas were chiefly in the muscles of the thigh or leg. Cutaneous receptive fields were classified by Schaibl et al. (1987) as 'low threshold' (cells excited best by innocuous intensities of mechanical stimulation), 'wide dynamic range' (cells activated by weak mechanical stimuli, but with their best responses to noxious stimuli) or 'high threshold' (innocuous stimuli had little effect, but noxious mechanical stimuli produced a vigorous discharge). Similarly, weak mechanical stimuli acting on the knee joint could excite some neurons, while others that could be activated by weak or strong articular stimuli, were excited best by noxious stimuli. Still other neurons were only activated by noxious stimuli. In several instances, contralateral receptive fields were noted in deep tissue or in the knee joint (Schaible et al., 1987). Thus stimuli from different receptive fields are integrated to a combined sensory response to limb position and motion, and it is important to remember that the role of joint receptors during locomotion cannot be considered in isolation.

PROPRIOCEPTION

In the experiments of Ferrell et al. (1985) on cat knee joints, injection of local anaesthetic produced gross abnormalities of posture and gait in half of the animals while all animals had reduced motor activities. Thus, nerve receptors around the joint seem to play a significant role in joint position sense and regulation of posture and movement – a hypothesis subsequently been confirmed by Ferrell and Smith (1987, 1989) in their clinical experiments on fingers. A digital nerve block impairs the ability to match the position of the target finger, and full extension of that finger leads to hyperextension of the anaesthetized digit. However the singular contribution of joint afferents to position sense is not clear. Meanwhile Ferrell et al. (1987) demonstrated a marked reduction in performance with joint anaesthesia only, suggesting that joint receptors alone can play an important role in proprioception, Clark et al. (1989) could not confirm these findings using a similar test protocol. On the other hand Edin and Johansson (1995) demonstrated that skin afferents alone give adequate information about joint position. It seems logical that the more numerous skin afferents would contribute more to joint position awareness than the few joint afferents.

EFFECTS OF SIGNALING ON TARGET ORGANS

MUSCLES

Joint afferents play a role in muscle activation pattern and motoneuron excitability (Baxendale et al., 1987) and contribute to postural reflex regulation of limb muscle tone

(Freeman and Wyke, 1966; Johansson *et al.*, 1991). Skeletomotor neurons (α moto-neurons) are only weakly influenced by low-threshold mechanoreceptors in knee ligaments, while the effects on the γ-muscle-spindle are so potent that even ligament stretches at low loads may induce major changes in the response of the spindle afferents (Johansson *et al.*, 1991). Since the primary afferents of muscle spindles play a role in regulating muscle stiffness, ligament receptors may contribute, via the γ-muscle-spindle system, to prepara-tory adjustment (presetting) of the stiffness of muscles around the knee joint, and thereby to joint stiffness and functional joint stability (Johansson *et al.*, 1991). Activation of joint afferents by joint movement has a positive feedback action on knee extensor and flexor muscles. According to Grigg *et al.* (1978) vasti motoneurons are excited and biceps/semitendinosus motoneurons inhibited by knee extension. Joint denervation disturbs quadri-ceps motoneurons activities for up to 1 year (Freeman and Wyke, 1966). These changes in hind-limb reflexes were found to be strictly ipsilateral following posterior articular neurec-tomy, but were sometimes bilateral after medial articular neurectomy. Massive injection of saline into the joint (200 ml) which stretches the joint capsule and thus activates its recep-tors, prevents patients from using quadriceps to lift the heel independent of pain (de Andrade *et al.*, 1965). With a lesser joint infusion (60 ml saline) a 30–50% inhibition of the reflex-evoked, quadriceps contraction was observed (Kennedy *et al.*, 1982). A linear correlation existed between the volume of fluid injected and the extent of inhibition. Inhibition was completely blocked by the intraarticular injection of 10 ml of Lidocaine. The most dramatic inhibition was observed in vastus medialis, where there the extent of inhibi-tion remained undiminished for 30 min after a 60 ml joint infusion (Kennedy *et al.*, 1982).

BONE

Osteoblasts are equipped with receptors to CGRP, VIP, noradrenaline (NA), and NPY and use cAMP as the transducer. The neurohormones stimulate or inhibit cyclic AMP-formation in osteoblasts and thus may have a role in regulating their activity (Bjurholm *et al.*, 1988b, 1992). CGRP has a dose-dependent osteogenic stimulating effect on bone marrow cells *in vitro* (Bernard and Shih, 1990). VIP and IL-1 enhance bone resorption *in vitro*, whereas CGRP inhibits resorption (Bjurholm, 1989). Significantly, IL-1 is also known to stimulate immune responses. Its presence in bone marrow nerves among immunocompe-tent cells may reflect a neuronal regulation of the immune system. The role of other trans-mitters identified in bone, i.e. SP, NPY and TH remains obscure and may be confined to sensory mediation and vasoregulation. However, the predominance of nerves in regions of high osteogenic activity, such as the epiphyseal osteochondral junction and the perios-teum may reflect neuronal involvement in bone differentiation and development (Bjurholm, 1989). Moreover, in osteoblastic cell lines, NPY inhibits cAMP formation induced by NA and parathormone, suggesting an interaction between local neuropeptides and a systemic calcium regulating hormone (Bjurholm, 1989; Bjurholm *et al.*, 1988b).

BLOOD CIRCULATION

Beta 1-adrenoreceptors in the joint capsule are involved in regulating the sympathetic control of blood flow in the rabbit knee joint (Najafipour and Ferrell, 1993). Section of the posterior articular nerve increases the blood flow to the posterior aspect of the joint capsule (Ferrell *et al.*, 1993). NPY and norepinephrine (NE) causes intraosseous vaso-constriction suggesting that they act as sympathetic neurotransmitters in the control of vascular tone in bone (Lindblad *et al.*, 1994).

NERVOUS FUNCTION IN INJURY AND DISEASE

Type II mechanoreceptors disappear gradually during the first 12 months after ACL rupture and no free nerve endings or mechanoreceptors are present in the ligament stump after 1 year (Denti *et al.*, 1994). Nevertheless, there is evidence that nerves reappear after ligament reconstruction (Aune *et al.*, 1996). During the first 2 weeks after replacing the rat ACL with a patellar tendon graft, the graft did not show any immunoreactivity for nerves. From 4–16 weeks, the insertions and superficial parts of the ligament showed immunore-activity for protein gene product 9.5, growth associated protein 43/B-50, and CGRP. Transection of the ACL, with the ensuing increase in joint laxity, had no immediate effect on the responsiveness of capsule afferents (Khalsa and Grigg, 1996), suggesting that liga-ment injury does not alter the nervous output of the joint. However, when articular nerves were also transected, osteoarthritic changes were more pronounced than after ACL tran-section alone (O'Connor *et al.*, 1992). Transection of articular nerves with an intact liga-ment did not cause knee joint osteoarthritis.

Nerve fibres immunoreactive to SP, CGRP, NPY and TH have been reported among differentiating chondroblasts at an early stage of ectopic bone formation (Bjurholm, 1989) and during fracture healing (Hukkanen *et al.*, 1993). IL-1 immunoreactive nerve fibres have also been observed during ectopic bone formation, especially in marrow and sur-rounding fibrous tissue (Kreicbergs *et al.*, 1995).

There is accumulating evidence that both the sensory and sympathetic nervous systems are affected in inflammatory joint disease, but some controversy whether their expression increases or decreases. Ahmed *et al.* (1995a,b) reported increased levels of SP, CGRP and NPY in synovium and bone marrow in adjuvant arthritis, but little change in the levels of VIP. In contrast, Da Silva *et al.* (1996) found levels of SP, CGRP, neuropeptide tyrosine, and TH in periarticular tissue, epiphysis and synovium significantly reduced in arthritic rats. After arthritis subsided, there was progressive reinnervation of all articular structures often beyond normal levels (Da Silva *et al.*, 1996). It is also unclear whether their change in number is a cause or rather a consequence of the disease.

SUMMARY

Most joint structures except for avascular cartilaginous tissues are richly innervated. With silver and gold stain techniques or other general neuronal markers, different mechano-receptors and free nerve endings can be differentiated in joint soft tissues. With immunohis-tochemical methods using antibodies against a number of neuropeptides, joints structures including bone have been shown to have a rich sensory (substance P, calcitonin gene-related peptide) and autonomic (tyrosine hydroxylase, vasoactive intestinal polypeptide) innerva-tion. There is evidence that joint sensory innervation plays a role in regulating muscle reflex activity, muscle and joint stiffness and the awareness of joint position, and thus is important in protecting synovial joints. Neuropeptides may also influence developmental processes at joint epiphyses and bone remodelling, but it is unclear whether they influence the structure of soft tissues such as cartilage, ligament, tendon and meniscus. Neuropeptide activity may also be involved in degenerative and inflammatory joint disease.

ACKNOWLEDGEMENTS

Supported by grants from the Swedish Medical Research Council (10396), the Swedish National Center for Research in Sports, and the Swedish Society for Medical Research.

REFERENCES

Ahmed, M., Bjurholm, A., Kreicbergs, A. and Schultzberg, M. (1993a) Sensory and autonomic innervation of the facet joint in the rat lumbar spine. *Spine*, **18**, 2121–2126.

Ahmed, M., Bjurholm, A., Kreicbergs, A. and Schultzberg, M. (1993b) Neuropeptide Y, tyrosine hydroxylase and vasoactive intestinal polypeptide-immunoreactive nerve fibres in the vertebral bodies, discs, dura mater, and spinal ligaments of the rat lumbar spine. *Spine*, **18**, 268–273.

Ahmed, M., Bjurholm, A., Schultzberg, M., Theodorsson, E. and Kreicbergs, A. (1995a) Increased levels of substance P and calcitonin gene-related peptide in rat adjuvant arthritis. A combined immunohistochemical and radioimmunoassay analysis. *Arthritis Rheum.*, **38**, 699–709.

Ahmed, M., Bjurholm, A., Theodorsson, E., Schultzberg, M. and Kreicbergs, A. (1995b) Neuropeptide Y- and vasoactive intestinal polypeptide-like immunoreactivity in adjuvant arthritis: Effects of capsain treatment. *Neuropeptides*, **29**, 33–43.

Albright, D., Zimny, M.L. and Dabezies, E. (1987) Mechanoreceptors in the human medial meniscus. *Anat. Rec.*, **218**, 6A–7A.

Aloisi, A.M., Carli, G. and Rossi, A. (1988) Response of hip joint afferent fibres to pressure and vibration in the cat. *Neuroscience Letters*, **90**, 130–134.

Andrew, B.L. (1954) The sensory innervation of the medial ligament of the knee joint. *J. Physiol.*, **123**, 241–250.

Andrew, B.L. and Dodt, E. (1953) The development of sensory nerve endings at the knee joint of the cat. *Acta. Phys. Scand.*, **28**, 287–296.

Aune, A.K., Hukkanen, M., Madsen, J.E., Polak, J.M. and Nordsletten, L. (1996) Nerve regeneration during patellar tendon autograft remodelling after anterior cruciate ligament reconstruction: An experimental and clinical study. *J. Orthop. Res.*, **14**, 193–199.

Baxendale, R.H., Ferrell, W.R. and Wood, L. (1987) The effect of mechanical stimulation of knee joint afferents on quadriceps motor unit activity in the decerebrated cat. *Brain Res.*, **415**, 353–356.

Bernard, G.W. and Shih, C. (1990) The osteogenic stimulating effect of neuroactive calcitonin gene-related peptide. *Peptides*, **11**, 625–632.

Biedert, R.M., Stauffer, E. and Friederich, N.F. (1992) Occurrence of free nerve endings in the soft tissue of the knee joint. A histologic investigation. *Am. J. Sports Med.*, **20**, 430–433.

Bjurholm, A. (1989) Neuroendocrine peptides in bone. Thesis, Stockholm.

Bjurholm, A., Kreicbergs, A., Brodin, E. and Schulzberg, M. (1988a) Substance P- and CGRP-immunoreactive nerves in bone. *Peptides*, **9**, 165–171.

Bjurholm, A., Kreicbergs, A., Schulzberg, M. and Lerner, U.H. (1988b) Parathyroid hormone and noradrena-line-induced enhancement of cyclic AMP in a cloned osteogenic sarcoma cell line (UMR 106) is inhibited by neuropeptide Y. *Acta. Physiol. Scand.*, **134**, 451–452.

Bjurholm, A., Kreicbergs, A., Terenius, L., Goldstein, M. and Schultzberg, M. (1988c) Neuropeptide Y-, tyrosine hydroxylase- and vasoactive intestinal polypeptide-immunoreactive nerves in bone and surrounding tissues. *J. Autonom. Nerv. Syst.*, **25**, 119–125.

Bjurholm, A., Kreicbergs, A., Schulzberg, M. and Lerner, U.H. (1992) Neuroendocrine regulation of cyclic AMP formation in osteoblastic cell lines (UMR-106-01, POS 17/2.8, MC3T3-E1, and Saos-2) and primary bone cells. *J. Bone Miner. Res.*, **7**, 1011–1019.

Bjurholm, A., Ahmed, M., Svensson, S.B., Kreicbergs, A. and Schultzberg, M. (1994) Interleukin-1 immuno-reactive nerve fibres in rat joint synovium. *Clin. Exp. Rheumatol.*, **12**, 583–587.

Boyd, I.A. (1954) The histological structure of the receptors in the knee joint of the cat correlated with their physiological response. *J. Physiol.* (*London*) **124**, 476–488.

Buma, P. (1994) Innervation of the patella. An immunohistochemical study in mice. *Acta Orthop. Scand.*, **65**, 80–86.

Burke, D., Gandevia, S.C. and Macefield, G. (1988) Responses to passive movement of receptors in joint, skin and muscle of the human hand. *J. Physiol.*, **402**, 347–361.

Clark, F.J., Grigg, P. and Chapin, J.W. (1989) The contribution of articular receptors to proprioception with the fingers in humans. *J. Neurophysiol.*, **61**, 186–193.

Da Silva, J.A., Fonseca, J.E., Graca, L., Moita, L. and Carmo-Fonseca, M. (1996) Reinnervation of post-arthritic joints in the rat. *Clin. Exp. Rheumatol.*, **14**, 43–51.

Day, B., MacKenzie, W.G., Shim, S.S. and Leung, G. (1985) The vascular and nerve supply of the human meniscus. *Arthroscopy*, **1**, 58–62.

De Andrade, J.R., Grant, C. and Dixon, A.St.-J. (1965) Joint distension and reflex muscle inhibition in the knee. *J. Bone Joint Surg.*, **47A**, 313–322.

Denti, M., Monteleone, M., Berardi, A. and Schiavone Panni, A. (1994) Anterior cruciate ligament receptors. Histologic studies on lesions and reconstruction. *Clin. Orthop.*, **308**, 29–32.

D'Sousa, M., MacIntyre, I., Girgis, S.I. and Mundy, G.R. (1986) Human synthetic calcitonin gene-related peptide inhibits bone resorption. *Endocrinology*, **119**, 58–61.

Edin, B.B. (1990) Finger joint movement sensitivity of non-cutaneous mechanoreceptor afferents in the human radial nerve. *Exp. Brain Res.*, **82**, 417–422.

Edin, B.B. and Abbs, J.H. (1991) Finger movement responses of cutaneous mechanoreceptors in the dorsal skin of the human hand. *J. Neurophysiol.*, **65**, 657–670.

Edin, B.B. and Johansson, N. (1995) Skin strain patterns provide kinaesthetic information to the human central nervous system. *J. Physiol.*, **487**, 243–251.

Ferrell, W.R. (1980) The adequacy of stretch receptors in the cat knee joint for signalling joint angle throughout a full range of movement. *J. Physiol.*, **299**, 85–99.

Ferrell, W.R., Baxendale, R.H., Carnachan, C. and Hart, I.K. (1985) The influence of joint afferent discharge on locomotion, proprioception and activity in conscious cats. *Brain Res.*, **347**, 41–48.

Ferrell, W.R., Gandevia, S.C. and McCloskey, D.I. (1987) The role of joint receptors in human kinaesthesia when intramuscular receptors cannot contribute. *J. Physiol.*, **386**, 63–71.

Ferrell, W.R., Khoshbaten, A., Angerson, W.J. and Najafipour, H. (1993) Localized neural control of blood flow in the posterior region of the knee joint in anaesthetized rabbits. *Exp. Physiol.*, **78**, 105–108.

Ferrell, W.R. and Smith, A. (1987) The effect of digital nerve block on position sense at the proximal inter-phalangeal joint of the human index finger. *Brain Res.*, **425**, 369–371.

Ferrell, W.R. and Smith, A. (1989) The effect of loading on position sense at the proximal interphalangeal joint of the human index finger. *J. Physiol.*, **418**, 145–161.

Freeman, M.A.R. and Wyke, B. (1966) Articular contribution to limb muscle reflexes. The effects of partial neurectomy of the knee-joint on postural reflexes. *Brit. J. Surg.*, **53**, 61–69.

Freeman, M.A.R. and Wyke, B. (1967) The innervation of the knee joint. An anatomical and histological study in the cat. *J. Anat.*, **101**, 505–532.

Gao, J., Öqvist, G. and Messner, K. (1994) The attachments of the rabbit medial meniscus. A morphological investigation using image analysis and immunohistochemistry. *J. Anat.*, **185**, 663–667.

Grigg, P. and Greenspan, B.J. (1977) Response of primate joint afferent neurons to mechanical stimulation of knee joint. *J. Neurophysiol.*, **40**, 1–8.

Grigg, P., Harrigan, E.P. and Fogarty, K.E. (1978) Segmental reflexes mediated by joint afferent neurons in cat knee. *J. Neurophysiol.*, **41**, 9–14.

Halata, Z. (1975) The mechanoreceptors of the mammalian skin: Ultrastructure and morphological classifi-cation. *Adv. Anat.*, **50**, 1–77.

Halata, Z. (1977) The ultrastructure of he sensory nerve endings in the articular capsule of the knee joint of the domestic cat (Ruffini corpuscles and Pacinian corpuscles). *J. Anat.*, **124**, 717–729.

Halata, Z., Badalamente, M.A., Dee, R. and Propper, M. (1984) Ultrastructure of sensory nerve endings in monkey (Macaca fascicularis) knee joint capsule. *J. Orthop. Res.*, **2**, 169–176.

Halata, Z. and Groth. H.-P. (1976) Innervation of the synovial membrane of cat joint capsule. *Cell Tiss. Res.*, **169**, 415–418.

Halata, Z. and Haus, J. (1989) The ultrastructure of sensory nerve endings in human anterior cruciate ligament. *Anat. Embryol.*, **179**, 415–421.

Halata, Z. and Munger, B.L. (1980a) Sensory nerve endings in rhesus monkey sinus hairs. *J. Comp. Neurol.*, **192**, 645–663.

Halata, Z. and Munger, B.L. (1980b) The sensory innervation of primate eyelid. *Anat. Rec.*, **198**, 657–670.

Halata, Z. and Munger, B.L. (1983) The sensory innervation of primate facial skin. II. Vermilion border and mucosa of the lip. *Brain Res. Rev.*, **5**, 81–107.

Hashimoto, T., Hamada, T., Sasaguri, Y. and Suzuki, K. (1994) Immunohistochemical approach for the investigation of nerve distribution in the shoulder joint capsule. *Clin. Orthop.*, **305**, 273–282.

Hedberg, A., Messner, K., Persliden, J. and Hildebrand, C. (1995) Transient local presence of nerve fibres at onset of secondary ossification in the rat knee joint. *Anat. Embryol.*, **192**, 247–255.

Hohmann, E.L., Levine, L. and Tashjian, A.H. Jr. (1983) Vasoactive intestinal peptide stimulates bone resorption via a cyclic adenosine 3',5'-monophosphate-dependent mechanism. *Endocrinology*, **112**, 1233–1239.

Hukkanen, M., Konttinen, Y.T., Santavirta, S., Paavolainen, P., Gu, X.-H., Terenghi, G. and Polak, J.M. (1993) Rapid proliferation of calcitonin gene-related peptide-immunoreactive nerves during healing of rat tibial fracture suggests neural involvement in bone growth and remodelling. *Neuroscience*, **54**, 969–979.

Iwasaki, A., Inoue, K. and Hukuda, S. (1995) Distribution of neuropeptide-containing nerve fibres in the synovium and adjacent bone of the rat knee joint. *Clin. Exp. Rheumatol.*, **13**, 173–178.

Johansson, H., Sjölander, P. and Sojka, P. (1991) Receptors in the knee joint ligaments and their role in the biomechanics of the joint. *Crit. Rev. Biomed. Engineering*, **18**, 341–368.

Kennedy, J.C., Alexander, I.J. and Hayes, K.C. (1982) Nerve supply of the human knee and its functional importance. *Am. J. Sports Med.*, **10**, 329–335.

Khalsa, P.S. and Grigg, P. (1996) Responses of mechanoreceptor neurons in the cat knee joint capsule before and after anterior cruciate ligament transection. *J. Orthop. Res.*, **14**, 114–122.

Klineberg, I., Greenfield, B.E. and Wyke, B. (1970) Afferent discharges from temporomandibular articular mechanoreceptors: An experimental study in the cat. *Arch. Oral. Biol.*, **15**, 935–952.

Krauspe, R., Schmidt, M. and Schaible, H.-G. (1992) Sensory innervation of the anterior cruciate ligament. *J. Bone Joint Surg.*, **74A**, 390–397.

Kreicbergs, A., Ahmed, M., Ehrnberg, A., Schultzberg, M., Svenson, S.B. and Bjurholm, A. (1995) Interleukin-1 immunoreactive nerves in heterotopic bone induced by DBM. *Bone*, **17**, 341–345.

Lindblad, B.E., Nielsen, L.B., Jespersen, S.M., Bjurholm, A., Bunger, C. and Hansen, E.S. (1994) Vasoconstrictive action of neuropeptide Y in bone. The porcine tibia perfused *in vivo*. *Acta Orthop. Scand.*, **65**, 629–634.

Lindström, S. and Takata, M. (1972) Monosynaptic excitation of dorsal spinocerebellar tract neurones from low threshold joint afferents. *Acta Physiol. Scand.*, **84**, 430–432.

Lundberg, A. and Oscarsson, O. (1960) Functional organization of the dorsal spino-cerebellar tract in the cat. VII. Identification of units by antidromic activation from the cerebellar cortex with recognition of five subdivisions. *Acta Physiol. Scand.*, **50**, 356–374.

Michelson, J.D. and Hutchins, C. (1995) Mechanoreceptors in human ankle ligaments. *J. Bone Joint Surg.*, **77B**, 219–224.

Millar, J. (1975) Flexion-extension sensitivity of elbow joint afferents in cat. *Exp. Brain Res.*, **24**, 209–214.

Najafipour, H. and Ferrell, W.R. (1993) Sympathetic innervation and beta-adrenoceptor profile of blood vessels in the posterior region of the rabbit knee joint. *Exp. Physiol.*, **78**, 625–637.

O'Connor, B.L. (1984) The mechanoreceptor innervation of the posterior attachments of the lateral meniscus of the dog knee joint. *J. Anat.*, **138**, 15–26.

O'Connor, B.L., Visco, D.M., Brandt, K.D., Myers, S.L. and Kalasinski, L.A. (1992) Neurogenic acceleration of osteoarthrosis. *J. Bone Joint Surg.*, **74A**, 367–376.

O'Connor, B.L. and McConnaughey, J.S. (1978) The structure and innervation of cat knee menisci, and their relation to a "sensory hypothesis" of meniscal function. *Am. J. Anat.*, **153**, 431–442.

Polacek, P. (1966) Receptors of the joints: Their structure, variability and classification. *Acta. Facultat. Med. Universität Brunensis*, **23**, 1–107.

Poyner, D.R. (1992) Calcitonin gene-related peptide: multiple actions, multiple receptors. *Pharmacol. Ther.*, **56**, 23–51.

Reimann, I. and Bach Christensen, S. (1977) A histological demonstration of nerves in subchondral bone. *Acta Orthop. Scand.*, **48**, 345–352.

Salo, P.T. and Tatton, W.G. (1993) Age-related loss of knee joint afferents in mice. *J. Neurosci. Res.*, **35**, 664–677.

Schaible, H.-G., Schmidt, R.F. and Willis, W.D. (1986) Responses of spinal cord neurones to stimulation of articular afferent fibres in the cat. *J. Physiol.*, **372**, 575–593.

Schaible, H.-G., Schmidt, R.F. and Willis, W.D. (1987) Convergent inputs from articular, cutaneous and muscle receptors onto ascending tract cells in the cat spinal cord. *Exp. Brain Res.*, **66**, 479–488.

Schutte, M.J., Dabezies, M.L., Zimny, M.L. and Happel, L.T. (1987) Neural anatomy of the human anterior cruciate ligament. *J. Bone Joint Surg.*, **69A**, 243–247.

Sharkey, K.A. and Bray, R.C. (1990) Innervation patterns of collateral knee ligaments as revealed by silver staining and immunohistochemistry. *Somatic and Visceral afferents III:* Soc. Neurosci. Abst., **16**, 882

Skoglund, S. (1956) Anatomical and physiological studies of knee joint innervation in the cat. *Acta Physiol. Scand.*, **36**, suppl. 124

Takahashi, S. (1995) Pacinian corpuscles in the articular capsule of the mouse knee joint, with special reference to postnatal development. *Hokkaido Jgaku Zasshi*, **70**, 159–173.

Wilson, A.S., Legg, P.G. and McNeur, J.C. (1969) Studies on the innervation of the medial meniscus in the human knee joint. *Anat. Rec.*, **165**, 485–492.

Wood, L. and Ferrell, W.R. (1984) Response of slowly adapting articular mechanoreceptors in the cat knee joint to alterations in intra-articular volume. *Ann. Rheuma. Dis.*, **43**, 327–332.

Zaidi, M., Fuller, K., Bevis, P.J.R., Gaines Das, R.E., Chambers, T.J. and MacIntyre, I. (1987a) Calcitonin gene-related peptide inhibits osteoclastic bone resorption: a comparative study. *Calcif. Tissue Int.*, **40**, 149–154.

Zaidi, M., Chambers, T.J., Gaines Das, R.E., Morris, H.R. and MacIntyre, I. (1987b) A direct action of human calcitonin gene-related peptide on isolated osteoclasts. *J. Endocrinol.*, **115**, 511–518.

Zimny, M.L.(1988) Mechanoreceptors in articular tissue. *Am. J. Anat.*, **182**, 16–32.

Zimny, M.L., Schutte, M. and Dabezies, E. (1986) Mechanoreceptors in the human anterior cruciate ligament. *Anat. Rec.*, **214**, 204–209.

Zimny, M.L. and St.Onge, M. (1987) Mechanoreceptors in the temporomandibular articular disc. *J. Dent. Res.*, **66**, 237.

Section 7
Clinical Aspects

26 An Anatomical Approach to the Understanding of Clinical Problems in the Shoulder

Richard L.M. Newell

Connective Tissue Biology Labs, Cardiff School of Biosciences,
University of Wales Cardiff, PO Box 911, Cardiff CF1 3US, UK

This contribution is designed to provide those readers whose background is non-medical with a practical introduction to clinical disorders commonly arising in major synovial joints and their surrounding tissues. The shoulder complex is used as the example. The approach is essentially anatomical, identifying common areas of pathological change. The clinical diagnosis and management of individual disorders are not discussed in depth, and less weighting is given to problems associated with acute injury – fractures, dislocations – than would be indicated by their clinical prevalence. The presentation is not intended as an exposition of new or original work.

THE EVOLUTIONARY AND FUNCTIONAL SIGNIFICANCE OF THE SHOULDER

In the Primates, one of the most important, if not *the* most important, musculoskeletal organ in the body is the hand. In terms of its relative physical size, the hand has a dispro-portionately large area of functional representation in both the motor and sensory areas of the cerebral cortex. Loss of a hand is a major deficit for any Primate, but is an espe-cially severe disability for humans. Taking a teleological point of view, the 'purpose' of a shoulder is to move the hand around freely in space and to provide a stable base while the hand is in use. Thus the importance of the shoulder, while secondary to that of the hand, is great, and differs markedly from that of the hip, whose function lies largely in bearing weight. Animals in which all four limbs have essentially the same function, as weight-bearing props, do not have 'hands' or 'shoulders' in the human sense.

THE ANATOMY OF THE 'SHOULDER COMPLEX'

When the human lower limb is moved as a whole in respect to the trunk, the movement may be considered for practical purposes as occurring at a single, large ball-and-socket synovial joint, the hip joint. Movement of the upper limb as a whole is different, as it must include movement of the components of the pectoral girdle – the clavicle (collar-bone) and the scapula (shoulder-blade). It is important to realise at the outset that the 'shoulder' in lay terms does not equate with the anatomical shoulder joint or gleno-humeral joint by which the 'ball', or head, of the humerus articulates with the 'socket' or glenoid fossa of the scapula. Movements which appear to take place 'at the shoulder' actually involve a complex of five functional 'joints'. Firstly there are the three true synovial joints of the pectoral girdle, represented in the human by the glenohumeral joint, between humerus and scapula, and the synovial joints at either end of the clavicle – the sternoclavicular and acromioclavicular joints. Secondly, there is movement of the body of the scapula (the actual shoulder 'blade') over the chest wall at the intermuscular plane which constitutes the scapulothoracic or axioscapular 'joint'. Finally, the non-articular part of the proximal humerus – the tubercles to which the smaller shoulder-muscles are attached – moves smoothly beneath a sleeve of larger muscles and beneath the acromion process of the scapula (felt as the bony 'point of the shoulder') as the limb is positioned in space. This movement takes place at the subacromial 'joint', a synovially-lined bursa. All of these components of the shoulder complex may be affected, separately or together, by disease or injury.

THE CLINICAL PRESENTATION OF
SHOULDER PROBLEMS

A patient may present for medical diagnosis and treatment in a variety of ways. These may largely be classified into acute or emergency presentation, often as a result of injury or medical 'collapse', and elective or non-emergency presentation in which the patient has time to think about the condition and formally to visit or consult the medical practitioner.

Patients commonly present electively to family physicians, orthopaedic surgeons, rheumatologists, and to a wide range of heterodox or alternative medical practitioners with symptoms arising in and around the shoulder. It is important to realise that though the patient may present with a "shoulder problem" – for example, pain in the shoulder – the causative pathology may in many cases be physically distant from the shoulder itself. Between a fifth and a quarter of patients presenting to specialist shoulder clinics turn out to have cervical spine (neck) problems, usually degenerative or osteoarthritic in nature. Pain can also be referred to the shoulder from thoracic and abdominal viscera, especially those structures anatomically related (lying next to) the diaphragm. However, the major-ity of patients who have located their problem in and around the shoulder are correct in this location, though the primary pathology usually lies in the musculoskeletal soft tissues of the region rather than in bone or cartilage.

TYPE OF PROBLEM – PATHOLOGICAL DIAGNOSIS

In basic terms, the pathological conditions which affect the shoulder joint are the same as those which can affect any synovial joint. It is the relative clinical importance of each condition which differs from joint to joint. For example, in quantitative terms, osteoarthritis is a major source of symptoms in both hip and knee, but a minor one in the shoulder.

Pathological conditions of any structure in the body can broadly be classified according to a useful working and teaching schema called 'the surgical sieve'. This is usually expressed thus:

1. Congenital conditions – present at birth
2. Acquired conditions – those not present at birth but acquired during post-natal life.
   These can be subdivided into:
   Traumatic
   Inflammatory
   Infective
   Neoplastic – benign and malignant
   Metabolic
   Degenerative
   Miscellaneous

Those groups of conditions *commonly* affecting the shoulder are highlighted.

MODE OF PRESENTATION

The symptoms with which patients complain of their "shoulder" may be grouped as shown below. The same grouping applies to patients presenting with acute injuries, though the time course and degree of urgency of presentation will differ according to circumstance:

Pain
Disorders of movement
– limited movement (stiffness)
– excessive movement (laxity)
– abnormal movement (instability)
Deformity

The three major groups may present singly or in combination. The absolute and relative severity of the symptoms, together with the natural history of their onset, will help determine the diagnosis in the individual case.

Let us pursue the commonest 'synovial joint' symptoms, pain and stiffness, in relation to the shoulder.

THE ANATOMICAL SOURCE OF THE PAIN

In any clinical problem, an accurate pathological diagnosis must be preceded by anatomical localisation of the symptoms. In general terms, if a patient complains of pain 'in the hip', once an anatomically remote source of pain (such as the spine) is excluded, then the cause of the pain is likely to be found within the hip joint itself and is likely directly to involve the articular surfaces. In the adult patient, the pathology is likely to be an 'arthritis', usually degenerative (osteoarthritis) or, much less commonly, inflammatory (rheumatoid arthritis). If the complaint is pain 'in the shoulder' however, then, again having excluded a remote source, the cause of the pain is much more likely to be found in the soft tissues which surround the glenohumeral joint than within the joint and directly involving articular cartilage and subchondral bone.

THE CAUSE OF THE STIFFNESS

The bony configuration of the shoulder joint is such that inherent skeletal stability is minimal. The socket is small and shallow when compared with the incomplete ball with which it articulates. Contrast the hip joint, in which a relatively small and complete ball is held very firmly in a deep bony socket – so deeply that a definite 'suction effect' comes into play. In the hip, osteoarthritis, often with concomitant peripheral osteophyte formation, is common, and the joint stiffens in part as a result of the ball becoming entrapped in the socket. This is especially the case in the *protrusio* configuration of arthritis of the hip. In the shoulder, though moderate osteoarthritic changes are often found radiologically or at post-mortem, the condition rarely presents as a clinical problem and the anatomical configuration of the joint is not conducive to osteophytic entrapment of the humeral head as a cause of stiffness.

Restriction of movement in the shoulder is much more likely to result from pathological changes in the collagenous structures which surround and form part of the glenohumeral joint, and in the tendons of muscles whose efficient working determines the functional integrity of the 'subacromial' joint. These changes are usually degenerative and inflammatory.

In order to understand this localisation of pathology more fully, one needs to appreciate the three-dimensional anatomy of the shoulder complex and in particular that of the glenohumeral joint.

ANATOMY FROM WITHOUT AND ANATOMY FROM WITHIN

Recent understanding of the anatomy of the shoulder complex in health and disease has advanced considerably as a result of the advent and development of new investigative techniques. These techniques are both non-interventional – such as modern imaging, especially using magnetic resonance (MRI) – and interventional or surgical, such as arthroscopy. The latter has also undergone rapid advance as a therapeutic technique, much shoulder surgery now being accomplished endoscopically.

Many anatomical structures within the glenohumeral and 'subacromial' joints have assumed new importance after many years of descriptive neglect in the anatomical texts.

MUSCLES WHICH MOVE THE SHOULDER COMPLEX

The clinical and functional understanding of these muscles owes much to the work of the late Lipmann Kessel of the Royal National Orthopaedic Hospital in London.

Kessel grouped the muscles acting on the shoulder into those concerned in the main with axioscapular movement – the rotation of the scapula on the chest wall – and those concerned primarily with glenohumeral movements. The muscles which act in concert to rotate the scapula as the limb is abducted (lifted away from the body) are the trapezius and the serratus anterior. These muscles may be involved in neuromuscular conditions, but are not directly involved in the more common degenerative and inflammatory disorders leading to pain and limitation of movement at the shoulder.

The muscles acting on the glenohumeral joint may be considered (Kessel) as two 'sleeves', the outer (more superficial) and larger being incomplete while the inner (deeper) and smaller sleeve is a complete one running from scapula to humerus. The movement of the outer sleeve over the inner depends upon the efficient action of the subacromial bursa in its rôle as a functional 'joint' of the shoulder complex. Thus any pathological condition which involves this bursa (subacromial bursitis, impingement syndromes) will adversely affect movement of the limb.

The outer, larger sleeve consists mainly of the deltoid muscle, while the inner musculotendinous sleeve constitutes the 'rotator cuff' of four scapulohumeral muscles. The supraspinatus runs superiorly to the head of the humerus, the subscapularis anteriorly, and the infraspinatus and teres minor muscles run posteriorly.

These four muscles work in a coordinated fashion both to move the humerus (three of them to rotate it, hence the 'rotator' cuff, while supraspinatus initiates abduction).

The superior part of this cuff – largely consisting of the supraspinatus tendon as it fuses with the joint capsule and with a superiorly-placed ligament, the coracohumeral ligament – is the site of some of the commonest degenerative pathology in the shoulder. As the tendon runs beneath the acromion process of the scapula it forms the 'floor' of the subacromial bursa. At this point the tendon is both mechanically vulnerable and subject to vascular compromise. There is said to be an area of limited vascular supply between those parts of the tendon supplied by the suprascapular artery and those supplied by the circumflex humerals. Codman termed this the 'critical area', and it is here that supraspinatus tendon rupture usually occurs.

Another muscle not to be neglected is biceps brachii, the tendon of whose long head runs right 'through' the glenohumeral joint on its way to the scapula. It travels in its own synovial sheath, and is tightly applied to the head of the abducted humerus helping to stabilise it superiorly. It forms an important arthroscopic 'landmark'. This tendon may be involved both in inflammatory and degenerative arthritides, and attrition rupture may occur where the tendon angles over the lateral margin of the head of the humerus. The tendon attaches proximally (at its scapular end) to the glenoid labrum, a fibrocartilaginous structure attached to the perimeter of the glenoid fossa, inside the capsular attachment. This labrum deepens the glenoid socket to some extent, thereby increasing glenohumeral stability. Traumatic tears of this labrum are responsible for the commonest form of recurrent dislocation of the shoulder.

THE GLENOHUMERAL CAPSULE AND ITS REINFORCING LIGAMENTS

As in all synovial joints, the articulating bones of the glenohumeral joint are connected by a fibrous capsule lined with synovium. This glenohumeral capsule is not of uniform thickness. It is thickest superiorly, where it is reinforced both by the supraspinatus tendon and by the coracohumeral ligament, and thinnest inferiorly where its relative laxity allows maximal abduction of the humerus. The capsule also has three variable thickenings anteriorly, the glenohumeral ligaments. It is increasingly believed that the primary pathology in the commonly occurring painful and stiff 'frozen shoulder' is a collagenous disorder causing contracture of this capsule. The rediscovery and further elucidation of the detailed anatomy of the capsule, the glenohumeral ligaments, and their attachments have led to the recent development of a reasoned and practical approach to the understanding of multidirectional shoulder instability.

DISORDERS OF SUBSIDIARY JOINTS OF THE SHOULDER COMPLEX

The clavicle articulates medially with the sternum or breastbone, and at its lateral end with the acromion process of the scapula. In each case a synovial joint, with the characteristic components of such a joint, is present. Both joints are subject to traumatic dislocation or subluxation (incomplete dislocation), the acromiothoracic more commonly than the sternoclavicular. Both may also be the site of degenerative and inflammatory arthritides which can present as painful limitation of shoulder movement.

FURTHER READING

Kessel, Lipmann (1982) *Clinical Disorders of the Shoulder.* Edinburgh: Churchill Livingstone.

27 Clinical Problems Associated with the Hand and Forearm

P.J. Mulligan

Research and Teaching Centre, Royal Orthopaedic Hospital,
The Woodlands, Northfield, Birmingham B31 2AP, UK

This chapter describes some of the clinical features of the rheumatoid hand and wrist determined by synovial change. In rheumatoid disease, tissue destruction in the hand leads to well recognised deformity. The intra-articular destruction of cartilage and the sub-condylar bone form the expected radiological changes. Much of the deformity is brought about by the attenuation and rupture of the joint capsule, ligaments and tendons. These structures both stabilise and mobilise, joints and thus the deformity is early, progressive and devastating. Much of it seems to occur with only minor intra-articular pathological change. Recognition of these destructive forces allows correction to be undertaken so that function can be maintained and deformity prevented. The functions of the wrist and finger joints are highly interdependent. There is a delicate balance of forces across the joint which, if disturbed, will lead to deformity and loss of function. This balance depends on the integrity of the capsule, ligaments and tendons that support the joint (Riordan and Fowler, 1958; Flatt, 1974; Clayton, 1989; Nalebuff, 1983).

From the clinical viewpoint, the patient may be aware of variable amounts of pain, weakness and the cosmetic effect of the deformity. The management of pain and synovial activity has become much more successful by the better application of drug therapy (Sones, 1971; Ferlic *et al.*, 1983). Loss of function and weakness impact strongly on the quality of daily life, and improving this is a major goal of surgery. The severity of the deformity can be well advanced and easily seen. Most rheumatoid patients have an understanding of their condition and do not ask for cosmetic improvement as a priority. If the appearance is bettered by the surgery, then this is also a pleasing feature and a well received bonus (Brewerton, 1971; Kucynski, 1971; Swanson *et al.*, 1973).

FINGER SYNOVITIS

Active synovitis cannot be cured by surgery. Surgery is for those tissues not responding to drug therapy, though occasionally, a single 'rogue' joint may fail to respond to therapy. Surgery is also necessary for reconstruction in the presence of imbalance and the stabilising or replacement of joints (Boyes, 1969; Brewerton 1971). In relation to imbalance, the metacarpophalangeal (MCP) joints are frequently recognised as a classic rheumatoid deformity. There is ulnar drift which can progress to volar subluxation of the proximal phalanges so that the metacarpal heads present their full contour and the fingers cannot function. The tendons crossing the joint have little effect on what will become floppy fingers. The attenuation of the capsule and collateral ligaments is only one of the factors. Synovitis in the joint disturbs the function of the dorsal hood of the extensor apparatus and the balance of extensor function is affected by neuropathy or ischaemia of the intrinsic muscles. The natural pull of the strong extensor and flexor tendons is towards ulnar drift and this is now uncontrolled in the rheumatoid hand (Flatt, 1966; Wilson and Carlbolm, 1989). The effect of this is enhanced by the frequent presence of radial-carpal tilt. This is subsequent to unconstrained tightness on the radial side of the carpus, and destruction of the ulnar restraining ligaments on the ulnar side is a common feature of the disease (Shapiro, 1968; Smith and Kaplan, 1967). Even before the skin is incised, the extensor tendon can be seen lying in the ulnar gutter rather than centrally across the metacarpal head (Smith and Kaplan, 1967; Stack and Vaughan-Jackson, 1971). As soon as this is recognised clinically, there is no possible correction other than surgical. Referral to a hand clinic should take place immediately and should not be delayed until the deformity is too severe. At operation, there is gross stretching of the dorsal radial capsule and hood. The proximal phalanges lie volar to the metacarpal heads and frequently there is secondary destruction of the dorsum of the proximal phalanges, adding to some of the difficulty in tightness in soft tissue reconstruction. Intrinsic muscles are tight and should be released and sometimes transferred. The standard procedure is to undertake joint replacements – the commonest is the sylastic Swanson replacement (Swanson, 1972; Millender and Nalebuff, 1973a) that has been available for 25 years or more and which produces good results. The amount of movement is variable, but that is not important if the strength, pain and deformity are corrected – as is frequently the case. Enhanced movement depends not only on the surgery but also on excellent post-operative rehabilitation.

It is interesting that besides the problems associated with the MCP joints, there is frequent deformity of the proximal interphalangeal (PIP) joints (Nalebuff, 1969a; Nalebuff and Potter, 1968). Some of these deformities are at an early stage and are secondary to the changes in the MCP joint. Correction of the deformity of the MCP joint can in itself correct the PIP joint deformity at an early stage. The reverse is never true. Swan's neck deformity has been described in several stages which are progressive. In the early condition the joint is still mobile and the deformity is secondary to loss of strength in the function of flexor digitorum superficialis or overtightness of the intrinsic tendon, or a combination of these. There are a number of other factors which are important as this deformity progresses (Nalebuff and Millender, 1975a; Gainor and

Hummel, 1985). In the early stage the release of the intrinsic tendons by manipulation or surgical release can be enough to correct the deformity. Further than this, surgical release and tenodesis of one lateral band is also helpful and can be very successful. When the deformity is fixed, then arthrodesis of the joints is the most usual outcome (Granowitz and Vainio, 1966). In general terms, the PIP joints in severe rheumatoid disease respond in function to arthrodesis. Joint replacement in the ring and little fingers can certainly be considered but are less successful. The reverse deformity of boutonniere, due to attenuation of the central slip of the extensor tendon, is also present in a number of patients, although less frequently (Souter, 1974; Nalebuff and Millender, 1975b). It is not often caught at an early stage but re-balancing surgery is less successful than it would be post-traumatically. Arthrodesis with the correction is a frequent outcome.

Synovitis along the course of the flexor tendons is common. Patients may present with pain in the hand, restriction of movement or triggering of fingers. It is due to abundant synovial change within the flexor digital sheath running from the head of the metacarpal down to the distal interphalangeal joint. In the early stages of the disease, simple but effective release of the A1 pulley and proximal synovectomy may be enough. Again, more extensive surgery is sometimes required. There is stiffness and the inability to flex the finger fully – either actively or passively. The stiffness can be confirmed by palpation along the length of the finger. Synovectomy is undertaken preserving and, if necessary, reconstructing the annular pulley systems in order to maintain the strength of the flexor pull. Gentle excision of the synovium as it erodes in the tendon and trimming of tendon nodules is also useful. Early and carefully monitored active flexion is required (Nalebuff, 1969b; Millis et al., 1976; Gray and Gottlieb, 1977; Ferlic and Clayton, 1978).

WRIST SYNOVITIS

FLEXOR TENDONS

Abundant synovium swathes the flexor tendons from the palm through the carpal tunnel to the wrist. Patients with wrist synovitis presents not only with pain but also with the symptoms of median nerve compression. Palpation proximal and distal to the carpal tunnel elicits the pain and swelling. It is now uncommon to undertake synovectomy in this area, because of the good response to drug therapy. Decompression of the carpal tunnel is undertaken. Release of the flexor retinaculum alone will bring about change in synovial activity. It is impossible to excise all the synovium present, in fact this is not necessary as good results are achieved without that. Ligament release is a worthwhile procedure and may be regarded as a prophylactic measure (Vainio, 1957; Barnes and Currey, 1967; Dell, 1979; Taleisnik, 1979). It is very rare that tendons which have undergone tenosynovectomy will subsequently rupture. In a number of cases tendons have already ruptured and so tendon graft or transfer can be undertaken, if necessary, to restore function. Rarely it affects only the STT joint (Kellgren and Ball, 1950; Nalebuff, 1975; Ertel et al., 1988).

EXTENSOR TENDONS

Most surgery for rheumatoid disease is undertaken on the dorsal rather than the flexor aspect of the wrist. There is frequent evidence of synovial activity in the wrist. A patient presenting with swelling due to synovitis might already have ruptured extensor tendons. This is well described and begins on the ulnar side of the carpus, involving the extensor tendons to the little and ring fingers and progressively moving across the hand to affect the other digits if left untreated (Nalebuff, 1975). Synovitis of extensor tendons frequently does not respond to drug therapy and if swelling persists for 6 months or more, surgery should be considered (Millender *et al.*, 1973). If there is weakness in the little finger then it is also important to undertake correction and prophylactic measures to prevent the other tendons from rupturing (Nalebuff, 1969c; Nalebuff and Patel, 1973). The surgery is available, interesting and successful. Another aspect of extensor wrist synovitis is the change which occurs in the distal radio-ulnar joint as a consequence of synovial destruction of the restraining ligaments and tendons that in turn leads to subluxation of the head of the ulna (Vaughan-Jackson, 1958). This sometimes leads to erosion in the dorsal capsule of the joint which directly affects the tendons. I think this is more common in osteoarthritis. In rheumatoid arthritis, the tendons have undergone change or progressive attrition and ischaemia. However, excision of the ulnar head is common (Smith Peterson *et al.*, 1943; Mikic and Helal, 1977; Newman, 1987). As a consequence, the supporting mechanism of the triangular fibrocartilage complex on the ulnar side of the carpus may be compromised. However, in most cases, the carpus will stabilise and will not undergo progressive ulnar translocation (Nanchahal *et al.*, 1996).

The synovium may also be active within the radiocarpal and intercarpal joints. Patients who present with swelling at the back of the wrist and deep pain, or even show radiological signs of intercarpal joint destruction, show secondary changes from the synovitis in these joints (Nalebuff and Garrod, 1984). At an early stage, radiological cystic change in the end of the radius or within the carpus indicates synovial activity in the recesses of ligament attachments. As this occurs, the ligaments become attenuated, particularly on the volar side, and there is progressive carpal collapse. The most severe example of this will be complete volar subluxation of the carpus and mid-carpal collapse. In some cases the joints undergo progressive ankylosis. There have been a number of staging classifications of these deformities. In the presence of such deformity, stabilisation of the radiocarpal joint is indicated, again as part of the procedure (Clayton, 1965; Mannerfelt and Malmsten, 1971; Millender and Nalebuff, 1973b). The patient, therefore, may undergo surgery at several levels. The surgery of the radiocarpal joint may be undertaken by a number of different procedures. Most frequently, I use the insertion of staples and this has been very successful (Shapiro, 1987). An assessment of the first 10 years of patients has shown extremely good results in terms of pain relief and function. There have been no serious complications. It allows the other tendon surgery and excision of the ulna head to be undertaken quickly and, under the same tourniquet, there may be time to do surgery to the fingers or the wrist. Rheumatoid patients have many operations (Baloch *et al.*, 1995) and it is good to avoid repetitive surgery. Because of this I think the inter-segmental arthrodesis around the carpus, which is very useful in other areas of carpal stability, is not applicable in rheumatoid disease. This is because further mid-carpal surgery is sometimes required later if a radiocarpal fusion alone is undertaken (Taleisnik, 1984, 1985). In the very unstable wrist, with considerable loss of bone stock, then intra-medullary rodding through the third metacarpal and across the carpus and radius is the procedure of choice. The important factor is to reduce pain and regain strength, and arthrodesis has been well known for this. Retaining wrist movement by wrist joint replacement has been fraught with danger. When successful it can be a happy outcome but because of the current risks of complication (either bio-mechanical failure or sylastic synovitis (Brase and Millender, 1986; Fatti et al., 1986; Menon, 1987), I would not advise this procedure.

The rheumatoid change, if understood and monitored, can present the opportunity for useful and well planned surgery. The presentation of staging of surgery to the rheumatoid patient has been well described. It is normal to do the wrist before the MCP joints and before the fingers. It is also important to plan a series of procedures that are likely to be successful, so that there is the confidence to proceed with the next as indicated. Careful planning and discussion with the patient would allow one to understand the special needs in each case and to offer appropriate surgery (Lipscomb, 1968; Souter, 1979).

REFERENCES

Baloch, K.G., Treacy, R.B.C., Waldram, M.A. and Mulligan, P.J. (1995) Radio-carpal fusion in rheumatoid arthritis. *J. Bone Joint Surg.*, **78B**, Suppl. 11, 146.

Barnes, C.G. and Currey, H.L.F. (1967) Carpal tunnel syndrome in rheumatoid arthritis. A clinical and electrodiagnostic survey. *Ann. Rheum. Dis.*, **26**, 226-233.

Boyes, J.H. (1969) The role of the intrinsic muscles in rheumatoid deformities. pp. 63–64. In: *La Main Rheumatoide.* (Tubiana, R. Ed), Expansion Scientifique Francaise, Paris.

Brase, D.W. and Millender, L.H. (1986) Failure of silicone rubber wrist arthroplasty in rheumatoid arthritis. *J. Hand Surg.*, **11A**, 175–183.

Brewerton, D.A. (1971) Pathological anatomy of rheumatoid finger joints. *Hand*, **3**, 121–124.

Clayton, M.L. (1965) Surgical treatment at the wrist in rheumatoid arthritis. A review of thirty-seven patients. *J. Bone Joint Surg.*, **47A**, 741–750.

Clayton, M.L. (1989) Historical perspectives on surgery of the rheumatoid hand. *Hand Clin.*, **5**, 111–114.

Dell, P. (1979) Compression of the ulnar nerve at the wrist secondary to a rheumatoid synovial cyst: Case report and review of the literature. *J. Hand Surg.*, **4**, 468–473.

Ertel, A.N., Millender, L.H., Nalebuff, E., McKay, D. and Leslie, B. (1988) Flexor tendon ruptures in patients with rheumatoid arthritis. *J. Hand Surg.*, **13A**, 860–866.

Fatti, J.F., Palmer, A.K. and Mosher, J.F. (1986) The long-term results of Swanson silicone rubber inter-positional wrist arthroplasty. *J. Hand Surg.*, **11A**, 166–175.

Ferlic, D.C. and Clayton, M.L. (1978) Flexor tenosynovectomy in the rheumatoid finger. *J. Hand Surg.*, **3**, 364–367.

Ferlic, D.C., Smyth, C.J. and Clayton, M.L. (1983) Medical considerations and management of rheumatoid arthritis. *J. Hand Surg.*, **8**, 662–666.

Flatt, A.E. (1966) Some pathomechanics of ulnar drift. *Plast. Reconstr. Surg.*, **37**, 295–303.

Flatt, A.E. (1974) *The Care of the Rheumatoid Hand.* 3rd ed. CV Mosby, St. Louis.

Gainor, B.J. and Hummel, G.L. (1985) Correction of rheumatoid swan-neck deformity by lateral band mobilization. *J. Hand Surg.*, **10A**, 370–376.

Granowitz, S. and Vainio, K. (1966) Proximal interphalangeal joint arthrodesis in rheumatoid arthritis. A follow-up study of 122 operations. *Acta Orthop. Scand.*, **37**, 301–310.

Gray, R.G. and Gottlieb, N.L. (1977) Hand flexor tenosynovitis in rheumatoid arthritis. Prevalence, distribution and associated rheumatic features. *Arthritis Rheum.*, **20**, 1003–1008.

Kellgren, J.H. and Ball, J. (1950) Tendon lesions in rheumatoid arthritis: A clinicopathological study. *Ann. Rheum. Dis.*, **9**, 48–65.

Kuczynski, K. (1971) The synovial structures of the normal and rheumatoid digital joints. *Hand*, **3**, 41–54.

Lipscomb, P.R. (1968) Surgery for rheumatoid arthritis – Timing and techniques: Summary. *J. Bone Joint Surg.*, **50A**, 614–617.

Mannerfelt, L. and Malmsten, M. (1971) Arthrodesis of the wrist in rheumatoid arthritis. A technique without external fixation. *Scand. J. Plast. Reconstr. Surg.*, **5**, 124–130.

Menon, J. (1987) Total wrist replacement using the modified Volz prosthesis. *J. Bone Joint Surg.*, **69A**, 998–1006.

Mikic, Z.D. and Helal, B. (1977) The value of the Darrach procedure in the surgical treatment of rheumatoid arthritis. *Clin. Orthop.*, **127**, 175–185.

Millender, L.H. and Nalebuff, E.A. (1973a) Metacarpophalangeal joint arthroplasty utilizing the silicone rubber prosthesis. *Orthop. Clin. North Am.*, **4**, 349–371.

Millender, L.H. and Nalebuff, E.A. (1973b) Arthrodesis of the rheumatoid wrist. An evaluation of sixty patients and a description of a different surgical technique. *J. Bone Joint Surg.*, **55A**, 1026–1034.

Millender, L.H., Nalebuff, E.A. and Holdsworth, D.E. (1973) Posterior interosseous nerve syndrome secondary to rheumatoid synovitis. *J. Bone Joint Surg.*, **55A**, 753–757.

Millis, M.B., Millender, L.H. and Nalebuff, E.A. (1976) Stiffness of the proximal interphalangeal joints in rheumatoid arthritis. The role of flexor tenosynovitis. *J. Bone Joint Surg.*, **58A**, 801–805.

Nalebuff, E.A. (1969a) Nature and management of flexor tendon nodules in the rheumatoid hand. In: *La Main Rheumatoide*, (Tubiana, R. Ed) pp. 123–128. Expansion Scientifique Francaise, Paris.

Nalebuff, E.A. (1969b) Surgical treatment of finger deformities in the rheumatoid hand. *Surg. Clin. North Am.*, **49**, 833–846.

Nalebuff, E.A. (1969c) Surgical treatment of tendon rupture in the rheumatoid hand. *Surg. Clin. North Am.*, **49**, 811–822.

Nalebuff, E.A. (1975) The recognition and treatment of tendon ruptures in the rheumatoid hand. In: *AAOS Symposium on Tendon Surgery in the Hand*. pp. 255–269. St. Louis, Mosby.

Nalebuff, E.A. (1983) Rheumatoid hand surgery – update. *J. Hand Surg.*, **8**, 678–682.

Nalebuff, E.A. and Garrod, K.J. (1984) Present approach to the severely involved rheumatoid wrist. *Orthop. Clin. North Am.*, **15**, 369–380.

Nalebuff, E.A. and Millender, L.H. (1975a) Surgical treatment of the swan-neck deformity in rheumatoid arthritis. *Orthop. Clin. North Am.*, **6**, 733–752.

Nalebuff, E.A. and Millender, L.H. (1975b) Surgical treatment of the boutonniere deformity in rheumatoid arthritis. *Orthop. Clin. North Am.*, **6**, 753–763.

Nalebuff, E.A. and Patel, M.R. (1973) Flexor digitorum sublimus transfer for multiple extensor tendon ruptures in rheumatoid arthritis. *Plast. Reconstr. Surg.*, **52**, 530–533.

Nalebuff, E.A. and Potter, T.A. (1968) Rheumatoid involvement of tendon and tendon sheaths in the hand. *Clin. Orthop.*, **59**, 147–159.

Nanchahal, J., Sykes, P.J. and Williams, R.L. (1996) Excision of the distal ulna in rheumatoid arthritis. *J. Hand Surg.*, **21B**, 189–196.

Newman, R.J. (1987) Excision of the distal ulna in patients with rheumatoid arthritis. *J. Bone Joint Surg.*, **69B**, 203–206.

Riordan, D.C. and Fowler, S.B. (1958) Surgical treatment of rheumatoid deformities of the hand. *J. Bone Joint Surg.*, **40A**, 1431–1431.

Shapiro, J.S. (1968) The etiology of ulnar drift: A new factor. *J. Bone Joint Surg.*, **50A**, 634.

Shapiro, J.S. (1970) A new factor in the etiology of ulnar drift. *Clin. Orthop.*, **68**, 32–43.

Shapiro, J.S. (1987) Power staple fixation in hand and wrist surgery: New applications of an old fixation device. *J. Hand Surg.*, **12A**, 218–227.

Smith, R.J. and Kaplan, E.B. (1967) Rheumatoid deformities at the metacarpophalangeal joints of the fingers. A correlative study of anatomy and pathology. *J. Bone Joint Surg.*, **49A**, 31–47.

Smith-Peterson, M.N., Aufranc, O.E. and Larson, C.B. (1943) Useful surgical procedures for rheumatoid arthritis involving joints of the upper extremity. *Arch. Surg.*, **46**, 764–770.

Sones, D.A. (1971) The medical management of rheumatoid arthritis and the relationship between the rheumatologist and the orthopaedic surgeon. *Orthop. Clin. North Am.*, **2**, 613–621.

Souter, W.A. (1974) The problem of boutonniere deformity. *Clin. Orthop.*, **104**, 116–133.

Souter, W.A. (1979) Planning treatment of the rheumatoid hand. *Hand*, **11**, 3–16.

Stack, H.G. and Vaughan-Jackson, O.J. (1971) The zigzag deformity in the rheumatoid hand. *Hand*, **3**, 62–67.

Swanson, A.B. (1972) Flexible implant arthroplasty for arthritic finger joints. Rationale, technique and results of treatment. *J. Bone Joint Surg.*, **54A**, 435–455.

Swanson, A.B., de Groot and Swanson, G. (1973) Pathogenesis and pathomechanics of rheumatoid deformities in the hand and wrist. *Orthop. Clin. North Am.*, **4**, 1039–1056.

Taleisnik, J. (1979) Rheumatoid synovitis of the volar compartment of the wrist joint: Its radiological signs and its contribution to wrist and hand deformity. *J. Hand Surg.*, **4**, 526–535.
Taleisnik, J. (1984) Subtotal arthrodesis of the wrist joint. *Clin. Orthop.*, **187**, 81–88.
Taleisnik, J. (1985) *The Wrist*. pp. 387–435. Churchill Livingstone, New York.
Vainio, K. (1957) Carpal canal syndrome caused by tenosynovitis. *Acta Rheum. Scand.*, **4**, 22–27.
Vaughan-Jackson, O.J. (1958) Attrition ruptures of tendons in the rheumatoid hand. *J. Bone Joint Surg.*, **40A**, 1431.
Wilson, R.L. and Carlbolm, E.R. (1989) The rheumatoid metacarpophalangeal joint. *Hand Clin.*, **5**, 223–237.

Index